T0249735

Neurologic Emergencies

Guest Editors

ALIREZA MINAGAR, MD, FAAN
ALEJANDRO A. RABINSTEIN, MD, FAAN

NEUROLOGIC CLINICS

www.neurologic.theclinics.com

Consulting Editor
RANDOLPH W. EVANS, MD

February 2012 • Volume 30 • Number 1

SAUNDERS an imprint of ELSEVIER, Inc.

W.B. SAUNDERS COMPANY
A Division of Elsevier Inc.

1600 John F. Kennedy Boulevard • Suite 1800 • Philadelphia, Pennsylvania 19103-2899

http://www.theclinics.com

NEUROLOGIC CLINICS Volume 30, Number 1
February 2012 ISSN 0733-8619, ISBN-13: 978-1-4557-3894-6

Editor: Donald Mumford

Neurologic Clinics (ISSN 0733-8619) is published quarterly by Elsevier Inc., 360 Park Avenue South, New York, NY 10010–1710. Months of issue are February, May, August, and November. Periodicals postage paid at New York, NY, and additional mailing offices. Subscription prices are $285.00 per year for US individuals, $470.00 per year for US institutions, $140.00 per year for US students, $359.00 per year for Canadian individuals, $564.00 per year for Canadian institutions, $397.00 per year for international individuals, $564.00 per year for international institutions, and $199.00 for Canadian and foreign students/residents. To receive student/resident rate, orders must be accompanied by name of affiliated institution, date of term, and the *signature* of program/residency coordinator on institution letterhead. Orders will be billed at individual rate until proof of status is received. Foreign air speed delivery is included in all *Clinics* subscription prices. All prices are subject to change without notice. **POSTMASTER:** Send address changes to *Neurologic Clinics*, Elsevier Health Sciences Division, Subscription Customer Service, 3251 Riverport Lane, Maryland Heights, MO 63043. **Customer Service: Telephone: 1-800-654-2452 (U.S. and Canada); 314-447-8871 (outside U.S. and Canada). Fax: 314-447-8029. E-mail: journalscustomerservice-usa@elsevier.com (for print support); journalsonlinesupport-usa@elsevier.com (for online support).**

Reprints. For copies of 100 or more of articles in this publication, please contact the Commercial Reprints Department, Elsevier Inc., 360 Park Avenue South, New York, New York, 10010-1710; Tel.: (+1) 212-633-3812; Fax: (+1) 212-462-1935, and E-mail: reprints@elsevier.com.

Neurologic Clinics is also published in Spanish by Nueva Editorial Interamericana S.A., Mexico City, Mexico.

Neurologic Clinics is covered in *Current Contents/Clinical Medicine, MEDLINE/PubMed (Index Medicus), EMBASE/Excerpta Medica, and PsycINFO, and ISI/BIOMED.*

Printed and bound by CPI Group (UK) Ltd, Croydon, CR0 4YY
Transferred to Digital Print 2012

Contributors

CONSULTING EDITOR

RANDOLPH W. EVANS, MD
Clinical Professor, Department of Neurology, Baylor College of Medicine, Houston, Texas

GUEST EDITORS

ALIREZA MINAGAR, MD, FAAN
Professor, Department of Neurology, Louisiana State University Health Sciences Center, Shreveport, Louisiana

ALEJANDRO A. RABINSTEIN, MD, FAAN
Professor, Department of Neurology, Mayo Clinic, Rochester, Minnesota

AUTHORS

MARIA I. AGUILAR, MD
Assistant Professor, Department of Neurology, Mayo Clinic Arizona, Phoenix, Arizona

NADEJDA ALEKSEEVA, MD
Department of Psychiatry, Overton Brooks VA Medical Center, Shreveport, Louisiana

ABDULNASSER ALHAJERI, MD
Endovascular Neuroradiologist, Assistant Professor, Division of Neuroradiology, Department of Radiology and Neurosurgery, University of Kentucky, Lexington, Kentucky

KELLY JO BALDWIN, MD
Resident, Department of Neurology, University of Pittsburgh Medical Center, Pittsburgh, Pennsylvania

REEM F. BUNYAN, MD
Department of Neurology, Mayo Clinic, Rochester, Minnesota

WALTER BUYLAERT, MD, PhD
Department of Emergency Medicine, Ghent University Hospital, Ghent, Belgium

RAUL CARDENAS, MD
Department of Neurosurgery, University of Texas Health Sciences Center in Houston, Houston, Texas

PRASHANT CHITTIBOINA, MD, MPH
Department of Neurosurgery, Louisiana State University Health Sciences Center in Shreveport, Shreveport, Louisiana

HUGO CUELLAR-SAENZ, MD
Division of Neuro-Interventional Surgery, Louisiana State University Health Sciences Center in Shreveport, Shreveport, Louisiana

FRANCISCO FERNANDEZ, MD
ChairPerson and Professor of Psychiatry, University of South Florida, Tampa, Florida

MARY FITZ-GERALD, MD
Department of Psychiatry, Louisiana State University Health Sciences Center, Shreveport, Louisiana

BRANDON FOREMAN, MD
Clinical Neurophysiology Fellow, Comprehensive Epilepsy Center, Neurological Institute of New York, Columbia University Medical Center, New York, New York

WILLIAM DAVID FREEMAN, MD
Assistant Professor, Departments of Neurology and Critical Care, Mayo Clinic Florida, Jacksonville, Florida

BENJAMIN W. FRIEDMAN, MD
Department of Emergency Medicine, Albert Einstein College of Medicine, Montefiore Medical Center, Bronx, New York

STEVEN L. GALETTA, MD
Van Meter Professor of Neurology; Director, Neuro-ophthalmology Division; Director, Neurological Training, Department of Neurology; Department of Ophthalmology, University of Pennsylvania School of Medicine, University of Pennsylvania, Philadelphia, Pennsylvania

FELIX GELLER, MD
Department of Psychiatry, Louisiana State University Health Sciences Center, Shreveport, Louisiana

HAROLD W. GOFORTH, MD
Assistant Professor of Internal Medicine & Psychiatry, Duke University Medical Center; Attending Physician, Durham Veterans Affairs Medical Center, GRECC, Durham, North Carolina

FERNANDO D. GOLDENBERG, MD
Assistant Professor, Department of Neurology, The University of Chicago Medical Center, Chicago, Illinois

EDUARDO GONZALEZ-TOLEDO, MD, PhD
Departments of Radiology and Neurology, Louisiana State University Health Sciences Center, Shreveport, Louisiana

RUSSELL GORE, MD
Department of Neurology, Emory University, Atlanta, Georgia

JENNIFER S. GRAVES, MD, PhD
Departments of Neurology and Ophthalmology, University of Pennsylvania School of Medicine, Philadelphia, Pennsylvania

BHARAT GUTHIKONDA, MD
Assistant Professor, Department of Neurosurgery, Louisiana State University Health Sciences Center in Shreveport, Shreveport, Louisiana

LAWRENCE J. HIRSCH, MD
Professor of Neurology, Chief of the Division of Epilepsy and EEG, Yale University School of Medicine, New Haven, Connecticut

SARA HOCKER, MD
Division of Critical Care Neurology, Mayo Clinic, Rochester, Minnesota

RITA HORTON, MD
Department of Psychiatry, Louisiana State University Health Sciences Center, Shreveport, Louisiana

ROGER E. KELLEY, MD
Professor and Chairman, Department of Neurology, Tulane University School of Medicine, New Orleans, Louisiana

SABINE LEMOYNE, MD
Department of Emergency Medicine, Ghent University Hospital, Ghent, Belgium

FRANK S. LIEBERMAN, MD
Associate Professor of Neurology, Director, Adult Neurooncology Program, Department of Neurology, Pittsburgh Cancer Institute, University of Pittsburgh Medical Center, Pittsburgh, Pennsylvania

RICHARD B. LIPTON, MD
Departments of Neurology, Epidemiology and Population Health, Montefiore Headache Center, Albert Einstein College of Medicine, Bronx, New York

SHERYL MARTIN-SCHILD, MD, PhD
Assistant Professor, Department of Neurology, Tulane University School of Medicine, New Orleans, Louisiana

ALIREZA MINAGAR, MD, FAAN
Endovascular Neuroradiologist, Assistant Professor, Division of Neuroradiology, Department of Radiology and Neurosurgery, University of Kentucky, Lexington, Kentucky

SAEED TALEBZADEH NICK, MD
Department of Neurology, Louisiana State University Health Sciences Center, Shreveport, Louisiana

CHRISTINA NOTARIANNI, MD
Department of Neurosurgery, Louisiana State University Health Sciences Center in Shreveport, Shreveport, Louisiana

PETER DE PAEPE, MD, PhD
Department of Emergency Medicine, Ghent University Hospital; Heymans Institute of Pharmacology, Ghent University, Ghent, Belgium

JAMES PATTERSON, MD, PhD
Department of Psychiatry, Louisiana State University Health Sciences Center, Shreveport, Louisiana

RODICA E. PETREA, MD
Assistant Professor, Department of Neurology, University of Kentucky College of Medicine, Lexington, Kentucky

AMY A. PRUITT, MD
Associate Professor of Neurology, Department of Neurology, University of Pennsylvania, Philadelphia, Pennsylvania

ALEJANDRO A. RABINSTEIN, MD, FAAN
Professor, Department of Neurology, Mayo Clinic, Rochester, Minnesota

KOUROSH REZANIA, MD
Assistant Professor, Department of Neurology, The University of Chicago Medical Center, Chicago, Illinois

BRADLEY J. ROBOTTOM, MD
Raleigh Neurology Associates, Durham, North Carolina

MOHAMMAD ALI SAHRAIAN, MD
Associate Professor of Neurology, Sina MS Research Center, Sina Hospital, Hassan Abad Square, Tehran, Iran

LISA M. SHULMAN, MD
Professor of Neurology, Co-Director of Maryland Parkinson's Disease and Movement Disorders Center, Department of Neurology, University of Maryland School of Medicine, Baltimore, Maryland

MARVIN SIH, MD
Neurophysiology Fellow, Department of Neurology, The University of Chicago Medical Center, Chicago, Illinois

JUNGER TANG, MD
Department of Neurology, Mayo Clinic, Rochester, Minnesota

RONALD J. TUSA, MD, PhD
Professor of Neurology, Emory University, Center for Rehabilitation Medicine, Atlanta, Georgia

WILLIAM J. WEINER, MD
Professor and Chairman of Neurology, Director of Maryland Parkinson's Disease and Movement Disorders Center, Department of Neurology, University of Maryland School of Medicine, Baltimore, Maryland

BRIAN WEINSHENKER, MD
Department of Neurology, Mayo Clinic, Rochester, Minnesota

STEVEN WHITE, MD
Professor, Department of Medicine, University of Chicago Medical Center, Chicago, Illinois

SAŠA A. ŽIVKOVIĆ, MD, PhD
Associate Professor of Neurology, Department of Neurology; Staff Neurologist, VA Pittsburgh Healthcare System, MSSL-Neurology, University of Pittsburgh Medical Center, Pittsburgh, Pennsylvania

Contents

The past 40 years have seen the evolution of acute ischemic stroke management from unproven therapies du jour, such as steroids, heparin for stroke in evolution, and hypervolemic-hemodilution, to more of a scientific basis for our decision-making process. This evolution is directly related to the advancements in imaging of stroke. It is also related to carefully designed, controlled clinical trials of potential therapies, which have led to the recognition of the benefits of thrombolytic therapy in the acute setting but have also caused confusion and frustration over the lack of benefit for potential neuroprotective agents that once seemed promising.

Intracranial hemorrhage (ICH) is defined as bleeding within the intracranial vault and has several subtypes depending on the anatomic location of bleeding. ICH is diagnosed through history, physical examination, and, most commonly, noncontrast CT examination of the brain, which discloses the anatomic bleeding location. Trauma is a common cause. In the absence of trauma, spontaneous intraparenchymal hemorrhage is a common cause associated with hypertension when found in the deep locations such as the basal ganglia, pons, or caudate nucleus. This article addresses the diagnosis and general management of ICH and discusses specialized management for select ICH subtypes.

This article reviews aspects of management of traumatic brain and spinal cord injury. A discussion of management of intracranial pressure after traumatic brain injury is followed by a discourse on cerebrovascular trauma and pediatric injuries. Specific management methods are discussed, including medical and surgical management in intracranial hypertension. A special attempt is made to include the current recommendations for management of brain and spinal cord injuries. Spinal cord injuries are discussed in the final section. With an increasing number of patients surviving after devastating spinal cord injuries, the special issues in their management are evaluated.

Neurologic effects of acute drug intoxication are varied. This article discusses the acute neurologic effects of certain drugs as well as associated treatments and guidelines to management.

Central nervous system (CNS) inflammatory demyelinating diseases are a group of disorders that include multiple sclerosis, acute disseminated

FORTHCOMING ISSUES

May 2012

Pregnancy and Neurologic Illness

Autumn Klein, MD,
Guest Editor

August 2012

EMG

Devon Rubin, MD,
Guest Editor

November 2012

Sleep Disorders

Bradley W. Vaughn, MD,
Guest Editor

RECENT ISSUES

November 2011

Disorders of Consciousness

G. Bryan Young, MD, *Guest Editor*

August 2011

Frontiers in Clinical Neurotoxicology

Michael R. Dobbs, MD, and
Daniel Rusyniak, MD, *Guest Editors*

May 2011

Multiple Sclerosis

Emmanuelle L. Waubant, MD, PhD,
Guest Editor

RELATED INTEREST
Neuroimaging Clinics, November 2010, (Volume 20, Issue 4)
Neuroradiology Emergencies
Alisa D. Gean, MD, *Guest Editor*
http://www.neuroimaging.theclinics.com/

Preface
Neurologic Emergencies

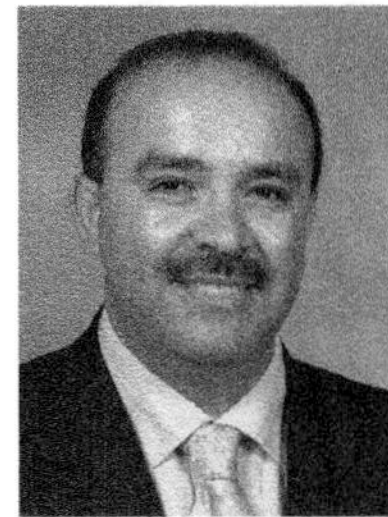
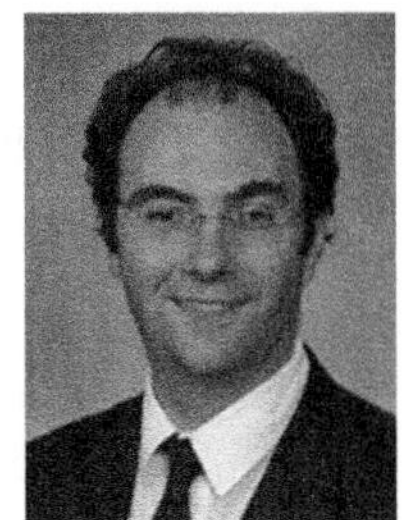

Alireza Minagar, MD Alejandro A. Rabinstein, MD
Guest Editors

Neurologists are often called to the emergency department to evaluate various acute primary central and peripheral nervous system disorders or neurological complications of multiple systemic illnesses. In these situations, prompt diagnosis can be lifesaving. Examples abound, but basilar thrombosis, aneurysmal subarachnoid hemorrhage, bacterial meningitis, and Guillain–Barre syndrome are just some illustrations. But the job of the neurologist is no longer restricted to being the master diagnostician. During the last three decades and with introduction of modern treatments, such as tissue plasminogen activator for treatment of acute ischemic stroke and the development of vascular interventional procedures, much can be offered to patients with acute neurological diseases in the emergency department.

This issue of *Neurologic Clinics* presents cutting-edge knowledge on the most common neurologic and psychiatric emergencies that can be encountered in the acute care setting. It contains 17 articles written by neurologists, psychiatrists, and neuroscientists with great expertise in each of these topics. Updated scholarly information is presented but the practical message is kept keenly in mind. Clinical advice for accurate diagnosis and effective management is highlighted. We hope that this issue will provide its readers with useful information and serve as a rich reference for their emergency room visits during in their daily neurology practice.

While editing this issue, we had the privilege of working with some of our finest academic peers. The superb quality of their contributions speaks for itself. Our greatest appreciation is due to these dedicated colleagues who spent their valuable time preparing their articles. We are confident that their efforts will be as highly valued by the readers of this issue as it was by us. We also appreciate the efforts of Mr Donald Mumford, Ms Diana Schaeffer, and the rest of the hardworking staff at Elsevier's

Neurol Clin 30 (2012) xiii–xiv
doi:10.1016/j.ncl.2011.10.001 **neurologic.theclinics.com**
0733-8619/12/$ – see front matter

publishing production team, who provided us with their constant support during the production of this issue.

Alireza Minagar, MD
Department of Neurology
Louisiana State University Health Sciences Center
1501 Kings Highway
Shreveport, LA 71130, USA

Alejandro A. Rabinstein, MD
Department of Neurology
Mayo Clinic
200 First Street SW-Mayo W8B
Rochester, MN 55905, USA

E-mail addresses:
aminag@lsuhsc.edu (A. Minagar)
rabinstein.alejandro@mayo.edu (A.A. Rabinstein)

Management of the Patient with Diminished Responsiveness

Sara Hocker, MD[a,*], Alejandro A. Rabinstein, MD[b]

KEYWORDS

• Coma • Encephalopathy • Management • Prognosis

Coma is an alteration of consciousness in which a person appears to be asleep, cannot be aroused, and has no evidence of awareness of the environment. Management of coma requires an organized and timely approach to determine the likely cause and initiate treatment. Coma often represents as a medical or surgical emergency that requires immediate action to preserve life or neurologic function. Examples include intoxications; acute metabolic derangements, such as diabetic ketoacidosis and fulminant hepatic failure; central nervous system (CNS) infections; basilar artery thrombosis; nonconvulsive status epilepticus; and acute cerebral mass lesions, such as intracerebral hemorrhage (**Fig. 1**) or large vessel territory ischemic stroke.

This article summarizes the main priorities in the acute treatment of comatose patients. A separate section addresses important factors in the long-term care of patients who remain in a prolonged state of unconsciousness and outcome prediction in patients who fail to awaken in the first days to early weeks. The evaluation and differential diagnosis of severe encephalopathy and coma are reviewed in a previous issue of *Neurologic Clinics*.

EMERGENCY MANAGEMENT

Coma is a neurologic emergency until proved otherwise. Evaluation and early intervention should proceed promptly and simultaneously. An organized protocol for urgent triage, evaluation, and management of coma is recommended (**Box 1**).

Management of the airway, ventilation, circulation, and sedation in patients with suspected or known neurologic injury requires understanding of the underlying issues

---

The authors have nothing to disclose.

[a] Division of Critical Care Neurology, Mayo Clinic, 200 First Street SW, RO_MA_08_WEST, Rochester, MN 55905, USA

[b] Department of Neurology, Mayo Clinic, 200 First Street SW - Mayo W8B, Rochester, MN 55905, USA

* Corresponding author.

E-mail address: Hocker.Sara@mayo.edu

Neurol Clin 30 (2012) 1–9
doi:10.1016/j.ncl.2011.09.009 **neurologic.theclinics.com**
0733-8619/12/$ – see front matter

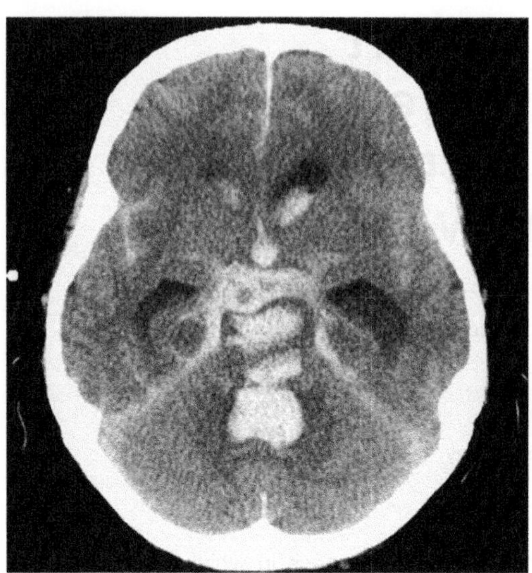

Fig. 1. An axial cut CT scan of the brain at the level of the temporal horns showing extensive subarachnoid hemorrhage and intraparenchymal hemorrhage within and extending through the dorsal pons into the fourth ventricle, with large amounts of blood also in the third and lateral ventricles, resulting from rupture of a distal basilar artery aneurysm. There is also obstructive hydrocephalus with dilation of the ventricles.

of elevated ICP, cerebral perfusion, neuromuscular status, and anatomy of the neuraxis.

Intubation is indicated in patients with hypoxia (Spo_2 <90%), hypoventilation or an inefficient respiratory pattern (ie, irregular or gasping), risk of aspiration as assessed by patient's ability to spontaneously swallow or swallow in response to suctioning, or anticipated deterioration. Cheyne-Stokes breathing and central neurogenic hyperventilation are not necessarily incompatible with normal gas exchange.

If patients are able to communicate verbally, the airway is not likely immediately jeopardized; however, patients presenting with alteration in the content or level of consciousness require repeated assessment of airway patency. A Glasgow Coma Scale score of 8 or less or the presence of nonpurposeful motor responses in a patient who has sustained head injury strongly suggests the need to establish a definitive airway.

If trauma is suspected, standard of care dictates that the cervical spine should be stabilized with a collar while securing the airway. If immobilization devices must be removed temporarily, direct laryngoscopy with manual in-line stabilization is standard of care for acute trauma patients with suspected cervical spine injury. The procedure was adopted because of weak empirical data and expert opinion; however, more recent data indicate that direct laryngoscopy and intubation are unlikely to cause clinically significant movement, may not immobilize injured segments, and degrade laryngoscopic view, which may cause hypoxia and worsen outcomes in traumatic brain injury.[1] It can be assumed that this may occur in any acutely brain-injured patient.

In cases of suspected elevated ICP, rapid sequence intubation is the preferred method of securing the airway because it provides protection against the reflex responses to laryngoscopy and resultant elevations in ICP. These reflexes occur

Box 1
Emergent management of coma in adults

Initial stabilization

Intubate if airway patency is compromised, gas exchange is inadequate, or respiratory pattern is inefficient.

Supplement oxygen.

Ensure adequate intravenous (IV) access.

Assess blood pressure and treat as indicated by the situation.

Obtain 12-lead ECG and initiate continuous cardiac monitoring.

Stabilize cervical spine if trauma suspected.

Treat witnessed seizures with lorazepam (2-4 mg IV), repeating every 5 minutes up to 8–16 mg depending on patient weight. Load with 20-mg/kg phenytoin equivalent fosphenytoin IV while administering the second or third dose of lorazepam.[20]

Initiate therapeutic hypothermia if postcardiac resuscitation encephalopathy is present.

Empiric interventions

Thiamine, 100 mg IV

Dextrose, 50% solution, 50 mL IV (after thiamine)

If ingestion is suspected, administer naloxone, 0.4–2 mg IV (may repeat in 2–3 minutes if inadequate response).

For suspected increased intracranial pressure (ICP), simultaneously hyperventilate and administer 1–2 g/kg IV 25% mannitol (or 30 mL 23% saline if central access is available) while obtaining a noncontrast CT scan of the head to determine if neurosurgical consultation is indicated

If infection is suspected, obtain blood cultures and administer dexamethasone and broad-spectrum antibiotics (third-generation cephalosporin, vancomycin, ampicillin, and acyclovir) while obtaining CT scan and lumbar puncture.

For suspected nonconvulsive SE, obtain emergent electroencephalogram. If suspicion is strong, start empiric treatment with lorazepam and fosphenytoin.

even in comatose patients without appropriate use of pretreatment and induction agents. The choice of medications is dependent on a patient's preintubation blood pressure (**Table 1**).

Once the airway is secured, oxygen saturation should be measured and supplemental oxygen provided. Adequacy of ventilation should be assessed by examination and arterial blood gases. Moderate hyperventilation (target $Paco_2$ 30–35 mm Hg) to lower ICP should be reserved for patients with increased ICP and considered a bridge therapy until osmotherapy can be administered or invasive treatment (such as placement of an external ventricular drain, in the case of obstructive hydrocephalus or hemicraniectomy, or suboccipital decompression, in the case of supratentorial or infratentorial mass lesions) can be performed. Routine hyperventilation may exacerbate cerebral ischemia by inducing cerebral vasoconstriction.

Appropriate IV access should be established with at least 2 large bore IVs and placement of a central line or intraosseous access if vasopressors are necessary.

All patients presenting with coma should receive thiamine and glucose without waiting for laboratory results or gathering of social history to treat potential hypoglycemia and avoid precipitating Wernicke encephalopathy. Although the use of a coma

Table 1
Pretreatment and induction agents in the neurologically injured patient

Normotensive or Hypertensive	Hypotensive
Intubation minus 3 minutes • Lidocaine, 1.5 mg/kg • Fentanyl, 2–3 -g/kg, to attenuate the reflex sympathetic response to intubation	Intubation minus 3 minutes • Fluids • Blood products • Inotropes • Pressors to maintain MAP >65 mm Hg
At time of intubation • Etomidate, 0.3 mg/kg, or propofol, 1.5 mg/kg • Succinylcholine,[a] 1.5 mg/kg, or rocuronium, 1.2 mg/kg	At time of intubation • Etomidate, 0.3 mg/kg, or ketamine, 0.5–1 mg/kg • Succinylcholine,[a] 1.5 mg/kg, or rocuronium, 1.2 mg/kg

[a] Succinylcholine should be avoided in patients who are very rigid because of the risk of inducing severe hyperkalemia.

cocktail, consisting of glucose, thiamine, naloxone, and flumazenil, is used frequently in patients presenting with an acute alteration of consciousness, a systemic review of trials considering outcome and adverse effects suggested that it is reasonable to use glucose and thiamine in all patients but that treatment with naloxone and flumazenil should be used only in the setting of known or strongly suspected drug overdose.[2] All comatose patients should have a baseline 12-lead ECG and have their cardiac rhythm monitored continuously for potentially life-threatening arrhythmias. Any witnessed seizures or signs of intracranial hypertension (ie, herniation syndrome is evident clinically or seems imminent based on CT findings) should be treated immediately (see **Box 1**). If patients have just undergone cardiopulmonary resuscitation after a witnessed ventricular fibrillation or ventricular tachycardia arrest, hypothermia should be initiated immediately while obtaining cardiology consultation.[3] Most hospitals now have protocols in place for therapeutic hypothermia after cardiac arrest. If there is no obvious cause for coma, a search should begin for historical or clinical findings. When a diagnosis is suspected, empiric treatments can be implemented while further diagnostic evaluation takes place (see **Box 1**).

PRINCIPLES OF SUPPORTIVE CARE—PREVENTING SECONDARY INJURY

Limiting secondary brain injury must be a priority in the initial management of coma because any additional insult in an acutely brain-injured patient directly worsens outcome and decreases the potential for functional recovery. Outcomes in patients with intracranial catastrophes are related to the ability to maintain cerebral oxygenation and perfusion, beginning with the initial evaluation in the field.[4]

Secondary injury can result from hypoxemia, hypotension, hyperthermia, or metabolic derangements. Hypoxia must be aggressively corrected; however, excessive oxygen supplementation may also worsen outcomes.[5,6] Hypercarbia should also be avoided because it can worsen intracranial hypertension.

Fluid resuscitation with isotonic solutions and, in refractory cases, infusion of vasopressors are indicated when systolic blood pressure is less than 90 mm Hg. Cerebral perfusion pressure, calculated by subtracting mean arterial pressure (MAP) from ICP, should remain above 60 mm Hg[7] in patients with ICP monitoring. In practice, however, the majority of comatose patients do not require ICP monitoring and in these patients the focus is should be on maintaining an adequate systemic blood pressure.

Extreme hypertension (MAP above 140 mm Hg) should be corrected with 10 mg IV labetalol, 10 mg IV hydralazine, or continuous infusion of IV nicardipine (starting at 5 mg/h). Sodium nitroprusside should be administered in refractory cases. It is prudent to withhold antihypertensive therapy in patients with less severe hypertension until the cause is known and further information is obtained because acutely lowering the blood pressure may compromise cerebral perfusion when intracranial hypertension is present.

For suspected or known elevation of ICP, pain and agitation should be treated with short-acting agents, hyperthermia and severe metabolic derangements should be corrected, and the head of the bed should be maintained at or above 30°.

MANAGEMENT OF SPECIFIC CAUSES OF COMA

After securing the airway, ensuring adequate ventilation and circulation, enacting appropriate measures of supportive care, and initiating empiric treatments based on available history and clinical signs, diagnostic evaluation may reveal a specific cause of coma. The following are generally accepted measures for treatable causes of coma not already addressed with emergency management:

- Correct severe hyponatremia with 3% hypertonic saline after placing a central venous catheter.
- Hypercalcemia may be treated with saline rehydration infusion followed by parenteral bisphosphonate pamidronate.
- Use available antidotes and consider hemodialysis for known ingestions.
- Aggressively hydrate patients with nonketotic hyperosmolality.
- Provide hydration and insulin for patients with diabetic ketoacidosis.
- Dialyze patients with acute renal failure.
- Administer corticosteroids for addisonian crisis.
- Give antithyroid drugs and β-blockers for thyrotoxicosis.
- Replace thyroid hormone for myxedema coma.
- Administer lactulose for acute liver failure or portosystemic encephalopathy.
- Give corticosteroids and obtain neurosurgical consultation for pituitary apoplexy.
- IV and/or intraarterial thrombolysis with or without mechanical thrombectomy may be instituted for acute basilar or carotid artery thrombosis (**Fig. 2**).
- Vasodilators should be given for hypertensive encephalopathy, but precipitous drop in blood pressure should be avoided.
- Treat cerebral venous and dural sinus thrombosis with heparin.
- Treat hydrocephalus with ventricular drainage.
- Mass lesions with signs of impending herniation should be treated with osmotherapy, corticosteroids (if vasogenic edema), hyperventilation, surgical resection, evacuation, or decompression.

LONG-TERM MANAGEMENT

Comatose patients may regain consciousness, remain unconscious, or lose all brain function (brain death). Most awaken within the first 2 weeks. Those who awaken may remain in a minimally conscious state (MCS) or in a persistent vegetative state (PVS) or they may become fully conscious but disabled or experience a complete recovery.

Treatment of patients in these categories is generally supportive and aimed at preventing complications related to chronic illness. Supportive care in the chronic critically ill may include tracheostomy, percutaneous gastrostomy, and bowel and

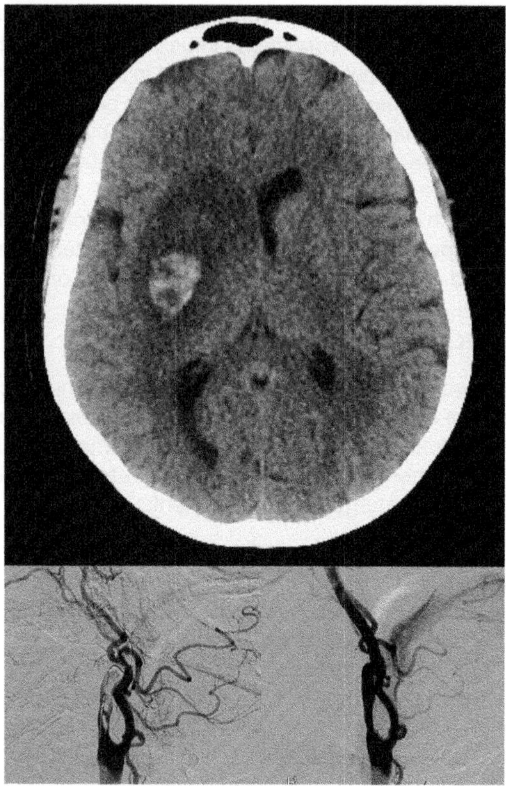

Fig. 2. (*Top*) Noncontrast CT scan showing hemorrhagic transformation of a striatocapsular infarct after revascularization of a right internal carotid artery occlusion through an endovascular procedure with Merci and Penumbra devices. (*Bottom left*) Diagnostic angiography with selective catheterization of the right internal carotid artery showing high-grade stenosis. (*Bottom right*) Right internal carotid artery post mechanical thrombectomy and stenting.

bladder care. Patients may be liberated from the ventilator and have their tracheostomy removed later if secretions are not a problem. Infection surveillance is important because colonization and infection with resistant bacteria are not uncommon. Although methicillin-resistant *Staphylococcus aureus* (MRSA) and vancomycin-resistant enterococci (VRE) may be reduced by strict isolation, meticulous hand hygiene by health care providers, and avoidance of multiple antibiotics, a recent large cluster-randomized trial found that surveillance for MRSA and VRE colonization and the expanded use of barrier precautions were not effective in reducing the transmission of MRSA or VRE, although the use of barrier precautions by providers was less than what was required.[8] Deep venous thrombosis prophylaxis is important in this population although thrombosis is less common in the chronic than in the acute phase of critical illness. Other complications in the long-term management of patients with impaired consciousness include contractures and decubitus skin ulcers. Contractures can be reduced by physical therapy. Decubitus skin breaks and ulcers can be prevented by special beds and monitoring of pressure sites along with frequent turning.

Neurostimulation is unproved in MCS and shown of no benefit in PVS. Dopaminergic agents, such as bromocriptine, zolpidem, and lamotrigine, are commonly used stimulant drugs in MCS but have not proved beneficial. Amantadine, a dopaminergic agonist and *N*-methyl-D-aspartic acid antagonist, was recently shown to improve both clinical signs of increased consciousness and functional behaviors during 4 weeks of treatment compared with placebo in a study presented at the 63rd annual meeting of the American Academy of Neurology.[9]

OUTCOME PREDICTION

Outcome prediction in acutely comatose patients is primarily influenced by the underlying cause and the degree of primary and secondary brain injury. To a lesser degree, outcome might be affected by physician expectation. When, in a physician's judgment, aggressive care would be futile and life-support measures are withdrawn, leading to death, this sequence of events could represent a self-fulfilling prophesy.[10] The true impact of this possibility in clinical practice is not known because most of the studies on predictors of poor outcome after acute brain insults have not taken into full account the potential influence of withdrawal of life-support measures. Therefore, it is prudent to acknowledge the limitations of prognostic models when discussing with families the possible outcome of a patient.[11]

Daily clinical examination is the most valuable prognostic tool. Confounding factors, such as sedatives and paralytic drugs, should be avoided to the extent possible to allow for careful examination.

Outcome after anoxic-ischemic brain injury in patients who have not been treated with therapeutic hypothermia is well studied. Four factors that predict poor outcome in this population include (1) absent pupillary light reflex, corneal reflexes, or motor responses at day 3, (2) absent somatosensory evoked potential cortical responses, (3) myoclonic status epilepticus, and (4) increased neuron-specific enolase (<33 ng/mL) at any time during the first 3 days. Current studies evaluating the validity of these factors in the hypothermia treated population are conflicting[12,13] and further research is needed in this area.

Outcome in CNS infections is affected by time to administration of antibiotic or antiviral drugs and corticosteroids.[14,15] With timely adequate antimicrobial and supportive therapy, prognosis can be favorable.

Outcome after traumatic brain injury is difficult to predict. Many young patients make a good recovery despite severe CT scan abnormalities and slow progress. Traumatic brain injury is a leading cause of death and disability worldwide, with most cases occurring in low-income to middle-income countries. Prognostic models, such as those developed from the Corticosteroid Randomization After Significant Head Injury trial[16] and the International Mission for Prognosis and Analysis of Clinical Trials in TBI database,[17] may improve predictions of outcome and help in clinical research. These prognostic models, which include simple variables, are available on the Internet (http://www.crash.lshtm.ac.uk/). The strongest predictors of outcome are age, motor score, pupillary reactivity, and CT characteristics, including the presence of traumatic subarachnoid hemorrhage.[18]

Surgery is no better than medical management in deep ganglionic hemorrhage but evacuation of cerebellar hematoma can result in dramatic improvement. Deteriorating patients with an expanding lobar hematoma may benefit from evacuation[19] but the degree of benefit is uncertain.

Outcome after aneurysmal subarachnoid hemorrhage (aSAH) is determined by initial clinical grade; 50% recover to a better grade and some patients may fully recover. Outcomes in aSAH have improved during the past 3 decades. The chance of a patient surviving an aSAH has increased by 17% during the past 3 decades and is approximately 65%, whereas incidence has remained stable at 3 per 100,000 patient-years. Two-thirds of aSAH survivors regain functional independence, half have cognitive impairments, half are dissatisfied with life, and only a third resume the same work as before the event.[20,21]

MCS may seem a better outcome for the family than PVS but may be a worse outcome for patients who could potentially have some awareness of devastating injury. Patients in MCS may further recover but no predictors are known.

Patients in PVS for less than 3 years may rarely partially recover, and when they do it is mostly after traumatic brain injury. Nonetheless, all patients remain severely disabled. Patients in PVS for 3 years or more do not recover; they have remarkable generalized brain atrophy on CT scan.

SUMMARY

- Acute coma must be considered a neurologic emergency.
- An organized protocol for urgent triage, evaluation, and management of coma is strongly recommended.
- The main priority after securing the airway and ensuring adequate ventilation and circulation is the limitation of secondary brain injury.
- The first priority with an acute structural cause of coma is treatment of increased ICP.
- The first priorities with a possible CNS infection are broad antibiotic and antiviral coverage and corticosteroids.
- Tracheostomy, percutaneous gastrostomy, bladder and bowel care, infection surveillance, and deep venous thrombosis prophylaxis are key components of longer-term care.
- The prognosis for neurologic recovery depends largely on cause and ranges from good prognosis for uncomplicated drug intoxications to poor prognosis for severe hypoxic ischemic injury.
- Outcome may be influenced by physician expectation.

REFERENCES

1. Manoach S, Paladino L. Manual in-line stabilization for acute airway management of suspected cervical spine injury: historical review and current questions. Ann Emerg Med 2007;50(3):236–45.
2. Hoffman RS, Goldfrank LR. The poisoned patient with altered consciousness. Controversies in the use of a 'coma cocktail'. JAMA 1995;274(7):562–9.
3. Chamorro C, Borrallo JM, Romera MA, et al. Anesthesia and analgesia protocol during therapeutic hypothermia after cardiac arrest: a systematic review. Anesth Analg 2010;110(5):1328–35.
4. Chesnut RM, Marshall LF, Klauber MR, et al. The role of secondary brain injury in determining outcome from severe head injury. J Trauma 1993;34:216–22.
5. Davis DP, Meade W, Sise MJ, et al. Both hypoxemia and extreme hyperoxemia may be detrimental in patients with severe traumatic brain injury. J Neurotrauma 2009;26(12):2217–23.
6. Kilgannon JH, Jones AE, Shapiro NI, et al, Emergency Medicine Shock Research Network (EMShockNet) Investigators. Association between arterial hyperoxia following resuscitation from cardiac arrest and in-hospital mortality. JAMA 2010;303(21):2165–71.
7. Dandapani BK, Suzuki S, Kelley RE, et al. Relation between blood pressure and outcome in intracerebral hemorrhage. Stroke 1995;26:21–4.

8. Huskins WC, Huckabee CM, O'Grady NP, et al. STAR*ICU Trial Investigators. Intervention to reduce transmission of resistant bacteria in intensive care. N Engl J Med 2011;364(15):1407–18.
9. Katz D, et al. The effectiveness of amantadine hydrochloride in improving level of consciousness and functional recovery in patients in the vegetative or minimally conscious state after traumatic brain injury [abstract]. Plenary session: contemporary clinical issues and case studies—63rd Annual Meeting of the American Academy of Neurology. April 9–16, Honolulu, Hawaii, 2011.
10. Becker KJ, Baxter AB, Cohen WA, et al. Withdrawal of support in intracerebral hemorrhage may lead to self-fulfilling prophecies. Neurology 2001;56(6):766–72.
11. Rabinstein AA. Ethical dilemmas in the neurologic ICU: withdrawing life-support measures after devastating brain injury. Continuum 2009;15(3):13–25.
12. Bisschops LL, van Alfen N, Bons S, et al. Predictors of poor neurologic outcome in patients after cardiac arrest treated with hypothermia: a retrospective study. Resuscitation 2011;82(6):696–701.
13. Fugate JE, Wijdicks EF, Mandrekar J, et al. Predictors of neurologic outcome in hypothermia after cardiac arrest. Ann Neurol 2010;68(6):907–14.
14. Tunkel AR, Hartman BJ, Kaplan SL, et al. Practice guidelines for the management of bacterial meningitis. Clin Infect Dis 2004;39(9):1267–84.
15. van de Beek D, de Gans J, McIntyre P, et al. Corticosteroids for acute bacterial meningitis. Cochrane Database Syst Rev 2007;1:CD004405.
16. Roberts I, CRASH trial management group. The CRASH trial: the first large-scale randomized controlled trial in head injury. Corticosteroid randomization after significant head injury. Natl Med J India 2002;15(2):61–2.
17. Roozenbeek B, Maas AI, Marmarou A, et al. IMPACT Study Group. The influence of enrollment criteria on recruitment and outcome distribution in traumatic brain injury studies: results from the impact study. J Neurotrauma 2009;26(7):1069–75.
18. Steyerberg EW, Mushkudiani N, Perel P, et al. Predicting outcome after traumatic brain injury: development and international validation of prognostic scores based on admission characteristics. PLoS Med 2008;5(8):e165 [discussion: e165].
19. Rabinstein AA, Atkinson JL, Wijdicks EF. Emergency craniotomy in patients worsening due to expanded cerebral hematoma: to what purpose? Neurology 2002; 58(9):1367–72.
20. Nieuwkamp DJ, Setz LE, Algra A, et al. Changes in case fatality of aneurysmal subarachnoid haemorrhage over time, according to age, sex, and region: a meta-analysis. Lancet Neurol 2009;8:635–42.
21. Rinkel GJ, Algra A. Long-term outcomes of patients with aneurysmal subarachnoid haemorrhage. Lancet Neurol 2011;10(4):349–56.

Epilepsy Emergencies: Diagnosis and Management

Brandon Foreman, MD[a], Lawrence J. Hirsch, MD[b,*]

KEYWORDS

• Epilepsy • Seizures • Status epilepticus • Coma
• Intensive care unit • Nonconvulsive seizures • Critical care

Emergencies in epilepsy may be encountered in the home, en route to a nearby hospital, in the emergency department (ED), in the hospital, or in an intensive care unit (ICU). Adequate and effective treatment delivered in a timely fashion is crucial to the successful management of these patients. This review addresses the diagnosis and management of acute seizures, status epilepticus, refractory status epilepticus, and seizures in the critically ill.

DEFINITIONS AND EPIDEMIOLOGY

Acute seizures (Szs) are the most common epilepsy emergency and comprise 1 million, or 1%, of all ED visits.[1] Szs are formally defined as transient occurrences of signs or symptoms related to abnormal synchronous neuronal activity.[2] The manifestations of Szs are protean. While in the acute setting, most Szs are identified by motor symptoms (especially clonic jerking, termed convulsive seizures [CSz]), it should be recognized that the majority of Szs in adults do not have prominent motor activity. If acute alteration of awareness occurs, these are known as complex partial seizures. For patients with impaired consciousness to begin with, Szs without prominent motor

Statement of disclosure: Dr Hirsch has received lecture fees from UCB-Pharma, Lundbeck, and GlaxoSmithKline; consulting fees from Lundbeck and Upsher-Smith; research funding from Lundbeck, Pfizer, Upsher-Smith, Eisai, and UCB-Pharma; and receives royalties from authoring chapters in *UpToDate: Neurology* as well as from coauthoring *Atlas of EEG in Critical Care* (Wiley, 2010). There are no disclosures related to stock ownership or options, or expert testimony. Dr Foreman has nothing to disclose.

[a] Comprehensive Epilepsy Center, Neurological Institute of New York, Columbia University Medical Center, 710 West 168th Street, New York, NY 10032, USA
[b] Division of Epilepsy and EEG, Yale University School of Medicine, PO Box 208018, New Haven, CT 06520, USA
* Corresponding author.
E-mail address: Lawrence.Hirsch@yale.edu

Neurol Clin 30 (2012) 11–41
doi:10.1016/j.ncl.2011.09.005 **neurologic.theclinics.com**

activity are typically referred to as nonconvulsive seizures (NCSzs). Typical seizures in ambulatory patients are self-limited and last less than 3 minutes.[3]

The annual incidence of Szs ranges from 70 to 100 in 100,000.[4] The annual cost of prehospital and ED care alone has been estimated at $1 billion.[5] More than half of patients with a first Sz will go on to have another. The occurrence of 2 or more unprovoked Szs constitutes a diagnosis of epilepsy.

When Szs are prolonged or recurrent without a return to baseline, they are referred to as status epilepticus (SE); the best studied form is convulsive SE (CSE). Most studies of SE use 30 minutes to define "prolonged," a classic distinction based on animal models of neuronal injury that originated with Gastaut.[6] Clinically, Szs do become self-sustaining with increased mortality when they last longer than 30 minutes,[7] but Szs lasting just 10 minutes are significantly more likely to extend into SE.[8] Further, despite clear guidelines that early treatment leads to better outcomes,[9] almost 60% of patients experience a delay of more than 30 minutes to treatment in hospitals.[10] Therefore, most neurologists use an operational definition of any Sz lasting more than 5 minutes, or 2 or more Szs between which the patient does not return to baseline, to facilitate more timely and therefore more effective treatment.[11] For practical purposes, SE should be diagnosed in "any patient that is still seizing."[12]

The definition of nonconvulsive status epilepticus (NCSE) has been more elusive. Electroencephalography (EEG) is required. The most common definitions include 30 to 60 minutes of impaired consciousness in conjunction with some form of Sz activity on EEG.[13] The eletrophysiologic definition of NCSE is beyond the scope of this article, but one definition has been suggested by Chong and Hirsch.[14]

SE complicates about 6% of Szs in the ED.[5] In the United States, the overall adjusted incidence of SE is 10.3 to 61 in 100,000.[15] Around a quarter are NCSE with a cumulative incidence of up to 14.1 in 100,000, although this is likely underascertained[13]; this means up to 152,000 individuals develop SE yearly[16] at a cost of around $4 billion.[17] Direct costs are between 60% and 90% higher for those with SE than for similar patients with intracerebral hemorrhage (ICH), myocardial infarction, or congestive heart failure without SE.[17]

Of those who develop SE, about a quarter develop refractory status epilepticus (RSE), a condition variably defined as SE wherein there is failure to respond to first-line and second-line antiepileptic drugs (AEDs).[18] Before EEG became a prominent tool in epilepsy emergencies, there were an estimated 2000 to 6000 cases per year; based on prospective data, this number is likely closer to 45,000 cases per year.[16,18] Up to a third of CSE patients continue to have continuous electrographic Sz activity after convulsive activity stops. When this is accompanied by periodic discharges on the EEG, it has been referred to as "subtle status epilepticus,"[18] or more recently as "status epilepticus terminans," a final stage of SE.[19] About a third of patients with RSE will have recurrence of Szs within 5 days of tapering an anesthetic medication, a condition referred to as "malignant" SE.[20]

Szs and SE are common among patients who are already hospitalized, although large prospective epidemiologic studies are lacking. The majority (about 75% overall in the literature, and up to 92% in one large series[21]) of critically ill patients with Szs have purely nonconvulsive Szs that cannot be recognized without continuous EEG monitoring (cEEG) (**Table 1**). Even after excluding those with prior clinical Sz activity or subtle motor signs, 8% of unexplained coma patients will have NCSE.[31] NCSzs have been documented in 19% of 570 inpatients with altered mental status in whom cEEG was requested.[21] In the neurologic ICU, 27% to 35% of patients undergoing cEEG will have NCSzs.[29,34] These statistics reflect a potentially huge number of patients for whom NCSzs or NCSE constitute a frequently delayed or misdiagnosed "brain-threatening emergency."[35]

Table 1
Prevalence of electrographic seizures and percentages that are clinically unrecognized

Study Population	EEG Type	Design	N	% of Patients with Any Seizures While on cEEG	% of Patients with Purely Nonconvulsive Seizures*	References
Altered consciousness or suspected subclinical seizures anywhere in medical center undergoing urgent routine EEG	Routine	Prospective	198	37	100 (32% had no subtle clinical signs)	Privitera et al[30]
Neuro-ICU	cEEG	Retrospective	124	35	74	Jordan[26]
Prior convulsive status epilepticus, altered consciousness without clinical seizure activity	cEEG	Prospective	164	48	100 (by definition)	DeLorenzo et al[24]
Moderate-to-severe traumatic brain injury, Neuro-ICU	cEEG	Retrospective	94	22	52	Vespa et al[32]
ICU, coma, without evidence of prior current clinical seizures	Routine	Retrospective	236	8	100 (by definition)	Towne et al[31]
Neuro-ICU with infarct or ICH	cEEG	Prospective	109	19% overall (Lobar ICH: 34% Deep ICH 21%)	79	Vespa et al[33]
All inpatients undergoing nonelective cEEG	cEEG	Retrospective	570	19	92	Claassen et al[21]
Neuro-ICU	cEEG	Retrospective	105	27	68	Pandian et al[29]
Under 18 years old, in an ICU	cEEG	Retrospective	117	44	75	Jette et al[25]
ICH	cEEG	Retrospective	102	31	58	Claassen et al[23]
Medical ICU patients without known acute brain injury	cEEG	Retrospective	201	10 (Sepsis: 16%)	67	Oddo et al[28]
All inpatients undergoing nonelective cEEG	cEEG	Retrospective	300	28	"Most"	Kilbride et al[27]
Pediatric ICU	cEEG	Prospective	100	46	70	Abend et al[22]

* This column refers to the following: Of all patients with seizures on cEEG, what percent of them had purely nonconvulsive seizures (ie, no clinically recognized ones) that could only be recognized with EEG.

Abbreviations: cEEG, continuous electroencephalographic monitoring; ICH, intracerebral hemorrhage; ICU, intensive care unit.

Data from Hirsch LJ. Urgent continuous EEG (cEEG) monitoring leads to changes in treatment in half of cases. Epilepsy Curr 2010;10(4):82–5; and Friedman D, Hirsch LJ. Diagnosing and monitoring seizures in the ICU: the role of continuous EEG for detection and management of seizures in critically ill patients. In: Varelas P, editor. Seizures in critical care: a guide to diagnosis and therapeutics. 2nd edition. New York: Humana Press; 2010. p. 23.

PRESENTATION AND CAUSE

"There are as many types of status as there are types of epileptic seizures"[6] and accordingly, they are both classified in similar terms (**Table 2**).[36] Both Szs and SE may be differentiated by their onset (focal or generalized) as well as the patient's level of awareness (simple or complex). CSz and CSE are clinically apparent, whereas NCSzs and NCSE may pose a diagnostic dilemma for the clinician (**Table 3**) and have not been adequately defined in terms of Sz subtype.

Szs are most commonly unprovoked or from progressive symptomatic causes.[37] SE, on the other hand, is most commonly from acute symptomatic etiology.[15] In hospitalized patients, the vast majority of Szs and SE have an acute symptomatic cause (**Box 1** and **Fig. 1**).[20,38]

MORBIDITY AND MORTALITY

Szs, and particularly SE, are significant sources of morbidity and mortality. For ambulatory patients with a single unprovoked Sz, more than half will go on to develop epilepsy and 3.4% will die over the next 30 days. An acute symptomatic Sz will only herald epilepsy 19% of the time, but 30-day mortality increases to 21%, almost 7 times as high as those with unprovoked Szs.[48] In the ED, around 1% of patients with Szs will require intubation and 23% are admitted to the hospital.[1]

SE will cause an estimated 42,000 deaths each year with a case-fatality rate ranging from 15% to 22%.[49] Age and etiology are the most consistent determinants; mortality is up to 34% in acute symptomatic SE and is between 38% and 67% in the elderly.[50] Mortality in SE after an anoxic event approaches 71%.[16] By itself, SE is sufficient to cause serious neuronal damage and mortality; in animals it has been shown that even if the systemic effects of SE are controlled, 30 minutes of SE may cause significant histologic damage.[51] Although the pathophysiology of SE is beyond the scope of this review, some of the broader concepts are represented in **Fig. 2**, and there are several excellent reviews.[52,55]

For those who survive SE, almost one-quarter will have a deterioration in their functional outcome[59] and 10% are left needing long-term care.[46] Around 6% develop an associated chronic encephalopathy.[39] 41% will go on to develop epilepsy.[60]

Table 2
Sample classification of status epilepticus

Type	Seizure Classification
Convulsive status epilepticus	Primary generalized Simple partial (SPSE or epilepsia partialis continua) Complex partial (CPSE with motor involvement) Secondarily generalized
Nonconvulsive status epilepticus in the ambulatory population (NCSE-A)	Primary generalized (eg, typical absence) SPSE CPSE Secondarily generalized
Nonconvulsive status epilepticus in the comatose or critically ill (NCSE-C)	Focal Bilateral/generalized
Myoclonic status epilepticus (MSE)	Primary MSE (in primary generalized epilepsy) Secondary MSE (in symptomatic generalized epilepsy) Symptomatic (eg, after cardiac arrest)

Abbreviations: CPSE, complex partial status epilepticus; SPSE, simple partial status epilepticus.

Table 3
Semiological spectrum of nonconvulsive seizures and nonconvulsive status epilepticus

Negative Symptoms	Positive Symptoms	
Anorexia	Agitation/aggression	Laughter
Aphasia/mutism	Automatisms	Nausea/vomiting
Amnesia	Blinking[a]	Nystagmus[a]
Catatonia	Crying	Eye deviation[a]
Coma	Delirium	Perseveration
Confusion	Delusions	Psychosis
Lethargy	Echolalia	Tremulousness
Staring	Facial twitching	Hippus[a]

[a] Applicable only to acute symptomatic comatose patients.

Data from Jirsch J, Hirsch LJ. Nonconvulsive seizures: developing a rational approach to the diagnosis and management in the critically ill population. Clin Neurophysiol 2007;118:1660–70; and Kaplan PW. Nonconvulsive status epilepticus in the emergency room. Epilepsia 1996;37(7):643–50.

There is significant debate over the morbidity and mortality of NCSzs and NCSE (**Fig. 3**). Studies have yielded inconsistent associations. For instance, generalized NCSE overall is associated with fairly high mortality[47]; yet there is stark contrast between the absence status of primary epilepsy, which leads to no measureable morbidity or mortality, and NCSE in comatose patients, which is associated with mortality rates of 51% to 65%.[18,24] Kaplan uses mental status as the major determinant of mortality in NCSE; in one study, death occurred in 39% who had severe mental status impairment compared with only 7% with mild impairment.[61] However, the vast majority of severely impaired patients die of their underlying comorbidities, leaving

Box 1
Some medications that lower the seizure threshold

- Analgesics: meperidine, fentanyl, tramadol
- Antiarrhythmics: mexiletine, lidocaine, digoxin
- Antibiotics: β-lactams (benzylpenicillin > semisynthetic penicillin; cefazolin; imipenem), quinolones, isoniazid, antimalarials (primaquine), metronidazole
- Antidepressants, especially bupropion and maprotiline
- AEDs: Phenytoin at supratherapeutic levels, tiagabine
- Baclofen
- Calcineurin inhibitors: cyclosporine, tacrolimus
- Chemotherapeutic agents: alkylating agents (chlorambucin, busulfan), α-interferons
- Neuroleptics, especially clozapine but also phenothiazines
- Lithium
- Multiple sclerosis medications: dalfampridine, 4-aminopyridine, β-interferons
- Radiographic contrast agents (intrathecal and intravenous)
- Theophylline
- Withdrawal from: opiates, alcohol, AEDs (especially benzodiazepines, barbiturates)

Data from Abou Khaled KJ, Hirsch LJ. Updates in the management of seizures and status epilepticus in critically ill patients. Neurol Clin 2008;26(2):385–408.

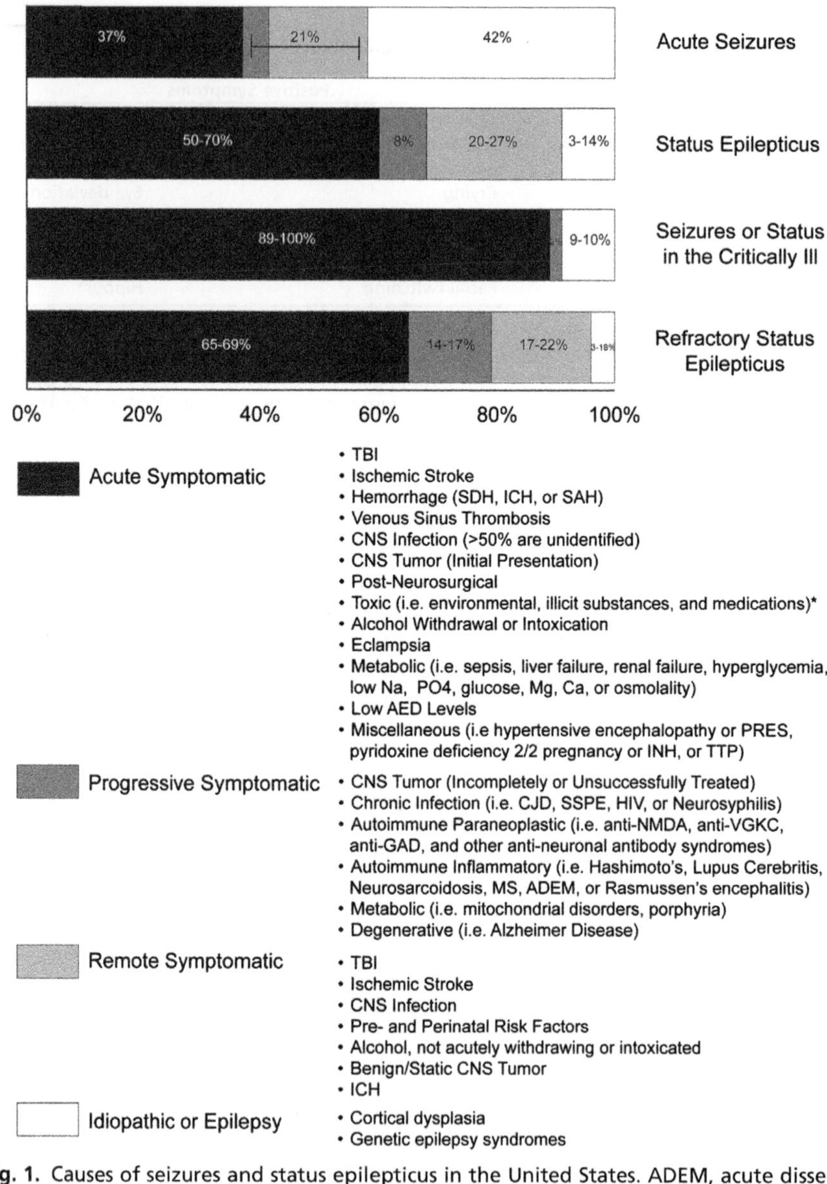

Fig. 1. Causes of seizures and status epilepticus in the United States. ADEM, acute disseminated encephalomyelitis; AED, antiepileptic drug; CJD, Creutzfeldt-Jakob disease; CNS, central nervous system; GAD, glutamic acid decarboxylase; HIV, human immunodeficiency virus; ICH, intracerebral hemorrhage; INH, isoniazid; MS, multiple sclerosis; NMDA, *N*-methyl-D-aspartate (receptor); PRES, posterior reversible leukoencephalopathy syndrome; SAH, subarachnoid hemorrhage; SDH, subdural hematoma; SSPE, subacute sclerosing panencephalitis; TBI, traumatic brain injury; TTP, thrombotic thrombocytopenic purpura; VGKC, voltage-gated potassium channel. *See **Box 1**. (*Data from* Refs.[16,20,37–47])

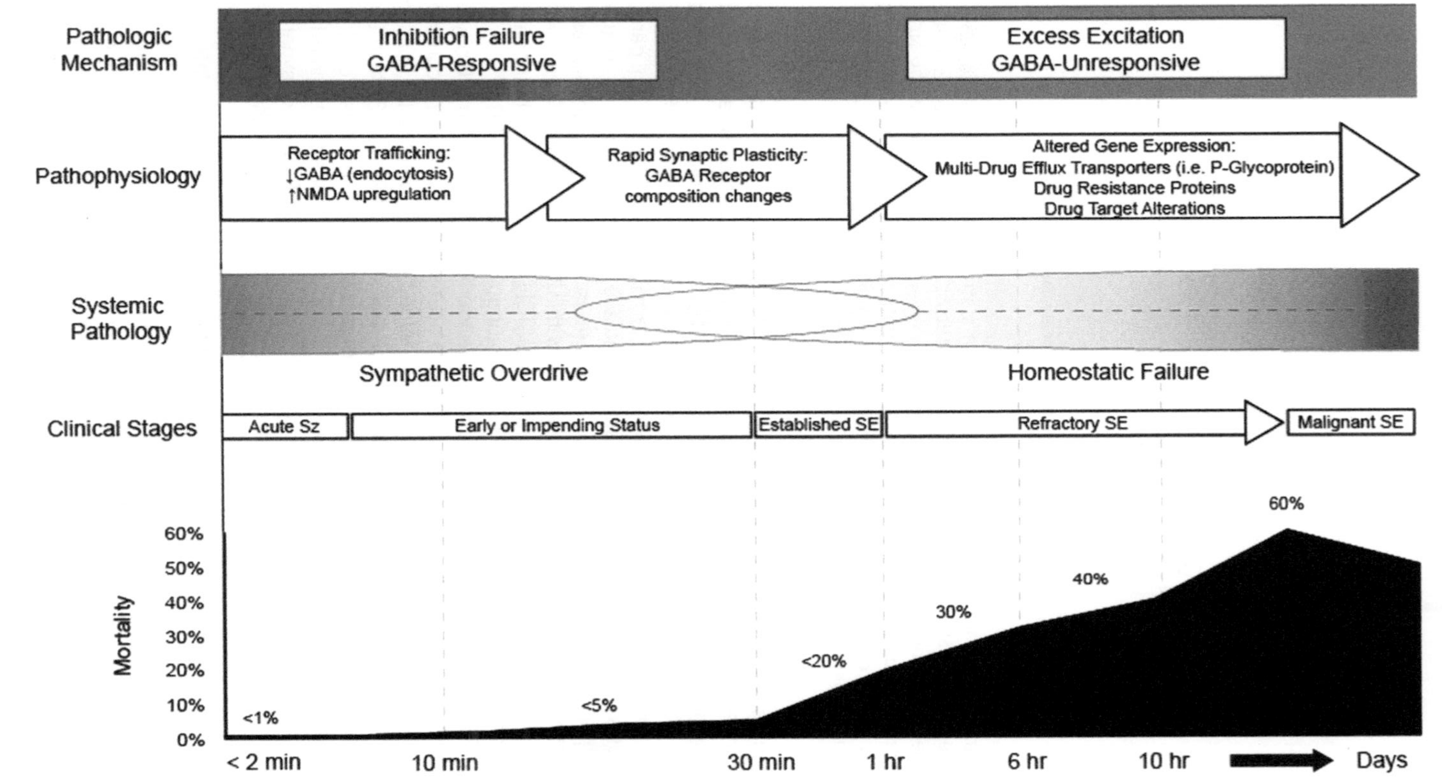

Fig. 2. The pathology of status epilepticus (SE). (*Data from* Refs.[3,7,16,18,20,46,47,49,52–58])

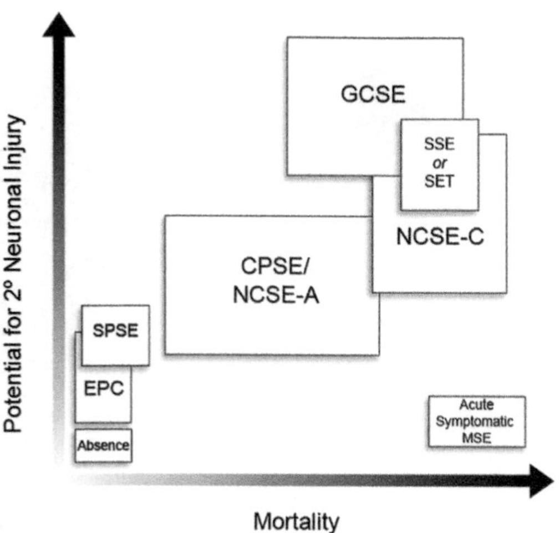

Fig. 3. Mortality and neuronal injury in subtypes of status epilepticus. Absence, absence status epilepticus; CPSE, complex partial status epilepticus; EPC, epilepsia partialis continua; GCSE, generalized convulsive status epilepticus; MSE, myoclonic status epilepticus; NCSE-A, nonconvulsive status epilepticus in the ambulatory patient; NCSE-C, nonconvulsive status epilepticus in the comatose or critically ill; SET, status epilepticus terminans; SPSE, simple partial status epilepticus; SSE, subtle status epilepticus.

a question as to the role of NCSE as an independent source of mortality. There are some compelling clinical data suggesting harmful effects of the Sz activity itself, including increased mortality when age and etiology are controlled[24]; associations between both the delay to diagnosis of NCSE and the duration of NCSE and mortality[62]; increased glutamate, glycerol, and lactate-pyruvate ratio on cerebral microdialysis[63]; increased neuron-specific enolase, a biomarker of neuronal damage[64]; increased glutamate, lactate-pyruvate ratio, and intracranial pressure during NCSzs compared with interictal periods within the same patient[65]; increased mass effect and shift on serial brain imaging after ICH[33]; and eventual hippocampal atrophy ipsilateral to NCSzs experienced after traumatic brain injury (TBI).[66]

Szs or SE in hospitalized patients is an independent risk factor for morbidity and mortality.[28,67] In one study of 41 hospitalized patients with SE, death occurred in 61% and only 1 in 5 returned to baseline on discharge.[42] In 201 medical ICU patients, Szs on cEEG were associated with death or poor outcome in 89% (vs 39% in those without Szs); Szs remained associated with worse outcome even when controlled for age, examination, and organ dysfunction.[28] In both medical and surgical ICUs, mortality associated with SE approaches 67%.[43] CSE and NCSE also act synergistically with acute brain pathology to worsen outcomes in situations such as stroke,[68] ICH,[33] subarachnoid hemorrhage (SAH),[69] and TBI.[32] Animal studies suggest this: for example, NCSzs in rat models of acute focal ischemia were associated with increased infarct size and higher mortality,[70] and a low-dose pilocarpine model of a single episode of NCSE in rats demonstrated permanent histologic, motor, and social behavior changes.[71] It stands to reason that treating Szs and SE quickly and effectively may potentially create better outcomes. Vespa's motto for cEEG monitoring in the ICU setting is: "to detect and protect."[72]

In the only prospective study of RSE, mortality was 39.3% despite a low percentage requiring intubation,[75] itself an independent risk factor for mortality in SE.[73] Rates of about 50% are more widely cited. Hospitalization is longer and there is a significant association with deterioration on functional measures[74]; only 20% return to baseline on discharge.[75]

The overall duration of SE may play a role in mortality. Studies stratifying duration[7,47,76] found a mortality of 2.7% at less than 30 minutes, 19% at less than 1 hour, 32% at over an hour, and logarithmically up to 6 hours thereafter. However, once RSE has become quite prolonged, duration may no longer be an independent predictor of outcome[54] even in RSE lasting longer than 7 days.[41]

PREHOSPITAL MANAGEMENT AND PRIMARY EVALUATION

An initial evaluation should take place either in the field or immediately on arrival to the ED in conjunction with medication administration (**Box 2**). As with any emergency, strict attention should be paid to the patient's airway, breathing, and circulation (the ABCs).

Treatment that is initiated early is much more likely to be effective[18] and improve outcomes.[77] Studies have reported that emergency medical services (EMS) may take 15 minutes to get to the ED[77]; only 41% of patients receive treatment before 30 minutes[10]; and delays to treatment of up to 50 minutes may occur despite established protocols.[78] When first-responders (ie, family members, EMS) are able to give medication, Sz time and recurrence decrease and patient outcomes are likely to improve.

Based on 11 randomized controlled studies, diazepam and lorazepam are clearly superior to placebo for stopping Szs and reducing the incidence of SE.[79] Their prompt prehospital administration actually leads to significantly decreased rates of intubation[77] compared with placebo. Intravenous (IV) lorazepam in particular has been shown to be superior to both diazepam alone and phenytoin (PHT) alone as first-line therapy in adults.[18,77] At times, IV access is not available. A variety of formulations of midazolam (intranasal, buccal, and intramuscular [IM]) have been used in children with prolonged Szs. Although buccal midazolam has been shown in a prospective randomized controlled trial to be more effective than rectal diazepam in aborting Szs in children,[80] the only approved non-IV benzodiazepine for adult patients remains rectal diazepam. A prospective study of adult prehospital IM versus IV benzodiazepine treatment is under analysis as of this review,[81] and the authors offer nasal midazolam,

Box 2
Initial steps in the prehospital management of seizures and status epilepticus

ABCs

Place in left-lateral decubitus position and remove any foreign objects from mouth (ie, dentures); no need for spinal precautions

Pulse oximetry and supplementary oxygen

Suction

Bag-valve mask or secure airway, as indicated

Cardiac monitoring

Insert peripheral intravenous line

Glucometer; if <80 mg/dL, administer 100 mg thiamine followed by 25–50 g dextrose 50%

Benzodiazepine administration based on availability

Data from Michael GE, O'Connor RE. The diagnosis and management of seizures and status epilepticus in the prehospital setting. Emerg Med Clin North Am 2011;29(1):29–39.

an effective and preferred route of administration,[82] to many of their patients at risk for Sz clusters or prolonged Szs to use at home.

Once the patient has arrived at the treating facility, the focus should remain basic and advanced life support measures, adequate monitoring of cardiopulmonary function, and rapid treatment. SE frequently occurs with systemic manifestations (**Table 4**). In addition, recognition of Szs or SE mandates an evaluation for its cause. An initial evaluation strategy is outlined in the first row of **Fig. 4**.

The value of imaging in the acute evaluation should be balanced against the risks of delaying treatment. Acute symptomatic causes should be urgently evaluated with noncontrast computed tomography in any patient without a known history of epilepsy or with focal findings on examination. EEG is an important tool to evaluate patients in SE. The resolution of clinical symptoms may belie 48% who are still having intermittent NCSzs in the subsequent 24 hours, and 14% still in NCSE after movements stop.[24] Similarly, Szs may occur in up to 34% of patients with acute brain injury,[34] and often manifests as a decrease in mental status out of proportion to the degree of injury. If the level of consciousness after a convulsive Sz of any duration does not improve by 20 minutes or normalize by 60 minutes, NCSE should be suspected[89] and an urgent EEG obtained.

Another consideration may include lumbar puncture if there is clinical suspicion for meningoencephalitis or SAH, but only once it is safe to do so and provided there is no delay to treatment of the Szs and possible infection. Empiric antibiotics should include 1 to 2 g ceftriaxone, 1 g vancomycin, and 10 mg/kg acyclovir. For the elderly, the addition of 30 mg/kg ampicillin may be warranted to cover for *Listeria* spp. In addition to cerebrospinal fluid, blood and urine should be concurrently evaluated for organisms.

PRIMARY MANAGEMENT OF SE

Just as in prehospital treatment, the authors' algorithm begins with use of γ-aminobutyric acid A ($GABA_A$) agonists: benzodiazepines (see **Fig. 4**). While multiple benzodiazepines will abort Szs with similar efficacy, Sz recurrence occurs less frequently with lorazepam than with diazepam owing to its decreased volume of distribution and long-lasting central nervous system (CNS) levels, up to 12 hours.[90] If diazepam or midazolam are used, a longer-acting maintenance AED, such as PHT or valproate (VPA), should be started concurrently. The response to lorazepam as a first-line agent falls between 59% and 89%.[18,77,90]

The choice of second-line agent has traditionally been PHT,[91] which works to prolong the recovery of voltage-gated sodium channels (see **Fig. 4**; **Table 5**). PHT is frequently underdosed[78] and should be based on weight. Complications from PHT include hypotension (27%–58%), respiratory depression (8%–10%), and cardiac arrhythmia (7%).[18] PHT may also impede motor recovery after stroke.[103] In addition, extravasation of IV PHT and its solvents (including propylene glycol) may cause soft tissue necrosis and/or distal ischemia as part of the "purple-glove syndrome." The incidence of this complication in one prospective study was 1.7%.[104] A safer but more expensive alternative is a water-soluble diphosphate sodium ester of PHT, fosphenytoin (FosPHT). Although FosPHT is a prodrug and must be converted to PHT, the conversion half-life is roughly 15 minutes, which is offset by faster infusion rates (about triple). Its primary benefit derives from avoiding hypotension and not having to slow down the infusion as often. Cardiac arrhythmia can still occur as FosPHT is converted to PHT,[105] and both cardiac and hemodynamic monitoring should continue for at least 15 minutes after the infusion of the prodrug is complete.

VPA acts on sodium channels, but has effects on calcium channels and $GABA_A$ as well. Two prospective, randomized trials have compared VPA with PHT for patients

Table 4
Systemic manifestations of status epilepticus

System	Effect	Result
Temperature	Increased systemic temperature due to sustained muscle activity; occurs in up to 83%	Neuronal injury, particularly in the cerebellum
Vascular	Blood pressure increases by up to 85 mm Hg systolic in the initial 30 min due to sympathetic overdrive; as cardiac output decreases with increasing mean arterial pressure, sudden loss of homeostatic mechanisms leads to hypotension as SE progresses >30 min	Hypertensive injury due to sympathetic tone followed by loss of perfusion to metabolically sensitive cortex
Cardiac	Potentially fatal cardiac arrhythmias occur in up to 58% Takotsubo cardiomyopathy and contraction band necrosis may occur due to endogenous catecholamines	Increased mortality
Cerebrospinal fluid	Pleocytosis; typically $<10 \times 10^6$/L, up to 80×10^6/L $\pm$ mild transient elevation in protein	Misdiagnosis of meningitis or encephalitis
Pulmonary	Elevated minute ventilation and pulmonary hypertension	Pulmonary edema
Other	Acidosis; pH <7.3 in up to 81% Rhabdomyolysis $\pm$ hyperkalemia[a] Hyperglycemia	Refractory hypotension, decreased respiratory drive Renal failure, cardiac arrhythmia Exacerbation of acidosis

[a] Depolarizing paralytics (ie, succinylcholine) are relatively contraindicated, as they may result in worsened muscle damage and hyperkalemia, thus facilitating cardiac arrhythmia.

Data from Refs.[39,55,83–88]

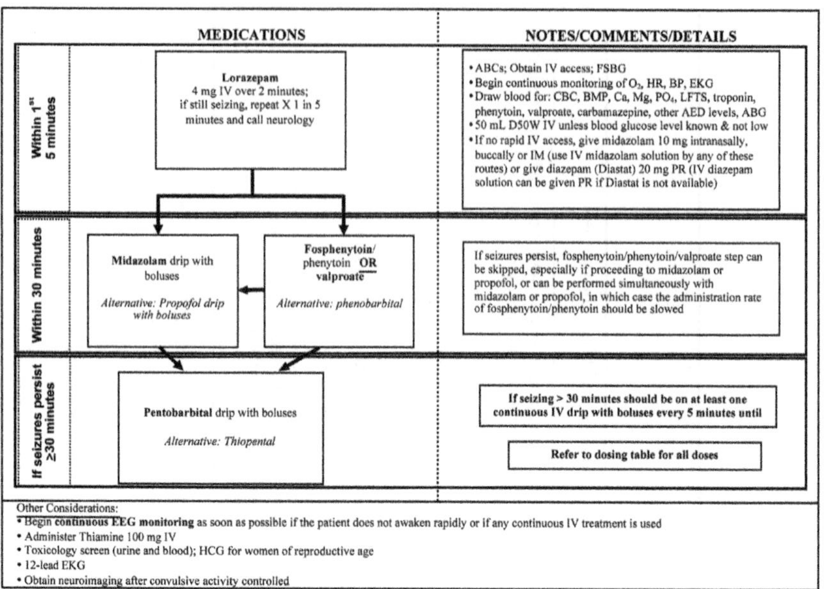

Fig. 4. Convulsive status epilepticus treatment algorithm in adults at Columbia University's Comprehensive Epilepsy Center. ABG, arterial blood gas; AED, antiepileptic drug; BMP, basic metabolic panel; BP, blood pressure; Ca, calcium; CBC, complete blood count; D50W, 50% dextrose in water; EKG, electrocardiogram; FSBG, finger stick blood glucose; HCG, human chorionic gonadotropin; HR, heart rate; IM, intramuscular; IV, intravenous; LFTs, liver function tests; Mg, magnesium; PO_4, phosphorus; PR, per rectum.

with SE. One study randomized 100 patients with SE refractory to diazepam to 20 mg/kg of either VPA or PHT, and found no difference in either efficacy or tolerability.[92] The second study used VPA (30 mg/kg) or PHT (18 mg/kg) as first-line treatment for SE using a crossover design. VPA was more effective in controlling SE both as the initial drug (66% vs 42%, $P = .046$) and as the second drug after the first had failed (79% vs 25%, $P = .004$).[100] Adverse effects associated with VPA based on studies in other scenarios include hyperammonemia, hepatic dysfunction, pancreatitis, parkinsonism, dose-dependent thrombocytopenia,[83] and other potential mechanisms that may lead to impaired coagulation such as lower platelet activation and prolonged thrombin time.[106] Of importance, there are few cardiovascular or mental status effects. One study reported loading doses of up to 32.7 mg/kg in elderly inpatients with no reported hypotension or arrhythmias.[107] This finding makes VPA a particularly attractive AED in the elderly, the critically ill, or those with advanced directives precluding intubation.

Two additional AEDs have recently been studied in SE. The first is levetiracetam (LEV), which is a synaptic vesicle (SV2A) ligand and inhibits high-voltage–gated calcium-channel currents. Adverse effects in two case series were limited to mild sedation (often when given close to benzodiazepines), mild nausea, transient asymptomatic thrombocytopenia, and a transient elevation in liver function tests.[94,99] Response varies: SPSE and CPSE were effectively treated by 1 to 2 g LEV as second-line therapy 60% to 79% of the time.[93,97] Generalized NCSE or subtle status responded 30% of the time, whereas none of the patients with GCSE in one series responded.[97] A small study of SE in elderly patients with medical comorbidities reported an 88% EEG response to 1.5 g IV bolus as first-line therapy.[108]

Table 5
Common medications in status epilepticus

Medication	Initial Dose	Clearance	Protein Binding	Maintenance	Level	Response
Non-cIV (Without Respiratory Depression, Except Phenobarbital)						
PHT	18–20 mg/kg IV up to 50 mg/min (25 mg/min for the elderly or patients with cardiovascular compromise)	Hepatic	90%	5–7 mg/kg PO/IV div up to TID; caution with tube feedings that decrease absorption	Total: 15–20 μg/mL Free: 1.5–2.5 μg/mL	37%–84%
FosPHT	18–20 PE/kg IV up to 150 mg/min	Same as PHT				
Valproate	20–40 mg/kg IV over 10 min	Hepatic	90%	1000 mg PO/IV q 6 h	80–140 μg/mL	79%–88%
Levetiracetam	2500 mg IV over 15 min (maximum bolus dose: 4 g)	Renal 67%, enzymatic hydrolysis 33%	<10%	2–12 g PO/IV div up to QID	25–60 mg/L	60%–90%
Lacosamide	300 mg IV over 30 min	Hepatic 60%, renal 40%	<15%[a]	200–300 mg PO/IV q 12 h	—	57%–60%
Phenobarbital	20 mg/kg IV up to 60 mg/min	Hepatic 75%, renal 25%	20%–45%	1–3 mg/kg/d PO/IV div BID or TID	20–50 mg/L	Equivalent to PHT/valproate
cIV (With Respiratory Depression)						
Midazolam	0.2 mg/kg IV q 5 min until Sz control or maximum dose 2 mg/kg	Hepatic; active metabolites excreted renally	95%	0.1–2.9 mg/kg/h cIV	—	Acute: 82% 48-h: 37% 7-d: N/A
Propofol	2 mg/kg IV q 5 min until Sz control or maximum dose 10 mg/kg	Hepatic	90%	2–15 mg/kg/h cIV (limited to 5 mg/kg/h for treatment >48 h)	—	Acute: 67%–73% 48-h: 54% 7-d: 43%
Pentobarbital	5 mg/kg IV up to 50 mg/min q 5 min until Sz control	Hepatic	35%–55%	1–10 mg/kg/h cIV	—	Acute: 92% 48-h: 57% 7-d: 22%
Ketamine	1.5 mg/kg IV q 5 min until Sz control or maximum 4.5 mg/kg	Hepatic	45%	1.2–7.5 mg/kg/h cIV	—	Unknown

Abbreviations: BID, Twice per day; cIV, continuous intravenous; div, divide; FosPHT, fosphenytoin; IV, intravenous; N/A, no data available; PE, phenytoin equivalents; PHT, phenytoin; PO, by mouth; q, every; QID, four times per day; Sz, seizure; TID, three times per day.

[a] New data suggest LCS may exhibit up to 90% protein binding.

Data from Refs.[74,92–102]

The second agent is the recently available AED lacosamide (LCS), which enhances the slow inactivation of voltage-dependent sodium channels. Similar to LEV and VPA, there are minimal if any effects on respiratory function, and cardiovascular effects are limited to potential PR interval prolongation. Although data on nonrefractory SE are limited, one case series of 39 patients has been published.[98] Dose ranges between 200 and 400 mg were given to patients, 85% of whom were in NCSE-A. Almost half of patients needed no further medication when LCS was used, and there were no adverse effects related directly to LCS.

PRIMARY MANAGEMENT OF RSE

Even prolonged RSE lasting months can resolve with good outcome.[41] Despite the incredible challenges of treating RSE and the lack of consensus on how to best to do so, it is crucial to establish a rapid, effective agent in patients who continue to have Szs. As only a minority of patients will respond to a third bolus AED,[18] a continuous IV (cIV) medication should be considered, either midazolam (MDZ) or propofol (PRO) initially (see **Fig. 4**). It should be emphasized that RSE is very often electrographic only, or has subtle clinical correlate, even after "successful" treatment of convulsions[18,24,74]; transfer to a unit or hospital with cEEG should be considered for the most effective use of these continuous drips.

MDZ is a rapid-acting benzodiazepine. Its major adverse effect is hypotension, often requiring pressors, and respiratory suppression. In addition, tachyphylaxis may occur and there is a theoretical concern of secondary downregulation of GABA receptors from either prolonged benzodiazepine use or SE. Because breakthrough Szs predict Sz recurrence after anesthetic weaning, in the authors' center MDZ infusion is now used at much higher doses than in the past, up to 2.9 mg/kg/h, 10 times higher than average rates in older studies. Sz suppression is typically maintained for 24 hours followed by slow weaning over 6 to 24 hours while on cEEG to evaluate for Sz recurrence.

PRO is a $GABA_A$ agonist with rapid onset (about 3 minutes) and easy reversibility. In addition, it inhibits *N*-methyl-D-aspartate (NMDA) and modulates calcium influx. Adverse effects include hypotension, respiratory suppression, transient movement disorders that may be misconstrued as Szs,[102] and the propofol infusion syndrome (PIS; **Box 3**). Originally described in children, PIS has been recognized in adults who receive propofol at more than 5 mg/kg/h for longer than 48 h, particularly after head injury.[109] A maximum of 5 mg/kg/h is recommended if PRO is to be maintained for more than 48 hours, and creatine kinase, lactic acid, pH, and triglycerides should be checked daily. To maintain efficacy while reducing the dose, some use an adjunctive "dose-sparing" cIV benzodiazepine.[102] As with MDZ, PRO is typically weaned over 6 to 24 hours.

Box 3
Propofol infusion syndrome: diagnostic criteria greater than 6 hours after initiation of propofol

Creatine kinase >2000 U/L

Triglycerides >500 mg/dL

Progressive lactic acidosis >2.5 mmol/L

+ Bicarbonate <20 mmol/L >6 hours after propofol infusion (not due to sepsis)

Data from Rossetti AO, Milligan TA, Vulliemoz S, et al. A randomized trial for the treatment of refractory status epilepticus. Neurocrit Care 2011;14:4–10.

For decades, the preferred anesthetic for ICU treatment of RSE has been barbiturates. In the United States this is typically pentobarbital, which acts on different GABA receptor isoforms than do benzodiazepines. While benzodiazepine-sensitive receptors are internalized in experimental models of SE, barbiturate-sensitive receptors maintain their responsiveness.[110] The adverse effects of pentobarbital are principally cardiovascular: cardiac depression, vasodilatation and hypotension, and poikilothermia.

MDZ, PRO, and barbiturates have been compared in a systematic review of 193 patients,[96] and more recently PRO and barbiturates have been compared in a prospective, randomized controlled trial of 23 patients.[101] In the systematic review, pressor-requiring hypotension occurred in about 30% of patients on MDZ, significantly fewer than with pentobarbital (77%). This result was likely related to dosing and goals of treatment: MDZ is typically titrated to Sz control whereas pentobarbital is titrated to background suppression. Related to this, MDZ was associated with significantly more breakthrough Szs (more than half) compared with PRO (15%) and pentobarbital (12%). However, cEEG was only performed in one-quarter of patients receiving pentobarbital (compared with 80% of those on MDZ), so it remains unclear if the rates of breakthrough Szs (usually NCSzs) were truly lower. Finally, doses of PRO averaging 3.2 mg/kg/h only succeeded in achieving burst suppression 38% of the time, much less often than with pentobarbital (96%). By contrast, the prospective trial randomized patients to either PRO or barbiturates with the goal of achieving background suppression. Seven-day Sz freedom rates after 36 to 48 hours of suppression-burst were similar between PRO and barbiturates, but patients receiving barbiturates experienced longer mechanical ventilation time than patients receiving PRO.

There does not appear to be any significant difference in mortality between MDZ, PRO, and barbiturates when used for RSE.[96,101] Mortality also remains the same when only one versus more than one anesthetic is administered.[111] Therefore, there are no clear guidelines as to which agent should be used first. Also, goals are not clear regarding titration of anesthetics to suppression burst versus Sz freedom, and for how long to do this. On one hand, barbiturate treatment seems to demonstrate significantly more suppression burst and possibly less Sz recurrence,[96] a predictor of relapse and subsequently mortality.[112] On the other hand, there is no clear difference in mortality between patients who achieve suppression burst and those who do not.[111] At least one organization has formally recommended 24 hours of suppression before medication weaning,[113] but data from a randomized prospective study found an overall Sz-free response rate of only 35% after suppression burst for 36 to 48 hours on cEEG.[101] Could longer durations therefore be required to establish efficacy of treatment? Older studies did not incorporate cEEG and therefore data are limited. Szs can still occur during suppression burst, and even during complete background EEG suppression.

MAINTENANCE THERAPY IN RSE

In RSE, maintenance AEDs facilitate continued Sz control after weaning from cIV medications. Agent(s) used in the initial treatment of SE should be maximized and continued, but additional AEDs are commonly required (see **Table 5**). PHT can be used IV or transitioned to oral administration. For patients receiving continuous tube feedings, dosing should remain IV to avoid a dramatic (up to 71%) decrease in absorption of PHT.[114] Daily total and free levels should be monitored. PHT is highly protein bound and hepatically cleared, thus free levels may be quite elevated in the setting of low protein binding or when using other highly protein-bound medications such as VPA or benzodiazepines. In critically ill patients on PHT plus full doses of VPA, the free PHT level is usually close to 3 times the expected level, that is, it is close to

30% of the total PHT rather than the usual 10%. In these patients, a total PHT level of 8 to 10 μg/mL will provide a high-therapeutic free level of 2.4 to 3.0 μg/mL. In some centers, free levels may take longer to report than total levels; if there is a predictable relationship between the two over several consecutive days of steady dosing, the total level may be used reliably.

VPA, like PHT, is highly protein bound and hepatically cleared. However, it is a cytochrome P450 inhibitor rather than inducer. Another interaction of particular concern has been the interaction between VPA and meropenem, and probably carbapenems as a class, which are widely used for resistant gram-negative infections. These antibiotics may dramatically reduce VPA levels, due to a variety of mechanisms involving decreased glucuronidation and increased renal excretion.[115]

LEV is only minimally protein bound and is cleared mostly by the kidneys. The significance of levels is not well established. Similarly, LCS is purported to have minimal protein binding, although a recent study demonstrated that perhaps 90% is protein bound.[116] LCS is both hepatically and renally cleared. Specifically for RSE, an uncontrolled, unblinded study reported that LCS has a response rate of 20%[98]; all 4 cases of refractory partial status responded to doses of 100 mg or less despite NCSE lasting up to 50 hours.[117] The authors' algorithm includes LEV and LCS as later add-on medication unless there are contraindications to PHT and VPA.

Phenobarbital, a barbiturate, may be used as a bolus for second-line or third-line treatment. Adverse reactions include respiratory depression, impaired mental status, hypotension, and rash. Like PHT, phenobarbital may affect motor recovery after stroke.[103] Phenobarbital can be useful in patients requiring cIV barbiturates, as phenobarbital reduces the risk of relapse even if levels are subtherapeutic.[112] It remains a reasonable alternative for the early treatment of SE, as it was not statistically inferior to lorazepam in the VA Cooperative study and did not have greater acute adverse events.[18] Because of hypotension, prolonged sedation, the need to load it fairly slowly, and its strong induction of P450 enzymes, the authors prefer other agents, but include phenobarbital as an option for select patients only.

Any oral agent may be used, such as topiramate (TPM), gabapentin (GPN), pregabalin (PGB), oxcarbazepine, or carbamazepine (CBZ). Two of these agents, PGB and TPM, have been studied in this setting. PGB was used in mostly partial RSE in 11 patients.[118] After a median of 5 days of RSE, 150 to 600 mg of PGB was given enterally in divided doses with Sz cessation within 24 hours in 5 patients for a response rate of 45%. TPM exhibits a variety of actions that may be helpful in SE including sodium-channel inhibition, GABA potentiation, high-voltage–gated calcium-channel inhibition, and antagonism of excitatory transmission. Rapid titration of up to 1600 mg/d (a very high dose) may be useful in treating RSE based on one series of 6 patients, although this has yet to be confirmed in further studies.[119] Animal studies suggest TPM may have neuroprotective properties, and may act synergistically with NMDA antagonists.[120] When using TPM, it should be kept in mind that it is a carbonic anhydrase inhibitor and may exacerbate acidosis. The authors avoid the use of TPM while using propofol, as it theoretically may exacerbate the acidosis associated with PIS. In addition, cases have been reported of acute hepatic failure associated with the use of TPM in combination with VPA.[121]

ALTERNATIVE MANAGEMENT OF RSE

As described, failure of an anesthetic agent or Sz recurrence after its withdrawal has been termed "malignant" status.[20] The authors might revise this definition as Sz recurrence at any time after a period of at least 24 hours of suppression burst on cEEG plus trials of at least 3 AEDs titrated to appropriate serum levels. Alternative strategies may need to be considered in these patients.

Ketamine is an NMDA antagonist that has been used by anesthesiologists for decades. In experimental models of prolonged SE, ketamine has been found to be less effective early, but is increasingly effective as Szs become self-sustained.[122] This process is the reverse of that of GABA agonists (including benzodiazepines and barbiturates), likely a result of internalization of GABA receptors during SE. Thus, glutamate blockade becomes more effective than GABA agonism in later stages of SE (see **Fig. 2**). In addition, because excitatory amino acid mediated toxicity is thought to underlie neuronal injury in SE, NMDA antagonism may be neuroprotective.[49] Animal models have suggested a synergistic effect when ketamine is used together with benzodiazepines in SE.[123] These models have also demonstrated potential ketamine toxicity, and a single anecdotal human case of cerebellar atrophy allegedly due to prolonged (72 hours) ketamine use in SE has been reported.[124]

Despite the theoretical benefits of ketamine and its short-term efficacy in aborting Szs, very few studies support its use. At the authors' center ketamine is used in conjunction with MDZ, often in the instance that maximal MDZ cIV has not resulted in Sz control on cEEG. It is also used as a bridge when tapering off of cIV barbiturates to limit withdrawal-associated Sz recurrence. Increased cardiovascular output, including tachycardia and hypertension, is both an adverse effect and a strength of ketamine, in contrast to the hypotension induced by other anesthetic agents used for treating RSE. Dissociative effects such as hallucinations or psychosis occur at subanesthetic dosing in awake patients, but are not a problem in this setting. Caution should be exercised prior to infusion in patients with elevated intracranial pressure; cardiovascular disease including hypertension; myocardial ischemia, or congestive heart failure; autonomic dysregulation; and TBI.

Inhaled anesthetics have been used with some success, but are impractical and have not demonstrated sustained benefit after cessation. Mirsattari and colleagues[125] reported a case series of isoflurane and desflurane in patients with RSE at end-tidal concentrations of 1.2% to 5%. Suppression burst was initiated within minutes and was maintained for a median period of 11 days while maintenance AEDs were optimized. Four of the 7 patients included in the study survived with good outcomes. Adverse effects included hypotension, along with ICU-associated problems such as atelectasis and ileus. With prolonged use of more than 30 days, thalamic and cerebellar hyperintensities on T2-weighted magnetic resonance imaging (MRI) may occur, indicating potentially reversible neurotoxicity.[126]

Lidocaine is a nonanesthetic class IB antiarrhythmic agent that has been used in cardiology for many years. It works by blocking sodium-channel conduction, attenuating depolarization, and decreasing automaticity. In addition, lidocaine has been used as a nonsedating, rapidly acting agent in SE. The largest prospective study comprised 36 chronic obstructive pulmonary disease patients with SE[127] in whom lidocaine given at cardiac doses led to immediate Sz cessation in almost three-quarters. Szs recurred quickly in more than half. Initial bolus is 1 to 3 mg/kg, and an infusion of up to 4 mg/kg/h is recommended to prevent recurrence.[128] Caution should be exercised in using lidocaine in patients with hepatic disease and the elderly, although it is noted that doses typically associated with hypotension or myocardial depression are about twice as high, and those associated with induction of Szs are about 3 times as high.[128]

Magnesium (Mg) is an important component of the NMDA receptor, effectively blocking transmission at membrane resting potential. Mg repletion may saturate NMDA receptors to restore tonic blockade. Its use is largely anecdotal in adults with the exception of eclampsia, in which it is the treatment of choice. The mechanism of action in eclampsia, however, is likely related to endothelial stabilization and therefore the treatment of the underlying condition, not the Szs directly. One recent study found Mg to be effective in 2 young adults with mitochondrial disease (POLG1 mutation).[129] Given the ever-growing spectrum of juvenile-onset and adult-onset presentations of mitochondrial disease, Mg should be considered in patients with cryptogenic RSE. Typical loading doses are 2 to 4 g IV, but optimal serum levels are not established.

Adjunctive medications may be useful; coadministration of benzodiazepines with PRO or ketamine has already been discussed. Pathologic studies have implicated drug efflux transporters such as P-glycoprotein (Pgp) in the refractory nature of prolonged RSE.[130] Verapamil, a calcium-channel antagonist and Pgp inhibitor, was used in one patient with recurrent Szs after prolonged RSE.[131] A dosage of 120 mg/d, roughly half the starting dose for cardiovascular indications, significantly reduced the burden of the patient's nocturnal Szs over the course of 2 weeks while levels of PHT and phenobarbital remained essentially constant. However, a recent animal study found no benefit of calcium-channel blockers for phenobarbital-resistant recurrent Szs, and 3 of the 11 animals actually developed Sz clusters.[132] Animal studies have also recently hinted at the use of HMG-CoA reductase inhibitors, or statins, in long-lasting SE.[133] Lovastatin decreased the expression of proinflammatory cytokine mRNA and body temperature in rats, which may provide neuroprotection. In addition, erythropoietin (EPO), a cytokine hormone with receptors located widely within the CNS, has been studied in low-dose pilocarpine rat models of SE. When administered after SE, EPO reduced blood-brain barrier disruption, decreased neuronal cell death, and attenuated microglial activation. Clinically, spontaneous recurrent Szs were less frequent during prolonged monitoring (>1 month).[134] Further studies will be required to test these agents for use in humans with SE.

There is a variety of nonpharmacologic interventions for RSE including hypothermia, electroconvulsive therapy (ECT), the ketogenic diet, and music therapy. Hypothermia, typically used in cardiac arrest patients, has been used for RSE in a small case series,[135] based on animal data[136] that suggests hypothermia has anticonvulsant and neuroprotective properties. Four patients refractory to MDZ and barbiturates received endovascular cooling to 31° to 33°C. cIV anesthetics were weaned, and after a 24-hour Sz-free period, 0.5°C rewarming every 4 hours to 36.5°C took place. RSE was stopped in all patients; 2 of the 4 remained Sz free. Adverse effects were prominent and included shivering, acidosis, coagulopathy, thrombosis (ie, deep vein thrombosis, pulmonary embolism), cardiac arrhythmia, and immunosuppression. Although these risks might be mitigated by a short duration of cooling, controlled studies are needed. ECT presumably increases endogenous anticonvulsant signaling pathways and induces a refractory period that aborts SE. One case series and review[137] suggests weaning all maintenance AEDs while on an anesthetic titrated to suppression burst followed by sessions of ECT for 3 to 8 days. If Szs recur, suppression can be resumed along with maintenance medications; however, 70% of the cases reported in the literature remained Sz free. Lastly, music has been reported to abort SE. Miranda and colleagues[138] have now reported two cases of RSE that spontaneously aborted within hours of continuously played classical music from Mozart and Bach.

The ketogenic diet (KD) is a carbohydrate-restricted diet with high fat content that induces ketosis and suppresses Szs. KD is typically used in children. In the ambulatory pediatric population, KD has been shown in a randomized controlled trial to effectively treat daily Szs (>90% reduction in Sz frequency in 7% vs 0% of controls and >50% reduction in Sz frequency in 38% vs 6% of controls).[139] Recently, KD has been used in two adult cases of RSE.[140] In both, KetoCal 4:1 tube feedings were gradually introduced to patients with malignant RSE. Ketosis was achieved in 8 to 10 days coincident with Sz control. There are a variety of adverse effects including hypoglycemia, gastrointestinal upset, and acidosis; long-term effects are not well reported, but include renal stones and growth delay. With the use of KD a nutritional specialist should be involved, a urinalysis should be checked for ketones daily, and serum β-hydroxybutyrate should be checked weekly.

Data on the effectiveness of epilepsy surgery for RSE are limited and are mostly from pediatric populations. Nonetheless, surgery may be considered in select patients with malignant RSE with evidence of one main Sz focus. One case series documented resection and multiple subpial transections in one patient with focal status and callosotomy in two patients with multifocal status, all with resolution of SE.[141] The patient with focal status continued to have "occasional brief partial seizures," one of the patients with multifocal status remained Sz free for 2 years, and the other had monthly Szs with one recurrence of treatable SE. A more recent case reported resection in one patient with focal status who remained Sz free at 16 months postsurgery.[142] Some investigators advocate for 2 weeks of failed treatment as a justification for surgery.[143] However, concordance is crucial for accurate localization, and MRI demonstrating focal restricted diffusion, ictal single-photon emission computed tomography (SPECT),[141] ictal ^{18}F-fluorodeoxyglucose positron emission tomography (PET),[142] or electrocorticography[141,142] may all be helpful. As RSE becomes malignant, physicians should consider acquiring data early so that surgical options become available. Other strategies that need further evaluation include vagus nerve stimulation and deep brain stimulation. The latter has been successfully used in intractable epilepsy to good effect,[144] but has been evaluated only in animal models of SE.[145]

RSE caused by CNS "infection" infrequently yields a proven pathogen.[40] A variety of autoimmune or paraneoplastic disorders may be implicated, although the incidence is unknown. It is reasonable, then, to consider steroids, adrenocorticotropic hormone, intravenous immunoglobulin, and/or plasma exchange to treat cryptogenic RSE in conjunction with other AEDs. It is even postulated that systemic exposure of brain tissue through damaged blood-brain barrier associated with prolonged Szs may induce a "secondary immune-mediated encephalitis,"[146] further justification for empiric immunomodulatory therapy in RSE.

TREATMENT CONSIDERATIONS IN THE COMATOSE OR CRITICALLY ILL

Szs and SE in the critically ill are largely nonconvulsive. As opposed to NCSE in the ambulatory population, the typical presentation of NCSE in the comatose or critically ill is nonlocalizing coma.[147] Despite more widely available cEEG, diagnosis is frequently delayed: by 24 hours in 16% of patients in the neuro-ICU,[62] by 48 hours in the medical ICU, and by 72 hours in the surgical ICU.[43] Routine EEG (20–60 minutes) will miss at least half of patients who are having NCSzs. In noncomatose patients, 24 hours of cEEG will identify up to 95% of patients with NCSzs. In comatose patients, only 80% will be diagnosed by 24 hours. Therefore, a full 48 hours of cEEG should be used in comatose patients to increase the sensitivity of NCSz detection to almost 90%.[21]

The critically ill will often do poorly regardless of the presence or absence of Szs. However, in multivariate analyses, NCSE,[18,24] delays to treatment,[62] duration of Szs,[24,62] and coma[54] portend worse prognosis. In the elderly, there is some retrospective evidence for increased mortality and longer hospitalization with IV benzodiazepine treatment,[148] but others suggest there were not adequate controls of dosage and timing in the study, and that "lack of clinical prudence [rather] than an inherent danger from the benzodiazepines" played a role.[35]

Complicating the diagnosis and management of Szs and SE in the critically ill are so-called boundary conditions,[13] whereby the EEG may appear potentially ictal yet does not strictly fulfill criteria for definite NCSzs or NCSE. In ambulatory patients, much of the differentiation between ictal and nonictal can be made based on mental status. In the critically ill, on the other hand, these conditions occur in the context of coma. Chong and Hirsch[14] provide a thorough review of patterns such as lateralized periodic discharges (LPDs), generalized periodic discharges (GPDs), and their potential clinical significance.

It is clear that LPDs are highly associated with Szs[149] and they may also be associated with worse outcomes after SE.[150,151] The authors' recent analysis of 200 patients with GPDs and a matched control group showed that GPDs are associated with NCSzs and NCSE but do not appear to be associated with worse outcome after thorough adjustment for age, neurologic examination, and etiology.[152] One subset of GPDs, triphasic waves, are seen in metabolic encephalopathy and degenerative diseases, but cannot be reliably distinguished from generalized epileptiform discharges or NCSE in a given individual based on EEG alone.[153,154] It should be noted that LPDs are occasionally ictal without question, for instance when they are associated with time-locked jerking on the contralateral side[14] or with aphasia that resolves along with the LPDs in response to AED.[155] At times, LPDs are associated with increased glucose metabolism on PET or increased cerebral blood flow on SPECT.[14] The authors view these periodic patterns as part of an ictal-interictal continuum, in an attempt to avoid the false dichotomy of interictal versus ictal EEG patterns in encephalopathic patients. Ongoing efforts are being made to define and therefore facilitate study of these and other confusing EEG phenomena.[156]

When there is reasonable suspicion for NCSE, an urgent EEG is indicated. A lack of rapid clinical response to an AED does not help rule out NCSE. In the VA Cooperative Study, 100% of the patients with subtle SE remained comatose 12 hours after treatment.[18] In another study, more than half of nonanoxic patients with NCSE in the ICU improved in alertness after treatment with AEDs, but the response was almost never immediate, sometimes only minimal, and not always sustained.[43] Yet if EEG is not available or the EEG findings lie along the ictal-interictal continuum, it may be useful to perform a trial of a rapid-acting AED at the bedside to evaluate for clinical improvement (**Box 4**). A major restriction of empiric AED trials in possible NCSE in the critically ill or comatose is that many EEG patterns resolve, leaving a comatose patient with diffuse slowing. Resolution of an abnormal pattern does not represent proof of its epileptic nature; for example, in patients believed to have pure metabolic encephalopathy without Szs, triphasic waves resolve with benzodiazepines as well.[153]

In the ICU most patients do not have a history of epilepsy, and new Szs may be the presenting symptom of a new cerebral insult.[45] For patients in whom the EEG is equivocal or clearly ictal, an assessment for acute brain injury (stroke, hemorrhage) or new systemic syndrome (hepatic failure, renal failure, sepsis), medication review, and consideration of lumbar puncture may be appropriate as treatment is initiated.[35] In patients with periodic discharges, equivocal patterns or only brief intermittent NCSzs, the authors generally try to avoid coma-inducing doses of medications, and typically start with IV PHT, VPA, or LEV, and possibly LCS.

In patients with frequent or periodic epileptiform discharges, cEEG monitoring is recommended for 48 hours, as these patients are more likely to have a delay before recording their first definite Sz.[27] The authors advocate a nonsedating AED for Sz prophylaxis for patients with frequent or periodic epileptiform discharges during the acute illness only (typically a couple of weeks) if there have been no definite Szs,

Box 4
Antiepileptic drug trial for diagnosis of suspected nonconvulsive status epilepticus

Indication:

Rhythmic or periodic focal or generalized epileptiform discharges on EEG with neurologic impairment

Contraindication:

Patients who are heavily sedated/paralyzed

Patients who have a clear reason for their level of consciousness

Monitoring:

EEG, pulse oximetry, blood pressure, electrocardiography, respiratory rate with dedicated nurse

Antiepileptic Drug Trial:

- Sequential small doses of rapidly acting short-duration benzodiazepine such as midazolam 1 mg per dose or nonsedating AED such as levetiracetam, valproate, phenytoin, or lacosamide
- Between doses, repeated clinical and EEG assessment
- Trial is stopped after any of the following
  - Persistent resolution of the EEG pattern (and examination repeated)
  - Definite clinical improvement
  - Respiratory depression, hypotension, or other adverse effect
  - A maximum dose is reached (such as 0.2 mg/kg midazolam, though higher may be needed if on chronic benzodiazepines)

Test is considered positive if there is resolution of the potentially ictal EEG pattern AND either an improvement in the clinical state or the appearance of previously absent normal EEG patterns (eg, posterior-dominant "alpha" rhythm). If EEG improves but patient does not, the result is equivocal.

Adapted from Jirsch J, Hirsch LJ. Nonconvulsive seizures: developing a rational approach to the diagnosis and management in the critically ill population. Clin Neurophysiol 2007;118:1660–70.

clinically or electrographically. If Szs develop, the authors typically treat with an AED for about 3 months, obtain another EEG, and re-assess at that point. There are minimal data to guide these decisions, but extensive experience with TBI, brain tumors, and other scenarios suggests that prolonged prophylactic AEDs in those without clear epilepsy (ie, recurrent unprovoked Szs, which excludes Szs during the acute illness) will not be effective and may cause unnecessary adverse effects.

SPECIAL SITUATIONS: ORGAN FAILURE

In patients with liver failure and Szs or SE, serum levels of hepatically metabolized medications will increase. In addition, decreased protein synthesis may lead to hypoalbuminemia, further increasing serum free (unbound) drug levels. Medications that are not hepatically metabolized and demonstrate minimal protein binding, such as LEV, GPN, or PGB, are easier to use in these settings.

Renal failure causes metabolic disturbances including hyponatremia, acidosis, and hypoalbuminemia. Medications that are renally cleared such as LEV, GPN, PGB, and to a lesser degree phenobarbital and TPM, should be dosed significantly lower and a dose should be given immediately following dialysis. Medications such as TPM and zonisamide have carbonic anhydrase activity, which can precipitate acidosis or renal calculi in patients with poor renal function. Highly protein-bound medications such as PHT, VPA, benzodiazepines, and possibly LCS[116] will experience higher-than-usual unbound levels for a given total serum level, but are only minimally dialyzed because protein-bound drug is not removed during dialysis.

SPECIAL SITUATIONS: ORGAN TRANSPLANTATION

Szs in transplant patients occur frequently in the context of the following: significant metabolic abnormalities, depending on the organ involved; infection or neurotoxicity from medications; and complications from surgery, such as hypoxia (**Table 6**). Liver transplant patients in particular appear to develop Szs 4 to 6 days postoperatively.[157] Abou Khaled and Hirsch[83] speculate that the cause may be withdrawal from high endogenous benzodiazepines as the new organ begins functioning. Patients on calcineurin inhibitors such as tacrolimus are at risk for the posterior reversible encephalopathy syndrome (PRES), characterized by Szs and cerebral edema associated with cortical blindness, aphasia, or altered mental status. Other factors implicated in the development of this syndrome include hypertension, hypomagnesemia, and supratherapeutic immunosuppressant levels.

Medications should not interfere with the new organ; for instance, certain AEDs (PHT, CBZ, and several others) can affect cardiac conduction and should be used judiciously after heart transplant. Similarly, barbiturates can cause myocardial depression. The choice of medication must also navigate the difficult interactions that often occur with transplant medications. Cyclosporine and methylprednisolone are metabolized through the cytochrome P450 pathway, thus inducers such as PHT, CBZ, and phenobarbital may increase clearance and reduce levels, sometimes quite dramatically.

SPECIAL SITUATIONS: PREGNANCY

As in the critically ill, Szs in a pregnant woman should warrant an evaluation for new acute brain injury, as only 15% to 30% of women with epilepsy develop increases in Sz frequency during pregnancy.[158] The reversible vasoconstriction syndrome (sometimes referred to as the Call-Fleming syndrome, or peripartum vasculopathy) may occur at any time during or even several weeks after pregnancy, and relative hypercoagulability increases the incidence of venous thrombosis. In addition, pregnancy-specific systemic illness such as hyperemesis gravidarum, the HELLP

Table 6
Incidence of clinical seizures (%) in organ failure or transplantation

Liver failure	2–33
Renal failure (on hemodialysis)	2–10
Transplant	
Liver	25–30
Kidney	1–31
Heart	2–15
Lung	22–27
Bone marrow	3–12.5
Pancreas	13

Data from Abou Khaled KJ, Hirsch LJ. Updates in the management of seizures and status epilepticus in critically ill patients. Neurol Clin 2008;26(2):385–408.

syndrome (hemolysis, elevated liver enzymes, and low platelets), and eclampsia may precipitate Szs. Eclampsia is the most common cause of Szs during pregnancy and may occur during or up to 3 weeks after pregnancy.[158] In patients with hypertension, Mg may be used to treat the underlying endothelial dysfunction in preeclampsia and eclampsia, and thereby help prevent Szs or SE.

A recent study group found that among pregnant women with epilepsy, SE occurred in 1.8% with no maternal mortality and one stillbirth related to CSE.[159] For a pregnant woman in SE, emphasis should be placed on positioning the woman into a left-lateral decubitus position if she is obviously gravid. Thiamine and glucose should be used empirically. Lorazepam should be used as a first-line agent to abort prolonged Szs, followed by Mg. A load of 2 to 4 g Mg may be given IV, but if Sz cessation is not prompt, alternative AEDs should be added according to the standard algorithm. It is important to recognize that unless a woman has previously been on VPA or phenobarbital with good control, it is not recommended to begin and maintain treatment with these medications.[160] In addition, hormone binding and increased renal and hepatic clearance of medications may lead to decreased drug concentrations, which will require close monitoring as Szs are controlled. Theoretical concerns for the fetus are derived from systemic effects of CSE such as hypoxia and lactic acidosis. If RSE develops, medications should be given aggressively as in nonpregnant patients, although boluses of anesthetic medications should perhaps be given somewhat more slowly and with fetal monitoring if possible. An obstetrics team should be closely involved to determine if and when the baby can be delivered to either treat (if eclamptic) or facilitate further treatment.

SUMMARY

Szs and SE are epilepsy emergencies with high morbidity and mortality. Early treatment is crucial, and the identification of an underlying etiology informs both continued treatment and prognosis. Many patients have underdiagnosed NCSzs or NCSE, particularly the comatose or critically ill, as well as those with acute or remote brain injury, prior convulsions, or sepsis. How aggressively to treat is controversial, but timely EEG can be useful for diagnosis, management, optimizing treatment response, and determining prognosis in these patients. Refractory conditions can be quite complicated, with limited evidence-based guidance, but treatment should not be restricted by nihilism even in the most prolonged cases, especially if there is not widespread irreversible brain injury. Further studies are needed to identify faster delivery mechanisms, appropriate monitoring, and more effective treatment in addition to clarifying our basic understanding of how these emergencies occur.

REFERENCES

1. Pallin DJ, Goldstein JN, Moussally JS, et al. Seizure visits in US emergency departments: epidemiology and potential disparities in care. Int J Emerg Med 2008;1(2):97–105.
2. Fisher RS, van Emde Boas W, Blume W, et al. Epileptic seizures and epilepsy: definitions proposed by the International League Against Epilepsy (ILAE) and the International Bureau for Epilepsy (IBE). Epilepsia 2005;46(4):470–2.
3. Theodore WH, Porter RJ, Albert P, et al. The secondarily generalized tonic-clonic seizure: a videotape analysis. Neurology 1994;44(8):1403–7.
4. Hauser WA, Beghi E. First seizure definitions and worldwide incidence and mortality. Epilepsia 2008;49(Suppl 1):8–12.

5. Martindale JL, Goldstein JN, Pallin DJ. Emergency department seizure epidemiology. Emerg Med Clin North Am 2011;29(1):15–27.
6. Gastaut H. Classification of status epilepticus. Adv Neurol 1983;34:15–35.
7. DeLorenzo RJ, Garnett LK, Towne AR, et al. Comparison of status epilepticus with prolonged seizure episodes lasting from 10 to 29 minutes. Epilepsia 1999;40(2):164–9.
8. Jenssen S, Gracely EJ, Sperling MR. How long do most seizures last? A systematic comparison of seizures recorded in the epilepsy monitoring unit. Epilepsia 2006;47(9):1499–503.
9. Treatment of convulsive status epilepticus. Recommendations of the Epilepsy Foundation of America's Working Group on Status Epilepticus. JAMA 1993; 270(7):854–9.
10. Pellock JM, Marmarou A, DeLorenzo R. Time to treatment in prolonged seizure episodes. Epilepsy Behav 2004;5(2):192–6.
11. Lowenstein DH, Bleck T, Macdonald RL. It's time to revise the definition of status epilepticus. Epilepsia 1999;40(1):120–2.
12. Hirsch LJ, Claassen J. The current state of treatment of status epilepticus. Curr Neurol Neurosci Rep 2002;2(4):345–56.
13. Shorvon S. The definition, classification and frequency of NCSE. In: Walker M, Cross H, Smith S, et al, editors. Nonconvulsive status epilepticus: Epilepsy Research Foundation Workshop Reports. Epileptic Disord 2005;7(3):253–96.
14. Chong DJ, Hirsch LJ. Which EEG patterns warrant treatment in the critically ill? Reviewing the evidence for treatment of periodic epileptiform discharges and related patterns. J Clin Neurophysiol 2005;22(2):79–91.
15. Chin RF, Neville BG, Scott RC. A systematic review of the epidemiology of status epilepticus. Eur J Neurol 2004;11(12):800–10.
16. DeLorenzo RJ, Hauser WA, Towne AR, et al. A prospective, population-based epidemiologic study of status epilepticus in Richmond, Virginia. Neurology 1996;46(4):1029–35.
17. Penberthy LT, Towne A, Garnett LK, et al. Estimating the economic burden of status epilepticus to the health care system. Seizure 2005;14(1):46–51.
18. Treiman DM, Meyers PD, Walton NY, et al. A comparison of four treatments for generalized convulsive status epilepticus. Veterans Affairs Status Epilepticus Cooperative Study Group. N Engl J Med 1998;339(12):792–8.
19. Claassen J, Hirsch LJ. Refractory status epilepticus. In: Sirven JI, Stern JM, editors. Atlas of video-EEG monitoring. 1st edition. New York: McGraw-Hill; 2011. p. 473–505.
20. Holtkamp M, Othman J, Buchheim K, et al. A "malignant" variant of status epilepticus. Arch Neurol 2005;62(9):1428–31.
21. Claassen J, Mayer SA, Kowalski RG, et al. Detection of electrographic seizures with continuous EEG monitoring in critically ill patients. Neurology 2004;62(10):1743–8.
22. Abend NS, Gutierrez-Colina AM, Topjian AA, et al. Nonconvulsive seizures are common in critically ill children. Neurology 2011;76(12):1071–7.
23. Claassen J, Jette N, Chum F, et al. Electrographic seizures and periodic discharges after intracerebral hemorrhage. Neurology 2007;69(13):1356–65.
24. DeLorenzo RJ, Waterhouse EJ, Towne AR, et al. Persistent nonconvulsive status epilepticus after the control of convulsive status epilepticus. Epilepsia 1998; 39(8):833–40.
25. Jette N, Claassen J, Emerson RG, et al. Frequency and predictors of nonconvulsive seizures during continuous electroencephalographic monitoring in critically ill children. Arch Neurol 2006;63(12):1750–5.

26. Jordan KG. Neurophysiologic monitoring in the neuroscience intensive care unit. Neurol Clin 1995;13(3):579–626.
27. Kilbride RD, Costello DJ, Chiappa KH. How seizure detection by continuous electroencephalographic monitoring affects the prescribing of antiepileptic medications. Arch Neurol 2009;66(6):723–8.
28. Oddo M, Carrera E, Claassen J, et al. Continuous electroencephalography in the medical intensive care unit. Crit Care Med 2009;37(6):2051–6.
29. Pandian JD, Cascino GD, So EL, et al. Digital video-electroencephalographic monitoring in the neurological-neurosurgical intensive care unit: clinical features and outcome. Arch Neurol 2004;61(7):1090–4.
30. Privitera M, Hoffman M, Moore JL, et al. EEG detection of nontonic-clonic status epilepticus in patients with altered consciousness. Epilepsy Res 1994;18(2):155–66.
31. Towne AR, Waterhouse EJ, Boggs JG, et al. Prevalence of nonconvulsive status epilepticus in comatose patients. Neurology 2000;54(2):340–5.
32. Vespa PM, Nuwer MR, Nenov V, et al. Increased incidence and impact of nonconvulsive and convulsive seizures after traumatic brain injury as detected by continuous electroencephalographic monitoring. J Neurosurg 1999;91(5):750–60.
33. Vespa PM, O'Phelan K, Shah M, et al. Acute seizures after intracerebral hemorrhage: a factor in progressive midline shift and outcome. Neurology 2003;60(9):1441–6.
34. Jordan KG. Continuous EEG and evoked potential monitoring in the neuroscience intensive care unit. J Clin Neurophysiol 1993;10(4):445–75.
35. Jordan KG, Hirsch LJ. In nonconvulsive status epilepticus (NCSE), treat to burst-suppression: pro and con. Epilepsia 2006;47(Suppl 1):41–5.
36. Engel J Jr. A proposed diagnostic scheme for people with epileptic seizures and with epilepsy: report of the ILAE Task Force on Classification and Terminology. Epilepsia 2001;42(6):796–803.
37. Hauser WA, Annegers JF, Kurland LT. Incidence of epilepsy and unprovoked seizures in Rochester, Minnesota: 1935-1984. Epilepsia 1993;34(3):453–68.
38. Annegers JF, Hauser WA, Lee JR, et al. Incidence of acute symptomatic seizures in Rochester, Minnesota, 1935-1984. Epilepsia 1995;36(4):327–33.
39. Aminoff MJ, Simon RP. Status epilepticus. Causes, clinical features and consequences in 98 patients. Am J Med 1980;69(5):657–66.
40. Bleck TP. Less common etiologies of status epilepticus. Epilepsy Curr 2010;10(2):31–3.
41. Cooper AD, Britton JW, Rabinstein AA. Functional and cognitive outcome in prolonged refractory status epilepticus. Arch Neurol 2009;66(12):1505–9.
42. Delanty N, French JA, Labar DR, et al. Status epilepticus arising de novo in hospitalized patients: an analysis of 41 patients. Seizure 2001;10(2):116–9.
43. Drislane FW, Lopez MR, Blum AS, et al. Detection and treatment of refractory status epilepticus in the intensive care unit. J Clin Neurophysiol 2008;25(4):181–6.
44. Hesdorffer DC, Logroscino G, Cascino G, et al. Incidence of status epilepticus in Rochester, Minnesota, 1965-1984. Neurology 1998;50(3):735–41.
45. Holtkamp M, Othman J, Buchheim K, et al. Predictors and prognosis of refractory status epilepticus treated in a neurological intensive care unit. J Neurol Neurosurg Psychiatry 2005;76(4):534–9.
46. Lowenstein DH, Alldredge BK. Status epilepticus at an urban public hospital in the 1980s. Neurology 1993;43(3 Pt 1):483–8.
47. Towne AR, Pellock JM, Ko D, et al. Determinants of mortality in status epilepticus. Epilepsia 1994;35(1):27–34.

48. Hesdorffer DC, Benn EK, Cascino GD, et al. Is a first acute symptomatic seizure epilepsy? Mortality and risk for recurrent seizure. Epilepsia 2009;50(5):1102–8.
49. Fountain NB. Status epilepticus: risk factors and complications. Epilepsia 2000; 41(Suppl 2):S23–30.
50. Logroscino G, Hesdorffer DC, Cascino G, et al. Short-term mortality after a first episode of status epilepticus. Epilepsia 1997;38(12):1344–9.
51. Meldrum BS, Vigouroux RA, Brierley JB. Systemic factors and epileptic brain damage. Prolonged seizures in paralyzed, artificially ventilated baboons. Arch Neurol 1973;29(2):82–7.
52. Chen JW, Wasterlain CG. Status epilepticus: pathophysiology and management in adults. Lancet Neurol 2006;5(3):246–56.
53. Costello DJ, Cole AJ. Treatment of acute seizures and status epilepticus. J Intensive Care Med 2007;22(6):319–47.
54. Drislane FW, Blum AS, Lopez MR, et al. Duration of refractory status epilepticus and outcome: loss of prognostic utility after several hours. Epilepsia 2009;50(6): 1566–71.
55. Fountain NB, Lothman EW. Pathophysiology of status epilepticus. J Clin Neurophysiol 1995;12(4):326–42.
56. Mazarati AM, Baldwin RA, Sankar R, et al. Time-dependent decrease in the effectiveness of antiepileptic drugs during the course of self-sustaining status epilepticus. Brain Res 1998;814(1–2):179–85.
57. Sisodiya SM, Thom M. Widespread upregulation of drug-resistance proteins in fatal human status epilepticus. Epilepsia 2003;44(2):261–4.
58. Wasterlain CG, Mazarati AM, Naylor D, et al. Short-term plasticity of hippocampal neuropeptides and neuronal circuitry in experimental status epilepticus. Epilepsia 2002;43(Suppl 5):20–9.
59. Claassen J, Lokin JK, Fitzsimmons BF, et al. Predictors of functional disability and mortality after status epilepticus. Neurology 2002;58(1):139–42.
60. Hesdorffer DC, Logroscino G, Cascino G, et al. Risk of unprovoked seizure after acute symptomatic seizure: effect of status epilepticus. Ann Neurol 1998;44(6): 908–12.
61. Shneker BF, Fountain NB. Assessment of acute morbidity and mortality in nonconvulsive status epilepticus. Neurology 2003;61(8):1066–73.
62. Young GB, Jordan KG, Doig GS. An assessment of nonconvulsive seizures in the intensive care unit using continuous EEG monitoring: an investigation of variables associated with mortality. Neurology 1996;47(1):83–9.
63. Vespa P, Prins M, Ronne-Engstrom E, et al. Increase in extracellular glutamate caused by reduced cerebral perfusion pressure and seizures after human traumatic brain injury: a microdialysis study. J Neurosurg 1998;89(6):971–82.
64. DeGiorgio CM, Heck CN, Rabinowicz AL, et al. Serum neuron-specific enolase in the major subtypes of status epilepticus. Neurology 1999;52(4):746–9.
65. Vespa PM, Miller C, McArthur D, et al. Nonconvulsive electrographic seizures after traumatic brain injury result in a delayed, prolonged increase in intracranial pressure and metabolic crisis. Crit Care Med 2007;35(12):2830–6.
66. Vespa PM, McArthur DL, Xu Y, et al. Nonconvulsive seizures after traumatic brain injury are associated with hippocampal atrophy. Neurology 2010;75(9):792–8.
67. Vignatelli L, Rinaldi R, Baldin E, et al. Impact of treatment on the short-term prognosis of status epilepticus in two population-based cohorts. J Neurol 2008;255(2):197–204.
68. Waterhouse EJ, Vaughan JK, Barnes TY, et al. Synergistic effect of status epilepticus and ischemic brain injury on mortality. Epilepsy Res 1998;29(3):175–83.

69. Dennis LJ, Claassen J, Hirsch LJ, et al. Nonconvulsive status epilepticus after subarachnoid hemorrhage. Neurosurgery 2002;51(5):1136–43 [discussion: 1144].
70. Williams AJ, Tortella FC, Lu XM, et al. Antiepileptic drug treatment of nonconvulsive seizures induced by experimental focal brain ischemia. J Pharmacol Exp Ther 2004;311(1):220–7.
71. Krsek P, Mikulecka A, Druga R, et al. Long-term behavioral and morphological consequences of nonconvulsive status epilepticus in rats. Epilepsy Behav 2004; 5(2):180–91.
72. Vespa P. Continuous EEG monitoring for the detection of seizures in traumatic brain injury, infarction, and intracerebral hemorrhage: "to detect and protect". J Clin Neurophysiol 2005;22(2):99–106.
73. Koubeissi M, Alshekhlee A. In-hospital mortality of generalized convulsive status epilepticus: a large US sample. Neurology 2007;69(9):886–93.
74. Mayer SA, Claassen J, Lokin J, et al. Refractory status epilepticus: frequency, risk factors, and impact on outcome. Arch Neurol 2002;59(2):205–10.
75. Novy J, Logroscino G, Rossetti AO. Refractory status epilepticus: a prospective observational study. Epilepsia 2010;51(2):251–6.
76. Waterhouse EJ, Garnett LK, Towne AR, et al. Prospective population-based study of intermittent and continuous convulsive status epilepticus in Richmond, Virginia. Epilepsia 1999;40(6):752–8.
77. Alldredge BK, Gelb AM, Isaacs SM, et al. A comparison of lorazepam, diazepam, and placebo for the treatment of out-of-hospital status epilepticus. N Engl J Med 2001;345(9):631–7.
78. Muayqil T, Rowe BH, Ahmed SN. Treatment adherence and outcomes in the management of convulsive status epilepticus in the emergency room. Epileptic Disord 2007;9(1):43–50.
79. Prasad K, Al-Roomi K, Krishnan PR, et al. Anticonvulsant therapy for status epilepticus. Cochrane Database Syst Rev 2005;4:CD003723.
80. McIntyre J, Robertson S, Norris E, et al. Safety and efficacy of buccal midazolam versus rectal diazepam for emergency treatment of seizures in children: a randomised controlled trial. Lancet 2005;366(9481):205–10.
81. Silbergleit R, Lowenstein D, Durkalski V. A double-blind randomized clinical trial of the efficacy of IM midazolam versus IV lorazepam in the pre-hospital treatment of status epilepticus by paramedics. In: Clinicaltrials.gov. Bethesda (MD): National Library of Medicine (US); 2000 [cited 6 Jun 2011]. Available at: https://clinitaltrials.gov/ct2/show/NCT00809146. Accessed June 6, 2011. NLM Identifier: 00809146.
82. Nocero M, Svoronos A, Arif H, et al. Nasal midazolam as a seizure-aborting therapy and comparison with oral and rectal benzodiazepines in adults [abstract S855.006]. Neurology Suppl 2011;76(9):A1–816.
83. Abou Khaled KJ, Hirsch LJ. Updates in the management of seizures and status epilepticus in critically ill patients. Neurol Clin 2008;26(2):385–408, viii.
84. Boggs JG, Painter JA, DeLorenzo RJ. Analysis of electrocardiographic changes in status epilepticus. Epilepsy Res 1993;14(1):87–94.
85. Legriel S, Bruneel F, Dalle L, et al. Recurrent takotsubo cardiomyopathy triggered by convulsive status epilepticus. Neurocrit Care 2008;9(1):118–21.
86. Manno EM, Pfeifer EA, Cascino GD, et al. Cardiac pathology in status epilepticus. Ann Neurol 2005;58(6):954–7.
87. Seow SC, Lee YP, Teo SG, et al. Takotsubo cardiomyopathy associated with status epilepticus. Eur J Neurol 2008;15(6):e46.

88. Willmore LJ. Epilepsy emergencies: the first seizure and status epilepticus. Neurology 1998;51(5 Suppl 4):S34–8.
89. Arif H, Hirsch LJ. Treatment of status epilepticus. Semin Neurol 2008;28(3): 342–54.
90. Leppik IE, Derivan AT, Homan RW, et al. Double-blind study of lorazepam and diazepam in status epilepticus. JAMA 1983;249(11):1452–4.
91. Claassen J, Hirsch LJ, Mayer SA. Treatment of status epilepticus: a survey of neurologists. J Neurol Sci 2003;211(1–2):37–41.
92. Agarwal P, Kumar N, Chandra R, et al. Randomized study of intravenous valproate and phenytoin in status epilepticus. Seizure 2007;16(6):527–32.
93. Aiguabella M, Falip M, Villanueva V, et al. Efficacy of intravenous levetiracetam as an add-on treatment in status epilepticus: a multicentric observational study. Seizure 2011;20(1):60–4.
94. Berning S, Boesebeck F, van Baalen A, et al. Intravenous levetiracetam as treatment for status epilepticus. J Neurol 2009;256(10):1634–42.
95. Claassen J, Hirsch LJ, Emerson RG, et al. Continuous EEG monitoring and midazolam infusion for refractory nonconvulsive status epilepticus. Neurology 2001; 57(6):1036–42.
96. Claassen J, Hirsch LJ, Emerson RG, et al. Treatment of refractory status epilepticus with pentobarbital, propofol, or midazolam: a systematic review. Epilepsia 2002;43(2):146–53.
97. Eue S, Grumbt M, Muller M, et al. Two years of experience in the treatment of status epilepticus with intravenous levetiracetam. Epilepsy Behav 2009;15(4):467–9.
98. Kellinghaus C, Berning S, Immisch I, et al. Intravenous lacosamide for treatment of status epilepticus. Acta Neurol Scand 2011;123(2):137–41.
99. Knake S, Gruener J, Hattemer K, et al. Intravenous levetiracetam in the treatment of benzodiazepine refractory status epilepticus. J Neurol Neurosurg Psychiatry 2008;79(5):588–9.
100. Misra UK, Kalita J, Patel R. Sodium valproate vs phenytoin in status epilepticus: a pilot study. Neurology 2006;67(2):340–2.
101. Rossetti AO, Milligan TA, Vulliemoz S, et al. A randomized trial for the treatment of refractory status epilepticus. Neurocrit Care 2011;14(1):4–10.
102. Rossetti AO, Reichhart MD, Schaller MD, et al. Propofol treatment of refractory status epilepticus: a study of 31 episodes. Epilepsia 2004;45(7):757–63.
103. Camilo O, Goldstein LB. Seizures and epilepsy after ischemic stroke. Stroke 2004;35(7):1769–75.
104. Burneo JG, Anandan JV, Barkley GL. A prospective study of the incidence of the purple glove syndrome. Epilepsia 2001;42(9):1156–9.
105. DeToledo JC, Ramsay RE. Fosphenytoin and phenytoin in patients with status epilepticus: improved tolerability versus increased costs. Drug Saf 2000; 22(6):459–66.
106. Zeller JA, Schlesinger S, Runge U, et al. Influence of valproate monotherapy on platelet activation and hematologic values. Epilepsia 1999;40(2):186–9.
107. Sinha S, Naritoku DK. Intravenous valproate is well tolerated in unstable patients with status epilepticus. Neurology 2000;55(5):722–4.
108. Fattouch J, Di Bonaventura C, Casciato S, et al. Intravenous levetiracetam as first-line treatment of status epilepticus in the elderly. Acta Neurol Scand 2010;121(6):418–21.
109. Vasile B, Rasulo F, Candiani A, et al. The pathophysiology of propofol infusion syndrome: a simple name for a complex syndrome. Intensive Care Med 2003; 29(9):1417–25.

110. Kapur J. Hippocampal neurons express GABA A receptor insensitive to diazepam in hyperexcitable conditions. Epilepsia 2000;41(Suppl 6):S86–9.
111. Rossetti AO, Logroscino G, Bromfield EB. Refractory status epilepticus: effect of treatment aggressiveness on prognosis. Arch Neurol 2005;62(11):1698–702.
112. Krishnamurthy KB, Drislane FW. Relapse and survival after barbiturate anesthetic treatment of refractory status epilepticus. Epilepsia 1996;37(9):863–7.
113. Meierkord H, Boon P, Engelsen B, et al. EFNS guideline on the management of status epilepticus in adults. Eur J Neurol 2010;17(3):348–55.
114. Bauer LA. Interference of oral phenytoin absorption by continuous nasogastric feedings. Neurology 1982;32(5):570–2.
115. Sander JW, Perucca E. Epilepsy and comorbidity: infections and antimicrobials usage in relation to epilepsy management. Acta Neurol Scand Suppl 2003;180: 16–22.
116. Greenaway C, Ratnaraj N, Sander JW, et al. Saliva and serum lacosamide concentrations in patients with epilepsy. Epilepsia 2011;52(2):258–63.
117. Koubeissi MZ, Mayor CL, Estephan B, et al. Efficacy and safety of intravenous lacosamide in refractory nonconvulsive status epilepticus. Acta Neurol Scand 2011;123(2):142–6.
118. Novy J, Rossetti AO. Oral pregabalin as an add-on treatment for status epilepticus. Epilepsia 2010;51(10):2207–10.
119. Towne AR, Garnett LK, Waterhouse EJ, et al. The use of topiramate in refractory status epilepticus. Neurology 2003;60(2):332–4.
120. Fisher A, Wang X, Cock HR, et al. Synergism between topiramate and budipine in refractory status epilepticus in the rat. Epilepsia 2004;45(11):1300–7.
121. Hamer HM, Knake S, Schomburg U, et al. Valproate-induced hyperammonemic encephalopathy in the presence of topiramate. Neurology 2000;54(1):230–2.
122. Borris DJ, Bertram EH, Kapur J. Ketamine controls prolonged status epilepticus. Epilepsy Res 2000;42(2–3):117–22.
123. Martin BS, Kapur J. A combination of ketamine and diazepam synergistically controls refractory status epilepticus induced by cholinergic stimulation. Epilepsia 2008;49(2):248–55.
124. Ubogu EE, Sagar SM, Lerner AJ, et al. Ketamine for refractory status epilepticus: a case of possible ketamine-induced neurotoxicity. Epilepsy Behav 2003;4(1):70–5.
125. Mirsattari SM, Sharpe MD, Young GB. Treatment of refractory status epilepticus with inhalational anesthetic agents isoflurane and desflurane. Arch Neurol 2004; 61(8):1254–9.
126. Fugate JE, Burns JD, Wijdicks EF, et al. Prolonged high-dose isoflurane for refractory status epilepticus: is it safe? Anesth Analg 2010;111(6):1520–4.
127. Pascual J, Ciudad J, Berciano J. Role of lidocaine (lignocaine) in managing status epilepticus. J Neurol Neurosurg Psychiatry 1992;55(1):49–51.
128. Walker IA, Slovis CM. Lidocaine in the treatment of status epilepticus. Acad Emerg Med 1997;4(9):918–22.
129. Visser NA, Braun KP, Leijten FS, et al. Magnesium treatment for patients with refractory status epilepticus due to POLG1-mutations. J Neurol 2011;258(2):218–22.
130. Loscher W. Mechanisms of drug resistance in status epilepticus. Epilepsia 2007;48(Suppl 8):74–7.
131. Schmitt FC, Dehnicke C, Merschhemke M, et al. Verapamil attenuates the malignant treatment course in recurrent status epilepticus. Epilepsy Behav 2010; 17(4):565–8.
132. Jambroszyk M, Tipold A, Potschka H. Add-on treatment with verapamil in pharmacoresistant canine epilepsy. Epilepsia 2011;52(2):284–91.

133. Gouveia TL, Scorza FA, Silva MJ, et al. Lovastatin decreases the synthesis of inflammatory mediators in the hippocampus and blocks the hyperthermia of rats submitted to long-lasting status epilepticus. Epilepsy Behav 2011;20(1):1–5.
134. Chu K, Jung KH, Lee ST, et al. Erythropoietin reduces epileptogenic processes following status epilepticus. Epilepsia 2008;49(10):1723–32.
135. Corry JJ, Dhar R, Murphy T, et al. Hypothermia for refractory status epilepticus. Neurocrit Care 2008;9(2):189–97.
136. Schmitt FC, Buchheim K, Meierkord H, et al. Anticonvulsant properties of hypothermia in experimental status epilepticus. Neurobiol Dis 2006;23(3):689–96.
137. Kamel H, Cornes SB, Hegde M, et al. Electroconvulsive therapy for refractory status epilepticus: a case series. Neurocrit Care 2010;12(2):204–10.
138. Miranda M, Kuester G, Rios L, et al. Refractory nonconvulsive status epilepticus responsive to music as an add-on therapy: a second case. Epilepsy Behav 2010;19(3):539–40.
139. Neal EG, Chaffe H, Schwartz RH, et al. The ketogenic diet for the treatment of childhood epilepsy: a randomised controlled trial. Lancet Neurol 2008;7(6):500–6.
140. Wusthoff CJ, Kranick SM, Morley JF, et al. The ketogenic diet in treatment of two adults with prolonged nonconvulsive status epilepticus. Epilepsia 2010;51(6):1083–5.
141. Ma X, Liporace J, O'Connor MJ, et al. Neurosurgical treatment of medically intractable status epilepticus. Epilepsy Res 2001;46(1):33–8.
142. Costello DJ, Simon MV, Eskandar EN, et al. Efficacy of surgical treatment of de novo, adult-onset, cryptogenic, refractory focal status epilepticus. Arch Neurol 2006;63(6):895–901.
143. Lhatoo SD, Alexopoulos AV. The surgical treatment of status epilepticus. Epilepsia 2007;48(Suppl 8):61–5.
144. Fisher R, Salanova V, Witt T, et al. Electrical stimulation of the anterior nucleus of thalamus for treatment of refractory epilepsy. Epilepsia 2010;51(5):899–908.
145. Hamani C, Hodaie M, Chiang J, et al. Deep brain stimulation of the anterior nucleus of the thalamus: effects of electrical stimulation on pilocarpine-induced seizures and status epilepticus. Epilepsy Res 2008;78(2–3):117–23.
146. Robakis TK, Hirsch LJ. Literature review, case report, and expert discussion of prolonged refractory status epilepticus. Neurocrit Care 2006;4(1):35–46.
147. Jordan KG. Nonconvulsive status epilepticus in acute brain injury. J Clin Neurophysiol 1999;16(4):332–40 [discussion: 353].
148. Litt B, Wityk RJ, Hertz SH, et al. Nonconvulsive status epilepticus in the critically ill elderly. Epilepsia 1998;39(11):1194–202.
149. Orta DS, Chiappa KH, Quiroz AZ, et al. Prognostic implications of periodic epileptiform discharges. Arch Neurol 2009;66:985–91.
150. Jaitly R, Sgro JA, Towne AR, et al. Prognostic value of EEG monitoring after status epilepticus: a prospective adult study. J Clin Neurophysiol 1997;14(4):326–34.
151. Nei M, Lee JM, Shanker VL, et al. The EEG and prognosis in status epilepticus. Epilepsia 1999;40(2):157–63.
152. Foreman B, Claassen J, Hirsch LJ. A controlled study of 202 patients with generalized periodic discharges (GPDs): relationship to seizures and outcome. New Orleans (LA): American Clinical Neurophysiology Society; 2011.
153. Fountain NB, Waldman WA. Effects of benzodiazepines on triphasic waves: implications for nonconvulsive status epilepticus. J Clin Neurophysiol 2001;18(4):345–52.

154. Brenner RP. Is it status? Epilepsia 2002;43(Suppl 3):103–13.
155. Ono S, Chida K, Fukaya N, et al. Dysphasia accompanied by periodic lateralized epileptiform discharges. Intern Med 1997;36(1):59–61.
156. Hirsch LJ, Brenner RP, Drislane FW, et al. The ACNS subcommittee on research terminology for continuous EEG monitoring: proposed standardized terminology for rhythmic and periodic EEG patterns encountered in critically ill patients. J Clin Neurophysiol 2005;22(2):128–35.
157. Wijdicks EF, Plevak DJ, Wiesner RH, et al. Causes and outcome of seizures in liver transplant recipients. Neurology 1996;47(6):1523–5.
158. Beach RL, Kaplan PW. Seizures in pregnancy: diagnosis and management. Int Rev Neurobiol 2008;83:259–71.
159. EURAP Study Group. Seizure control and treatment in pregnancy: observations from the EURAP epilepsy pregnancy registry. Neurology 2006;66(3):354–60.
160. Meador K, Reynolds MW, Crean S, et al. Pregnancy outcomes in women with epilepsy: a systematic review and meta-analysis of published pregnancy registries and cohorts. Epilepsy Res 2008;81(1):1–13.

Headache Emergencies: Diagnosis and Management

Benjamin W. Friedman, MD[a,*], Richard B. Lipton, MD[b,c]

KEYWORDS

• Headache • Emergency • Diagnosis • Management

Headaches are a common reason for visiting a neurologist, a primary care provider, or an emergency department. Most headaches that cause a medical visit are benign in nature in that the pain is self-limited and mortality or irreversible morbidity is unlikely. These benign headaches may be one of the primary headache disorders, such as migraine, tension-type headache, or cluster headache, or a secondary cause of headache, such as viral rhinosinusitis or cervicogenic headache. For most of these benign headaches, pain and other symptoms can be treated with over-the-counter or prescription medication. Occasionally, the pain from the benign headaches can be so severe and unremitting as to constitute a true emergency. This subject will be discussed later. At times, headaches are symptomatic of an underlying process that requires prompt diagnosis and urgent treatment to reduce threats to life or limb. Suspicion of these disorders mandates emergent diagnostic testing to exclude the disease. In this article, the authors review the 6 most common presentations for worrisome headaches and briefly discuss the differential diagnosis. The authors then review the specific etiologic categories of headaches most commonly sought in the differential diagnosis of a worrisome headache.

CLINICAL PRESENTATIONS OF CONCERN

In this section, the authors describe a series of relatively common headache presentations that raise the specter of worrisome headache. These presentations may occur

[a] Department of Emergency Medicine, Albert Einstein College of Medicine, Montefiore Medical Center, 111 East 210th Street, Bronx, New York 10467, USA

[b] Department of Neurology, Montefiore Headache Center, Albert Einstein College of Medicine, Bronx, 1300 Morris Park Avenue, Bronx, NY 10461, USA

[c] Department of Epidemiology and Population Health, Montefiore Headache Center, Albert Einstein College of Medicine, Bronx, 1300 Morris Park Avenue, Bronx, NY 10461, USA

* Corresponding author.

E-mail address: bwfriedmanmd@gmail.com

Neurol Clin 30 (2012) 43–59

doi:10.1016/j.ncl.2011.09.008

neurologic.theclinics.com

in isolation or in various combinations. For example, progressive headache may develop with evolving focal features in a worrisome combination.

First, Worst, or Sudden Onset

Most patients who present to a clinician with a new-onset headache will have a benign cause. However, the physician should be cautious about attributing the headache to a benign syndrome without a well-defined headache history. A low threshold for diagnostic imaging is warranted in patients who present with a new headache type, even though many of these will prove to be either self-limited or one of the defined recurrent headache syndromes.

The headaches of cerebrovascular catastrophes are often described as abrupt onset or the worst headache of the patients' life. The differential diagnosis for sudden-onset headache is broad and includes benign causes, such as migraine. However, a "worst headache of my life" or a sudden-onset headache should cause the clinician to consider hemorrhagic stroke, including aneurysmal subarachnoid hemorrhage, cervical artery dissection, venous sinus thrombosis, pituitary apoplexy, and other forms of intracranial hemorrhage.

Progressive Headache

A progressive, gradually worsening subacute headache raises concern for an enlarging space-occupying lesion. Intracranial mass lesions often produce focal signs and symptoms. Masses located outside the substance of the brain or in selected intraparenchymal regions, such as the anterior frontal lobe, cerebellum, or intrahemispheric fissure, may grow large without producing focal features. Neuroimaging is warranted to exclude a primary or metastatic tumor, subdural hematoma, hydrocephalus, abscess, and other intracranial mass lesions.[1] Although many patients will ultimately be given a benign diagnosis, such as transformed migraine, medication overuse headache, or new daily persistent headache, these diagnoses require the exclusion of space-occupying lesions.

Headache Associated with Focal Signs and Symptoms

Headaches associated with focal signs and symptoms require a thorough work-up to exclude mass lesions, ischemic or hemorrhagic stroke, a vascular pathologic condition, or infection. The differential diagnosis of headache plus focal findings is broad and work-up should be guided by the patients' profile of other risk factors. Symptomatic malignancy is usually visualized on routine noncontrast head computed tomography (CT). Cervical artery dissection requires dedicated imaging of the cervical arteries, whereas cerebral venous sinus thrombosis requires dedicated imaging of the cerebral venous system. Idiopathic intracranial hypertension requires the measurement of cerebral spinal fluid pressure. Infections, such as cryptococcal meningitis or Lyme meningitis, require spinal fluid analysis. Risk factors for these various illnesses and the appropriate work-up are discussed later.

Headache Associated with Fever and Stiff Neck

Meningitis classically presents with fever, meningismus, and altered mental status.[2] Patients with meningitis and an intact sensorium usually report headache. Pyogenic or sterile meningitis must be considered in patients who present with a headache, fever, or stiff neck. Less commonly, encephalitis, brain abscess, collagen vascular disease, and carcinomatous meningitis may cause these symptoms.

New-Onset Headache after 55 Years of Age

Beginning in the sixth decade of life, giant cell arteritis begins to emerge on the differential diagnosis of headaches. Concern for malignancy and atherosclerotic vascular disease also increases. Clinicians should consider ordering serum markers of inflammation, such as an erythrocyte sedimentation rate and a C-reactive protein, and neuroimaging in patients aged older than 55 years with a new-onset headache.[3]

New-Onset Headache in a Person with Cancer, HIV, or Immunosuppression

Rarer infectious causes of headaches are a concern in immunosuppressed patients. Cryptococcal meningitis may present with nothing more than an indolent headache. Toxoplasmosis usually causes focal neurologic symptoms along with the headache, whereas patients with a brain abscess often will not seem toxic. Mycobacterium, syphilis, and HIV itself may also cause headaches.[4] HIV is a risk factor for central nervous system (CNS) lymphoma. Patients with known malignancy are at risk for CNS metastases, particularly from primary malignancies of the lung, breast, and gastrointestinal tract.[5]

CAUSES OF CONCERN: HEADACHE AND CEREBROVASCULAR EMERGENCIES

Aneurysmal Subarachnoid Hemorrhage

Cerebrovascular aneurysms are present in 2% of the population,[6] whereas national data reveal that 30,000 Americans suffer a subarachnoid hemorrhage each year.[7] Aneurysmal subarachnoid hemorrhage is a devastating illness, with mortality rates approaching 50% and substantial morbidity.[7] Patients suffering from subarachnoid hemorrhage who have the best prognosis are those who are diagnosed while neurologically intact.[8] Because the rebleed rate is substantial, it is essential to diagnose and treat these patients emergently. In patients who are obtunded or present with focal neurologic impairment, the indication for head imaging is obvious. The difficulty arises in determining which neurologically intact patients who present with headache require an emergent and complete work-up.

Some authorities advocate casting a very wide net in the pursuit of aneurysmal subarachnoid hemorrhage.[8] Conducting a work-up of all patients who present with a first, worst, or changed headache will make missing subarachnoid hemorrhage unlikely and may be appropriate for a practice that sees mostly high-acuity patients or sees headaches only infrequently. Risk stratifying based on features of the headache history may also be a reasonable strategy. For example, the headache of subarachnoid hemorrhage usually peaks in intensity rapidly. Headaches that take more than several minutes to peak in intensity are substantially less likely to be a subarachnoid hemorrhage.[9] Unlike the primary headache disorders, subarachnoid hemorrhage is less common in patients younger than 45 years.[10] Clinical decision rules can be used to help decide which patients who present to an emergency department with acute-onset headache require an emergent work-up (**Box 1**). Although severe pain, occipital location, vomiting, elevated blood pressure, and neck symptoms in conjunction with headache have been identified as high-risk features, the absence of any one of these does not preclude the disease.[10]

A noncontrast head CT will diagnosis most cases of subarachnoid hemorrhage, particularly if performed soon after the ictus. The sensitivity of head CT for subarachnoid blood decreases with time because the hemoglobin within the cerebrospinal fluid (CSF) is metabolized and diluted. If performed within 6 hours, the sensitivity of head CT approaches 100%, although this diminishes to the low 90s by 24 hours and less than 75% within several days.[11] To exclude the diagnosis of subarachnoid hemorrhage

Box 1
Clinical decision rules for the diagnosis of nontraumatic subarachnoid hemorrhage

Canadian subarachnoid decision rule

Each of these 3 rules were 100% sensitive for identifying subarachnoid hemorrhage in a population of patients with nontraumatic headache that peaked in intensity within 1 hour. These rules have yet to be validated in a distinct population.

Rule 1

- Aged older than 40 years
- Complaint of neck pain or stiffness
- Witnessed loss of consciousness
- Onset with exertion

Rule 2

- Arrival by ambulance
- Aged older than 45 years
- Vomiting at least once
- Diastolic blood pressure greater than 100 mm Hg

Rule 3

- Arrival by ambulance
- Systolic blood pressure greater than 160 mm Hg
- Complaint of neck pain or stiffness
- Aged 45 to 55 years

Perry JJ, Stiell IG, Sivilotti ML, et al. High risk clinical characteristics for subarachnoid haemorrhage in patients with acute headache: prospective cohort study. BMJ 2010;341:c5204. doi: 10.1136/bmj.c5204.

Clinical predictors associated with any bad outcome

Taken together, these 3 clinical features identified 98.6% of all pathologic headaches that presented to one emergency department over a 14-month period.

- Aged older than 50 years
- Sudden-onset headache
- Any neurologic abnormality on physical examination

From Perry JJ, Stiell IG, Sivilotti ML, et al. High risk clinical characteristics for subarachnoid haemorrhage in patients with acute headache: prospective cohort study. BMJ 2010;341:c5204; with permission.

definitively, a spinal fluid analysis is required in which the evidence of bleeding is sought. This evidence may be in the form of red blood cells not attributable to trauma from the lumbar puncture itself or xanthochromia, the yellowish tinge that CSF acquires from the metabolism of red blood cells. As a cautionary note, xanthochromia may take hours to develop, so a lumbar puncture within several hours of the bleed may not demonstrate xanthochromia. Alternatively, rather than a lumbar puncture, a CT angiogram or magnetic resonance (MR) angiogram may be used to evaluate for a causative aneurysm. Although these imaging modalities are not 100% sensitive for causative aneurysms, the combination of either of these tests with a normal noncontrast head CT is sufficiently sensitive, given that the first test is searching just for blood and the second is searching for an aneurysm.[11] Because a causative aneurysm is managed differently than a small incidentally discovered aneurysm, an abnormal CT or MR angiogram should be followed with a lumbar puncture if there is no evidence of bleeding on imaging.

Definitive treatment of a leaking aneurysm involves identifying the aneurysm and excluding it from the circulatory system. For aneurysms that are amenable to neurosurgical and cerebrovascular interventional procedures, the latter results in better long-term outcomes, assuming sufficient local expertise.[12] Nimodipine, a calcium channel blocker, should be started soon after a diagnosis of aneurysmal subarachnoid hemorrhage is made to lessen the likelihood of vasospastic-induced ischemic outcome.[13] Antifibrinolytics (eg, aminocaproic acid) do not improve the overall outcome because the reduction in the rate of rebleeding is offset by an increase in poor outcome caused by cerebral ischemia.[14] Similarly, corticosteroids have not been demonstrated to be of benefit.[15] The ideal management of blood pressure is not clearly understood, although some amount of blood pressure modulation is likely to be of benefit. Opioid analgesia and antiemetics should be used to make patients comfortable. Clinically evident seizures should be treated with anticonvulsants but the prophylactic use of these drugs is controversial.[16]

Cervical Artery Dissection

Carotid and vertebral artery dissections are a rare cause of stroke and an even rarer cause of isolated headache,[17] although they should be considered higher in the differential diagnosis of nonelderly patients who present with headache, neck, or facial pain with neurologic deficits. Classically, carotid artery dissection will present with a partial Horner syndrome, retinal or cerebral ischemic symptoms, pulsatile tinnitus, or cranial neuropathies in patients with a history of minor neck trauma or Valsalva maneuvers.[18] Vertebral artery dissection is more likely to cause brain stem ischemic symptoms.[18] However, the presentation or cervical artery dissections can be quite variable. This disease may present with little more than a headache, facial pain, or carotidynia. Spontaneous, atraumatic dissections are common. Therefore, cervical artery dissection should be on the differential diagnosis of any patient with a new-onset cluster headache or trigeminal neuralgia.

The prevalence of this disease is probably underappreciated because patients who present with pain but no focal neurologic impairment are less likely to receive an aggressive work-up. There is often a delay of at least 1 day between the time of the injury and the presentation to a physician,[19,20] suggesting that the progression or persistence of symptoms result in a visit rather than the initial symptoms and that some patients may improve spontaneously. Pain may precede neurologic findings by days in patients who ultimately develop ischemic symptoms.[20,21] The headache has been described as a pulsating pain and as a steady or constrictive pain.[20] It can be sudden or acute onset, progressive, or intermittent. It may be associated with nausea and vomiting.[17]

Diagnosis is readily made with CT or MR angiography. Ultrasonography lacks the sensitivity of these other imaging modalities but can be used to confirm the diagnosis when it is clinically apparent.[22]

Prognosis is generally good and associated with both traditional cerebrovascular risk factors and neurologic impairment at diagnosis.[23,24] Ischemic or hemorrhagic stroke can occur. It is unclear how common these outcomes are in carotid dissection because diagnosis is often contingent on the presence of focal neurologic signs and symptoms. Most ischemic strokes in the setting of carotid dissection are thought to be embolic, although watershed ischemia and low-flow strokes can also occur. Patients are usually treated with anticoagulation or antiplatelet therapy. Randomized comparative studies do not exist, therefore, it is impossible to be certain which therapy is preferable. However, a Cochrane synthesis of the literature suggests anticoagulants may be more effective at preventing death and disability than antiplatelet agents.[25] The role of endovascular stenting is ill defined.[26]

Cerebral Venous Sinus Thrombosis

Cerebral venous sinus thrombosis is a rare cause of stroke with neurologic symptoms that often presage the headache. It is eminently treatable, although diagnosis may be difficult because of a subtle or indolent presentation. Risk factors for this illness are those that predispose patients to thromboembolic disease. Thus, patients with venous sinus thrombosis are substantially younger than other patients who suffer ischemic or hemorrhagic stroke and have a different set of comorbidities than patients with traditional atherosclerotic stroke. Specifically, the use of oral contraceptives; the puerperium; genetic mutations associated with thrombophilia, such as factor V Leiden deficiency; and medical illness associated with thrombophilia, such as systemic lupus erythematosus or inflammatory bowel disease; place patients at risk of venous sinus thrombosis. Also, the extension of head and face infections as well as neurosurgical procedures can cause the sinus thrombosis to develop.[27]

Cerebral venous sinus thrombosis may present with a thunderclap headache, although the headache is more commonly gradual in onset.[28] Seizure and focal neurologic signs and symptoms develop as intracranial pressure increases. Papilledema may also be present as the disease progresses.

Diagnosis is often difficult because the disease is rare, the headache may be nonspecific, and the pathologic condition is not readily apparent on routine head imaging. To be assured of excluding the diagnosis, imaging of the cerebral sinuses is required; this is most commonly done with MR venography. Serum markers of fibrinolysis, specifically the D dimer, may be used to exclude thromboembolic processes in patients at low risk of disease, particularly if the symptoms are of shorter duration.[29,30]

Treatment of this disease includes addressing the acute thrombus; addressing the symptoms caused by the thrombus, such as headache, nausea, and seizures; identification of the factors that placed patients at risk of thrombus development; and optimizing therapy to prevent future thromboembolic events. Anticoagulation is considered standard therapy for this disease, although there is an associated risk of intracranial hemorrhage. For most patients, the benefit of therapy with unfractionated or low-molecular-weight heparin outweighs the risk. Thrombolysis, particularly local thrombolysis achieved by the administration of the thrombolytic directly to the thrombus, may be useful, although it also carries the associated risk of hemorrhage.[31]

Giant Cell Arteritis

Giant cell arteritis (or temporal arteritis) is a disease exclusively of patients in the second half of life, can cause permanent visual loss and, thus, needs to be excluded as the diagnosis in all patients aged older than 50 years who present with new-onset headache. Visual loss in this disorder is usually caused by anterior optic neuropathy but posterior optic neuropathy, central retinal artery, and cortical blindness may occur. This disease is an inflammatory arteriopathy affecting the aorta, occasionally the vertebral arteries, and branches of the external carotid artery, most notably the temporal artery. The specific cause or inciting event is currently unknown. The inflammatory infiltration of blood vessel walls leads to luminal narrowing and ischemic events downstream.[32] Giant cell arteritis is comorbid with polymyalgia rheumatica.

Headache is present in 75% of patients with temporal arteritis and is frequently the presenting chief complaint. The headache of temporal arteritis is variable. It may affect just the temple but it may also extend to the occiput or generalize.[33] It may be isolated to the occipital area.[34] It is often described as achy and persistent. New-onset stabbing headache has also been described.[35] International Headache Society criteria attribute the headache to temporal arteritis only if the headache responds to corticosteroid therapy.[36]

Jaw claudication (pain in the proximal jaw most notable with vigorous chewing) is an uncommon but highly suggestive feature. Diplopia and ophthalmoparesis may occur. The absence of visual symptoms or of headache does not rule out the disease.[37] On physical examination, beading, prominence, engorgement, or tenderness of the temporal artery are predictive of a positive biopsy result.[37]

The American College of Rheumatology diagnostic criteria are standard and require 3 of the following 5 items: greater than or equal to 50 years of age; a new headache type; temporal artery abnormalities, including tenderness or decreased pulsations not attributable to atherosclerosis; a Westergren erythrocyte sedimentation rate greater than or equal to 50 mm/h; and a biopsy specimen showing vasculitis characterized by a predominance of mononuclear cell infiltration or granulomatous inflammation. Based on these criteria, patients can be diagnosed with temporal arteritis without a biopsy result. Furthermore, a positive biopsy by itself does not define the disease without the other criteria.[38]

Giant cell arteritis can largely be excluded from diagnostic consideration with normal blood tests. Although neither a normal erythrocyte sedimentation rate nor a normal C-reactive protein excludes the diagnosis definitely, the combination of 2 normal results makes the diagnosis substantially less likely.[39,40] Patients who remain at high suspicion for disease despite normal laboratory values should still be referred for temporal artery biopsy.

Patients with giant cell arteritis are at high risk of permanent visual loss in 1 or both eyes and, therefore, corticosteroid therapy should be initiated promptly. The optimal agent, dose, and route of delivery of corticosteroids is not established, although high doses of oral agents are commonly used. Earlier initiation of therapy improves outcomes.[41]

Reversible Cranial Vasoconstriction Syndrome

Reversible cranial vasoconstriction syndrome has been known by a variety of names over the years, including Call-Fleming syndrome, postpartum angiopathy, and migrainous vasospasm. It is characterized by discrete areas of vasoconstriction within the cerebral vasculature that normalize within 3 months. On imaging studies, the cerebral vasculature assumes a sausage-on-a-string or beads-on-a-string appearance representing multiple discrete areas of vasoconstriction. Reversible cranial vasoconstriction syndrome is thought to cause a recurrent thunderclap headache and is associated with ischemic and hemorrhagic stroke. The true population prevalence is unknown; it is only identified in patients who have suffered a stroke or in patients who have experienced a thunderclap headache and receive a thorough work-up. For most patients with a thunderclap headache, a specific cause is not discovered[42]; this syndrome may be the cause of many of them. On the other hand, this syndrome could be rare; case series may be the result of thorough work-ups in regional referral centers.

A severe acute-onset headache is the predominant symptom of reversible cranial vasoconstriction syndrome. Some patients experience neurologic symptoms, including transient or lasting focal deficits and seizures, or recurrent thunderclap headaches. The headache is usually bilateral. Associated symptoms included nausea, vomiting, agitation, and photophobia. An antecedent use of vasoactive substances, including cannabis, selective serotonin-norepinephrine reuptake inhibitors, and nasal decongestants, is commonly reported.

It is currently uncertain how to manage this disease once it is diagnosed. By definition, the disease is self-limited, although transient ischemia or hemorrhage leaves a minority of patients with permanent focal deficits or cognitive impairment. Calcium channel blockers are used to decrease vasospasm and, thereby, presumably improve outcomes. Glucocorticoids also have been used to treat patients. The population at risk of poor outcome and, therefore, whom to treat has not yet been defined.[43,44]

CAUSES OF CONCERN: HEADACHE AND SPACE-OCCUPYING LESIONS

Intracranial Neoplasm

Brain tumor is often on the mind of patients who present to a clinician with a new mild or moderate headache. For many of these patients, clear reassurance that they do not have a brain tumor is as important as a specific diagnosis and treatment.[3] A multitude of different types of tumors can cause a headache. Secondary headache may be caused by neoplasms that originate from the brain, meninges, or skull, or may have metastasized from a more distant location, most commonly lung, breast, gastrointestinal tract, or kidneys.[5]

Intracranial neoplasms commonly present with headache along with focal neurologic deficits, seizures, or neurocognitive deficits. It is less common for patients to present with an isolated headache and no other neurologic complaints, although this becomes more common in the geriatric population because brain atrophy allows more space for a malignancy to grow asymptomatically. Classically, brain neoplasm present with a nocturnal headache that awakens patients from sleep, morning headaches, vomiting, and headaches that worsen with the Valsalva maneuver. This classic presentation is uncommon and should not be relied on. The headache of brain neoplasms may be quite variable; it has been described as throbbing, pressurelike, and shooting. Commonly, these headaches are not constant, severe, or progressive.[45]

The diagnosis of intracranial neoplasm is often readily apparent on routine noncontrast head CT, although sometimes contrast is needed to identify or delineate the primary process. The question for the physician invariably is how aggressively to pursue neuroimaging in patients with a new headache and a normal neurologic examination. Some expert opinion and guideline statements recommend imaging all patients with a new headache type and certainly those patients aged older than 50 years.[1,8]

Symptoms usually respond to corticosteroids, such as dexamethasone, which are quite effective at decreasing the resultant edema. Definitive treatment depends on tumor size, type, location, and overall patient prognosis. Antiepileptic drugs are reserved for patients who develop seizures and should not be administered prophylactically.[46]

Posttraumatic Hematoma

A headache in the setting of blunt head trauma raises the concern of an intracranial hematoma, particularly if the trauma was of sufficient severity to cause alterations in level of consciousness. Blood may collect in the brain parenchyma, the subarachnoid space, the subdural space, or the epidural space. In addition, minor head trauma may also result in a postconcussive syndrome consisting of headache, neurocognitive deficits, and dizziness. However, the focus here is on the identification of patients who require emergent neurosurgical intervention. A noncontrast head CT is a highly sensitive test for identifying clinically significant posttraumatic hematomas. The challenge with this illness is to identify which patients require emergent neuroimaging.

A common clinical scenario is the patient who complains of headache in the immediate posttraumatic period. Most patients who experience minor or minimal head trauma will have a normal head CT and will not require neurosurgical intervention. Headache itself in the setting of minor head trauma does not help discriminate between those patients with a normal versus abnormal head CT.[47] Two high-quality competing clinical decision rules have been published that identify a low-risk population of patients who are exceedingly unlikely to require neurosurgical intervention (**Box 2**).[48,49] The New Orleans criteria is the more conservative of the two rules, requiring imaging in all victims on minor blunt head trauma with a Glasgow Coma Scale of less than 15, with a headache, or with any stigmata of trauma above the clavicles.[49] As a result, this clinical decision rule requires more head CTs to be performed; application of this rule in an emergency department population would allow CT to be avoided in only 10% of patients.[47] The Canadian CT head rule potentially allows 50% of head CTs to be avoided, although its sensitivity may be less than 85% in

Box 2
Clinical decision rules for the diagnosis of clinically important neurotraumatic processes

New Orleans criteria

- All patients with positive CT scans had at least 1 of the following:
  - Headache
  - Vomiting
  - Aged older than 60 years
  - Drug or alcohol intoxication
  - Deficits in short-term memory
  - Physical evidence of trauma above the clavicles
  - Seizure

Canadian CT head rule

- CT head is only required for patients with minor head injuries with any 1 of the following:
  - GCS score less than 15 at 2 hours after injury
  - Suspected open or depressed skull fracture
  - Any sign of basal skull fracture (hemotympanum, raccoon eyes, CSF otorrhea/rhinorrhea, Battle sign)
  - Vomiting 2 episodes or more
  - Aged 65 years or older
  - Amnesia before impact greater than or equal to 30 minutes
  - Dangerous mechanism (pedestrian struck by motor vehicle, occupant ejected from motor vehicle, fall from height more than 3 ft or 5 stairs)

From Haydel MJ, Preston CA, Mills TJ, et al. Indication for computed tomography in patients with minor head injury. N Engl J Med 2000;343:100–5; with permission.

a population of very high-risk head trauma patients.[50] Although not tested in an outpatient setting, the Canadian rule supports infrequent neuroimaging in a population of neurologically intact victims of minor head trauma who walk into a clinic and whose symptomatology includes only mild or moderate headache.

Pituitary Apoplexy

A Hemorrhagic infarct of the pituitary may cause a devastating presentation of headache, bitemporal visual field deficits, ophthalmoplegia, and cardiovascular collapse. A headache, usually sudden onset, is a prominent feature in patients who have not lost mental status.[51] Pituitary apoplexy occurs most often within an abnormal pituitary, often because of an adenoma. A precipitating factor may be identified, such as initiation or withdrawal of medical pituitary therapy, major surgery, parturition, anticoagulant therapy, or head trauma.[52] A history of pituitary adenoma is a feature of the past medical history that can help the clinician arrive at the correct diagnosis; however, for most patients with pituitary apoplexy, the apoplexy is the presenting event.[53] A noncontrast head CT can usually visualize large pituitary adenomas, although magnetic resonance imaging optimizes sensitivity. Emergency medical management is directed toward replacement of corticosteroids to ensure hemodynamic stability. Emergent neurosurgical decompression is often performed to restore lost or worsening vision.[54]

CAUSES OF CONCERN: HEADACHE AND INCREASED INTRACRANIAL PRESSURE WITHOUT A MASS LESION

Idiopathic Intracranial Hypertension

Compared with other headache disorders, idiopathic intracranial hypertension (IIH) is a relatively uncommon neurologic disease seen primarily in young obese women of childbearing age. Because the headache pattern is chronic and because visual complaints are common, the headache may be carelessly ascribed to chronic migraine with aura. However, visual loss with this disease can be dramatic, rapidly progressive, and irreversible, so this diagnosis cannot be missed.[55]

A headache is the most prominent symptom of IIH. The headache is often nonspecific or may mimic migraine. Visual complaints are common but may be fleeting or waxing and waning. Patients also may complain of pulsatile tinnitus. As the disease progresses, the physical examination will reveal papilledema and visual field defects, including an enlarged blind spot initially, followed by loss of peripheral vision.

A thorough neurologic examination searching for papilledema, visual field deficits, and ophthalmoplegias will identify most cases of IIH. The finding of papilledema then warrants neuroimaging to ensure no intracranial mass is causing the papilledema and a lumbar puncture to measure the opening pressure of the cerebral spinal fluid. Pressures more than 220 mm are consistent with IIH. Cerebral venous sinus imaging will ensure that the elevated opening pressure is not caused by impaired venous return.

Symptomatic treatment includes lowering intracranial pressure and relieving the headache. Lumbar puncture is the mainstay for accomplishing this goal, although long-term management goals include minimizing the number of lumbar punctures performed. Visual loss may be ameliorated with optic nerve sheath fenestration or CSF diversion. Acetazolamide is used to mitigate chronic symptoms. Some data indicate good long-term outcomes in those patients who continue to use acetazolamide, although clinical trial data are not yet available.[56] Corticosteroids also have been used, although rebound headache may occur when doses are tapered.

CAUSES OF CONCERN: HEADACHE AND SYSTEMIC ILLNESS

Hypertensive Headache

The link between hypertension and headache is well established in the public mind, although epidemiologic studies do not support this association.[57] No data are available to support or refute the common practice of using antihypertensives for patients with elevated blood pressure who present to a physician with an acute headache. It is clear, however, that certain antihypertensives, such as the beta-blockers and angiotensin receptor blockers, decrease the frequency of headaches when used prophylactically in patients with frequent disabling migraines.[58,59] Similar uncertainty surrounds the common clinical scenario of patients who present with a headache, an elevated blood pressure, and no history of hypertension. The International Headache Society defines a hypertensive headache as one in which there is a paroxysmal increase in systolic or diastolic blood pressure to greater than 160 mm HG or 120 mm HG, respectively.[36] The headache must be either bilateral or pulsating or precipitated by physical activity. It must develop during the hypertensive period and resolve within 1 hour after normalization of blood pressure. Absent the signs of encephalopathy, it is unclear if these patients should be treated with analgesics, antimigraine medication, or with antihypertensive medication. One treatment option the authors have found useful is to use intravenous (IV) metoclopramide, a medication with both antimigraine and antiheadache efficacy, which is also known to lower blood pressure.

CAUSES OF CONCERN: HEADACHE AND INFECTION

Meningitis/Encephalitis

CNS infections run the gamut from severe and life threatening to self-limited and benign. The diagnosis at times may be obvious based on physical appearance of patients and other times may present with little more than a subacute headache or a fever. A spinal fluid analysis is the definitive test to diagnose meningitis but it is not always necessary to perform a lumbar puncture to dictate management; at times, treatment must be initiated before the definitive diagnosis is available.

Bacterial meningitis is a life-threatening illness that requires early suspicion and prompt antimicrobial therapy. Classically, bacterial meningitis presents with fever, nuchal rigidity, and altered mental status, although the presence of the complete triad is variable and in some cohorts has been present in fewer than 50% of patients.[2,60] Headache is a common feature of bacterial meningitis, but no classic headache pattern has been described.

Lyme meningitis is a subtle illness. Therefore, practitioners in endemic regions need to maintain an awareness of the typical presentation to ensure that the diagnosis will be made. Headache and meningismus may be no worse than moderate. Arthralgias and malaise may be the most prominent symptoms. A history of erythema migraines is usually present. Neuropathic or radicular sensory symptoms and cranial neuropathies, particularly facial nerve palsy, may be present.[61]

Cryptococcal meningitis is, for the most part, a disease of the immunocompromised, although occasional cases in immunocompetent patients are reported. One needs to have a high index of suspicion for this illness as T cells decrease because the initial presentation can be nonspecific, often no more than a mild headache with low-grade fevers and malaise. As the illness progresses, nuchal rigidity, cranial neuropathies, and altered mental status occur. Patients using immunotherapy for solid organ transplant or on chronic corticosteroids are also at risk of cryptococcal infection.[62,63]

Viral meningitis can be a painful and functionally disabling illness but is unlikely to be life threatening in immunocompetent adults without evidence of encephalitis or myelitis. Common causes are enteroviruses, herpes simplex viruses, and varicella-zoster virus. When headache is a prominent component of what otherwise seems like an acute viremia, a spinal fluid analysis may not influence management, although it is often difficult to exclude bacterial meningitis on clinical grounds alone. Unlike in bacterial meningitis whereby alterations in consciousness are a prominent component of the patients' presentation, headache is usually the most prominent feature of viral meningitis. Hospital admission may be required for pain control, antiemetics, and IV fluid therapy.

EMERGENCY PRESENTATIONS OF PRIMARY HEADACHE DISORDERS

Status Migrainosus

Although status migrainosus does not threaten life or limb, this unremitting, unbearable headache should be treated expeditiously and effectively. For some of these patients, oral, inhaled, or rectal medications will suffice. Others should be referred to an infusion center or an emergency department for parenteral treatment. While treating the patients' pain, the clinician should be sure to eliminate secondary headache from the differential diagnosis. Gradual onset of the patients' typical migraine, which ultimately was simply not responsive to the patients' usual medication, is a reassuring history. However, a new headache type in a known migraineur should not be automatically attributed to migraine.

A wide variety of parenteral medications are available to treat status migrainosus (**Table 1**), although no high-quality evidence for the treatment of status migrainosus has been published. Treatment decisions are based on open-label studies or on randomized, double-blind trials of therapies for acute migraine. The Raskin protocol has long been used with success.[64] This combination of IV dihydroergotamine and metoclopramide administered every 8 hours is used successfully in many inpatient headache units. The antiemetic dopamine antagonists droperidol and prochlorperazine are highly effective and can be substituted for metoclopramide.[65] Corticosteroids

Table 1
Intravenous medications that may be used for status migrainosus

Medication	Dose	Cautions/Side Effects
Dihydroergotamine	1 mg	Administer with antiemetic; contraindicated in patients with severe hypertension, coronary artery disease, pregnancy, recent use of sumatriptan, or currently using macrolide antibiotics or retroviral therapy
Metoclopramide	10 mg to be infused over 15 min	Akathisia may be treated with diphenhydramine or midazolam
Prochlorperazine	10 mg to be infused over 15 min	Akathisia may be treated with diphenhydramine or midazolam
Droperidol	2.5 mg to be infused over 15 min	Akathisia may be treated with diphenhydramine or midazolam; may cause QT prolongation, which can lead to clinically significant arrhythmia
Ketorolac	30 mg IV push	Caution in patients with chronic kidney disease or peptic ulcer disease
Valproic Acid	1 mg to be infused over 10–15 min	Contraindicated in pregnancy, use cautiously in patients with liver disease
Dexamethasone	10 mg slow IV push	

decrease the recurrence of headache after initial successful parenteral treatment[66] and, barring contraindications, should be used in patients with migraines of sufficient severity to require hospitalization. Parenteral nonsteroidal antiinflammatory drugs, such as ketorolac, can be coadministered with dihydroergotamine and the dopamine-antagonists. IV valproic acid may also have a role for some patients with unremitting migraine.[67] Finally, aggressive IV fluid rehydration, particularly in migraineurs suffering substantial nausea and vomiting, may be effective.

If relief has not been obtained from any of the therapies listed previously, opioids are a reasonable last resort. Opioids are effective, safe, and well-tolerated analgesics. They are generally avoided as initial migraine therapy for fear of exacerbating the underlying migraine disorder but should not be withheld on principle when patients are suffering.

AN APPROACH TO HEADACHE WORK-UP

Most headaches that present de novo in any practice setting will be benign. For most patients, management should consist of identifying the headache disorder and providing patients with a specific diagnosis, identifying causative or contributing factors, and initiating appropriate treatment. For some patients, the headache is a warning sign of a more ominous underlying disorder. The astute clinician needs to diagnose the malignant secondary causes of headache without unnecessarily exposing every headache patient to the expense, inconvenience, and side effects of a full work-up; postlumbar puncture headache is common, contrast-induced nephropathy or allergic complications of CT scans with contrast can be serious, and our understanding of long-term medical imaging–induced radiation toxicity is evolving. Furthermore, excess diagnostic testing leads to the discovery of incidental findings or equivocal results, which can only be addressed with further testing. Thus, diagnostic testing should not be undertaken lightly.

On the other hand, the differential diagnosis of headache is finite, and most pathologic causes of headache can be diagnosed with neurovascular imaging and a few well-chosen blood tests, such as an erythrocyte sedimentation rate, a C-reactive protein, and a D dimer. In patients who, based on history and physical examination, are at high risk of secondary headaches, the complete work-up should be pursued emergently.

A middle-of-the-road approach is to perform a noncontrast head CT followed by a lumbar puncture in all neurologically intact patients who present with a first, worst, or changed headache, plus an erythrocyte sedimentation rate and a C-reactive protein in patients aged 50 years and older. This pathway will identify all but the rarest of the secondary headaches.

Practice patterns should depend on the case mix at individual sites and characteristics of the individual patient. Practices that see predominantly high-acuity patients need to have streamlined pathways to facilitate a diagnostic work-up. Clinicians who see predominantly low-acuity patients need to maintain the diseases discussed in this article within their differential diagnoses.

SUMMARY

In conclusion, headache may be a warning sign of a wide variety of malignant processes. Careful attention to the patients' history and physical examination and a thoughtful approach to the differential diagnosis will help guide diagnostic work-up and management. Although benign causes of headaches are more common than malignant secondary processes, appropriate management of the headache depends on excluding malignant secondary processes.

REFERENCES

1. Edlow JA, Panagos PD, Godwin SA, et al. Clinical policy: critical issues in the evaluation and management of adult patients presenting to the emergency department with acute headache. Ann Emerg Med 2008;52(4):407–36.
2. Attia J, Hatala R, Cook DJ, et al. The rational clinical examination. Does this adult patient have acute meningitis? JAMA 1999;282(2):175–81.
3. Frishberg BM. The utility of neuroimaging in the evaluation of headache in patients with normal neurologic examinations. Neurology 1994;44(7):1191–7.
4. Gladstone J, Bigal ME. Headaches attributable to infectious diseases. Curr Pain Headache Rep 2010;14(4):299–308.
5. Kirby S, Purdy RA. Headache and brain tumors. Curr Neurol Neurosci Rep 2007; 7(2):110–6.
6. Rinkel GJ, Djibuti M, Algra A, et al. Prevalence and risk of rupture of intracranial aneurysms: a systematic review. Stroke 1998;29(1):251–6.
7. Bederson JB, Connolly ES Jr, Batjer HH, et al. Guidelines for the management of aneurysmal subarachnoid hemorrhage: a statement for healthcare professionals from a special writing group of the Stroke Council, American Heart Association. Stroke 2009;40(3):994–1025.
8. Edlow JA, Caplan LR. Avoiding pitfalls in the diagnosis of subarachnoid hemorrhage. N Engl J Med 2000;342(1):29–36.
9. Linn FH, Rinkel GJ, Algra A, et al. Headache characteristics in subarachnoid haemorrhage and benign thunderclap headache. J Neurol Neurosurg Psychiatry 1998;65(5):791–3.
10. Perry JJ, Stiell IG, Sivilotti ML, et al. High risk clinical characteristics for subarachnoid haemorrhage in patients with acute headache: prospective cohort study. BMJ 2010;341:c5204.
11. McCormack RF, Hutson A. Can computed tomography angiography of the brain replace lumbar puncture in the evaluation of acute-onset headache after a negative noncontrast cranial computed tomography scan? Acad Emerg Med 2010; 17(4):444–51.
12. van der Schaaf I, Algra A, Wermer M, et al. Endovascular coiling versus neurosurgical clipping for patients with aneurysmal subarachnoid haemorrhage. Cochrane Database Syst Rev 2005;4:CD003085.
13. Dorhout Mees SM, Rinkel GJ, Feigin VL, et al. Calcium antagonists for aneurysmal subarachnoid haemorrhage. Cochrane Database Syst Rev 2007;3: CD000277.
14. Roos Y, Rinkel G, Vermeulen M, et al. Antifibrinolytic therapy for aneurysmal subarachnoid hemorrhage: a major update of a Cochrane review. Stroke 2003; 34(9):2308–9.
15. Feigin VL, Anderson N, Rinkel GJ, et al. Corticosteroids for aneurysmal subarachnoid haemorrhage and primary intracerebral haemorrhage. Cochrane Database Syst Rev 2005;3:CD004583.
16. Riordan KC, Wingerchuk DM, Wellik KE, et al. Anticonvulsant drug therapy after aneurysmal subarachnoid hemorrhage: a critically appraised topic. Neurologist 2010;16(6):397–9.
17. Arnold M, Cumurciuc R, Stapf C, et al. Pain as the only symptom of cervical artery dissection. J Neurol Neurosurg Psychiatry 2006;77(9):1021–4.

18. Schievink WI. Spontaneous dissection of the carotid and vertebral arteries. N Engl J Med 2001;344(12):898–906.
19. Ahmad HA, Gerraty RP, Davis SM, et al. Cervicocerebral artery dissections. J Accid Emerg Med 1999;16(6):422–4.
20. Silbert PL, Mokri B, Schievink WI. Headache and neck pain in spontaneous internal carotid and vertebral artery dissections. Neurology 1995;45(8):1517–22.
21. Campos CR, Evaristo EF, Yamamoto FI, et al. Spontaneous cervical carotid and vertebral arteries dissection: study of 48 patients. Arq Neuropsiquiatr 2004; 62(2B):492–8 [in Portuguese].
22. Nebelsieck J, Sengelhoff C, Nassenstein I, et al. Sensitivity of neurovascular ultrasound for the detection of spontaneous cervical artery dissection. J Clin Neurosci 2009;16(1):79–82.
23. Fischer U, Ledermann I, Nedeltchev K, et al. Quality of life in survivors after cervical artery dissection. J Neurol 2009;256(3):443–9.
24. Lee VH, Brown RD Jr, Mandrekar JN, et al. Incidence and outcome of cervical artery dissection: a population-based study. Neurology 2006;67(10):1809–12.
25. Lyrer P, Engelter S. Antithrombotic drugs for carotid artery dissection. Cochrane Database Syst Rev 2010;10:CD000255.
26. Pham MH, Rahme RJ, Arnaout O, et al. Endovascular stenting of extracranial carotid and vertebral artery dissections: a systematic review of the literature. Neurosurgery 2011;68(4):856–66.
27. Ferro JM, Canhao P, Stam J, et al. Prognosis of cerebral vein and dural sinus thrombosis: results of the International Study on Cerebral Vein and Dural Sinus Thrombosis (ISCVT). Stroke 2004;35(3):664–70.
28. de Bruijn SF, Stam J, Kappelle LJ. Thunderclap headache as first symptom of cerebral venous sinus thrombosis. CVST Study Group. Lancet 1996;348(9042):1623–5.
29. Crassard I, Soria C, Tzourio C, et al. A negative D-dimer assay does not rule out cerebral venous thrombosis: a series of seventy-three patients. Stroke 2005; 36(8):1716–9.
30. Kosinski CM, Mull M, Schwarz M, et al. Do normal D-dimer levels reliably exclude cerebral sinus thrombosis? Stroke 2004;35(12):2820–5.
31. Einhaupl K, Stam J, Bousser MG, et al. EFNS guideline on the treatment of cerebral venous and sinus thrombosis in adult patients. Eur J Neurol 2010;17(10): 1229–35.
32. Nordborg E, Nordborg C. Giant cell arteritis: epidemiological clues to its pathogenesis and an update on its treatment. Rheumatology (Oxford) 2003;42(3): 413–21.
33. Solomon S, Cappa KG. The headache of temporal arteritis. J Am Geriatr Soc 1987;35(2):163–5.
34. Pfadenhauer K, Weber H. Giant cell arteritis of the occipital arteries–a prospective color coded duplex sonography study in 78 patients. J Neurol 2003;250(7):844–9.
35. Rozen TD. Brief sharp stabs of head pain and giant cell arteritis. Headache 2010; 50(9):1516–9.
36. International Headache Society Classification Subcommittee. The international classification of headache disorders- 2nd edition. Cephalalgia 2004;24(Suppl 1): 1–151.
37. Smetana GW, Shmerling RH. Does this patient have temporal arteritis? JAMA 2002;287(1):92–101.
38. Hunder GG, Bloch DA, Michel BA, et al. The American College of Rheumatology 1990 criteria for the classification of giant cell arteritis. Arthritis Rheum 1990; 33(8):1122–8.

39. Parikh M, Miller NR, Lee AG, et al. Prevalence of a normal C-reactive protein with an elevated erythrocyte sedimentation rate in biopsy-proven giant cell arteritis. Ophthalmology 2006;113(10):1842–5.
40. Walvick MD, Walvick MP. Giant cell arteritis: laboratory predictors of a positive temporal artery biopsy. Ophthalmology 2011;118(6):1201–4.
41. Gonzalez-Gay MA, Blanco R, Rodriguez-Valverde V, et al. Permanent visual loss and cerebrovascular accidents in giant cell arteritis: predictors and response to treatment. Arthritis Rheum 1998;41(8):1497–504.
42. Savitz SI, Levitan EB, Wears R, et al. Pooled analysis of patients with thunderclap headache evaluated by CT and LP: is angiography necessary in patients with negative evaluations? J Neurol Sci 2009;276(1–2):123–5.
43. Calabrese LH, Dodick DW, Schwedt TJ, et al. Narrative review: reversible cerebral vasoconstriction syndromes. Ann Intern Med 2007;146(1):34–44.
44. Chen SP, Fuh JL, Wang SJ. Reversible cerebral vasoconstriction syndrome: an under-recognized clinical emergency. Ther Adv Neurol Disord 2010;3(3):161–71.
45. Valentinis L, Tuniz F, Valent F, et al. Headache attributed to intracranial tumours: a prospective cohort study. Cephalalgia 2010;30(4):389–98.
46. Tremont-Lukats IW, Ratilal BO, Armstrong T, et al. Antiepileptic drugs for preventing seizures in people with brain tumors. Cochrane Database Syst Rev 2008;2: CD004424.
47. Stiell IG, Clement CM, Rowe BH, et al. Comparison of the Canadian CT Head Rule and the New Orleans Criteria in patients with minor head injury. JAMA 2005;294(12):1511–8.
48. Stiell IG, Wells GA, Vandemheen K, et al. The Canadian CT Head Rule for patients with minor head injury. Lancet 2001;357(9266):1391–6.
49. Haydel MJ, Preston CA, Mills TJ, et al. Indications for computed tomography in patients with minor head injury. N Engl J Med 2000;343(2):100–5.
50. Smits M, Dippel DW, de Haan GG, et al. External validation of the Canadian CT Head Rule and the New Orleans Criteria for CT scanning in patients with minor head injury. JAMA 2005;294(12):1519–25.
51. Randeva HS, Schoebel J, Byrne J, et al. Classical pituitary apoplexy: clinical features, management and outcome. Clin Endocrinol (Oxf) 1999;51(2):181–8.
52. Semple PL, Jane JA Jr, Laws ER Jr. Clinical relevance of precipitating factors in pituitary apoplexy. Neurosurgery 2007;61(5):956–61 [discussion: 961–2].
53. Sibal L, Ball SG, Connolly V, et al. Pituitary apoplexy: a review of clinical presentation, management and outcome in 45 cases. Pituitary 2004;7(3):157–63.
54. Ayuk J, McGregor EJ, Mitchell RD, et al. Acute management of pituitary apoplexy–surgery or conservative management? Clin Endocrinol (Oxf) 2004; 61(6):747–52.
55. Friedman DI. Idiopathic intracranial hypertension. Curr Pain Headache Rep 2007; 11(1):62–8.
56. Kesler A, Hadayer A, Goldhammer Y, et al. Idiopathic intracranial hypertension: risk of recurrences. Neurology 2004;63(9):1737–9.
57. Weiss NS. Relation of high blood pressure to headache, epistaxis, and selected other symptoms. The United States Health Examination Survey of Adults. N Engl J Med 1972;287(13):631–3.
58. Hansson L, Smith DH, Reeves R, et al. Headache in mild-to-moderate hypertension and its reduction by irbesartan therapy. Arch Intern Med 2000;160(11): 1654–8.
59. Evers S, Afra J, Frese A, et al. EFNS guideline on the drug treatment of migraine–revised report of an EFNS task force. Eur J Neurol 2009;16(9):968–81.

60. van de Beek D, de Gans J, Spanjaard L, et al. Clinical features and prognostic factors in adults with bacterial meningitis. N Engl J Med 2004;351(18):1849–59.
61. Pachner AR, Steiner I. Lyme neuroborreliosis: infection, immunity, and inflammation. Lancet Neurol 2007;6(6):544–52.
62. Jarvis JN, Harrison TS. HIV-associated cryptococcal meningitis. AIDS 2007; 21(16):2119–29.
63. Pappas PG, Perfect JR, Cloud GA, et al. Cryptococcosis in human immunodeficiency virus-negative patients in the era of effective azole therapy. Clin Infect Dis 2001;33(5):690–9.
64. Raskin NH. Repetitive intravenous dihydroergotamine as therapy for intractable migraine. Neurology 1986;36(7):995–7.
65. Kelly AM, Walcynski T, Gunn B. The relative efficacy of phenothiazines for the treatment of acute migraine: a meta-analysis. Headache 2009;49(9):1324–32.
66. Colman I, Friedman BW, Brown MD, et al. Parenteral dexamethasone for acute severe migraine headache: meta-analysis of randomised controlled trials for preventing recurrence. BMJ 2008;336(7657):1359–61.
67. Leniger T, Pageler L, Stude P, et al. Comparison of intravenous valproate with intravenous lysine-acetylsalicylic acid in acute migraine attacks. Headache 2005;45(1):42–6.

Dizziness and Vertigo: Emergencies and Management

Ronald J. Tusa, MD, PhD[a,*], Russell Gore, MD[b]

KEYWORDS

• Vertigo • Dizziness • Vestibular • Imbalance
• Emergency room • Nystagmus

A 49-year-old woman is brought to the emergency room (ER). For the past two days, she has had a sense of rotation and imbalance. The goal of the ER evaluation is to

- Quickly identify if the problem is peripheral (inner ear or vestibular nerve) or central
- Determine if the patient needs to be admitted to the hospital or referred to a specialty clinic
- Offer initial management of the problem.

There are three key features in the history and five key elements of clinical examination that can be used to make these decisions.

THREE KEY ITEMS IN THE HISTORY

The history is by far the most important part of the evaluation. Unfortunately, taking a good history can be extremely tedious because complaints are often vague and frequently filled with anxiety-provoked symptoms. The three key items to obtain from the history are tempo, symptoms, and circumstances (**Table 1**). Determine if the patient has an acute attack of dizziness (3 days or fewer), chronic dizziness (more than 3 days), or spells of dizziness. If the patient suffers from spells, try to determine the average duration of the spells in seconds, minutes, or hours. Defining and expanding on the patient's vague report of dizziness is critical when describing the patient's symptoms. Dizziness is an imprecise term used to describe a variety of symptoms, each of which has a different pathophysiologic mechanism. A careful history can differentiate disequilibrium, primarily a balance problem, from the

The authors have nothing to disclose.
[a] Center for Rehabilitation Medicine, Emory University, 1441 Clifton Road NE, Atlanta, GA 30322 USA
[b] Department of Neurology, Emory University, Atlanta, GA 30322, USA
* Corresponding author.
E-mail address: rtusa@emory.edu

Neurol Clin 30 (2012) 61–74
doi:10.1016/j.ncl.2011.09.006
neurologic.theclinics.com
0733-8619/12/$ – see front matter

Table 1
Key items in the history of the dizzy patient

Disorder	Tempo	Symptoms	Circumstances
Acute Vestibular Neuritis	Acute (<3 d)	Vertigo, disequilibrium, N/V, oscillopsia	Spontaneous, exacerbated by head movements
Wallenberg Infarct	Acute	Vertigo, disequilibrium, N/V, tilt, lateropulsion, ataxia, crossed sensory loss, oscillopsia	Spontaneous, exacerbated by head movements
Anxiety or Depression	Chronic	Lightheaded, floating, or rocking	Induced by eye movements with head still
Benign Paroxysmal Positional Vertigo	Spells: s	Vertigo, lightheaded, nausea	Positional: lying down, sitting up or turning over in bed, bending forward
Orthostatic Hypotension	Spells: s	Lightheaded	Positional: standing up
Transient Ischemic Attack	Spells: min	Vertigo, lightheaded, disequilibrium	Spontaneous
Migraine	Spells: min	Vertigo, dizziness, motion sickness	Usually movement-induced

Abbreviation: n/v, nausea and vomiting.

subjective sensation of dizziness in the head. If dizziness is primarily in the head, the physician must determine if the sensation is lightheadedness (presyncope, rocking, or swaying) or vertigo (the abnormal sensation of rotation, linear movement, or tilt). Finally, associated symptoms of nausea and vomiting, vertical diplopia, tinnitus, hearing loss, or oscillopsia (the illusion of visual motion) must be elicited in the history. Knowledge of the circumstances triggering or exacerbating symptoms often helps to elucidate the mechanism behind dizziness. Is symptoms onset spontaneous or are symptoms triggered by movements, an event, or clustered during a specific time of day? If it is reported that movements exacerbate symptoms, it is important to differentiate whether the movements are primarily head movements, body movements or postural changes, or eye movements. Using the history of the 49-year-old woman given above, acute vestibular loss on one side (vestibular neuritis) is the most likely diagnosis (see **Table 1**). The clinical examination will help confirm this diagnosis.

FIVE KEY ELEMENTS OF THE CLINICAL EXAMINATION

The five key elements in the clinical examination of a dizzy patient are assessment of the vestibule-ocular reflex (VOR), spontaneous nystagmus, positional nystagmus, the Romberg test, and gait. **Table 2** lists the most common findings in normal individuals, individuals with acute unilateral peripheral vestibular loss (the case example), benign paroxysmal positional vertigo (BPPV), and central vestibular problems. Techniques to assess each of these examination elements in a normal individual are described below.

Vestibular-Ocular Reflex

The intact VOR compensates for head movements by moving the eyes in the opposite direction to head movements, thus fixing the eyes with respect to the world (**Fig. 1**). Examine the VOR using the head thrust. Have the patient fixate a target and observe the eyes after passive head thrusts horizontally and vertically. After the head thrust, the eyes of the patient should remain stable and focused on the target. This indicates

Table 2
Key items in the clinical examination of the dizzy patient

Examination	Normal	Acute Vestibular Neuritis	BPPV	Central
VOR Assessed by Head Thrust	Normal (no corrective saccade)	Corrective saccade needed after head thrust done in direction of defective inner ear	Normal	Normal
Spontaneous Nystagmus Assessed by Ophthalmoscope	None	Horizontal and mild torsional enhanced with fixation blocked	None	May or may not be present; often vertical or gaze evoked
Positional Nystagmus or Vertigo Assessed with Dix-Hallpike or Supine	None	Does not enhance vertigo, may enhance nystagmus	Transient upbeat and torsional nystagmus during Dix-Hallpike	None, or may have sustained or transient nystagmus with or without vertigo
Romberg	Negative	Negative	Negative	Often positive
Gait	Normal	Slow, cautious, wide-based, robotic	Normal	Often impaired

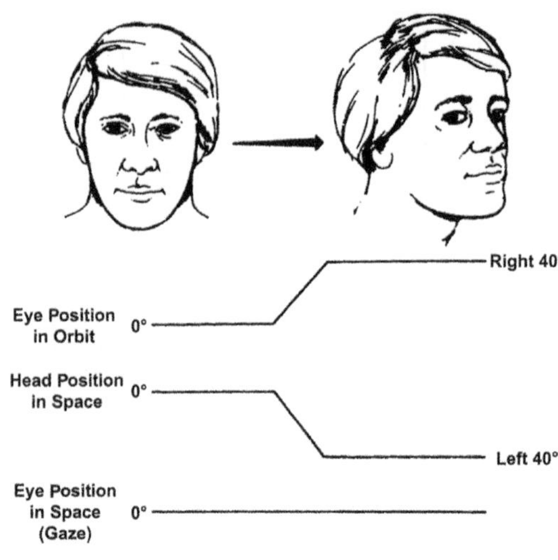

Fig. 1. The VOR in a normal individual. Top row shows the head moving quickly from center (0°) to left 40°, and it shows what happens to the eyes. The next three rows in the figure graphically show eye position in the orbit, head position in space, and eye position in space during this head movement. (*Adapted from* Leigh RJ, Zee DS. The neurology of eye movements. New York: Oxford Univ Press; 1999; with permission.)

a normal VOR. If the VOR is impaired, the eyes of the patient will not remain stable and a corrective, refixation saccade back to the target is observed.[1,2]

Presence of Spontaneous Nystagmus in Light With and Without Fixation Blocked

Normal individuals have no spontaneous nystagmus in the light (fixation present) or in the dark (fixation blocked) (see **Table 2**). The presence of spontaneous nystagmus should be assessed with and without fixation because peripheral causes of nystagmus usually can be suppressed with fixation, whereas central causes cannot be suppressed. An easy way to test this is during the ophthalmoscopic examination with the other eye fixating a target.[3] During this procedure, the optic nerve is visualized and assessed for spontaneous nystagmus with the unobscured eye fixating on a distant target. The examiner then covers the fixating eye with the hand and assesses the optic nerve for an unchanged nystagmus, suggesting a central cause, or an increase in nystagmus, suggesting a peripheral cause. During this examination, the optic nerve head should not show any oscillation. If it does, determine the direction of the quick phases. Remember, the direction of movement of the disk will be opposite to what is occurring.

The Presence of Positional Nystagmus

Positional nystagmus and vertigo is best assessed using the Dix-Hallpike test (**Fig. 2**). Normally, there is no nystagmus or vertigo with this maneuver. A positive Dix-Hallpike will result in transient symptoms of vertigo and torsional nystagmus, generally after a 30-second delay, with the head turned toward the affected ear. When normal individuals sit up, they may complain of lightheadedness due to a transient blood pressure drop.

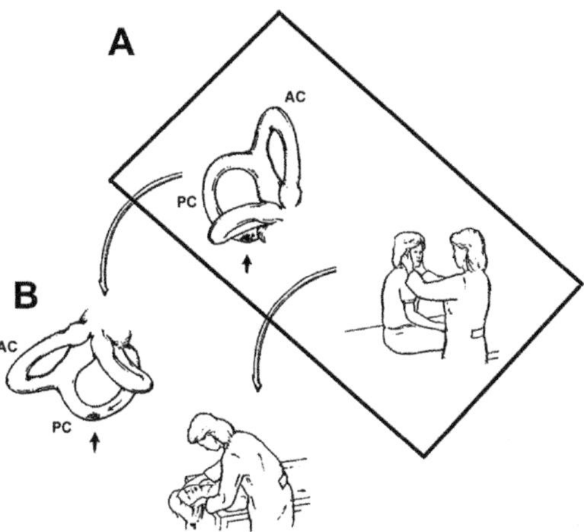

Fig. 2. Dix-Hallpike test for BPPV. (*A*) The patient sits on the examination table and the head is turned 45° horizontally. (*B*) The head and trunk are quickly brought straight back "en bloc" so that the head is hanging over the edge of the examination table by 20°. Nystagmus is looked for and the patient is asked if they have vertigo. Although not shown in the figure, the patient is then brought up slowly to a sitting position with the head still turned 45° and nystagmus is looked for again. This test is repeated with the head turned 45° in the other direction. This figure also shows movement of free-floating otoconia in the right posterior SCC (*large black arrows*) during the Dix-Hallpike test. In this example, the patient would have nystagmus and vertigo when the test is done on the right side, but not when the test is done on the left side. AC, anterior semicircular canal; PC, posterior semicircular canal. (*Data from* Herdman SJ, Tusa RJ, Zee DS, et al. Single treatment approaches to benign paroxysmal positional vertigo. Arch Otolaryngol Head Neck Surg 1993;119:450–4.)

Romberg Test

In the Romberg test, the patient is asked to stand with feet slightly apart, first with eyes open, and then closed. The patient is asked to fold her or his arms across the chest for 30 seconds eyes open, and then 30 seconds eyes closed. A positive Romberg is one in which the patient is stable with eyes open, but loses balance with eyes closed. A positive Romberg may be found in patients with proprioceptive defects from a peripheral neuropathy, dorsal root ganglia, or dorsal column disease. It is rarely found in individuals with acute vestibular loss.

Gait

The patient should be asked to walk at a comfortable pace for about 20 ft in one direction, and then to turn and come back. Features to look for are gait speed, the base width, step length, arm swing, minimal gyration of trunk and deviation of path, and movement of the head especially during turns (the head usually turns before the body).

IMAGING AND LABORATORY TESTS

Vertigo and dizziness can be effectively evaluated in the acute setting primarily based on clinical presentation and examination. However, additional testing may be required to confirm the diagnosis. From a diagnostic standpoint, differentiating peripheral and central causes for these symptoms is paramount to manage the condition appropriately and avoid overlooking a central condition. **Table 3** summarizes some the hallmark examination features differentiating peripheral and central vertigo. The

Table 3
Features that distinguish peripheral from central causes of vertigo

Findings	Peripheral Cause	Central Cause
Direction of Nystagmus	Usually mixed plane (horizontal and torsional)	Usually single plane (horizontal, torsional, or vertical)
Effect of Gaze on Nystagmus	Nystagmus increases with gaze toward direction of quick phase	Nystagmus does not change or reverses direction
Effect of Fixation on Nystagmus	Nystagmus decreases	Nystagmus does not change or increases
Ice-water Caloric Test	Spontaneous nystagmus does not change when affected ear is irrigated; nystagmus decreases or reverses direction when nonaffected side is irrigated	Spontaneous nystagmus increases when affected ear is irrigated; nystagmus reverses direction when nonaffected side is irrigated
Balance	If patient is younger than age 50 years, balance is normal except no sharpened Romberg test; if older than age 50 years, may have positive Romberg test	May have severe defect regardless of age (positive Romberg, patient veers when walking with eyes open)

differential diagnosis of dizziness and vertigo always includes infarcts or hemorrhage in the cerebellum, thalamus, or brainstem. The presentation of dizziness is associated with stroke in an estimated 3% to 4% of cases presenting to ERs.[4] Concern for stroke often leads to imaging studies in the acute setting; however, recent work has demonstrated superior sensitivity with oculomotor examination compared with early MRI.[4,5] When a central cause for dizziness and vertigo is suspected based on the clinical examination, imaging is certainly warranted. Based on the location of lesions likely to result in dizziness and vertigo stroke syndromes and with the acute onset of such symptoms, diffusion-weighted MRI is preferred over CT scan. Unnecessary tests are frequently performed when benign, peripheral causes for vertigo, such as BPPV, are demonstrated by clinical examination.[6] When a peripheral cause for dizziness and vertigo is suggested by clinical examination, additional testing is warranted. Viral cultures are not necessary because they do not alter treatment. Blood work should include fluorescent treponemal antibody absorption, rheumatoid factor, antinuclear antibody, and erythrocyte sedimentation rate to screen for otic syphilis and vasculitis. An audiogram should be obtained if the patient complains of hearing loss. A bedside caloric can be done immediately to help distinguish a peripheral from a central defect. A quantified caloric study, or electronystagmography (ENG), should be obtained several days after onset to document the extent of vestibular defect. Only admit the patient to the hospital if extreme dehydration is present from vomiting (rarely necessary) or if a central disorder is suspected. The patient should return in a few days to make certain the symptoms are resolving. It is then important to refer them promptly for vestibular rehabilitation.

CLINICAL CASE EXAMPLES

Acute Unilateral Peripheral Vestibular Loss

Acute vestibular neuritis: history and clinical exam

This disorder presents with intense vertigo, nausea, oscillopsia (illusion of movement of the visual world due to spontaneous movement of the eyes), and disequilibrium that persists for days. The vertigo is quite severe and patients prefer to lie quietly. Thus, the vertigo, nausea, and oscillopsia are occurring spontaneously, but they are exacerbated by head movements. Within a few days these symptoms begin to resolve and the patient is left with a dynamic deficit (vertigo and disequilibrium induced by rapid head movements), which can last for weeks to months until central compensation occurs. Thus, the tempo is acute; the symptoms include vertigo, imbalance, nausea, and oscillopsia; and the circumstances are that the vertigo is continuous and exacerbated with head movements. Based on these key items in the history, acute vestibular neuritis is likely (see **Table 1**).

The clinical examination for acute vestibular neuritis is detailed in **Table 2**. Examine the VOR using head thrust. Have the patient fixate a target and observe the eyes after thrusting the head horizontally at an angle of approximately 20°. After the head thrust, a saccadic eye movement will occur about 250 milliseconds after the head thrust. This saccade allows the patient to refixate on the target. It occurs because the VOR is impaired in the direction that the head was thrust.[1] Next, look for the presence of spontaneous nystagmus, with and without fixation, using an ophthalmoscope. It is important to do this with fixation blocked because peripheral vestibular loss causes nystagmus that can be suppressed with fixation. Acute, unilateral, vestibular loss causes a horizontal jerk nystagmus in which the quick phases are directed toward the normal ear. In addition, there is usually a torsional nystagmus in which the quick phases move the superior pole of each eye toward the normal ear. Thus, if the individual has a right vestibular loss, a left beat nystagmus and left torsional nystagmus will occur (the direction of the nystagmus is labeled based on the direction of the quick phase). Next, look for the presence of positional nystagmus. In vestibular neuritis, the spontaneous nystagmus may be enhanced during positional testing but there is usually no increase in vertigo. Next, examine Romberg and gait. The Romberg is negative; that is, there is no falling, sidestepping, or eye opening for 30 seconds. The gait will be slow, cautious, wide-based, and robotic with no movement of the head on body, especially during turns.

Pathophysiology and cause

Vestibular neuritis is preceded by a common cold 50% of the time. The prevalence of vestibular neuritis peaks at age 40 to 50 years.[7,8] Vestibular neuritis behaves similar to Bell palsy and is thought to frequently represent a reactivated dormant herpes infection in the Scarpa ganglia.[9] Vestibular neuritis primarily affects the superior division of the vestibular nerve, which innervates the anterior and lateral semicircular canals (SCCs).[10]

Management, including laboratory tests

Vestibular neuritis is diagnosed based primarily on the clinical presentation. Viral cultures are not necessary because they do not alter treatment. The differential diagnosis includes infarcts or hemorrhage in the cerebellum, or in the brainstem distribution of the posterior inferior cerebellar artery and anterior inferior cerebellar artery. Additional imaging, specialized tests, such as ENG, or hospital admission may be indicated if a central cause is suspected.

Management of acute vertigo from vestibular neuritis varies depending on how many days have elapsed since the onset (**Table 4**). Only admit the patient to the hospital if extreme dehydration is present from vomiting (rarely necessary) or if a central disorder is suspected. Blood work should include fluorescent treponemal antibody absorption, rheumatoid factor, antinuclear antibody, and erythrocyte sedimentation rate to screen for otic syphilis and vasculits. An audiogram should be

Table 4
Management of acute vertigo from vestibular neuritis

Days One to Three	After Day Three
Administer vestibular suppressants (Phenergan, Antivert, or Valium)	Stop vestibular suppressants
Administer prednisone	Taper over the course of 10 d
Prescribe bed rest (hospitalize if patient dehydrated or central defect suspected)	Prescribe vestibular adaptation exercises
Perform laboratory tests If central defect is suspected, obtain CT scan or MRI of head	Perform laboratory tests Audiogram (obtain immediately if Meniere disease suspected) Electronystagmography (limited) Blood work (rheumatoid factor, sedimentation factor, antinuclear antibody, fluorescent treponemal antibody absorption)

obtained if the patient complains of hearing loss. A minimal ice-water caloric test may be a suitable procedure for bedside assessment of vestibular function.[11] In this test, 0.5 to 1 mL of ice water is inserted into the external auditory canal and allowed to sit for 40 seconds before it is removed. The number of quick phases of nystagmus over the course of 15 seconds are counted, preferably with fixation blocked. Peripheral vestibular loss will results in reduced nystagmus on that side. A quantified caloric study (ENG) should be obtained several days after onset to document the extent of vestibular defect. By this time, the spontaneous nystagmus should be significantly decreased. A variety of vestibular suppressant medications can be employed for symptomatic treatment. These should be used for 1 week or less because the acute phase is a self-limited disorder. The authors use intramuscular Phenergan (25–50 mg) at the onset of severe vertigo, and then send the patient home for 3 days of bed rest with Phenergan suppositories to be taken as needed. This medication is causes sedation and reduces nausea. The patient returns in a few days to make certain the symptoms are resolving. It is then important to stop the medication and refer them promptly for vestibular rehabilitation. Prednisone (1 mg/kg) during the first 10 to 20 days of the attack may shorten the course of the illness.[12–15]

Spells of Dizziness

BPPV; history and clinical examination

There are several causes of spells of dizziness, but the most common cause is BPPV. Patients with BPPV usually complain of vertigo that lasts less than 1 minute. It usually occurs in the morning when they get up or turn over in bed. It may also occur when they lie down in bed or move their head back. After a bad attack, they frequently complain of disequilibrium that lasts for several hours. Therefore, the tempo is spells lasting seconds, the symptoms are vertigo and nausea, and the circumstances are positional when lying down, sitting up, or bending over (see **Table 1**). The diagnosis of BPPV is secured by the clinical examination. All key elements of the clinical examination are usually normal except for the positional test (Dix-Hallpike test; see **Table 2**). This test elicits a torsional-upbeat nystagmus associated with vertigo when the affected ear is inferior. The nystagmus usually has a latency of 3 to 20 seconds, fatigues less than 1 minute, and habituates with repeat maneuvers. If nystagmus and vertigo persist while the patient is in this position, and is not present while sitting, a central disorder (central positional vertigo) should be considered, although there are exceptions.[16]

Pathophysiology and cause

BPPV is usually idiopathic, but can also occur after head trauma, labyrinthitis, and ischemia in the distribution of the anterior inferior cerebellar artery. The pathophysiological mechanism for BPPV is usually due to canalithiasis; that is, portions of otoconia from the utricle that are misplaced and free-floating in the posterior SCC (see **Fig. 2**). This condition inappropriately causes the afferents from the posterior SCC to discharge when the head stops moving after head rotation.

Management, including laboratory tests

BPPV is a clinical diagnosis based on the history and the Dix-Hallpike test. No special testing is required.[6] BPPV is best treated by a maneuver that moves the debris out of the posterior SCC and back into the utricle. The authors primarily use a single-treatment approach modified from Epley,[17] which is now generally referred to as the canalith-repositioning maneuver (CRM) (**Fig. 3**). The authors found total remission or significant improvement from BPPV in 90% of patients treated using this maneuver.[18] Complications from the CRM are rare.[19] During the CRM, a Dix-Hallpike maneuver is first performed toward the side of the affected ear and the head is kept down for

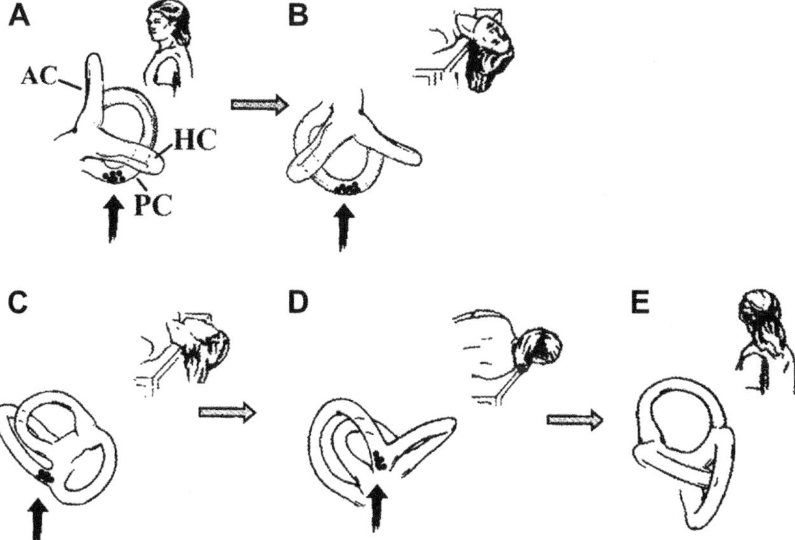

Fig. 3. Canalith repositioning maneuver for treatment of BPPV. Filled arrows indicate location of the posterior SSC. The patient is first moved from sitting (*A*) into the Dix-Hallpike position with the head turned 45° toward the affected side (*B*). After a few minutes, the patient's head is turned so the opposite ear is down (*C*) and then is rolled onto that shoulder with the nose pointed 45° down (*D*). After a few minutes, the patient sits up, keeping the head turned while coming into the sitting position (*E*). Because the debris will move whenever the head is moved during this maneuver, the patient should be advised to expect vertigo to occur several times during the treatment. Some patients only experience vertigo during the initial movement into the Dix-Hallpike position. (*Data from* Herdman SJ, Tusa RJ, Zee DS, et al. Single treatment approaches to benign paroxysmal positional vertigo. Arch Otolaryngol Head Neck Surg 1993;119:450–4.)

2 minutes. Then the head is rotated toward the unaffected side and the patient is rolled over onto this side until the face is pointed down. This position is maintained for 2 minutes. With the head deviated toward the unaffected side, the patient slowly sits up. To make certain the debris does not move back toward the cupula, the patient is asked to sit with the head upright for 20 minutes. A consensus paper that summarizes the best controlled studies on treatment of several types of BPPV was published in 2008.[20] It is unclear what happens to the free-floating otoconia after the treatment, but, presumably, it is reabsorbed into the calcium matrix in the utricle. The patient should have follow-up after the ER with a clinic familiar with BPPV to be certain the treatment worked. Vestibular suppressant drugs do not have a role in the treatment of BPPV unless the patient refuses to do the treatment due to excessive vertigo and nausea.

Central Dizziness and Vertigo

Stroke and vertebral basilar ischemia: history and clinical examination

The central causes of dizziness seen in the ER are extensive. A couple of the most common are reviewed here. The most worrisome central cause of dizziness is acute ischemic event in the posterior fossa. The symptoms and signs vary depending on the location of the ischemic event (**Table 5**). Vertigo is among the initial symptoms in 48% of patients with stroke; however, stroke is diagnosed in fewer than 5% of patients presenting with dizziness.[4,21] A small percentage of patients with vertebral basilar ischemia may present with isolated spells of vertigo, presumably due to ischemia in the distribution of the anterior vestibular artery, a branch from the anterior inferior cerebellar artery (AICA) (see **Table 5**). This small artery perfuses the anterior and lateral SCC and the utricular maculae, and spares the cochlea. The clinical examination of central vestibular defects is detailed in **Table 2**. The VOR using the head thrust test is normal for all central defects unless the peripheral vestibular system is involved (infarct in the dorsolateral pons-AICA). Look for spontaneous nystagmus due to central defects with the eyes looking straight ahead, to the left, and to the right. Do this also using the ophthalmoscope to block fixation. Selective lesions in the central vestibular pathways result in spontaneous nystagmus due to unopposed higher spontaneous neural activity in the intact vestibular pathways (**Table 6**). Unlike spontaneous nystagmus from peripheral vestibular lesions, those from central vestibular lesions are not readily suppressed with fixation. Look for central positional vertigo when laying the patient supine or during the Dix-Hallpike test. This is a transient or sustained downbeat nystagmus with severe vertigo and is due to lesions that disrupt the pathways between the midline cerebellar structures and vestibular nucleus (see **Table 6**).[22] A positive Romberg test may be found in patients with proprioceptive defects from dorsal root ganglia or dorsal column disease. Gait is very helpful test to assess patients with central defect because it often is impaired even when few additional findings are noted. The gait may be spastic, ataxic, halting, or freezing. Romberg and gait assessment are also helpful in identifying a functional component.[23]

Pathophysiology and cause

The central vestibular structures are perfused by several vessels within the vertebral-basilar system. **Table 5** describes the structures and resulting signs from ischemic events and strokes.

Dorsolateral pontine infarct The AICA perfuses the lateral cerebellum (cerebellar branch), the dorsolateral pons (pontine branch), and the labyrinth (labyrinth artery). Vertigo can occur from infarcts in either the pontine branch or labyrinth artery. The AICA syndrome may present with just peripheral signs if the labyrinth artery is solely

Table 5
Symptoms and signs from stroke in the posterior fossa

Region	Vessel and Structure	Symptoms and Signs
Dorsolateral Pons	AICA	
	Cerebellar branch	
	Lateral cerebellum	Ipsilateral dysmetria
	Pontine branch	
	CN V and VII	Vertigo, ipsilateral pain, and temp loss (face), peripheral VII loss, dysarthria
	Sympathetic CN III fibers, middle cerebellar, peduncle, paramedian pontine reticular formation	Ipsilateral Horner, dysmetria, saccade palsy
	Spinothalamic tract	—
	Labyrinthine artery branch	
	Cochlea and labyrinth	Contralateral loss pain and temp (body)
	Anterior vestibular artery subbranch	
	Horizontal SCC, anterior SCC, utricle	Vertigo, imbalance, nausea, vomiting, absent ipsilateral VOR
	Posterior vestibular artery subbranch	
	Posterior SCC, saccule, cochlea	Vertigo, ipsilateral sensorineural hearing loss, tinnitus, normal VOR
Dorsolateral Medulla (Wallenberg Syndrome)	Posterior inferior cerebellar artery	
	Cerebellar branch	
	Posterior inferior cerebellum	Imbalance, ipsilateral ataxia
	Medullary branch	
	V nucleus-tract, IX nucleus-tract, X nucleus-tract, sympathetic tract	Ipsilateral pain and temp loss (face), decreased gag, vocal cord paresis, ipsilateral Horner
	Inferior cerebellar peduncle, vestibular otolith	Ipsilateral ataxia, lateropulsion, ocular tilt
	Lateral spinothalamic tract	Contralateral loss pain and temp (body)
	Vestibular VIII nucleus	Vertigo, nausea, vomiting, nystagmus (pure torsional or vestibular with reversal on gaze toward lesion side)
Medial Medulla (Lower Medulla)	Penetrator from anterior spinal artery	
	XII nucleus, pyramidal tract, medial meniscus	Ipsilateral tongue weakness, contralateral weakness (body), decreased vibration and proprioception (body)
	Nucleus intercalatus	Vertigo, nausea, vomiting, upbeat nystagmus, truncal ataxia

Abbreviations: cn, cranial nerve; temp, temperature.

Table 6
Vestibular nystagmus due central lesions

Nystagmus	Pathology	Possible Mechanism
Torsional Nystagmus	Dorsolateral medulla lesion	Decreased tonic neural activity to the INC from anterior and posterior SCC on one side.
Downbeat Nystagmus	Cerebellar flocculus lesion or floor of fourth ventricle lesion	Decreased tonic neural activity to the INC from posterior SCC on both sides
Central Positional Nystagmus or Vertigo	Midline vestibular cerebellum	Disruption between cerebellar nodulus and vestibular nucleus
Upbeat Nystagmus	Brachium conjunctivum lesion Dorsal upper medulla lesion	Decreased tonic neural activity to INC from central anterior SCC on both sides.
Seesaw Nystagmus	Unilateral lesion of INC	Unilateral inactivation of INC on one side
Periodic Alternating Nystagmus	Cerebellar nodulus lesions	Unstable (high gain) neural activity in the medial vestibular nucleus.

Abbreviation: INC, interstitial nucleus of Cajal.

involved (vertigo, nausea, vomiting, hearing loss, and tinnitus) or may include more central signs if the dorsolateral pons is involved (dysarthria, peripheral facial palsy, trigeminal sensory loss, Horner syndrome, dysmetria, contralateral temperature, and pain sensory loss).[24] The labyrinthine artery originates directly from the basilar artery in approximately 15% of patients.

Dorsolateral medulla infarct The posterior inferior cerebellar artery perfuses the posterior inferior cerebellum (cerebellar branch) and the dorsolateral medulla. Vertigo can occur from infarcts in the lateral medulla (Wallenberg syndrome) due to involvement of the vestibular nucleus. Characteristic signs include crossed sensory signs, ipsilateral lateropulsion, ataxia, and Horner sign. Nystagmus may be pure torsion, or mixed torsion and horizontal. When the nystagmus contains a horizontal component, it reverses direction on gaze toward the lesion side, unlike nystagmus from peripheral vestibular lesions.

Medial medulla infarct The upper medial medulla is usually perfused by a penetrating vessel from the vertebral artery and the lower medial medulla is perfused by a branch from the anterior spinal artery. Infarcts in the latter may result in vertigo from involvement of the intercalatus nucleus.[25] The physiologic role of the intercalatus nucleus is poorly understood, but it is thought to be involved with the vertical neural integrator. Characteristic signs include ipsilateral tongue weakness, contralateral body weakness, sensory loss, and upbeat nystagmus.

Management, including laboratory tests

There are only anecdotal comments about the effectiveness of treatment of vertigo from cerebrovascular disorders. Ondansetron (Zofran) may be appropriate for severe vertigo and nausea from stroke.[26] Coumadin and transluminal angioplasty of vertebral artery stenosis and, occasionally, aspirin or ticlopidine have been found to be effective in stopping spells of central vertigo from vertebrobasilar artery insufficiency.[27–30] Treatment includes reduction of risk factors for cerebrovascular disease and antiplatelet therapy. These patients usually have known cerebrovascular disease or risk factors for this disease. Magnetic resonance arteriography can be performed to assess posterior circulation vessels and transcranial Doppler may detect decreased flow in the basilar artery.

SUMMARY

The causes of dizziness in patients seen in the ER can usually be determined by a focused evaluation that consists of identifying three key features in the history five key elements of the clinical examination.

REFERENCES

1. Halmagyi GM, Curthoys IS. A clinical sign of canal paresis. Arch Neurol 1988;45: 737–9.
2. Leigh RJ, Zee DS. The neurology of eye movements. New York: Oxford Univ Press; 1999.
3. Zee DS. Ophthalmoscopy in examination of patients with vestibular disorders. Ann Neurol 1978;3:373–4.
4. Newman-Toker DE, Kattah JC, Alvernia JE, et al. Normal head impulse test differentiates acute cerebellar strokes from vestibular neuritis. Neurology 2008;70: 2378–85.
5. Kattah JC, Talkad AV, Wang DZ, et al. HINTS to diagnose stroke in the acute vestibular syndrome: three-step bedside oculomotor examination more sensitive than early MRI diffusion-weighted imaging. Stroke 2009;40:3504–10.
6. Polensek SH, Tusa R. Unnecessary diagnostic tests often obtained for benign paroxysmal positional vertigo. Med Sci Monit 2009;15(7):MT89–94.
7. Coats AC. Vestibular neuronitis. Acta Otolaryngol Suppl (Stockh) 1969;251:5–32.
8. Sekitani T, Imate Y, Noguchi T, et al. Vestibular neuronitis: Epidemiological survey by questionnaire in Japan. Acta Otolaryngol Suppl (Stockh) 1993;503:9–12.
9. Furuta Y, Takasu T, Sato KC, et al. Latent herpes simplex virus type 1 in human vestibular ganglia. Acta Otolaryngol (Stockh) 1993;(Suppl 503):85–9.
10. Fetter M, Dichgans J. Vestibular neuritis spares the inferior division of the vestibular nerve. Brain 1996;119:755–63.
11. Schmäl F, Lübben B, Weiberg K, et al. The minimal ice water caloric test compared with established vestibular caloric test procedures. J Vestib Res 2005;15(4):215–24.
12. Ariyasu L, Byl FM, Sprague MS, et al. The beneficial effect of methylprednisolone in acute vestibular vertigo. Arch Otolaryngol Head Neck Surg 1990;116:700–3.
13. Ohbayashi S, Oda M, Yamamoto M, et al. Recovery of vestibular function after vestibular neuronitis. Acta Otolaryngol Suppl (Stockh) 1993;503:31–4.
14. Strupp M, Zingler VC, Arbusow V, et al. Methylprednisolone, valacyclovir, or the combination for vestibular neuritis. N Engl J Med 2004;351(4):354–61.
15. Shupak A, Issa A, Golz A, et al. Prednisone treatment for vestibular neuritis. Otol Neurotol 2008;29(3):368–74.
16. Baloh RW, Yue Q, Jacobson K, et al. Persistent direction-changing positional nystagmus: another variant of benign positional vertigo. Neurology 1995;45:1297–301.
17. Epley JM. The canalith repositioning procedure: for treatment of benign paroxysmal positional vertigo. Otolaryngol Head Neck Surg 1992;107:399–404.
18. Herdman SJ, Tusa RJ, Zee DS, et al. Single treatment approaches to benign paroxysmal positional vertigo. Arch Otolaryngol Head Neck Surg 1993;119: 450–4.

19. Herdman SJ, Tusa RJ. Complications of the canalith repositioning procedure. Arch Otolaryngol 1996;122:281–6.
20. Fife TD, Iverson DJ, Lempert T, et al. Quality Standards Subcommittee, American Academy of Neurology. Practice parameter: therapies for benign paroxysmal positional vertigo (an evidence-based review): report of the Quality Standards Subcommittee of the American Academy of Neurology. Neurology 2008;70(22): 2067–74.
21. Grad A, Baloh RW. Vertigo of vascular origin. Arch Neurol 1989;46:281–4.
22. Brandt T. Positional and positioning vertigo and nystagmus. J Neurol Sci 1990;95: 3–25.
23. Lempert T, Brandt T, Dieterich M, et al. How to identify psychogenic disorders of stance and gait. J Neurol 1991;238:140–6.
24. Oas JG, Baloh JG. Vertigo and the anterior inferior cerebellar artery syndrome. Neurology 1992;42:2274–9.
25. Munro NA, Gaymard B, Rivaud S, et al. Upbeat nystagmus in a patient with a small medullary infarct. J Neurol Neurosurg Psychiatry 1993;56:1126–8.
26. Rice GP, Ebers GC. Ondansetron for intractable vertigo complicating acute brainstem disorders. Lancet 1995;345:1182–3.
27. Gomez CR, Cruz-Flores S, Malkoff S, et al. Isolated vertigo as a manifestation of vertebrobasilar ischemia. Neurology 1996;47:94–7.
28. Fife TD, Baloh RW, Duckwiler GR. Isolated dizziness in vertebrobasilar insufficiency: clinical features, angiography and follow-up. J Stroke Cerebrovasc Dis 1994;4:4–12.
29. Crawley F, Clifton A, Brown MM. Treatable lesions demonstrated on vertebral angiography for posterior circulation ischemic events. Br J Radiol 1998;852: 1266–70.
30. Strupp M, Planck JH, Arbusow V, et al. Rotational vertebral artery occlusion syndrome with vertigo due to labyrinthine excitation. Neurology 2000;54:1376–9.

Acute Visual Loss and Other Neuro-Ophthalmologic Emergencies: Management

Jennifer S. Graves, MD, PhD[a,b,*], Steven L. Galetta, MD[b,c]

KEYWORDS

• Vision loss • Double vision • Papilledema • Optic neuropathy

Neuro-ophthalmologic findings have exquisite localizing value to clinicians. They can guide emergency room providers in the management of acute visual complaints and alert them to other neurologic emergencies, such as hydrocephalus and transtentorial herniation. This article outlines the symptoms and signs of specific neuro-ophthalmic disorders and their association with neurologic emergencies.

SYMPTOMS AND SIGNS OF NEURO-OPHTHALMOLOGIC DISORDERS

Acute Visual Loss

The most important first step in evaluating acute visual loss is to establish whether the underlying cause is neurologic or optic. A readily available test in the emergency room is the pinhole examination (**Fig. 1**). Visual acuity should be tested for each eye separately. If the acuity improves with pinhole, then it is likely that the symptoms are optic. Common causes for this include uncorrected refractive error, lens or corneal opacity, and vitreous disease. If the acuity does not improve with pinhole, then the symptoms may be from neurologic visual loss either from optic nerve or retinal disease.

Dr Graves has nothing to disclose.
Dr Galetta has received honoraria and consulting fees from Biogen-Idec, Novartis, and Teva.

[a] Department of Neurology, University of Pennsylvania School of Medicine, 3 East Gates Building, 3400 Spruce Street, Philadelphia, PA 19104, USA
[b] Department of Ophthalmology, University of Pennsylvania School of Medicine, Philadelphia, PA, USA
[c] Neuro-ophthalmology Division, Department of Neurology, University of Pennsylvania School of Medicine, University of Pennsylvania, 3 East Gates Building, 3400 Spruce Street, Philadelphia, PA 19104, USA
* Corresponding author. Department of Neurology, University of Pennsylvania School of Medicine, 3 East Gates Building, 3400 Spruce Street, Philadelphia, PA 19104.
E-mail address: jennifer.graves@uphs.upenn.edu

Neurol Clin 30 (2012) 75–99
doi:10.1016/j.ncl.2011.09.012 **neurologic.theclinics.com**
0733-8619/12/$ – see front matter

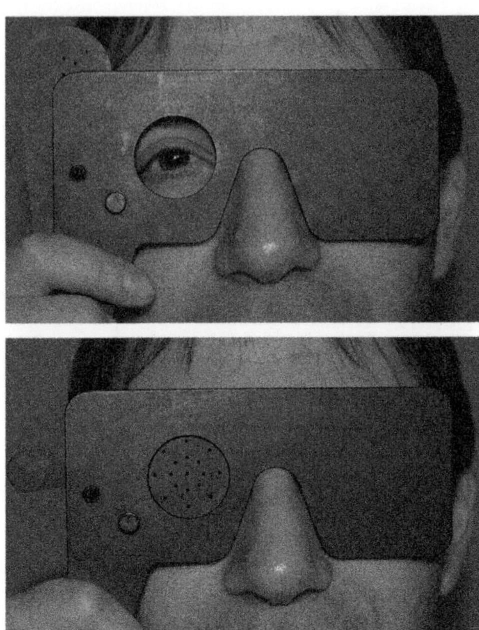

Fig. 1. Pinhole testing may help distinguish whether the visual loss is neurologic or optic. (*Top*) Occluder for testing vision one eye at a time. By convention the right eye is tested first. (*Bottom*) Occluder with pinholes. If the visual acuity is subnormal but can be improved with pinholes, refractive error or media opacities should be suspected. (*Adapted from* Liu GT, Volpe NJ, Galetta SL. Neuro-opthalmology: diagnosis and management. 2nd edition. Philadelphia: W. B. Saunders Company; 2010; Elsevier with permission.)

When there is suspicion for neurologic visual loss, localization may be provided by the swinging flashlight test, color vision evaluation, fundoscopic examination, and visual field testing. The swinging flash light test is used to determine the presence of a relative afferent pupillary defect (RAPD) and is performed by brisk and alternate stimulation of the eyes with a bright light source (**Fig. 2**). If there is pupillary dilatation in response to direct stimulation (the consensual response is greater than the direct response), then the patient has an RAPD. This finding is strongly suggestive of an optic neuropathy in the eye with the impaired direct response. Severe retinal disease may also produce an RAPD but it is less common and usually does produce the magnitude of the afferent pupillary defect (APD) that is associated with an optic neuropathy. Color vision loss further supports a diagnosis of optic nerve disease. This can be tested formally with a color plate book or by subjective comparison of colors, most commonly red, between the two eyes.

Funduscopic examination is helpful in identifying optic nerve and retinal disorders. Optic disc abnormalities can be seen in inflammatory, infiltrative, infectious, or ischemic disorders (discussed later). Although an MRI may demonstrate enhancement of the optic nerve in cases of acute idiopathic demyelinating optic neuritis, the fundoscopic examination is frequently unremarkable.[1] There is mild swelling in approximately one-third of patients. Conversely, the majority of patients with ischemic optic neuropathies have disc swelling and hemorrhages acutely. In ischemic optic neuropathy, the disc swelling may be segmental and this can be a clue to the mechanism of

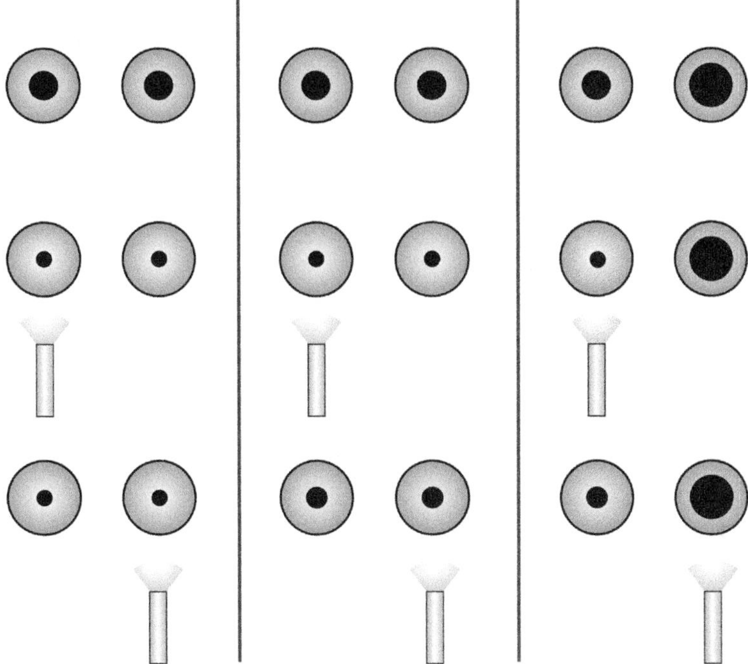

Fig. 2. Swinging flashlight test and the APD. (*Left panel*) Normal swinging flashlight test, in which light directed in either eye elicits the same amount of pupillary constriction. (*Middle panel*) Swinging flashlight test revealing a left RAPD in the hypothetical setting of visual loss in the left eye due to an optic neuropathy. Pupillary sizes are equal at rest in ambient lighting. Light stimulation of the good right eye results in brisk bilateral pupillary constriction. Light stimulation of the visually impaired left eye produces comparatively weaker pupillary constriction, and both pupils dilate. (*Right panel*) Left third nerve palsy and optic neuropathy. The left pupil is fixed and dilated. When the light is shone into the good right eye, the right pupil constricts normally. When the light is shone into the left eye, however, the right pupil dilates because of the left optic neuropathy. (*Adapted from* Liu GT, Volpe NJ, Galetta SL. Neuro-opthalmology: diagnosis and management. 2nd edition. Philadelphia: W.B. Saunders Company; 2010; Elsevier with permission.)

the visual loss. Infectious and infiltrative causes of optic neuropathy may also have significant optic disc elevation and edema. A chronic optic neuropathy may result in a pale appearance of the optic disc and the presence of shunt vessels on the disc may signify an underlying mass lesion compressing the optic nerve.

Visual field testing lends additional information to the localization of the visual loss (**Table 1**). Optic neuritis typically presents with central or centrocecal scotomas, although other patterns, such as generalized depression and altitudinal or arcuate defects, are seen.[1] Anterior ischemic optic neuropathy (AION) often presents with altitudinal defects. Abrupt onset of complete unilateral visual field loss is suggestive for a vascular process (central retinal artery or ophthalmic artery occlusion). Bitemporal field loss is characteristic of a compressive lesion in the region of the optic chiasm. Anterior chiasmal lesions may present with findings of an ipsilateral optic neuropathy and a temporal field deficit in the contralateral eye signifying injury to the junction of the optic nerve and the crossing fibers in the optic chiasm. Damage to the optic tract may manifest as an incongruous homonymous hemianopsia. Patients with an optic tract

Table 1
Causes of vision loss

Lesion	Cause	Findings
Optic	Refractive error, media opacities, vitreous abnormalities	No APD; usually unilateral; improvement with pinhole
Optic nerve	Inflammatory lesions (MS, sarcoid); ischemia (atherosclerotic, hypoperfusion, vasculitic); infiltrative/infectious (neoplastic, cytomegalovirus, syphilis)	APD present; central, centrocecal, arcuate, or wedge field defect with apex at blind spot; disc swelling may be if papillitis is due to inflammatory, ischemic, or infiltrative lesion
Chiasm	Parasellar mass (pituitary adenoma, craniopharyngioma, meningioma, aneurysm); chiasmal neuritis	Bitemporal hemianopsia, may be asymmetric; junctional lesion may cause ipsilateral APD, central or centrocecal scotoma, and contralateral superior temporal defect
Optic tract	Neoplastic, inflammatory, ischemic, infectious	APD variable; incongruous hemianopsia; bow-tie disc atrophy if long standing
Lateral Geniculate	Infarction, arteriovenous malformation, neoplastic	Incongrous hemianopsia, optic atrophy late; horizontal sectoranopsia or quadruple quadrantanopia suggestive of infarction
Optic radiations (parietal)	Neoplastic, inflammatory, ischemic, infectious	No APD; inferior contralateral quadrantanopia; ipsilateral smooth pursuit abnormalities; spasticity of conjugate gaze
Optic radiations (temporal)	Neoplastic, inflammatory, ischemic, infectious	No APD; superior contralateral quadrantanopia, may be slightly incongruous
Occipital	Ischemic, neoplastic, infectious, inflammatory	No APD; congruous contralateral hemianopsia; macular sparing and Riddoch phenomena may be present

Data from Laskowitz D, Liu GT, Galetta SL. Acute visual loss and other disorders of the eyes. Neurol Clin 1998;16:323–53.

lesion frequently have an RAPD on the side with greater field loss. Moreover, optic atrophy associated with a homonymous field deficit indicates injury of the optic tract or the lateral geniculate body.

Homonymous quadrantanopsia is characteristic of lesions to the optic radiations. A superior quadrantanopsia results from damage to the temporal geniculocalcarine radiations (Meyer loop) and an inferior quadrantanopsia from injury to the parietal radiations. Often associated with parietal lesions are an ipsilateral disorder of smooth pursuit and spasticity of conjugate gaze. The latter refers to deviation of the eyes superiorly and away from the side of the lesion during eye closure as opposed to the normal Bell phenomenon (each eye typically deviates superiolaterally). Homonymous congruous lesions reflect occipital lobe disease. Common causes include ischemic, neoplastic, infectious, and inflammatory disorders. Due to a dual blood supply, the occipital poles are often spared in ischemic lesions and, therefore, macular (central) vision on the side of the hemianopsia may be preserved. Management of acute visual loss depends on the localization and cause of the disorder but most cases require neuroimaging and computerized visual field perimetry (**Fig. 3**).

Other causes of acute vision loss may need to be considered in the differential diagnosis of patients. Central serous retinopathy and other maculopathies may mimic optic neuropathy and present with edema of the macula and central vision loss. These patients typically do not have an APD unless the vision loss is severe and describe a distortion of images (metamorphopsia) not present in optic neuropathies. Retinal vascular insult or insufficiency causes acute vision loss. A central retinal artery occlusion is an emergency, although the efficacy of available treatments is debated ,with a recent prospective, randomized trial of thrombolytic therapy demonstrating poor efficacy and potential harm.[2,3] Patients present with sudden, typically unilateral vision loss with whitening of the retina, highlighting the cherry-red spot of the macula, which is devoid of overlying ganglion cells. Other associated findings may include optic nerve swelling or pallor, visible emboli, and boxcarring of vessels.[4] Visual outcome is often poor. A branch retinal artery occlusion is associated with less severe visual loss and whitening along a branch artery, most commonly a temporal branch. Etiologies for these vascular insufficiencies include various types of emboli, local thrombosis, underlying infectious or inflammatory disorder, vasospasm, or hypoperfusion. Venous vascular insufficiency may also occur. Central retinal venous occlusion classically presents with a dramatic "blood and thunder" appearance of the fundus with dilated tortuous retinal veins, extensive retinal edema, and intraretinal hemorrhages in all 4 quadrants. There may be optic nerve swelling. Complications of central retinal venous occlusion include macular edema and management may involve laser coagulation, intraocular steroid injection, and anti–vascular endothelial growth factor medications.[5]

Specific management of 2 common entities associated with acute vision loss is discussed.

Giant cell arteritis

Classically, giant cell arteritis (GCA) is strongly suggested when an older patient presents with headache, sudden visual loss, and jaw claudication. Unfortunately for diagnosticians, many patients present with occult signs of the disease, and vigilance must be maintained when considering this diagnosis. Patient demographics are an important factor in determining the level of clinical suspicion because the disease is rarely seen under age 60. GCA is more common in white patients and in women and may have both a genetic and environmental basis of pathogenesis.[6–8]

Depending on the extent of ophthalmic and retinal artery involvement, there may or may not be changes seen on the eye examination. The most common cause of

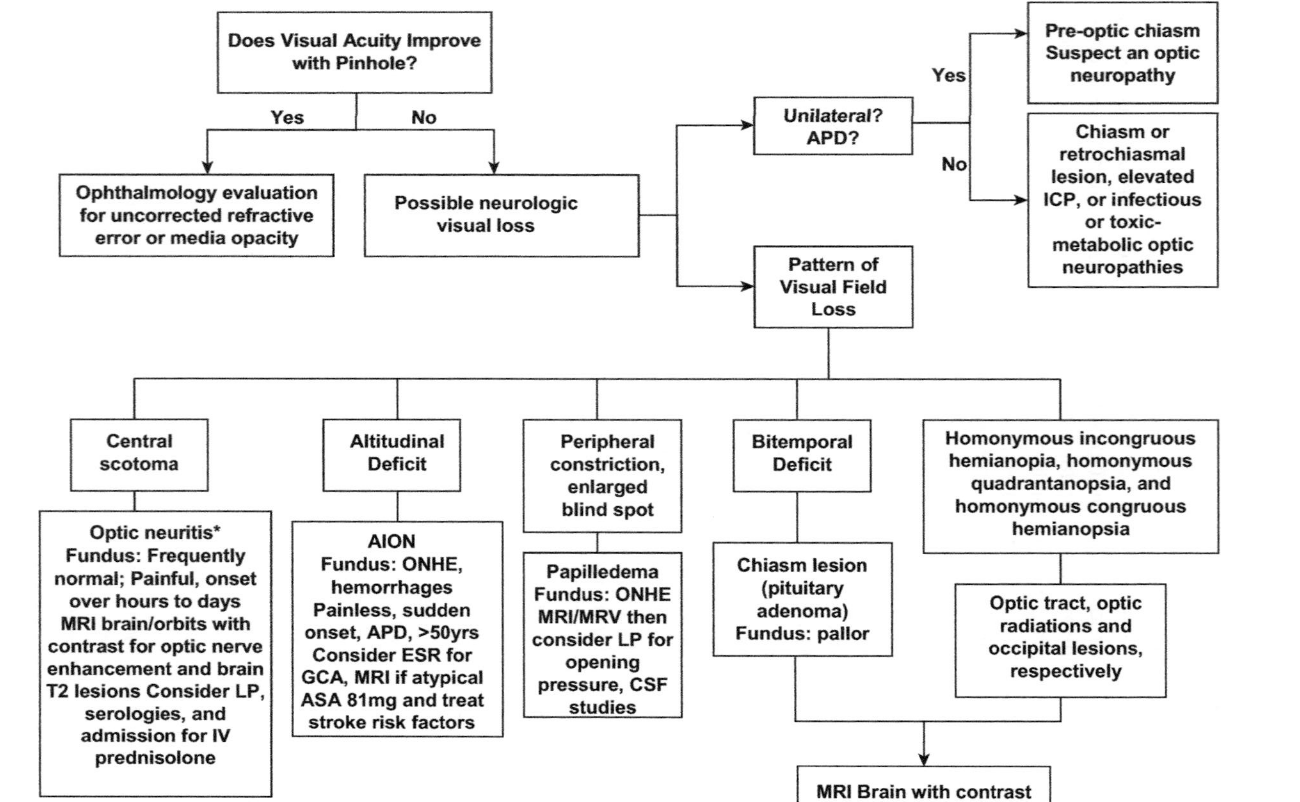

Fig. 3. Management of acute vision loss. he evaluation of acute vision loss that may present in the emergency room. Common causes are highlighted. ASA, aspirin; ICP, intracranial pressure; ONHE, optic nerve head edema. *Although central scotomas are the most common deficit seen in optic neuritis, other patterns may be seen as well.

GCA-related vision loss is arteritic AION. In this case, patients may have findings of decreased vision on examination consistent with an optic neuropathy, including an APD, and on fundus examination may have a chalky white optic disc with edema. Laboratory tests readily available in the emergency room that may aid in the diagnosis of GCA include an erythrocyte sedimentation rate (ESR) or C-reactive protein. Although nonspecific, elevation of either value may add to the clinical suspicion for GCA.[9–11] To make a definitive diagnosis, a biopsy is required.

The treatment of GCA is steroids and these should be initiated while awaiting an expeditious biopsy. Although the need for intravenous versus oral steroids remains controversial in the literature, the authors recommend for patients with visual symptoms that intravenous methylprednisolone (1 g total per day for 3 days) be given followed by prednisone (60 mg daily) until further follow-up.[11,12] **Box 1** summarizes the diagnostic features and acute management of GCA associated with visual complaints.

Acute demyelinating optic neuritis

Acute demyelinating optic neuritis is often associated with multiple sclerosis (MS) and presents with vision loss over hours to days (**Box 2**). Typically, retro-orbital pain worse with eye movements is present.[1] Patients may describe a central blur although any field loss may be observed. Patients usually complain of impaired color vision and images are described as dim or less bright. The most common demographic for this disorder is young women, but optic neuritis can be seen at any age, including children and older adults. If available, an MRI of the brain should be obtained to assess the risk of developing MS and an orbital MRI can be obtained to confirm the diagnosis. Orbital imaging should be strongly considered when the features of the event are atypical, including absence of pain, progressive visual loss, or failure to have some improvement in vision. Management in the emergency setting includes documentation of an eye examination with visualization of the fundus, initiation of intravenous steroids if appropriate, and ophthalmologic consultation or outpatient referral for computerized visual fields.

The Abnormal Optic Disc

Evaluation of neuro-ophthalmic complaints in the emergency room should always include a fundus examination. Direct visualization with an ophthalmoscope is the

Box 1
Evaluation and management of giant cell arteritis

Clinical Features

Sudden transient or persistent vision loss associated with headache or scalp tenderness in patients over age 50. Most prevalent in white women. History of jaw claudication and polymyalgia rheumatica strongly associated with GCA. May also more rarely present as an isolated third, fourth, or sixth nerve palsy or ocular muscle weakness.

Diagnostic Testing

ESR

C-reactive protein

Fluorescein angiography

Temporal artery biopsy

Treatment

Intravenous Solu-Medrol (1 g daily $\times$ 3 days) if visual symptoms present

Oral prednisone (60 mg daily) until follow-up

Box 2
Evaluation and management of acute demyelinating optic neuritis

Clinical Features

Onset over hours to days of vision loss

Retro-orbital pain worse with eye movements

Most common <50 years, women

Diagnostic Testing

MRI brain and orbits

Consider lumbar puncture, visual evoked potential

Computerized visual fields (outpatient)

Serologic studies if atypical

Treatment

Intravenous methylprednisolone (1 g daily × 3 days) if acute, followed by oral prednisone taper

Outpatient follow-up in 4 weeks; if no improvement, reconsider other diagnoses

Referal for consideration of disease-modifying therapy if high risk for MS[a]

[a] Patients with 2 or more lesions on their MRI of the brain have a high risk of conversion to clinically definite MS.

Data from Beck RW, Trobe JD, Moke PS, et al. High- and low-risk profiles for the development of multiple sclerosis within 10 years after optic neuritis: experience of the optic neuritis treatment trial. Arch Ophthalmol 2003;121:944–9.

most frequently used technique in this setting. A recently introduced supplementary tool is the nonmydriatic fundus camera, which allows a nonspecialist to have vivid views of the optic nerve and to provide a recording of the nerves' appearance for future follow-up with a neuro-ophthalmologist.[13] Disc swelling from elevated intracranial pressure, papilledema, indicates a medical emergency and requires immediate work-up and therapy. There are many other causes, however, of the abnormal-appearing optic disc (**Fig. 4**; **Table 2**).

Papilledema is a term often misapplied. This term should be used to describe swollen-appearing nerves associated with elevated intracranial pressure. A swollen appearance may also be caused by congenital anomalies, infection, inflammatory processes, and ischemia. In these cases (except congenital anomalies), *optic nerve head edema* is a better term to describe the swollen appearance. History is helpful in determining the likelihood for elevated intracranial pressure. The presence of headache, nausea, tinnitus, transient visual obscurations, double vision, or other neurologic deficits raises clinical suspicion. On examination, papilledema is typically bilateral. In the early stages, the swelling begins in the superior-inferior axis. The disc is hyperemic and there is obscuration of the retinal vessels as they leave the disc. The cup is preserved. As the papilledema progresses, exudates, cotton-wool spots, and hemorrhages often appear. Spontaneous venous pulsations are not typically present. Visual acuity and color vision are preserved until the late stage of papilledema. Mild swelling and decreased central vision should raise suspicion for a different cause of optic nerve head edema. The most common visual deficits associated with papilledema are an enlarged blind spot and peripheral field constriction.

Once suspected, papilledema requires immediate evaluation and neuroimaging. A mass lesion, severe cerebral edema, venous thrombosis, and hydrocephalus must

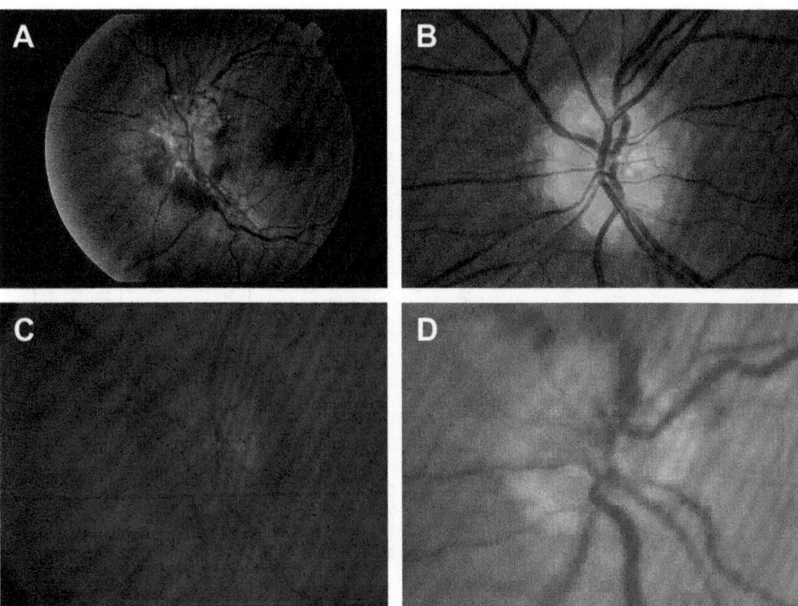

Fig. 4. Images of the abnormal optic disc. Fundus photos of the optic disc. (*A*) Acute papilledema with disc swelling, exudates, and hemorrhages. (*B*) Pseudopapilledema with optic nerve head drusen. (*C*) Acute optic neuritis with mild disc edema without hemorrhages. (*D*) Acute AION disc swelling with hemorrhages seen superiorly.

be ruled out. In the absence of lesions that might be associated with herniation, a lumbar puncture with opening pressure measurement should be performed. The diagnosis of pseudotumor cerebri (idiopathic intracranial hypertension) is suggested when neuroimaging studies and cerebrospinal fluid (CSF) examination are normal except for an elevated CSF opening pressure (**Box 3**). Pseudotumor cerebri is associated with obesity, anemia, and the prior use of glucocorticoids, vitamin A products, tetracycline derivatives, or synthetic growth hormones.[11,14–23] Often, patients report a recent weight gain. The disease is less common in thin men. Obstructive sleep apnea may be an important risk factor in men.[24] After diagnosis, baseline computerized visual fields should be performed. Treatment with acetazolamide may improve the papilledema, visual complaints, and headache.[25] If this medication is not successful, other diuretics and carbonic anhydrase inhibitors may be considered, such as furosemide and topiramate.[26] In obese patients, long-term therapy involves a weight loss program.[27,28] Progressive or severe vision loss, however, warrants more aggressive initial therapy. These patients may need to be hospitalized, administered glucocorticoids acutely, and evaluated for a surgical procedure, such as ventriculoperitoneal shunt or optic nerve fenestration.[29,30] The former is usually performed when the predominant complaint is headache.

A diagnosis frequently confused with papilledema, optic nerve drusen give the appearance of an elevated swollen nerve, though there is no acute edema. Termed *pseudopapilledema*, the appearance of this congenital abnormality is typified by glistening hyaline bodies, an absent cup, and anomalous but unobscured retinal vessels. These vessels seem to originate from the center of the disc and may have trifurcations. There are no cotton wool spots, exudates, or hemorrhages. The border of the disc may

Table 2
Differential diagnosis of the abnormal optic disc

Cause	History	Fundoscopic Appearance	Visual Examination	Ancillary Diagnostic Tests
Increased ICP (papilledema)	Morning headache, tranisent visual obscurations, double vision, tinnitus, nausea	Usually bilateral; disc hyperemia, cup preserved (early), cotton wool spots, exudates, obscuration of retinal vessels, absence of SVPs	No APD, central acuity spared, no color loss, enlarged blind spot, visual field constriction, and inferior nasal defect	MRI/MRV of head; lumbar puncture (document OP, rule out infection)
Drusen (pseudopapilledema)	Usually asymptomatic	Glistening hyaline bodies, absence of disc hyperemia, hemorrhage, or exudate; anomalous retinal vessels with central origination and trifurcations, irregular disc border, absent cup	Normal examination or irregular peripheral field constriction, enlarged blind spot; normal visual acuity	CT or orbital ultrasound may visualize calcified hyaline bodies
Optic neuritis	History of MS (or other inflammatory disorder); retro-orbital pain on eye movement, if demyelinating may worsen with heat (Uhthoff phenomenon)	Variable disc swelling, typically mild (retrobulbar involvement has normal disc appearance); unilateral in adults	APD; loss of central acuity and color discrimination; central or centrocecal scotoma	MRI for evidence of demyelination; CSF for pleocytosis and oligoclonal bands
Ischemia (AION)	Sudden painless loss of vision; >50 years of age; hypertension, diabetes, history of hypotensive episode	Usually unilateral; segmental disc edema; other eye may show absent cup	Variable field abnormality; often altitudinal; acuity variably affected; APD common	Work-up for hypertension, diabetes, vasculitis, GCA (glucose, BP, ESR, RPR)
Infection	History of known infection or compromised immune status, systemic symptoms, such as fever, meningismus, other focal neurologic deficits	May be bilateral or assymetric disc swelling with or without exudates, may also be associated with a macular star		Head CT or MRI, infectious work-up, including serologic and CSF studies (HIV, RPR, Lyme disease, cat scratch, and other as appropriate)
Infiltrative	History of neoplasm, sarcoid, or other infiltrative disease	Possible disc elevation and swelling; pallor	Variable field abnormality and acuity loss	MRI of the brain and orbits; CSF for pleocytosis and cytology

Abbreviations: BP, blood pressure; ICP, intracranial pressure; OP, opening pressure; RPR, rapid plasma reagin; SVPs, spontaneous venous pulsations.
Data from Laskowitz D, Liu GT, Galetta SL. Acute visual loss and other disorders of the eyes. Neurol Clin 1998;16:323–53.

Box 3
Evaluation and management of pseudotumor cerebri

Clinical Features

Headache, transient visual obscurations, double vision (if abducens affected), nausea, tinnitus. History of recent weight gain or obesity common. Typically bilateral papilledema. Central acuity preserved until late stages.

Diagnostic Testing

MRI and magnetic resonance venography (MRV) of the brain

Lumbar puncture with opening pressure recorded

Computerized perimetry

Treatment

Mild vision loss

Acetazolamide (furosemide, Topamax)

Weight loss

Severe or progressive vision loss

Prednisolone or prednisone

Ventriculoperitoneal shunt or optic nerve fenestration

be irregular due to the hyaline deposits. These patients rarely complain of visual symptoms. Pseudopapilledema is often observed in patients evaluated for other ocular or neurologic complaints. Computerized visual fields may reveal subtle deficits from the drusen, but significant visual loss is not seen. An orbital ultrasound can demonstrate the presence of the calcified drusen and establish the absence of true edema.[31] The drusen may also be seen on CT scan with cuts through the orbit.

There are several disease processes that can result in optic nerve head edema without elevated intracranial pressure. One-third of patients with acute demyelinating optic neuritis (discussed previously) demonstrate mild swelling (**Box 2**).[1] Hemorrhages in these patients are rare. They present with visual loss associated with retro-orbital pain with eye movements. In contrast, the majority of patients with AION present with acute optic nerve head edema, exudates, and hemorrhages. These patients tend to be over age 50, have painless sudden vision loss, and are less likely to recover their vision compared with those with optic neuritis.[32,33] Eyes at risk for AION are those with a small cup-to-disc ratio.[34] Often this finding is seen in the unaffected eye of patients suspected to have unilateral acute vision loss from AION. Due to the superior and inferior divisions of the retinal vasculature, the optic nerve swelling may be sectoral with corresponding altitudinal defects on visual field examination. Currently there are no approved therapies for AION. The use of steroids is controversial.[3] There is an approximately 15% risk of developing AION in the fellow eye.[35] Aggressive treatment of predisposing risk factors, diabetes, hypertension, and underlying collagen vascular disorders should be administered but it is unclear whether any measure affects the natural history of AION. Most patients with AION are given aspirin (81 mg daily) as a preventative agent. There is no long-term evidence that aspirin is effective in preventing fellow eye involvement. Owing to concern for nocturnal hypotension contributing to the ischemia, blood pressure medication dosing may need to be shifted to earlier times in the day.[36] GCA should be considered in all cases of AION (discussed previously), in particular those older patients with scalp tenderness, headache, and jaw claudication (**Box 1**).

Infections or infiltrative processes may also cause optic disc swelling. Patients may or may not have prior history of systemic symptoms, or other neurologic findings. When presenting with only visual complaints, a thorough evaluation with neuroimaging, serologies, and CSF may be required. Possible infections include HIV, syphilis, or Lyme disease. Common infiltrative processes include sarcoid, lymphoma, and other cancers. Inflammatory disorders other than MS can be associated with optic neuritis, including neuromyelitis optica and systemic lupus erythematosis.

Optic neuritis, ischemic optic neuropathy, toxic metabolic disorders, and compressive and hereditary optic neuropathies may all cause optic nerve pallor or atrophy. Although less likely to present in an emergency room, compressive optic neuropathies should be considered if a patient's visual complaints are longstanding or progressive. A complete review of optic neuropathies and causes of optic nerve atrophy is beyond the scope of this article.

Double Vision

Double vision is a common complaint in neuro-ophthalmologic emergencies and there are many potential causes. It first should be established whether the double vision is monocular or binocular. This is most readily evaluated by asking a patient if the double vision resolves when he or she covers one eye. If it does not improve, then the origin of the visual defect is not in the binocular misalignment of the two eyes. Monocular double vision is rarely associated with neurologic disease. It is often secondary to refractive error or media opacity and in these settings improves when a pinhole is placed over the affected eye. If the double vision is binocular and improves with one eye covered, then it should be asked whether the images are deviated horizontally or vertically and in what direction of gaze the divergence is greatest. These details help to localize the nerve or muscle affected. History of timing of onset, association with pain or headache, and fluctuation of symptoms may also be critical in establishing the correct diagnosis. For example, painless diplopia worsened by fatigue raises the clinical suspicion for myasthenia gravis. Most cases of ocular misalignment are due to cranial nerve palsy, restriction of one or more of the extraocular muscles, or brainstem disease causing internuclear ophthalmoplegia or skew deviation. Forced duction testing, involving the direct pushing of an anesthetized eye with a cotton-tipped applicator, can help distinguish nerve palsy versus muscle restriction. Inability to move the eye manually indicates a restrictive process, such as thyroid eye disease or muscle entrapment. The presence of other brainstem neurologic findings supports the diagnosis of a supranuclear cause of diplopia.

The third cranial nerve innervates the superior, medial, and inferior recti and inferior oblique as well as the levator and pupil. A complete third nerve palsy presents with ptosis, pupillary dilation, and an eye positioned out and down. Many third nerve lesions, however, present with partial findings, with or without pupillary involvement. The third nerve may be damaged anywhere along its course from the nucleus through the cavernous sinus and superior orbital fissure. There are many causes of third nerve palsies (**Table 3**). Of most concern in the emergency room is the presence of an aneurysm compressing the nerve. Another common cause of third nerve dysfunction is microvascular ischemia. Care must be taken to complete a thorough evaluation of patients to determine if urgent imaging must be obtained to avoid a life-threatening complication.

Emergency room history and examination for a new-onset third nerve palsy aids in the localization and the differential diagnosis of the lesion. Special attention should be

Table 3
Differential diagnosis of third nerve palsy

Differential Diagnosis	History	Signs	Diagnostic Tests
Aeurysmal compression	Retro-orbital pain, headache, stiff neck	Pupillary involvement common; aberrant regeneration may be present	MRI and MRA of the head or CTA; if negative consider conventional angiogram
Uncal herniation	Trauma, intracranial hemorrhage, neoplasm	Altered mentation, pupillary involvement, ipsilateral hemiparesis	Neuroimaging (MRI, CT)
Vasculopathic	Over age 50; diabetes, hypertension, headache, retroorbital pain may be indistinguishable from aneurysm	No aberrant regeneration, pupil usually spared	ESR, RPR, BP glucose
Chronic meningitis	Immunocompromised, constitutional symptoms, meningismus	Other cranial nerves may be involved	Neuroimaging (CT or MRI), then lumbar puncture; MRI may show nerve or meningeal enhancement
Cavernous sinus neoplasm	Retro-orbital pain	Pupil may be spared; CSS	MRI
Cavernous-carotid fistula	Vasculopathy, trauma	Mastoid or orbital bruit, CSS, chemosis, exophthalmos	MRI, MRA
Cavernous aneurysm	Vasculopathy, trauma	Pupil may be spared; CSS	MRI, MRA
Cavernous sinus inflammation (Tolosa-Hunt syndrome)	Retro-orbital pain; may be associated with collagen-vascular disease	Pupil may be spared; CSS	MRI may document cavernous sinus enhancement
Pituitary apoplexy	Severe headache, meningismus, visual loss	CSS, ophthalmoparesis (may be bilateral), visual field loss	MRI (CT may miss apoplexy), lumbar puncture may document RBC, WBC
GBS (Miller Fisher variant)	Preceding viral illness; painless	Areflexia, ataxia, extremity numbness or weakness	Lumbar puncture may demonstrate cytoalbuminologic dissociation; electrodiagnostic studies; MRI to exclude other etiologies
Myasthenia gravis	Painless, fluctuates with fatigue; dysarthria or dysphagia	Pupil spared, ptosis, orbicularis weakness, fatigue with 1 min of upgaze, curtaining	Serum Ach-R antibody level, electrodiagnostic studies
Midbrain lesion (infarct, tumor, demyelination)	Hypertension, DM, cardiogenic emboli, MS	Contralareral hemiparesis, rubral tremor	MRI
Wernicke encephalopathy	Alcohol abuse, or other nutritional deficiency	Nystagmus, abduction deficit, ataxia, confusion	Improvement with thiamine (give before glucose)

Abbreviations: Ach-R, acetylcholine receptor; BP, blood pressure; CSS, cavernous sinus syndrome; DM, diabetes mellitus; RBC, red blood cell count; RPR, rapid plasma reagin; WBC, white blood cell count.

Data from Laskowitz D, Liu GT, Galetta SL. Acute visual loss and other disorders of the eyes. Neurol Clin 1998;16:323–53.

given to any additional neurologic deficits, status of the pupil, and presence or absence of aberrant regeneration. In third nerve nuclear lesions, for example, brainstem infarctions or masses, the contralateral superior rectus muscle is weak (innervation of the superior rectus is crossed) and there is bilateral ptosis (levator complex is midline). The third nerve fascicle travels ventrally and depending on its rostral-caudal position, lesions to the fascicle may also be associated with contralateral ataxia (Claude syndrome), contralateral rubral tremor (Benedikt syndrome), or contralateral hemiparesis (Weber syndrome). The nerve is susceptible to diseases of the subarachnoid space and in cases of CSF inflammation, infection, or malignancy, there may be other signs of neurologic imvolvement, such as other cranial nerve palsies or weakness. As the nerve passes freely in the subarachnoid space, it is subject to compression against the free tentorial edge, as in the case of impending uncal herniation. Context is important in evaluating the likelihood of herniation as a cause of third nerve dysfunction. An awake alert patient sitting upright in the emergency room is likely to have another cause for the palsy, whereas an intensive care unit patient who is obtunded or has a history of trauma or mass lesion is at much higher risk. Additional dysfunction of the fourth, sixth, or the first or second divisions of the fifth cranial nerve indicates the site of the lesion may be in the cavernous sinus (discussed later). Loss of vision or signs on examination of optic pallor or visual field deficits suggests involvement at the orbital apex or a rapidly expanding sellar lesion as may occur in pituitary apoplexy. The latter may also present as a cavernous sinus syndrome.

The presence or absence of pupillary dilation may help distinguish between aneurysmal compression and microvascular ischemia as causes of third nerve palsies. Aneurysms in the subarachnoid space compress the superficial parasympathetic fibers traveling along the third nerve and lead to early pupillary involvement. In contrast, ischemic palsies involve the pupillary fibers in approximately a third of patients.[37] These patients tend to have the risk factors of age over 50, diabetes, and hypertension. Patients with partial third nerve palsies, however, may initially present with pupil sparing but then develop pupil involvement as the lesion (ie, aneurysm) enlarges. Careful and expedient follow-up is required for these patients and they should undergo neuroimaging. The authors prefer CT angiography (CTA) imaging in evaluating patients with isolated third nerve palsies, but magnetic resonance angiography (MRA) imaging also has good sensitivity in detecting aneurysms.[38,39] Although the sensitivity of MRA and CTA for detecting aneurysms is in the 90% to 98% range (depending on the size of the aneurysm), these results are dependent on the skills of the neuroradiologist and the quality of the imaging.[39–41] Thus, if there is any doubt about the presence of an aneurysm, the authors suggest conventional angiography. A complete third nerve palsy without pupillary involvement is unlikely to be from a compressive aneurysm, but in the authors' experience it is prudent to consider imaging in any patient with an isolated ocular motor nerve palsy. Vascular palsies on average improve or resolve within 3 months.[42] In the absence of improvement, neuroimaging is required.

Aberrant regeneration refers to the chronic denervation and reinervation with misdirection of third nerve fibers. On adduction or depression of the eye there is often eyelid retraction. Alternatively, retraction of the globe may occur on attempted vertical gaze or pupillary constriction with adduction. Aberrant regeneration is a sign of a chronic compressive lesion, such as a slow growing aneurysm or tumor. It almost never occurs in ischemic lesions.

The fourth cranial nerve innervates the superior oblique muscle, responsible for intortion and depression of the eye in adduction. A patient with injury to this nerve has vertical double vision worse in contralateral gaze and ipsilateral head tilt

(**Box 4**). The most common reason for acute acquired fourth nerve palsy is trauma. Microvascular disease and inflammatory disease of the subarachnoid space may also cause fourth nerve injury. Neoplasm rarely affects the fourth nerve in isolation. Decompensation of a congenital fourth nerve palsy is typically insidious in onset and more frequently presents in the clinic than the emergency room. The 3-step test for diagnosing a fourth nerve palsy is as follows: identify the hypertropic (higher) eye, establish whether the hypertropia increases in right or left gaze, and similarly tilt the head to the right and left to determine if there is worsening of double vision and alignment (Bielschowsky test). A typical fourth nerve palsy worsens with contralateral gaze and ipsilateral head tilt but improves with contralateral head tilt. Patients may not be aware that are holding their head in a contralateral tilt as compensation for the nerve palsy.

The sixth cranial nerve innervates the lateral rectus. Palsies of the sixth nerve present with horizontal double vision that worsens when gazing in the ipsilateral direction. On examination, evaluation of a patient's eye movements reveals a deficit in abduction, unless the palsy is subtle, in which case measurements of eye alignment are required to localize the injury. Using alternate cover or Maddox rod testing, an esophoria, greater in the ipsilateral direction, defines an abduction deficit. Care must be taken, however, to differentiate between a sixth nerve palsy and a restrictive process, such as thyroid disease involvement of the medial rectus. The sixth nerves are vulnerable to compression in cases of increased intracranial pressure as they ascend and then bend along the clivus to enter the Dorello canal. Trauma, microvascular disease, and neoplasm may cause sixth nerve palsies (**Table 4**). The sixth nerve's prolonged course through the subarachnoid space makes it susceptible to traumatic injury. Ischemic injury is also common. Timely imaging is warranted, however, even in patients with isolated sixth nerve palsies and vascular risk factors, because brain lesions may present in this setting. As in suspected cases of vascular

Box 4
Fourth nerve palsy

Action of Fourth Nerve

Incyclotorsion

Depresses the eye in adducton

Clinical Presentation

Vertical diplopia

Posttrauma

Microvascular risk factors

Positional head tilt

Three-Step Test

Identify which eye is hypertropic

Determine if hypertropia is worse in right versus left gaze

Bielschowsky head tilt test—tilt head to right and left

Diagnosis

Hypertropia worse in contralateral gaze and ipsilateral head tilt; improved alignment and vision in contralateral head tilt

Table 4
Differential diagnosis of abduction deficits

Differential Diagnosis	History	Additional Signs	Diagnostic Tests
Brainstem disease (infarction, tumor, demyelination)	Vertigo, dysarthria, perioral numbness	Ipsilateral gaze paresis, INO, facial paresis, contralateral hemiparesis	MRI brain
Meningitis (carcinomatous, TB, fungal, sarcoid, Lyme disease, syphilis)	Systemic/constitutional symptoms, headache meningismus; history of TB, syphilis, or malignancy	Other cranial nerves involved	MRI brain may show leptomeningeal and nerve enhancement; lumbar puncture, including cytology and microbiology studies
Increased intracranial pressure	Headache, nausea, ataxia	Papilledema, enlarged blind spots; often bilateral	CT head, lumbar puncture
Trauma	History of trauma	Vision loss, other ocular motility abnormalities with orbital trauma, Battle sign, CSF otorrhea, hemotympanum, VII or VIII deficits with a fracture of middle cranial fossa (petrous apex)	CT head and orbits, consider angiogram if chemosis, exophthalmos to rule out a carotid-cavernous fistula
Microvascular	Over age 50, diabetes, hypertension, ± headache	Unilateral isolated	RPR, ESR (GCA can cause an isolated cranial nerve palsy), BP, glucose
Neoplasm	Progressive diplopia, facial weakness or numbness, hearing loss	Isolated abduction deficit or multiple cranial neuropathies, papilledema, ataxia	MRI brain
Thyroid eye disease	Progessive, may be worse in mornings, symptoms of hyperthyroidism	Proptosis, eyelid retraction and lag, restriction on forced duction	CT or MRI orbits to rule out entrapment or mass, orbital ultrasound, thyroid function tests
Cavernous sinus inflammation (Tolosa-Hunt syndrome)	Retro-orbital pain; may be associated with collagen-vascular disease	Cavernous sinus syndrome	MRI may document cavernous sinus enhancement
Convergence spasm	Report bilateral eye crossing	Symptoms improve when distracted, fluctuating esotropia, miosis	Oculocephalics
Myasthenia gravis	Fluctuates with fatigue; dysarthria or dysphagia	Ptosis, orbicularis weakness, fatigue with 1-min upgaze, curtaining	Serum Ach-R antibody level, Tensilon test, electrodiagnostic studies
Wernicke encephalopathy	Alcohol abuse or other nutritional deficiency	Nystagmus, bilateral abduction deficit, ataxia, confusion	Improvement with thiamine (give before glucose)

Abbreviations: Ach-R, acetylcholine receptor; BP, blood pressure; INO, internuclear ophthalmoplegia; RPR, rapid plasma reagin; TB, tuberculosis.

third nerve palsies, if there is no improvement in three months, neuroimaging is required.

Neoplasms of the skull base, such as meningiomas, nasopharyngeal carcinomas, chondromas, or cordomas, may compress the sixth nerve at the clivus, resulting in insidious onset of double vision and progressive esophoria and abduction deficit. Because it is the only cranial nerve not fixed to the wall of the cavernous sinus, it may be the first to be compressed by a cavernous sinus neoplasm or cavernous carotid aneurysm.

The presence of other findings on the examination aids to localize and differentiate the causes of sixth nerve palsies. An abduction deficit, ipsilateral facial weakness, and contralateral hemiparesis localizes to the ventral pons (Millard-Gubler syndrome).[43,44] A sixth nerve palsy associated with headache, nausea, fever, meningismus, and other cranial nerve involvement is concerning for basilar meningitis from tuberculosis, sarcoid, or fungal infections. Bilateral sixth nerve palsies must be imaged urgently to rule out states of elevated intracranial pressure or neoplasm. Other causes of bilateral sixth abduction deficits include ocular myasthenia, Miller Fisher variant of Guillain-Barré syndrome (GBS), and restrictive disease, such as thyroid eye disease or entrapment of the medial rectus.

Bilateral ophthalmoplegia involving any of the ocular motor nerves may indicate a condition requiring immediate work-up and treatment in the emergency room (**Box 5**). If there is a history of alcohol use, bariatic surgery, or other nutritional deficiency, Wernicke disease should be considered and thiamine given before any glucose solutions. A thiamine level before administration and response to the vitamin confirm the diagnosis. Typically, these patients also present with altered mental status, nystagmus, and ataxia. A brainstem stroke with bilateral ocular motor involvement is acute in onset and commonly associated with other localizing symptoms, such as loss of consciousness, other cranial nerve involvement, weakness, or ataxia. Pituitary apoplexy may result in blood or infarcted tissue expanding into unilateral or

Box 5
Causes of bilateral ophthalmoparesis

Wernicke encephalopathy

History of alcohol abuse or nutritional deficiency, confusion, ataxia; treat with thiamine

Brainstem stroke

Stroke risk factors, other brainstem symptoms; emergent MRI brain

Pituitary apoplexy

Severe headache, meningismus; cranial nerve III, IV, V1 or V2 involvement; emergent MRI

Botulism

Anorexia, vomiting, dilated unreactive pupils, bradycardia; electrodiagnostic studies and serum bioassay

Myasthenia gravis

Painless, fluctuates with fatigue, ptosis, orbicularis weakness, dysarthria, pupil spared; evaluate respiratory status, anti-acetylcholinereceptor antibody, electrodiagnostic tests, Tensilon test

GBS (Miller Fisher variant)

Preceding gastrointestinal or upper respiratory illness, areflexia, ataxia, extremity numbness or weakness; lumbar puncture, electromyogram/nerve conduction studies bilateral cavernous sinuses. Botulism presents with bilateral duction deficits and must be managed urgently in the emergency room. Other neuromuscular diseases, myasthenia gravis, or less commonly Miller Fisher variant of GBS may also present acutely. In addition to neurologic evaluation, respiratory function must be evaluated in these conditions. Thyroid eye disease may produce bilateral ophthalmoplegia but the onset is typically more insidious.

Lastly, a skew deviation causes vertical misalignment of the eyes and double vision. Most commonly it occurs from acute brainstem dysfunction but can result from peripheral vestibular or cerebellar lesions. Other signs of brainstem injury help distinguish a skew deviation from a third or fourth nerve palsy. The examination also suggests a likely skew deviation when the eye movements and alignment do not support either of these cranial nerve palsies and there is no evidence for myasthenia gravis or thyroid disease.

The combination of a skew deviation with ocular torsion and a head tilt is referred to as the ocular tilt reaction. This triad of signs is typically observed with lesions of the lateral pontomedullary junction or the paramedian thalamic-mesencephalic region and results from dysfunction of the utricular pathways that begin in the labyrinths and terminate in the rostral brainstem.[45] The utricular pathway mediating vertical gaze synapses at the vestibular nuclei and crosses to ascend in the medial longitudinal fasciculus. In the rostral brainstem, it connects to the nuclei that activate the 4 vertically acting muscles: the superior rectus, superior oblique, inferior rectus, and inferior oblique. Although the exact pathways that mediate a skew deviation and ocular tilt reaction are unknown, clinical observation has demonstrated the localizing value of a skew deviation (**Table 5**).[46] Helpful in relating the site of the lesion and the neuro-ophthalmologic findings is remembering that the superior rectus subnucleus and trochlear nucleus control contralateral superior rectus and superior oblique muscles, respectively. This means that a lesion of the right utricular nerve or caudal brainstem causes left hypertropia from impaired left inferior rectus and right superior rectus function. In contrast, a rostral lesion after the crossing in the medial longitudinal fasciculus results in ipsilateral hypertropia.

The most common causes of a skew deviation are brainstem stroke and neoplasm, emphasizing the need for expedient imaging in these patients.

NEURO-OPHTHALMOLOGIC SIGNS OF NEUROLOGIC EMERGENCIES

Increased Intracranial Pressure

Neuro-ophthalmic findings alert an emergency room provider to increased intracranial pressure, even before ventricular changes are seen on neuroimaging (**Box 6**).[47,48]

Table 5
Localizing value of skew deviation

Lesion Location	Type of Skew	Associated Signs
Lateral pontomedullary	Contralateral hypertropia	Ipsilateral excyclotorsion; ipsilateral facial numbness; ipsilateral Horner; lateropulsion
Midline cervicomedullary junction	Bilateral inferior rectus	Downbeat nystagmus
Medial longitudinal fasciculus	Ipsilateral hypertropia	Internuclear ophthalmoplegia
Rostral midbrain	Ipsilateral hypertropia	Vertical gaze palsy; conjugate cyclotorsion, eyelid retraction

Box 6
Neuro-ophthalmic signs of increased intracranial pressure

Dorsal midbrain syndrome

Impaired upgaze, pupillary light-near dissociation, eyelid retraction, convergence retraction nystagmus

Ocular motility deficit

Bilateral abduction deficit or divergence insufficiency; rarely fourth nerve palsy

Papilledema

Bilateral, may be assymetric, optic nerve head edema; enlarged blind spot; peripheral constriction; late stage with central vision loss

Early hydrocephalus may present with a dorsal midbrain syndrome (Parinaud syndrome) or ocular motility abnormalities. In Parinaud syndrome, the dorsal midbrain is compressed by ventricular dilatation. It must be differentiated from other causes of midbrain compression, such as a tumor. Bilateral upgaze is impaired. A patient's eyes may drift downward after an initial attempt to look up or there may be complete paresis of upgaze. Commonly, light-near dissociation is observed, with poor pupillary response to light but an intact response to near. Other features of the dorsal midbrain syndrome are eyelid retraction and convergence retraction nystagmus (saccades). The eyelid retraction (Collier sign) may be subtle or prominent, and the nystagmus refers to the periodic retraction of the eyes back into the orbit with attempted upgaze. The latter can be elicited with a downward moving optokinetic strip or drum, driving the patient to attempt upward saccades.

In addition to the dorsal midbrain syndrome, bilateral abduction deficits may be seen in early hydrocephalus due to brainstem compression and stretching of the sixth cranial nerves. Patients complain of horizontal double vision and in early stages only at distance. Mild esotropias are well tolerated at near. Thus, early hydrocephalus can mimic divergence insufficiency and care must be taken to look for other signs and symptoms of elevated intracranial pressure. Fourth nerve dysfunction has been reported in hydrocephlus but is rare.[49,50] Third nerve palsy in this setting is uncommon and should raise suspicion for a cause other than hydrocephalus.

As discussed previously, papilledema is optic nerve head swelling in the setting of raised intracranial pressure. It is the most common cause of visual loss in hydrocephalus and spares central vision until the late stages. The first deficit is typically an enlarged blind spot, followed by peripheral visual field constriction. Patients often describe vague blurry vision, transient visual obscurations, or peripheral vision loss. Depending on the cause of the increased intracranial pressure, shunting or shunt repair may be necessary urgently to preserve vision.

Herniation Syndromes

A feared emergency in the ICU setting, brain herniation is catastrophic and, depending on the structures compressed, associated with specific neuro-ophthalmic signs. The most familiar to clinicians, uncal herniation results in compression against the free tentorial edge of the parasympathetic fibers traveling on the third nerve. In early stages there may be ipsilateral pupillary dilation with sluggish response to light and in later stages with further compression of the third nerve and midbrain and a complete third nerve palsy as well as ipsilateral or contralateral hemiparesis. Ultimately, the vestibular ocular response disappears with worsening brainstem ischemia and the contralateral pupil also dilates.

Subfalcian herniation may compress the ipsilateral anterior cerebral artery causing frontal lobe ischemia with isilateral gaze deviation and leg weakness. Central transtentorial herniation compresses the diencephalon with resultant progressive lethargy. Initially the pupils are small and reactive. Roving eye movements and oculocephalic reflexes indicate the midbrain is intact. With continued compression, the pupils dilate to midposition and become fixed, the third nerve pressed against the clivus or petroclinoid ligament. With midbrain ischemia, the pupils may become irregular and the oculocephalic reflexes difficult to elicit. Patients may develop midbrain hyperventilation and decerebrate rigidity. Autonomic dysfunction and death occur when the compression reaches the caudal brainstem.

Occipital infarction and cortical vision loss occur in transtentorial herniation when the posterior cerebral artery is compressed against the free edge of the tentorium. Either right or left artery may be involved and the infarction may be unilateral or bilateral in this setting. Given the depressed mental status in this setting, the vision loss likely is undetected acutely.

Vascular Lesions

Carotid dissection

Patients with a carotid dissection typically have a history of trauma affecting the cervical region or a history of connective tissue disease making them susceptible to vessel wall tears. They present with unilateral neck pain and headache and half present with a Horner syndrome from damage to the sympathetic fibers traveling in the pericarotid plexus.[51] Horner syndrome consists of miosis, ptosis, and, depending on the location of the injury to the sympathetc fibers, ipsilateral anhidrosis. The ptosis of Horner syndrome tends to be mild. Patients may also describe tinnitus or a rushing sound in the ipsilateral ear. Of concern in a carotid dissection is embolization of clot to distal arteries and resultant ischemic stroke, amaurosis fugax, or central retinal or ophthalmic artery occlusion. Ischemic optic neuropathy and orbital ischemia are also reported.[52,53]

Cavernous sinus syndrome

The cavernous sinus is a collection of venous channels posterior to the orbit and lateral to the pituitary fossa. It is encapsulated by dura and not contiguous with the subarachnoid space. Through the right and left cavernous sinuses traverse the carotid siphons, oculosympathetic fibers, and cranial nerves III, IV, VI, V1, and V2. All of the cranial nerves except the sixth are fixed along the lateral wall of the sinus. Depending on the location of the lesion, any of these structures may be involved in a cavernous sinus syndrome. A complete syndrome would consist of ophthalmoplegia, ptosis, mydriasis, hypesthesia of V1 and V2, and orbital pain. Partial syndromes that can be seen include an isolated third or sixth nerve palsy or a combination of a sixth nerve palsy and Horner syndrome.

Mass lesions in the cavernous sinus may cause the insidious onset of diplopia and facial numbness. Meningiomas are the most common neoplasms arising from the cavernous sinus.[54,55] Metastases and contiguous head and neck cancers, such as nasopharyngeal carcinoma, also cause cavernous sinus syndromes. A slow-growing cavernous carorid aneurysm may present with compressive symptoms. These aneurysms are not typically life threatening because hemorrhages are contained within the sinus and dura. They are not causes of subarachnoid bleeding but are treated for their neuro-ophthalmic symptoms.

Acute causes of a cavernous sinus syndrome that require immediate recognition and treatment include a cavernous sinus thrombosis and high-flow carotid cavernous fistula. Septic cavernous sinus thrombosis typically involves extension of a facial or sinus infection into the cavernous sinus and if untreated may lead to meningitis and infarction. The most common organisms involved are staphylococcus and streptococcus and the mainstay of treatment is antibiotics.[56,57] Fungal infections are more rare but, when present, often require surgery in addition to amphotericin. The use of anticoagulants is controversial.[56,58] A carotid cavernous fistula may present with a triad of a painful red eye with chemosis, pulsatile exophthalmus, and an ocular bruit.[59] An examiner may note arteriolization of the episclerotic vessels. Double vision and motility deficits are not uncommon and vision loss may occur from elevated intraocular pressure, optic neuropathy, or retinopathy.[60]

An idiopathic granulomatous inflammatory reaction (Tolosa-Hunt syndrome) and pituitary apoplexy may also cause a cavernous sinus syndrome. The former is a diagnosis of exclusion and is treated acutely with corticosteroids. Orbital inflammation may be evident on MRI. Pituitary apoplexy is discussed below.

Pituitary Apoplexy

Pituitary apoplexy refers to the hemorrhagic infarction of the pituitary gland. It can be life threatening and must be recognized in the emergency room. Often it occurs in the setting of a previously undetected pituitary lesion. Patients present with headache and commonly neuro-ophthalmic signs. If there is an underlying large lesion or extension of the hemorrhage superiorly, bitemporal visual field loss or a junctional scotoma may be present from compression of the crossing nasal fibers in the chiasm and junction of the optic nerve and chiasm, respectively. Lateral extension may involve the cavernous sinus and cause a third nerve (located superiorly in the sinus) palsy or other variation of a cavernous sinus syndrome. These patients may have meningismus from subarachnoid blood and chemical meningitis. Red blood cells and polymorphonuclear cells may be present in the spinal fluid. Care must be taken to differentiate pituitary apoplexy from subarachnoid hemorrhage because CT scans of the head and vasculature may be unremarkable. Similarly, this dangerous condition may also be mistaken for viral or bacterial meningitis. Clinicians must have suspicion for this diagnosis, with the neuro-ophthalmic examination often providing important clues, and if the head CT is negative, pursue an MRI of the brain in the emergency setting. Treatment involves immediate supplementation with hydrocortisone to avoid life-threatening hemodynamic instability and neurosurgical consultation.[61]

Other Neurologic Emergencies with Neuro-ophthalmic Signs

Neuro-ophthalmic findings may provide localizing information for neurovascular injuries. Frontal lobe infarctions and hemorrhages are associated with a contralateral gaze palsy. An acute frontal hemorrhage, however, may cause wrong-way eyes or forced contralateral gaze from the irritating effects of the hemorrhage. Parietal damage may incur inferior field cuts and smooth pursuit abnormalities. There are multiple neuro-ophthalmic findings associated with thalamic hemorrhages. The most common is an esotropia caused by bilateral pseudo-sixth nerve palsies with downward gaze deviation, presumably due to the loss of projections that inhibit convergence. Pontine hemorrhages may cause pinpoint reactive pupils or ocular bobbing.

Ocular motility deficits are common in several neuromuscular emergencies. Almost all patients with myasthenia gravis have ptosis and extraocular motor palsies during the course of their disease. Evidence for myasthenia on examination should prompt immediate assessment of breathing, swallowing, and weakness to determine if treatment should be pursued as inpatient or outpatient and whether immediate breathing support is required. The Miller Fisher variant of GBS, with features of ophthalmoplegia, areflexia, and ataxia, or typical GBS must also be considered in patients with bilateral ocular motility deficits.[62] Urgent evaluation of these patients also includes a respiratory and swallowing assessment. The most common neuro-ophthalmic finding is bilateral abduction deficits.[63] Botulism, another neuromuscular emergency, presents with extraocular muscle weakness, ptosis, and poorly reactive dilated pupils. Early on, the condition may be confused with myasthenia gravis, but the pupillary abnormalities are distinctive.

Trauma causes many neuro-ophthalmic disorders. Compression or severing of the optic nerve causes acute vision loss and treatment is controversial. The acute use of steroids has not been well supported by the literature.[64] Surgical intervention is also controversial and depends on the nature of the injury.[65] Orbital fractures may result in entrapment of the extraocular muscles and motility deficits. Forced ductions help distinguish entrapment from traumatic cranial nerve palsies. In the setting of trauma, fourth nerve palsies are the most common and when bilateral are usually accompanied by loss of consciousness.[66] Severe head trauma with neurologic injury may cause cortical blindness. The most common neuro-ophthalmic complaint after trauma is convergence insufficiency.[67] Patients report difficulty with seeing objects at near and on examination may have abnormal accommodation. This issue tends to improve over time without intervention, but orthoptic exercises, prisms, and surgery may be helpful in persistent cases.

REFERENCES

1. The clinical profile of optic neuritis. Experience of the Optic Neuritis Treatment Trial. Optic Neuritis Study Group. Arch Ophthalmol 1991;109:1673–8.
2. Schumacher M, Schmidt D, Jurklies B, et al. Central retinal artery occlusion: local intra-arterial fibrinolysis versus conservative treatment, a multicenter randomized trial. Ophthalmology 2010;117:1367–75, e1.
3. Hayreh SS. Vascular disorders in neuro-ophthalmology. Curr Opin Neurol 2011; 24:6–11.
4. Hayreh SS, Zimmerman MB. Fundus changes in central retinal artery occlusion. Retina 2007;27:276–89.
5. Wong TY, Scott IU. Clinical practice. Retinal-vein occlusion. N Engl J Med 2010; 363:2135–44.
6. Galetta SL, Raps EC, Wulc AE, et al. Conjugal temporal arteritis. Neurology 1990; 40:1839–42.
7. Gonzalez-Gay MA. Genetic epidemiology. Giant cell arteritis and polymyalgia rheumatica. Arthritis Res 2001;3:154–7.
8. Mitchell BM, Font RL. Detection of varicella zoster virus DNA in some patients with giant cell arteritis. Invest Ophthalmol Vis Sci 2001;42:2572–7.
9. Hunder GG, Bloch DA, Michel BA, et al. The American College of Rheumatology 1990 criteria for the classification of giant cell arteritis. Arthritis Rheum 1990;33: 1122–8.
10. Hayreh SS, Podhajsky PA, Raman R, et al. Giant cell arteritis: validity and reliability of various diagnostic criteria. Am J Ophthalmol 1997;123:285–96.
11. Liu GT, Volpe NJ, Galetta SL. Neuro-opthalmology: diagnosis and management. 2nd edition. Philadelphia: W.B. Saunders Company; 2010.

12. Chan CC, Paine M, O'Day J. Steroid management in giant cell arteritis. Br J Ophthalmol 2001;85:1061–4.
13. Bruce BB, Lamirel C, Wright DW, et al. Nonmydriatic ocular fundus photography in the emergency department. N Engl J Med 2011;364:387–9.
14. Radhakrishnan K, Ahlskog JE, Cross SA, et al. Idiopathic intracranial hypertension (pseudotumor cerebri). Descriptive epidemiology in Rochester, Minn, 1976 to 1990. Arch Neurol 1993;50:78–80.
15. Daniels AB, Liu GT, Volpe NJ, et al. Profiles of obesity, weight gain, and quality of life in idiopathic intracranial hypertension (pseudotumor cerebri). Am J Ophthalmol 2007;143:635–41.
16. Galvin JA, Van Stavern GP. Clinical characterization of idiopathic intracranial hypertension at the Detroit Medical Center. J Neurol Sci 2004;223:157–60.
17. Biousse V, Rucker JC, Vignal C, et al. Anemia and papilledema. Am J Ophthalmol 2003;135:437–46.
18. Friedman DI. Medication-induced intracranial hypertension in dermatology. Am J Clin Dermatol 2005;6:29–37.
19. Liu GT, Kay MD, Bienfang DC, et al. Pseudotumor cerebri associated with corticosteroid withdrawal in inflammatory bowel disease. Am J Ophthalmol 1994;117:352–7.
20. Quinn AG, Singer SB, Buncic JR. Pediatric tetracycline-induced pseudotumor cerbri. J AAPOS 1999;3:53–7.
21. Fraunfelder FW, Fraunfelder FT, Corbett JJ. Isotretinoin-associated intracranial hypertension. Ophthalmology 2004;111:1248–50.
22. Malozowski S, Tanner LA, Wysowski DK, et al. Benign intracranial hypertension in children with growth hormone deficiency treated with growth hormone. J Pediatr 1995;126:996–9.
23. Malozowski S, Tanner LA, Wysowski D, et al. Growth hormone, insulin-like growth factor I, and benign intracranial hypertension. N Engl J Med 1993;329:665–6.
24. Fraser JA, Bruce BB, Rucker J, et al. Risk factors for idiopathic intracranial hypertension in men: a case-control study. J Neurol Sci 2010;290:86–9.
25. Wandstrat TL, Phillips J. Pseudotumor cerebri responsive to acetazolamide. Ann Pharmacother 1995;29:318.
26. Finsterer J, Foldy D, Fertl E. Topiramate resolves headache from pseudotumor cerebri. J Pain Symptom Manage 2006;32:401–2.
27. Kupersmith MJ, Gamell L, Turbin R, et al. Effects of weight loss on the course of idiopathic intracranial hypertension in women. Neurology 1998;50:1094–8.
28. Johnson LN, Krohel GB, Madsen RW, et al. The role of weight loss and acetazolamide in the treatment of idiopathic intracranial hypertension (pseudotumor cerebri). Ophthalmology 1998;105:2313–7.
29. Liu GT, Glaser JS, Schatz NJ. High-dose methylprednisolone and acetazolamide for visual loss in pseudotumor cerebri. Am J Ophthalmol 1994;118:88–96.
30. Banta JT, Farris BK. Pseudotumor cerebri and optic nerve sheath decompression. Ophthalmology 2000;107:1907–12.
31. Kurz-Levin MM, Landau K. A comparison of imaging techniques for diagnosing drusen of the optic nerve head. Arch Ophthalmol 1999;117:1045–9.
32. Optic nerve decompression surgery for nonarteritic anterior ischemic optic neuropathy (NAION) is not effective and may be harmful. The Ischemic Optic Neuropathy Decompression Trial Research Group. JAMA 1995;273:625–32.
33. Hayreh SS. Anterior ischemic optic neuropathy. Clin Neurosci 1997;4:251–63.
34. Beck RW, Servais GE, Hayreh SS. Anterior ischemic optic neuropathy. IX. Cup-to-disc ratio and its role in pathogenesis. Ophthalmology 1987;94:1503–8.

35. Newman NJ, Scherer R, Langenberg P, et al. The fellow eye in NAION: report from the ischemic optic neuropathy decompression trial follow-up study. Am J Ophthalmol 2002;134:317–28.
36. Hayreh SS. Management of ischemic optic neuropathies. Indian J Ophthalmol 2011;59:123–36.
37. Jacobson DM. Pupil involvement in patients with diabetes-associated oculomotor nerve palsy. Arch Ophthalmol 1998;116:723–7.
38. Numminen J, Tarkiainen A, Niemela M, et al. Detection of unruptured cerebral artery aneurysms by MRA at 3.0 tesla: comparison with multislice helical computed tomographic angiography. Acta Radiol 2011;52(6):670–4.
39. Chaudhary N, Davagnanam I, Ansari SA, et al. Imaging of intracranial aneurysms causing isolated third cranial nerve palsy. J Neuroophthalmol 2009;29:238–44.
40. Elmalem VI, Hudgins PA, Bruce BB, et al. Underdiagnosis of posterior communicating artery aneurysm in noninvasive brain vascular studies. J Neuroophthalmol 2011;31:103–9.
41. Hacein-Bey L, Provenzale JM. Current imaging assessment and treatment of intracranial aneurysms. AJR Am J Roentgenol 2011;196:32–44.
42. Capo H, Warren F, Kupersmith MJ. Evolution of oculomotor nerve palsies. J Clin Neuroophthalmol 1992;12:21–5.
43. Matlis A, Kleinman Y, Korn-Lubetzki I. Millard-Gubler syndrome. AJNR Am J Neuroradiol 1994;15:179–81.
44. Casero. The Millard-Gubler syndrome. Am J Ophthalmol 1948;31:344.
45. Dieterich M, Brandt T. Wallenberg's syndrome: lateropulsion, cyclorotation, and subjective visual vertical in thirty-six patients. Ann Neurol 1992;31:399–408.
46. Brandt T, Dieterich M. Skew deviation with ocular torsion: a vestibular brainstem sign of topographic diagnostic value. Ann Neurol 1993;33:528–34.
47. Chou SY, Digre KB. Neuro-ophthalmic complications of raised intracranial pressure, hydrocephalus, and shunt malfunction. Neurosurg Clin N Am 1999;10:587–608.
48. Corbett JJ. Neuro-ophthalmologic complications of hydrocephalus and shunting procedures. Semin Neurol 1986;6:111–23.
49. Cobbs WH, Schatz NJ, Savino PJ. Midbrain eye signs in hydrocephalus. Trans Am Neurol Assoc 1978;103:130.
50. Guy JR, Friedman WF, Mickle JP. Bilateral trochlear nerve paresis in hydrocephalus. J Clin Neuroophthalmol 1989;9:105–11.
51. Hart RG, Easton JD. Dissections of cervical and cerebral arteries. Neurol Clin 1983;1:155–82.
52. Rivkin MJ, Hedges TR 3rd, Logigian EL. Carotid dissection presenting as posterior ischemic optic neuropathy. Neurology 1990;40:1469.
53. Galetta SL, Leahey A, Nichols CW, et al. Orbital ischemia, ophthalmoparesis, and carotid dissection. J Clin Neuroophthalmol 1991;11:284–7.
54. Thomas JE, Yoss RE. The parasellar syndrome: problems in determining etiology. Mayo Clin Proc 1970;45:617–23.
55. Sekhar LN, Sen CN, Jho HD, et al. Surgical treatment of intracavernous neoplasms: a four-year experience. Neurosurgery 1989;24:18–30.
56. Cannon ML, Antonio BL, McCloskey JJ, et al. Cavernous sinus thrombosis complicating sinusitis. Pediatr Crit Care Med 2004;5:86–8.
57. DiNubile MJ. Septic thrombosis of the cavernous sinuses. Arch Neurol 1988;45:567–72.
58. Bhatia K, Jones NS. Septic cavernous sinus thrombosis secondary to sinusitis: are anticoagulants indicated? A review of the literature. J Laryngol Otol 2002;116:667–76.

59. Kupersmith MJ, Berenstein A, Choi IS, et al. Management of nontraumatic vascular shunts involving the cavernous sinus. Ophthalmology 1988;95:121–30.
60. Leonard TJ, Moseley IF, Sanders MD. Ophthalmoplegia in carotid cavernous sinus fistula. Br J Ophthalmol 1984;68:128–34.
61. Murad-Kejbou S, Eggenberger E. Pituitary apoplexy: evaluation, management, and prognosis. Curr Opin Ophthalmol 2009;20:456–61.
62. Fisher CM, Adams RD. Diphtheritic polyneuritis; a pathological study. J Neuropathol Exp Neurol 1956;15:243–68.
63. Lee SH, Lim GH, Kim JS, et al. Acute ophthalmoplegia (without ataxia) associated with anti-GQ1b antibody. Neurology 2008;71:426–9.
64. Yu-Wai-Man P, Griffiths PG. Steroids for traumatic optic neuropathy. Cochrane Database Syst Rev 2011;1:CD006032.
65. Yu Wai Man P, Griffiths PG. Surgery for traumatic optic neuropathy. Cochrane Database Syst Rev 2005;4:CD005024.
66. Sydnor CF, Seaber JH, Buckley EG. Traumatic superior oblique palsies. Ophthalmology 1982;89:134–8.
67. Lepore FE. Disorders of ocular motility following head trauma. Arch Neurol 1995;52:924–6.

Neurologic Emergencies in Patients Who Have Cancer: Diagnosis and Management

Kelly Jo Baldwin, MD[a], Saša A. Živković, MD, PhD[b,*], Frank S. Lieberman, MD[c]

KEYWORDS

- Leptomeningeal carcinomatosis • Cerebral edema • Seizure
- Metastasis • Compressive myelopathy • Hydrocephalus
- Stroke • Paraneoplastic

The central and peripheral nervous systems can be significantly affected by cancer. Neurologic signs and symptoms are present in about 30% to 50% of oncologic patients presenting to the emergency department or in neurologic consultation at teaching hospitals.[1,2] Neurologic emergencies in patients who have cancer frequently require (neuro)surgical intervention, and prompt diagnosis and effective collaborative effort with neurosurgeons are essential to improve the outcomes. There are many neurologic emergencies that can occur from direct or indirect involvement of cancer in the brain and spinal cord, and in the peripheral nervous system. The direct effects of cancer on the central nervous system (CNS) include brain metastases, cerebral edema, seizure, spinal cord compression, hydrocephalus, and leptomeningeal carcinomatosis. Indirect complications include stroke, cerebral venous sinus thrombosis, infectious disease, and paraneoplastic encephalitis. Different modalities of cancer treatment are also associated with various neurologic complications and emergencies (**Box 1**). Such a wide spectrum of neurologic emergencies causes significant morbidity

---

The authors have nothing to disclose.

[a] Department of Neurology, University of Pittsburgh Medical Center, 337C Scaife Hall, 200 Lothrop Street, Pittsburgh, PA 15213, USA
[b] Department of Neurology, VA Pittsburgh Healthcare System, MSSL-Neurology, University of Pittsburgh Medical Center, University Drive C, 10E Room 133, Pittsburgh, PA 15240, USA
[c] Adult Neurooncology Program, Department of Neurology, Pittsburgh Cancer Institute, University of Pittsburgh Medical Center, UPMC Cancer Pavilion, Room 567, 5150 Centre Avenue, Pittsburgh, PA 15232, USA
* Corresponding author.
E-mail address: zivksx@upmc.edu

Neurol Clin 30 (2012) 101–128
doi:10.1016/j.ncl.2011.09.004
0733-8619/12/$ – see front matter Published by Elsevier Inc.

Box 1
Iatrogenic neurologic emergencies caused by treatment of cancer

Seizures caused by chemotherapeutic agents (ifosfamide, busulfan)

Cerebrovascular complications

- Intracranial hemorrhage (thrombocytopenia caused by chemotherapy)
- Cerebral venous sinus thrombosis (asparaginase)

Leukoencephalopathy (intrathecal methotrexate, etanercept)

Visual loss (vincristine, cisplatin)

Hearing loss (cisplatin)

Peripheral neuropathy (vincristine, cisplatin, bortezomib, thalidomide, paclitaxel, oxaliplatin)

Ataxia (cytarabine, cisplatin)

Aseptic meningitis (cytarabine, methotrexate)

Opportunistic CNS infections (related to immunosuppression and neurosurgical procedures)

- Viral encephalitis, bacterial and fungal meningitis
- Progressive multifocal leukoencephalopathy (PML)

Radiation necrosis

- Brain and spinal cord edema (acute)
- Radiation myelopathy and motor neuron injury (delayed)
- Radiation vasculopathy (delayed)

and mortality for patients who have cancer and requires prompt diagnostic and treatment measures. This article reviews the most common neurologic emergencies affecting patients who have cancer and discusses their epidemiology, clinical presentation, diagnosis, and treatment modalities.

BRAIN METASTASES

Brain metastases seem to be increasingly diagnosed in patients who have cancer as a result of advances in diagnostics and probably also because of improving outcomes and longer survivals. If left untreated, brain metastases typically lead to progressive neurologic deterioration. Many patients with cerebral metastases and primary brain tumors develop other neurologic complications such as cerebral edema and seizures.

Epidemiology

Epidemiologic studies documented symptomatic brain metastases in 8% to 10% of patients who have cancer.[3,4] Metastatic brain disease is overall tenfold more common than primary brain tumors.[5] Autopsy studies suggest that another third of patients with metastasis may have asymptomatic lesions. The most common malignancies to metastasize to the brain include lung (16%–19%), breast (5%), renal cell (6%–10%), melanoma (7%), and colorectal carcinoma (2%).[6] Depending on molecular and histopathology profile, different neoplasm subtypes metastasize to the brain with varying frequencies.[7] In breast cancer, HER-2 overexpression is associated with a significantly higher risk of brain metastases.[8] Lung adenocarcinoma subgroup of non–small cell lung cancer is also more likely to metastasize than other types of lung cancer.[4]

Clinical Presentation and Diagnosis

Brain metastases may present with symptoms of increased intracranial pressure, focal neurologic deficits, or they may be asymptomatic. Typically, patients present with signs and symptoms of increased intracranial pressure such as altered mental status, headache, or vomiting. They may also exhibit focal neurologic signs such as hemiparesis, aphasia, or seizures. When a patient with cancer presents with an acute neurologic decline, the initial imaging modality is usually noncontrast head computed tomography (CT), which allows for rapid diagnosis of intracranial hemorrhage, hydrocephalus, herniation syndromes, and large-vessel ischemia.[9] In a nonemergent setting, magnetic resonance imaging (MRI) of brain with and without contrast is the study of choice for evaluating possible primary brain neoplasm or metastases (**Fig. 1**).[10,11]

The results of brain MRI largely predict the next step in diagnosis and management. Although the presence of a solitary contrast-enhancing lesion may not always indicate a brain metastasis, a single contrast-enhancing lesion was reported to be a metastasis in more than 90% of patients.[11] Differential diagnosis also includes

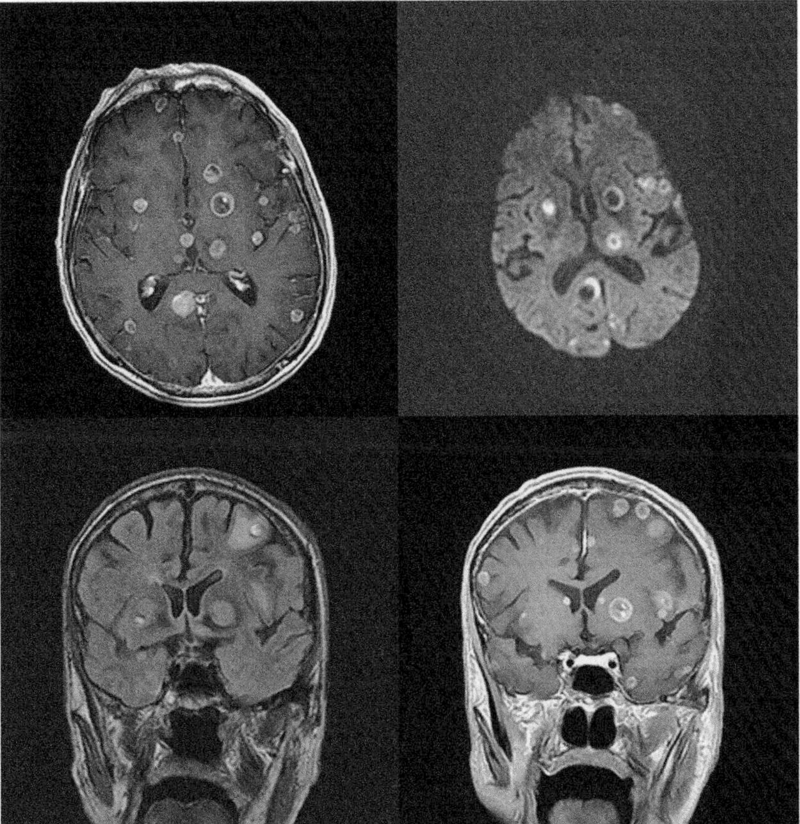

Fig. 1. Multiple brain metastases in a 73-year-old patient with adenocarcinoma of the lung (MRI of brain; *top left* and *bottom right*, contrast-enhanced axial and coronal T1-weighted images; *top right*, diffusion-weighted imaging; *bottom left*, coronal fluid-attenuated inversion recovery [FLAIR]).

abscess, granuloma, and primary brain neoplasm. In a patient with an existing primary cancer, brain biopsy may not be necessary. It has been recommended to monitor small (<1 cm) asymptomatic lesions instead of pursuing more aggressive therapy or invasive diagnostic methods.[12] In a patient with widespread metastatic disease and multiple brain lesions on MRI (see **Fig. 1**), further invasive testing is often deferred. If diagnosis remains uncertain, or when there is no primary malignancy identified, histopathologic analysis and biopsy remain the gold standard for diagnosis of intracranial lesions.[9]

Management

Treatment of brain metastases depends on location and characteristics of the metastases and the individual patient's features. Untreated brain metastases may lead to increased intracranial pressure and death within 1 to 2 months. Treatment options include surgical resection, whole-brain radiation, stereotactic radiosurgery, and chemotherapy. Treatment of brain metastases also includes symptomatic treatment of seizures and brain edema. Neurosurgical evaluation and decisions on treatment steps for metastatic brain lesions are based on number of lesions, location, and performance status.[9,13] In patients with solitary lesions in noneloquent brain regions with good performance status and known primary tumor, surgical resection possibly followed by radiation therapy is generally preferred (class I evidence).[14] If a lesion is located in an eloquent area, radiation therapy is preferred, especially for patients with poor performance status. Whole-brain radiation therapy (WBRT) is usually the treatment of choice for multifocal symptomatic brain metastases. Although treatment is often effective and relieves symptoms, the prognosis still remains poor and almost half of affected patients die from further CNS progression. In combination with WBRT, surgical resection may improve outcomes for selected patients with good functional status.[14] Chemotherapy is usually considered as adjunctive therapy in treatment of brain metastases and its routine use is not recommended.[15] Germ cell tumors and non-Hodgkin lymphoma with CNS involvement are treated with chemotherapy. In contrast, brain metastases from melanoma and renal cell carcinoma typically do not respond to chemotherapy.[9] Despite aggressive therapy for brain metastases, many patients suffer from malignant cerebral edema and seizure. Adequate diagnosis and treatment of these overlying problems is important to reduce the morbidity and improve quality of life for patients.

Cerebral Edema

Metastatic brain disease precipitates cerebral edema through several mechanisms. Metastases cause direct disruption of the blood-brain barrier. In addition, tumor cells secrete various cytokines and growth factors including vascular endothelial growth factor (VEGF), which promotes angiogenesis.[16] VEGF stimulates the creation of endothelial gaps, fragmentations, and fenestrations in the endothelium, which leads to degeneration of the basement membrane. These changes lead to leakage of fluid from the intravascular compartment to the parenchyma, and increased interstitial fluid pressure with vasogenic edema. Peritumoral edema eventually leads to signs and symptoms related to mass effect and increased intracranial pressure. Corticosteroids remain the backbone of treatment protocols for managing malignant cerebral edema, and dexamethasone is the recommended choice.[17] Overall, in most patients, low-dose dexamethasone (4 or 8 mg/d) is as effective as a higher dose (16 mg/d), which is associated with more side effects, without additional clinical benefit.[18] However, for patients with more severe symptoms, higher doses should be considered.[17] Subsequently, corticosteroids are gradually tapered off over 2 weeks or longer.[17]

Chronic steroid treatment is associated with multiple complications, including immunosuppression, increased risk of opportunistic infections, and hyperglycemia. Hyperventilation may decrease increased intracranial pressure promptly, but its effectiveness is limited by short duration of action. Hypertonic saline and mannitol may be helpful to reverse impeding cerebral herniation and decrease intracranial pressure.[19] In an emergent setting, biologic therapies are not used (yet), but their effects improve understanding of the underlying pathophysiology. Antiangiogenic therapy with VEGF tyrosine kinase inhibitor cediranib showed encouraging results, with improved vasogenic edema, reduction of steroid dosage, and better short-term outcome (lack of progression at 6 months).[20] A similar effect was also observed with bevacizumab (monoclonal antibody targeting VEGF-A) in glioblastoma multiforme.[21] At this time, antiangiogenic therapies are not a standard of care for brain edema, especially in an emergent setting.

SEIZURES

Seizures related to brain metastases and primary brain tumors are a frequent neurologic complication and may manifest as simple or complex partial seizures, generalized seizures, or even status epilepticus. Prompt diagnosis and treatment are essential to avoid morbidity associated with prolonged convulsive seizures and status epilepticus. Seizures are more common with primary brain tumors, and up to 40% of patients with brain metastases develop seizures as well. Local milieux in tumors and peritumoral tissue may also increase susceptibility to seizures.[22] Concurrent parenchymal metastases and neoplastic meningitis further increase the risk of seizures. In addition, paraneoplastic encephalitis may precipitate seizures or status epilepticus, and patients with systemic cancer without evidence of direct CNS involvement may also develop seizures.[23,24]

Epidemiology

The frequency of seizure depends on the type of primary neoplasm and the location of the tumor. Seizures can present as focal, generalized, or nonconvulsive. Glioneural tumors may also exhibit intrinsic epileptogenicity. Seizure is more common with low-grade primary brain tumors and low-grade gliomas, and oligodendroglioma are associated with seizures about 60% to 80% of the time. The higher prevalence of seizures in low-grade gliomas is probably partly related to a longer survival.[25] Low-grade gliomas also decrease seizure threshold by disrupting normal networks in cortical regions and white matter.[22] High-grade gliomas have a lower incidence of seizures (about 30% to 50%). Typically, high-grade gliomas induce seizures by abrupt tissue damage caused by necrosis, hemorrhage, or edema. Tumor location in an epileptogenic area, such as the mesial temporal lobe and insular cortex, is more likely to be associated with intractable epilepsy. Cortical tumors are more likely to result in epilepsy than subcortical tumors. Glioneural tumors occur more commonly in the temporal lobe, which may in part explain their epileptogenic potential. Seizures may also occur in patients with systemic cancer and without evidence of brain metastases or neoplastic meningitis.[23] Other causes of seizures in patients with cancer include neurotoxicity of chemotherapy and other medications (eg, busulfan, ifosfamide), ischemic and hemorrhagic strokes, opportunistic CNS infections, brain radiation injury, transient metabolic disturbances (eg, hypoglycemia), paraneoplastic disorders, and worsening of preexisting epilepsy (**Box 2**).[25]

Box 2
Causes of seizures in patients who have cancer

1. Tumor-related causes
   - Brain parenchymal metastases and primary brain tumors
   - Neoplastic meningitis
   - Paraneoplastic limbic encephalitis
2. CNS infections
   - Meningoencephalitis
   - Abscess
3. Treatment-related causes
   - Toxicity of medications
     - Chemotherapy (busulfan, ifosfamide, cisplatin)
     - Other medications (cephalosporins, imipenem)
   - Radiation necrosis
4. Cerebrovascular complications
   - Cerebral venous sinus thrombosis
   - Ischemic stroke
   - Intracranial hemorrhage (coagulopathy, thrombocytopenia)
5. Metabolic disturbances
   - Hypoglycemia/hyperglycemia
   - Hyponatremia
   - Hypocalcemia
6. Other causes
   - Posterior reversible encephalopathy syndrome
   - Worsening of preexisting epilepsy

Diagnosis and Management

Diagnosis of seizure disorder is supported by clinical history and electroencephalogram. E Electroencephalography (EEG) shows focal epileptiform changes localizing to the area of brain metastases. However, EEG may disclose electrographic seizures in the absence of a clinical equivalent or nonconvulsive status epilepticus, which can present with nonspecific impairment of alertness and may easily be missed if not clinically suspected. Treatment of tumor-associated epilepsy uses a combined approach with treatment of seizure origin (eg, resection of tumor) and symptomatic treatment with antiepileptic medications. Total tumor resection may provide relief with seizure freedom at 6 months after resection in up to 89% of patients with primary brain tumors, compared with resolution of seizures in 57% with subtotal tumor resection.[26] However, other studies report lack of correlation with completeness of tumor resection.[27] Emergent treatment of status epilepticus in patients who have cancer does not differ from standard treatment protocols,[28] but the subsequent choice of maintenance antiepileptic treatment is more complex because older-generation antiepileptics such as phenytoin, carbamazepine, and phenobarbital are enzyme inducers and interact with chemotherapy regimens. Enzyme-inducing antiepileptic medications may accelerate metabolism of corticosteroids and commonly used chemotherapeutics metabolized through the cytochrome P450 system, complicating the dosing and potentially decreasing the effectiveness of chemotherapy protocols. A recent study showed improved outcomes of patients with glioblastoma treated with chemotherapy and enzyme-inducing antiepileptic medications.[29] Newer classes of antiepileptics have less metabolic and pharmacokinetic interactions, and thus are frequently preferred in patients who have cancer. Levetiracetam does not inhibit the P450 enzyme system, it has no active metabolites, and it exhibits almost no protein binding. Other options include gabapentin, pregabalin, lamotrigine, and lacosamide. Topiramate is frequently avoided in patients who have cancer at risk of cachexia because of its appetite-suppressing properties. Side effects of levetiracetam are mild in most patients, and most commonly include somnolence, fatigue, and dizziness. However, levetiracetam may also precipitate potentially severe behavioral abnormalities requiring discontinuation in up to 7% of treated patients.[30]Up to 37% of patients report negative behavioral changes including aggression, loss of self-control, and sleep problems.[31] Up to 60% of patients with cerebral metastases remain seizure-free with antiepileptic medications,[13] and most other patients have a decrease in seizure frequency. However, routine prophylactic use of anticonvulsant medications for patients with brain tumors without a history of clinical seizure is not well established.[32] In adults with brain metastases without prior history of clinical seizures, routine prophylactic use of anticonvulsants is not recommended (class III evidence).[33] Antiepileptic treatment may be further complicated by expression of multidrug-resistance proteins in tumor cells decreasing the local concentration and effectiveness of antiseizure medications.[34]

Nonconvulsive status epilepticus (NCSE) is easily overlooked, especially in encephalopathic or comatose patients with other possible causes of altered mental status, and may be difficult to diagnose even with EEG.[35] NCSE has been described in oncologic patients with neoplastic meningitis, with primary brain tumors and brain metastases but also occurs in patients with systemic cancer in the absence of evidence of CNS metastases.[23,36,37] Seizure treatment becomes important in end-of-life care for patients with high-grade glioma because more than 50% of patients suffer from seizures during end-of-life care, with a third of patients experiencing seizures 1 week before death.[38]

ACUTE OBSTRUCTIVE HYDROCEPHALUS

Hydrocephalus and increased content of cerebrospinal fluid (CSF) occurs as a result of discrepancy between cerebrospinal production and absorption, leading to enlargement of the ventricles. Prompt evaluation and timely intervention by a neurosurgeon are essential in reducing the morbidity associated with hydrocephalus.

Epidemiology

Hydrocephalus is a frequent concern and major neurologic emergency in patients with cancer, and carries a significant morbidity. Generally, hydrocephalus is classified as either obstructive or nonobstructive. Obstructive or noncommunicating hydrocephalus results when CSF cannot freely traverse the ventricular system, commonly because of an intraventricular mass. Nonobstructive or communicating hydrocephalus is caused by impairment of CSF reabsorption. Obstructive hydrocephalus can be a result of an intraventricular tumor, such as a colloid cyst, ependymoma, intraventricular meningioma, choroid plexus papilloma, or posterior fossa tumor. In adult oncologic patients, obstructive hydrocephalus is frequently caused by bulky leptomeningeal carcinomatosis or metastases with intraventricular extension. In pediatric patients with posterior fossa tumors, hydrocephalus is common. Nonobstructive hydrocephalus in patients who have cancer is typically caused by impaired venous drainage from cerebral sinus venous thrombosis, infectious meningitis, metastatic seeding, or subarachnoid hemorrhage.

Clinical Presentation

Acute obstructive hydrocephalus develops rapidly over several hours, and reaches 80% of maximal ventricular dilatation by 6 hours. Tumors that interfere with CSF flow of the third and fourth ventricle may produce a ball-valve effect; this results in periodic increases in intracranial pressure (plateau waves of Lundberg). Symptoms largely depend on the length of time that the hydrocephalus has developed. Symptoms of rapidly occurring acute hydrocephalus include headache, double vision, transient visual obscurations, decreased mental status, ataxia, and vomiting. About 50% of patients with brain tumors complain of headache throughout their disease. Headaches related to increased intracranial pressure are classically occipital in location, worsened by Valsalva maneuver, and are often associated with nausea or vomiting.

Diagnosis and Management

Diagnosis of acute hydrocephalus should be considered in any patient who presents with altered mental status, headache, and vomiting. Fundoscopy shows papilledema, and focal neurologic signs may develop as well. Imaging by noncontrast head CT can give a rapid and accurate assessment of ventricular size. Obstructive hydrocephalus classically displays ventriculomegaly proximal to the site of obstruction with periventricular edema.

Acute hydrocephalus is a life-threatening emergency and, if quickly recognized, can be effectively treated. An emergency ventriculostomy can be performed by a neurosurgeon within minutes. Other neurosurgical options include ventricular shunting, endoscopic ventriculostomy, aqueductoplasty (for aqueductal stenosis), and septostomy (for isolated lateral hydrocephalus). In some patients, tumor debulking may be necessary to improve CSF flow, and prompt neurosurgical evaluation is necessary. A recent retrospective study showed the third ventriculostomy as a safe and effective procedure in controlling hydrocephalus related to posterior fossa tumors, which can relieve symptoms quickly in the perioperative period.[39] In cases of hydrocephalus caused by leptomeningeal carcinomatosis or metastatic seeding of the CSF, most patients are managed with radiation therapy and chemotherapy. Another option is ventriculoperitoneal shunting.[40]

SPINAL METASTASES AND COMPRESSIVE MYELOPATHY

In patients who have cancer, a new onset of back pain raises the concern of possible spinal metastases and should be promptly evaluated to avoid severe morbidity associated with untreated vertebral metastases. Timely evaluation and treatment are essential to reduce morbidity and maintain neurologic function.

Epidemiology

Spinal metastases are common and their incidence has been estimated at 5% in all patients who have cancer.[41] The vertebral column is the most common site for osseous metastasis, and, in general, the spine is the third most common location for metastasis after the liver and lungs.[42] Direct metastasis to spinal cord is rare. It is estimated that 70% of patients who die with cancer have spinal metastasis at autopsy; however, only 14% of these have clinically apparent disease. Up to 20% of patients presenting with spinal metastases do not have prior diagnosis of cancer.[43] The most common types of tumor to have spinal involvement include prostate, breast, and lung, followed by lymphoma, renal cell carcinoma, and multiple myeloma. Most commonly, spinal metastases involve the thoracic spine (70%), then lumbar (20%), followed by cervical spine (10%).[41] In addition, lung and breast carcinoma more commonly metastasize to thoracic spine, whereas colon and pelvic neoplasm usually involve lumbosacral spine. Spinal involvement of systemic cancer typically arises by 2 mechanisms: hematogenous spread or direct extension. The seeding of tumor cells via hematogenous spread occurs via the Baston venous plexus to the vertebral column. Malignant invasion of the vertebral bodies is destructive and invariably leads to vertebral collapse. Less commonly, paravertebral malignancy can directly invade the spinal canal by destroying the vertebral body or by entrance through the vertebral foramen. Parenchymal metastases to spinal cord are rare. Regardless of the route of spinal entry, epidural spinal compression becomes the ultimate neurologic emergency. Epidural spinal cord compression affects 5% of all patients who have cancer. It is imperative to recognize the signs and symptoms of spinal cord compression, because early treatment can significantly improve morbidity and mortality. If spinal cord compression is not promptly treated, the patient will suffer cord edema followed by white matter ischemia and irreversible cord infarction.[44]

Clinical Presentation

Pain is the most common presenting symptom in patients with spinal metastasis and may be further characterized as progressive and unrelenting, worsened when laying flat, thoracic predominance, with direct tenderness to palpation.[45] The most important management principle is the necessity to carefully evaluate any new complaint of back pain in a patient with cancer. Mechanical back pain may represent spinal instability and impending collapse, as well as acute-on-chronic pain from compression fractures.[44] Radicular symptoms may also be present, and this symptom in a patient with known cancer demands expeditious evaluation to determine the cause. Although pain generally precedes neurologic symptoms, many patients go undiagnosed until weakness ensues. About 70% of patients have bilateral lower extremity weakness by the time of diagnosis. Sensory symptoms and bowel or bladder dysfunction are also common, but frequently occur late in the course.[1]

Diagnosis

Diagnosis begins with an accurate history and physical examination. New onset of back pain or focal neurologic symptoms in a patient with diagnosed malignancy should be further evaluated with imaging. MRI of the entire spine remains the most sensitive and specific imaging modality for diagnosis of spinal metastasis (with reported 93% sensitivity and 97% specificity) (**Fig. 2**).[1] This imaging modality is also useful for planning of radiotherapy and surgical resection. A radiologic study of 57 patients with cancer compared use of T1-weighted MRI alone versus combined T1-weighted and T2-weighted imaging for presence of vertebral metastasis, epidural metastasis, and spinal cord compression. The study found that, if used alone, T1-weighted sagittal MRI of the spine failed to detect 13% of the vertebral metastases that were detectable with comprehensive imaging protocol.[46] In most patients with a known primary malignancy, diagnosis of spinal metastasis is based on imaging and does not require biopsy. If MRI is not obtainable (eg, pacemaker), CT myelography may provide diagnostically useful information. In patients without a previous

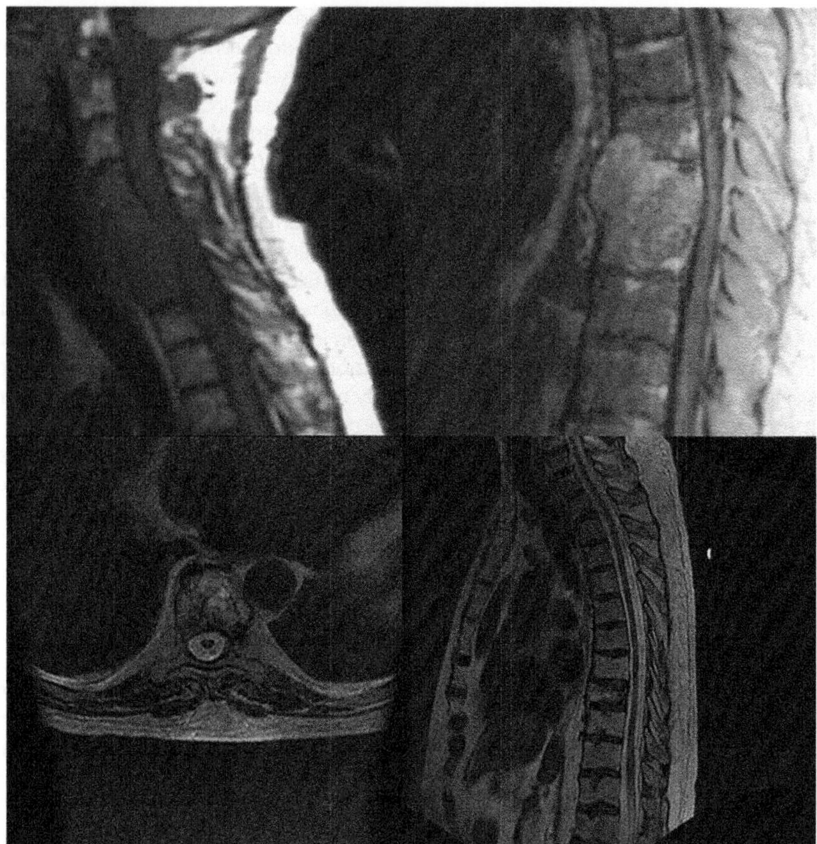

Fig. 2. Vertebral metastases and epidural compressive myelopathy. *Top left*, epidural metastasis from renal cell carcinoma with cervical spinal cord compression in 64-year-old man on MRI, T1-weighted image; *top right*, epidural thoracic spine metastasis from breast adenocarcinoma with thoracic spinal cord compression in 61-year-old woman on MRI, T1-weighted image; *bottom*, vertebral metastasis associated with thyroid carcinoma in 52-year-old woman on MRI, T2-weighted images. (*Courtesy of* Dr P Gerszten. University of Pittsburgh and Pittsburgh Cancer Institute, Pittsburgh, PA.)

diagnosis of cancer, further work-up, including whole-body imaging, is required to identify potential primary tumor, and the optimal site to biopsy for diagnosis.[47]

Management

Treatment of spinal metastases is mostly palliative and is based on preservation of neurologic function.[48] Treatment options consist of corticosteroids, radiation therapy, chemotherapy, surgical decompression, and emerging minimally invasive interventions.[47] Epidural spinal metastatic disease with compressive myelopathy is a neurologic emergency in which early recognition and intervention determines whether neurologic catastrophe would follow. The most important predictor of outcome in epidural cord compression from metastatic disease is the severity of deficit when the treatment is instituted. It is incumbent on the physician to recognize the warning sign, expeditiously obtain definitive imaging, and institute treatment. Indications to proceed with surgical decompression include acute cord compression, spinal instability, and unrelenting pain from pathologic fractures. Following onset of compressive myelopathy, rapid progression is common, and 30% of patients with weakness progress to paraplegia within 1 week. Functional recovery is unlikely if paraplegia is present for more than 24 hours.

Corticosteroids are the initial symptomatic treatment of epidural spinal cord compression. Mechanism of action is thought to involve reduction of vasogenic edema, stabilization of membranes, and decreased local inflammation. In specific tumor types such as multiple myeloma, prostate cancer, and lymphoma, there is also a direct tumorlytic effect. Multiple randomized controlled trails of high-dose intravenous steroids before radiotherapy show improvement in patient ambulation at 6 months. Dosing for dexamethasone typically starts with a 100-mg intravenous loading dose followed by 96 mg orally daily for 3 days, then rapid taper is instituted.[49] Surgery is the optimal therapy for appropriately selected patients (class I evidence). The first decision step is neurosurgical evaluation. Patients with radiosensitive tumors, minimal signs or symptoms, or limited functional status or limited survival are exceptions to this general rule.

A landmark study by Patchell and colleagues[50] in 2005 analyzed treatment outcomes in 101 patients with epidural spinal cord compression restricted to a single area and at least 1 neurologic symptom or sign. Half of the study participants (50/101) were treated with decompressive surgery followed by radiotherapy, and the remaining 51 participants were treated with radiotherapy alone. The surgical group showed improved survival, longer time with neurologic improvement, continence, and ambulatory status.[50] However, this study excluded the patients with radiosensitive tumors. Minimally invasive procedures, including vertebroplasty and kyphoplasty for malignant compression fractures, may provide significant pain relief in more than 80% of treated patients.[51] A prospective trial with 139 male veteran participants with initial spinal epidural metastases showed that treatment with glucocorticoid therapy and radiotherapy was as likely to maintain ability to walk as combined surgical decompression of the spinal cord with radiotherapy and glucocorticoid therapy.[52] This population was largely limited to prostate cancer (55%) or lung cancer (37%).

As with surgery, the primary goal of radiation therapy is to protect neurologic function and decrease pain. Lymphoma and primary germ cell tumors are most radiosensitive. Breast, prostate, and lung cancer are considered intermediately sensitive. Melanoma, osteosarcoma, and renal cell carcinoma are generally radioresistant.[53] The seminal study that showed efficacy of radiation therapy showed pain relief in 71% of patients and 76% preserved or regained ambulatory status.[54] About 36% to 40% of paraparetic patients and 13% to 15% of paralyzed patients become ambulatory after radiation.[55] Radiation treatment typically targets 1 to 2 vertebral bodies above and below the site, and the standard therapy consists of 30 Gy divided in 10 fractions.

Chemotherapy has a limited role in selected responsive tumors without malignant compression, but, even with careful selection, response to chemotherapy remains unpredictable and slow. These tumors include Hodgkin and non-Hodgkin lymphoma, germ cell tumors, breast or prostate, or neuroblastoma.

LEPTOMENINGEAL CARCINOMATOSIS/LYMPHOMATOSIS

Leptomeningeal carcinomatosis/lymphomatosis (LMC) or lymphomatous/carcinomatous meningitis is defined as malignant seeding or infiltration of the leptomeninges. In patients with leukemias, the term leukemic meningitis is frequently used.

Epidemiology

Leptomeningeal progression is most common with hematologic malignancies (5%–15% of patients), followed by solid tumors (1%–5%) and primary brain tumors (1%–2%).[56] Autopsy studies revealed that up to 19% of patients who have cancer with neurologic symptoms may also have leptomeningeal disease.[57] Malignant cells gain access to the subarachnoid space by 2 mechanisms: direct extension and hematogenous dissemination.[58,59] Direct extension mainly occurs in primary intracranial neoplasm and metastases from solid tumors. Primary intracranial tumors such as medulloblastoma, ependymoma, choroid plexus carcinoma, primary CNS lymphoma, and malignant cerebellar astrocytoma are particularly prone to LMC. Metastatic brain tumors and cancers of the head and neck can also directly invade the CSF by making direct contact with the meninges and disrupting the subarachnoid and ventricular spaces.[59]

Clinical Presentation

Signs and symptoms affecting multiple areas of the neuraxis simultaneously are typical of leptomeningeal carcinomatosis. Symptoms occur because of the involvement of the brain hemispheres, brainstem and cranial nerves, and spinal cord and roots.[59] The most common neurologic signs include a triad of symptoms that suggest brain hemisphere disturbance (eg, headache and encephalopathy), multiple cranial nerve deficits (eg, diplopia), and spinal root involvement (eg, weakness and pain following radicular distribution).[59] Cranial nerve signs also include trigeminal neuropathy, facial weakness, and hearing loss, and some patients may also manifest meningeal signs including nuchal rigidity. Leptomeningeal carcinomatosis may precipitate obstructive hydrocephalus, particularly with bulky disease of the CNS. Radionucleotide scans reveal limitation of CSF flow in about 70% of patients with LMC.

Diagnosis

Diagnosis of LMC is made by clinical examination, CSF analysis, and radiologic data. Repeated lumbar punctures may be needed, and opening pressure, protein and glucose content, cell count, and cytology should be routinely evaluated. Common findings include increased protein (75%), increased opening pressure (50%), leukocytosis (64%), and low glucose (40%).[59] Flow cytometry improves the sensitivity of diagnosis for leukemic meningitis. The sensitivity of a single large-volume lumbar puncture is 38% to 66%, and performing 3 large-volume lumbar punctures increases the sensitivity to 90%.[57] Gadolinium-enhanced MRI has replaced CT as the imaging modality of choice for diagnosing LMC. The sensitivity of nonenhanced MRI in identifying patients with LMC is about 70%. However, because these MRI findings are not specific for LMC, imaging alone should not be used to establish the diagnosis. Typical imaging features of LMC include contrast enhancement of the meninges, cortical convexities, basilar cistern, and cauda equina.[60] Meningeal biopsy of contrast-enhancing lesions remains the gold standard for definite diagnosis of leptomeningeal carcinomatosis/lymphomatosis.[59]

Management

The primary goal of early diagnosis and treatment is to stabilize, and possibly improve, neurologic symptoms. Without treatment, overall survival is typically 4 to 6 weeks secondary to neurologic decline. With aggressive treatment, survival generally improves by 1 to 3 months, but there are only a few reported cases of long-term survivors. Treatment of LMC includes focal radiotherapy for bulky disease, local chemotherapy, and systemic chemotherapy. Combination treatment strategies with radiotherapy and chemotherapy may be necessary when managing bulky disease with compromised flow of CSF. Intrathecal chemotherapy showed clinical improvement or stabilization in 50% of patients, with median survival of 5.8 months after diagnosis, but the poor long-term prognosis remained unchanged.[61]

ISCHEMIC STROKE AND INTRACRANIAL HEMORRHAGE

Ischemic stroke and intracranial hemorrhages are major sources of morbidity and mortality in patients who have cancer. In addition to typical risk factors for stroke, direct and indirect effects of neoplasm and side effects of treatment must be considered.

Epidemiology

Neoplastic diseases increase the risk of ischemic and hemorrhagic stroke compared with the general population. Large autopsy studies indicate that up to 15% of patients who have cancer have evidence of prior ischemic infarcts, and only half of these patients had symptomatic lesions at some point during their illness.[62] Conversely, in a large retrospective study of 1274 patients who presented with stroke, 12% of patients had a secondary diagnosis of cancer. In that study, 86% of strokes were ischemic and the remaining 14% were hemorrhagic.[63] In another retrospective study of patients who had cancer with acute stroke, 30% had lung cancer, 9% primary brain tumors, 9% prostate, and 6% each of breast, hematologic, gynecologic, and gastrointestinal neoplasms.[64] In addition to the usual stroke risk factors (eg, hypertension, hypercholesterolemia), there are multiple other direct and indirect mechanisms that lead to an increased risk of stroke in patients who have cancer. These mechanisms can be divided into direct tumor effect, coagulopathies, and consequences of therapy.[65] Typical stroke risk factors such as hypertension, hyperlipidemia, and tobacco use do not seem to be significantly different in patients with stroke who have cancer versus patients with stroke who do not have cancer.[66] The frequency of intratumoral cranial hemorrhages varies among different cancer types, and more frequent occurrences were reported with melanoma metastases and glial and germ cell primary brain tumors. Intracranial hemorrhage related to tumor must be distinguished from other causes, including hypertension, cerebral aneurysms, and arteriovenous vascular malformations.

Direct Tumor Effects

Tumors can also damage the cerebral vasculature directly. For example, primary brain neoplasms can directly compress or invade surrounding vessels. Cardiac and pulmonary tumors, such as atrial myxomas, can also directly cause stroke by embolizing to the large intracranial vessels. Hematologic malignancies can also directly cause stroke via hyperviscosity associated with polycythemia vera and hyperleukocytosis from acute leukemia, which may impair cerebral perfusion, resulting in ischemia. Hyperleukocytosis can also manifest as altered mental status, seizure, and sudden death. There is a fourfold increase in the incidence of stroke in hyperleukocytosis (>100,000) compared with patients with normal white blood cell counts. Fatal intracranial hemorrhage occurs in more than 5% of patients with acute leukemias, especially acute myelogenous leukemia (AML).[67] Cerebrovascular complications are less common with lymphomas than with leukemias. Primary intravascular neoplasms such as intravascular lymphomatosis have a predilection for cerebral vessels and can cause cerebral infarction.

Coagulopathies

More common than cancer directly causing a stroke are the indirect effects of malignancy on the coagulation pathways. In general, solid tumors are more associated with venous thrombosis and hematologic malignancies with bleeding diathesis. Two distinct mechanisms have been proposed: disseminated intravascular coagulation (DIC) and nonbacterial thrombotic endocarditis. In DIC, there is a disruption in balance of thrombus formation and thrombolysis, resulting in microthrombi formation in small vessels, and thrombocytopenia causing hemorrhage in other areas. DIC is more common in hematologic malignancies than in primary solid tumors. DIC is diagnosed in approximately 15% of patients with acute leukemia, and bleeding manifestations prevail rather than thrombosis.[68] Nonbacterial thrombotic endocarditis (NBTE) can occur in association with DIC, which may predispose cardiac valves to edema and degeneration. Subsequently, platelets and thrombin are deposited on the valves. Embolic strokes from NBTE are one of the most common mechanisms for stroke in patients who have cancer.[65] Autopsy studies find that up to 27% of strokes in patients who have cancer may be related to NBTE.[62] This condition seems to be more common in patients with mucin-producing adenocarcinoma of the lung and gastrointestinal tract, pancreatic adenocarcinoma, and lymphoma. However, other studies reported conflicting results, suggesting that only 1% to 3% of patients with stroke who have cancer are a result of NBTE.[63,64] Such discrepancies with autopsy studies may be attributable to diagnostic difficulties when clinicians try to establish diagnosis of NBTE with certainty.[64]

There have been several other proposed mechanisms to explain a relative prothrombotic state in patients who have cancer that predispose them to cerebral infarction. It is well established that many patient have increased D-dimer levels, protein S and C deficiency, activated protein C resistance, antiphospholipid antibodies, hyperfibrinogenemia, thrombocytosis, and a general state of inflammation. The exact mechanism for a hypercoagulable state in most patients who have cancer is poorly understood. Transcranial Doppler has been used to monitor the risk of embolic strokes in patients who have cancer, and embolic signal was observed in patients with ischemic stroke who have cancer, particularly in those without conventional stroke risk factors.[69] This study also found that increased D-dimer levels were independently correlated with embolic signal, which greatly decreased with anticoagulation.[69]

Treatment Effects

Cancer treatment protocols using techniques such as cranial/neck radiation and chemotherapy can also predispose patients to stroke. Postradiation vasculopathy can damage the intracranial and extracranial vessels and lead to stroke. Typically, this affects the large vessels of the head and neck, leading to stenosis at about 3 to 5 years after radiation therapy.[70] Studies indicate that 12% to 60% of patients with a history of neck radiation develop internal carotid artery stenosis.[71] A recent study of risk factors in carotid stenosis showed that a history of radiation alone was comparable with having a history of hypertension, hyperlipidemia, diabetes, or coronary artery disease. Radiation-associated carotid stenosis was associated with lesions that were much longer, at atypical sites, and had more aggressive plaques. Because of the unusual and long segments of artery involved, this study suggested the use of carotid stenting rather than carotid endarterectomy in the prevention of ischemic infarction.[71] This recommendation was supported in another study comparing patients with stenosis from radiation versus no radiation for durability of carotid angioplasty and stenting. This study found that freedom from restenosis did not differ significantly between the 2 groups.[72] Prior history of brain irradiation increases the risk of ipsilateral stroke and is reported in up to 25% of patients with stroke who have cancer.[73] Increased risk of stroke was also reported with chemotherapy protocols with cisplatin.[74] Other chemotherapeutic agents that have been reported to cause cerebrovascular events include intrathecal methotrexate, L-asparaginase, and intra-arterial chemotherapy regimens.

Diagnosis and Recommendations

Diagnosis of stroke is made by clinical examination and imaging of the brain parenchyma and the intracranial and extracranial arteries. In the acute setting with a convincing clinical history and examination, CT head and CT angiogram may be more accessible to establish the diagnosis in a timely manner. MRI of the brain with diffusion-weighted imaging sequences is another option for diagnosing acute stroke, and is helpful in evaluation of suspected brain metastases or leptomeningeal carcinomatosis. In the acute setting, without known brain metastases, a patient who has cancer may be a candidate for intravenous thrombolysis. However, clinic trials of stroke treatment in patients who have cancer are lacking. Recent small case series reported successful treatment of stroke in 3 patients who had cancer with intravenous tissue plasminogen activator.[75] However, thrombolytic therapy may also precipitate intratumoral bleeding.[76] Standard anticoagulation may not prevent recurrent strokes in some patients with possible hypercoagulable states.[77] Standard evaluation of patients with stroke should include echocardiogram (at least transthoracic) to investigate possible intracardiac thrombus, tumor, or vegetation. Although there are several proposed mechanisms of hypercoagulability, there are still no established guidelines for when to perform comprehensive laboratory analysis of hypercoagulable state. Although not established by class I evidence, clinical experience suggests that secondary stroke prevention in a patient with NBTE should use low-molecular-weight heparinoids rather than warfarin or antiplatelet agents.

Cerebral Venous Sinus Thrombosis

Cerebral venous sinus thrombosis (CVST) in patients who have cancer can be caused by direct compression from primary brain malignancies or from secondary hypercoagulability. Other risk factors include dehydration and infections. The most common malignancy associated with CVST is acute lymphoblastic leukemia. CVST can progress to both ischemic and hemorrhagic venous infarctions with an atypical anatomic distribution, different than with arterial strokes. Clinical features of headache, altered consciousness, focal neurologic deficit, and seizure are frequent with CVST. Conventional brain imaging alone is of little diagnostic value in CVST, because it usually shows nonspecific lesions, such as hemorrhage, infarct, or edema, and is normal in up to 25% of cases. Prompt diagnosis should be made by pursuing detailed imaging of the venous vascular system. The 2 most common imaging modalities to evaluate CVST remain CT venogram and magnetic resonance (MR) venogram, whereas conventional angiograms are now infrequently used. The main limitation of these imaging techniques is their inability to differentiate thrombosis and hypoplasia, a frequent diagnostic dilemma for the lateral venous sinuses. MRI sequence with T2 susceptibility-weighted imaging may be of additional diagnostic value in evaluation of CVST, particularly during the acute phase of CVST when the sensitivity of the other sequences is incomplete, and may reveal isolated cortical venous thrombosis.[78]

Treatment of CVST includes supportive or symptomatic measures such as hydration, appropriate antimicrobials, control of seizures with anticonvulsants, and control of intracranial pressure with neurosurgical procedures. Antithrombotic treatments include unfractionated and low-molecular-weight heparin, oral anticoagulants, thrombolysis, and endovascular approaches. A randomized double-blind placebo-controlled trial showed safety and effectiveness with the use of heparin in the treatment of CVST, and showed that limited intracerebral hemorrhage is not a definitive contraindication for anticoagulation.[79] A randomized, placebo-controlled trial of subcutaneous low-weight-molecular heparin in adults showed a trend for better outcome in the treated group.[80] Therefore, subcutaneous (low-molecular-weight) and intravenous (unfractionated) heparin are commonly considered as a first-line treatment of CVST, even in the presence of hemorrhagic infarction. If the patient deteriorates despite supportive care and heparin treatment, selective catheter-guided local thrombolysis may be an option, if available.[81] Randomized trials investigating interventional techniques for CVST in patients with or without cancer are needed, and there is still no consensus on available treatment options, although anticoagulation is generally considered as a safe treatment with potential reduction of mortality and morbidity.[82] Despite treatment, mortality from CVST remains at 8%, and patients with underlying malignancy may have worse outcomes.[83,84]

CNS INFECTIONS

Infections involving the CNS cause significant morbidity and mortality in patients with cancer, and their manifestations may mimic cancer recurrence, treatment-related toxicities, and paraneoplastic encephalitis. In addition, cancer treatment and neurosurgical procedures increase the risk of CNS infections, and careful and timely evaluation and treatment are needed to reduce associated morbidity and mortality.

Epidemiology

It has been estimated that 16% of CNS infections may occur in patients with an underlying CNS malignancy.[85] The risk of opportunistic CNS infection is determined by the extent of immunosuppression and intensity of exposure to infectious agents. There are several participating mechanisms proposed to explain the pathophysiology of infection in patients with cancer, including neutrophil disruption and bone marrow suppression, which are common in patients with lymphoma and leukemia. Iatrogenic factors contributing to blood-brain barrier disruption include central lines and CNS ports or reservoirs, and neurosurgical procedures can also predispose patients who have cancer to CNS infection.[86] Immunosuppression may also occur with lymphocyte and immunoglobulin dysfunction in chronic lymphocytic leukemia, multiple myeloma, or patients with splenectomy. Impaired T cell function is significantly affected by chemotherapy and corticosteroids and increases the risk of infection. Each of these mechanisms impairs patients' ability to protect themselves from common infections, and puts them at risk for developing opportunistic infections. Overall risk of CNS infections is mostly determined by the extent of immunologic compromise and intensity of (environmental) exposure to specific pathogens. Meningitis, encephalitis, brain abscesses, and catheter-related or shunt-related infections are the most common neurologic infections in patients who have cancer.[87] Neurosurgical procedures are associated with an increased risk of CNS infections, and prior neurosurgical procedures were reported in 78% of patients who have cancer with bacterial or fungal meningitis.[86] Meningitis associated with external ventricular shunts typically present within a month from surgery.[88]

CNS infections in patients who have cancer are caused by a wide array of bacterial, viral, and fungal pathogens, and infections with multiple pathogens (simultaneous or sequential) are common.[85–87]

Diagnosis

There are several diagnostic challenges in diagnosing patients who have cancer with CNS infections. Many patients do not display the characteristic signs and symptoms for meningitis, such as fever, nuchal rigidity, or headache because of their diminished immune response. Coexisting conditions such as encephalopathy, metabolic derangements, CNS involvement of cancer, seizures, aseptic meningitis, and treatment side effects may also precipitate new symptoms mimicking a CNS infection. Diagnostic procedures such as lumbar puncture may be dangerous to complete because of thrombocytopenia or coagulopathies. Both typical and atypical infectious agents may not have typical presentations in an immunocompromised patient. Diagnosis of CNS infection is made by clinical history, laboratory studies (including CSF analysis), and imaging. Subacute presentation may be more suggestive of a fungal process, whereas an acute meningoencephalitis would suggest a more probable bacterial or viral cause. A focal neurologic deficit typically involves a bacterial or fungal abscess, whereas diffuse encephalitis is more likely to be viral.[87]

CSF analysis obtained via lumbar puncture is helpful in identifying the causative organism. The classic CSF abnormalities in bacterial meningitis include increased opening pressure, polymorphonuclear leukocytosis of more than 100 cells/mm^3, glucose less than 40 mg/dL or less than 30% of serum glucose, and protein greater than 45 mg/dL. CSF Gram stain and culture should also be obtained. CSF findings may be deceiving with catheter-associated ventriculitis because up to 22% of patients may have normal cell counts with positive cultures.[89] In viral meningitis, opening pressure is normal, and there is lymphocytic pleocytosis, with normal glucose, and normal or slightly increased protein content. There is also a growing number of new diagnostic tests using immunology and molecular diagnostics to rapidly identify specific pathogens that may be difficult to culture. Molecular diagnostic testing using polymerase chain reaction analysis is more widely available for herpes viruses 1, 2, and 6, cytomegalovirus, Epstein-Barr virus, varicella zoster virus, John Cunningham (JC) virus, and enteroviruses. Additional testing for emerging infectious agents is available through research and commercial laboratories. Neuroimaging studies, including CT or MRI brain, may be helpful in identifying ring-enhancing or discrete focal lesions concerning for abscess or metastases, but are usually not sufficient to distinguish CNS infections from their mimics. Definitive diagnosis for solitary brain lesions is provided by histopathologic analysis of specimens obtained by image-guided or open biopsy. Clinicians must maintain a high index of suspicion for CNS infection in any patient with an underlying malignancy who presents with new onset of focal or nonlocalizing neurologic signs or symptoms.

Management

Early in the course, before cause has been established, broad-spectrum empiric treatment is started. Empiric therapy for community-acquired bacterial meningitis includes dexamethasone, a third-generation or fourth-generation cephalosporin, and vancomycin.[90] Ampicillin is added to the empiric regimen for coverage of *Listeria monocytogenes* in an individual with impaired cell-mediated immunity, and metronidazole is added in individuals with the predisposing conditions of otitis, mastoiditis, and sinusitis, and also in neurosurgical patients, especially those with ventriculostomies. Adjunctive dexamethasone improves the prognosis of pneumococcal meningitis (class III evidence).[91] Amphotericin B and flucytosine are used in the treatment of infections caused by *Cryptococcus neoformans* and *Aspergillus*, and other antifungal treatment options include voriconazole, itraconazole, and ketoconazole. Treatment options for viral infections are largely limited to acyclovir (for herpes simplex virus [HSV] and varicella zoster virus infections) and ganciclovir (cytomegalovirus and human herpesvirus 6). Less commonly, foscarnet and cidofovir are used. It is imperative to use a targeted therapy as soon as the causative organism is identified.

PARANEOPLASTIC LIMBIC ENCEPHALITIS

Once considered a rare syndrome, paraneoplastic limbic encephalitis is now recognized as a diverse, clinically and immunobiologically heterogeneous group of disorders with relevance to the differential diagnosis of acute neurologic, psychiatric, autonomic, and epileptic disorders (**Table 1**).[92] Early description of cases of limbic encephalitis (LE) showed frequent association of increased titers of anti-Hu antibodies in serum and CSF and the presence of small cell lung carcinoma (SCLC).[93] Subsequently, a different antibody was described in patients with testicular cancer. In a series of 13 patients with testicular cancer and LE, 10 of them had increased titers of antibodies targeting another onconeural antigen named Ma-2.[94] Less commonly, LE has been described in patients with other types of cancer and with other paraneoplastic antibodies including Ta, Tr, CV-2/CRMP-5, and Ri antibodies.[95–97] In addition to paraneoplastic syndromes associated with solid tumors, LE has also been described in patients with Hodgkin and non-Hodgkin lymphoma.[98,99] More recently, additional variants of paraneoplastic LE have been described and characterized by the presence of increased autoantibody titers in serum and CSF of autoantibodies directed against synaptic proteins, including the *N*-methyl-D-aspartate receptor (NMDAR), 2-amino-3-(5-methyl-3-oxazol-4-yl) propanoic acid receptor (AMPAR), γ-aminobutyric acid-B receptor (GABAbR), leucine-rich glioma-inactivated (LGi-1) protein, contactin-associated protein 2 (CASPR-2), and voltage-gated potassium channel (VGKC); these define LE variants that are distinct from anti-Hu–associated LE.[100]

A spectrum of autoantibody-associated variants of LE continues to evolve and, in many cases, eradication of the underlying neoplasm may produce strong recovery (for the paraneoplastic forms). There is also increasing evidence that immunotherapy may be effective in specific clinical settings.[100,101]

Epidemiology

There are no reliable epidemiologic estimates of LE frequency, but it is probably underdiagnosed. In the PNS Euronetwork Database, LE has been reported in 10% of patients with paraneoplastic neurologic syndromes (PNS).[102] If this is extrapolated to the estimate of prevalence of paraneoplastic disorders at 3%,[103] it may be that 0.3% of patients who have cancer may develop paraneoplastic LE. However, reports in the literature are not as numerous. A recent review by Dalmau and colleagues[100] suggests that recently described anti-NMDAR-LE (133 cases reported per year) may be more common than anti-Hu (15 cases/y) and anti–voltage-gated potassium channel antibody encephalitides (83 cases/y).

Most patients with NMDAR-LE are women (80%), usually younger than 40 years, and tumors are rare in patients younger than 7 years or older than 40 years. Only 5% of affected men older than 18 years have an underlying neoplasm.[100] Typically, AMPAR-LE has been described in middle-aged women.[104,105]

Table 1
Paraneoplastic limbic encephalitides

Antigen	% Women; Median Age (y)	Most Common Tumor Types	Typical Symptoms	Other Paraneoplastic and Autoimmune Syndromes
Hu/Anna-1	25; 63	SCLC (NSCLC, neuroendocrine tumor, ovarian dysgerminoma)	Memory loss, confusion, seizures	Sensory neuropathy, cerebellar ataxia
Ma-2	32; 64	Testicular Ca (NSCLC, lymphoma	Memory loss, confusion, seizures	Brainstem and diencephalic encephalopathy
Tr/PCA-Tr	Rare	Hodgkin lymphoma	—	Cerebellar degeneration
Ri	Rare	Breast Ca	—	Brainstem encephalitis, opsoclonus myoclonus,
CV-2/CRMP-5	24; mean 63	SCLC (thymoma, breast Ca)	Memory loss, confusion, seizures	Neuropathy, cerebellar ataxia, chorea, dysautonomia
NMDAR	80–90; 23	Ovarian teratoma (lymphoma, neuroblastoma, breast Ca)	Psychiatric symptoms, abnormal movements	—
AMPAR	90; 60	Thymoma (breast Ca, SCLC, NSCLC)	Psychiatric symptoms, memory loss, confusion, seizures	Stiff-person syndrome
GABAbR	47; 62	SCLC[a]	Seizures, memory loss, confusion	—
CASPR-2	Rare	(Thymoma)[b]	—	Neuromyotonia, myasthenia
LGi-1	35; 60	Thyroid Ca, renal cell Ca, NSCLC, ovarian teratoma[c]	Memory loss, myoclonus, seizures	—

Abbreviations: Ca, carcinoma; NSCLC, non–small cell lung carcinoma; SCLC, small cell lung carcinoma.
[a] Tumor reported in 40% of cases.
[b] Most reported cases of LE were nonparaneoplastic.
[c] Tumors present in 11% to 20% of cases.
Data from Refs.[93,97,100,104,109,110,116]

Clinical Presentation

The first clinical and immunobiologic variant of LE associated with anti-Hu antibodies was described in the early 1990s.[93,106] The clinical presentation of LE may be mistaken for HSV encephalitis, with symptoms of memory disturbance, agitation, and seizures. Variants of LE have been defined by the presence of specific autoantibodies, and some patients may simultaneously have increased titers of several paraneoplastic antibodies. LE associated with anti-Hu antibodies may present as an isolated neurologic syndrome or in the context of a more widespread neurologic syndrome with involvement of cerebellum, brainstem, and spinal cord (paraneoplastic encephalomyelitis).[93] Paraneoplastic encephalomyelitis is less common in the absence of anti-Hu antibodies. Depression, anxiety, and hallucinations have been reported in patients with anti-Hu-associated LE, but these symptoms are not as prominent as with LE associated with anti-NMDAR antibodies.[107]

Patients with the anti-NMDAR variant of LE commonly present with rapidly developing psychiatric symptoms including anxiety, insomnia, fear, grandiose delusions, hyperreligiousity, mania, and paranoia.[108] Other symptoms may include alterations of consciousness (even coma), abnormal movements (especially dyskinesias), seizures, and autonomic instability. Central hypoventilation may occur when consciousness is still preserved. Generalized or complex partial seizures typically develop at an early stage.

The initial differential diagnosis in early stages mimics primary psychiatric disorders. In later stages, possible viral encephalitis, neuroleptic malignant syndrome, and the other forms of LE are the important differential diagnostic considerations.

Anti-AMPAR-LE also presents with acute limbic dysfunction, and is frequently associated with prominent psychiatric symptoms.[104] Most patients described so far have been middle-aged women, but the number of described cases with this variant of LE is small and the spectrum of clinical presentations continues to evolve.[105] About 70% of these patients have an underlying tumor of the lung, breast, or thymus. More frequently than with anti-NMDA-LE, other autoimmune disorders are also present, including diabetes, stiff-person syndrome, and hypothyroidism, as well as Raynaud syndrome.

Anti-GABAb LE involves both sexes equally, with the median age being 62 years.[109] Other autoantibodies may be present concomitantly, including anti-GAD antibodies. In about 40% to 50% of these patients, an SCLC or neuroendocrine cancer of the lung is found.

A lower occurrence of tumors has also been reported for 2 other LE syndromes previously ascribed to anti-VGKC that are now shown to be associated with antibodies targeting other specific synaptic function modulating proteins: anti-LGi1 and anti-CASPR-2. In anti-LGi-1 LE, memory disorder, confusion, and seizures dominate the clinical presentation.[110,111] Short tonic seizures and rapid eye movement sleep behavior disorders, as well as hyponatremia, have been reported. Only 11% to 20% of patients have an underlying tumor, usually thymoma or SCLC. Mutations of LGi-1 have been associated with autosomal dominant lateral temporal lobe epilepsy.[112] In anti-CASPR-2 LE, encephalitis and peripheral nerve hyperexcitability are usually present.[113] Some patients concurrently suffer myasthenia gravis with either anti-acetylcholine receptor or MuSK antibodies, and increased titers of anti-CASPR-2 antibodies have been described in patients with thymoma.[114] Some patients have presented with predominantly peripheral neuromuscular symptoms prompting the differential diagnosis of variant forms of motor neuron disease.

Diagnosis and Management

Compared with other paraneoplastic syndromes, LE may be one of the more treatable paraneoplastic disorders. Removal of the underlying neoplasm is usually more effective than immunosuppression. LE associated with anti-Ma2 antibodies seems to have a better prognosis with orchiectomy and aggressive treatment of residual disease, and patients with NMDAR-LE may improve with removal of teratoma.

Diagnosis of specific variants of LE is based on finding increased titers of specific autoantibodies in the serum and CSF. Additional testing should include investigations of possible mimics of paraneoplastic LE (especially CNS infections), and neuroimaging studies and EEG should be considered as well.

In NMDAR-LE, neuroimaging findings are usually nonspecific, and MRI may be normal in up to 50% of cases.[100] Functional neuroimaging with MR spectroscopy, PET, and single-photon emission computed tomography may show fluctuating multifocal abnormalities involving cortical and subcortical structures that may change during the course of the disease. EEGs are usually abnormal, and EEG may reveal underlying NCSE. However, most often EEG shows only nonspecific slowing.

As with other paraneoplastic disorders, CSF analysis in paraneoplastic LE is usually abnormal with mild lymphocytic pleocytosis, normal or mildly increased protein, and CSF-specific oligoclonal bands being found in approximately 60% of patients.[100,115] Most patients with NMDAR-LE have evidence of intrathecal synthesis of anti-NMDAR antibodies and, in patients who had a protracted course or who had been treated with plasma exchange or intravenous immunoglobulin (IVIG), anti-NMDAR antibody was detected only in CSF.[100] Persistence of antibody titers in CSF seems to correlate with ongoing symptomatic disease activity, but persistent serum antibody without evidence of intrathecal synthesis may be found in patients who have been successfully treated. The most useful screening studies for ovarian teratoma include MRI, CT scan, and pelvic and abdominal ultrasound. Serologic tumor markers seem unhelpful.

Management of paraneoplastic LE is based on the combination of tumor removal, immunotherapy, and symptomatic treatment (eg, treatment of seizures). Results of immunotherapy with corticosteroids, chemotherapy, plasma exchange, and biologic agents are frequently unsatisfying. However, LE associated with anti-NMDAR antibodies seems to be more responsive and treatment should include both immunotherapy and the search for an underlying tumor. Treatment options include corticosteroids, IVIG, or plasma exchange as the first phase of treatment, and this may be sufficient in some patients when an underlying teratoma is identified and removed.[100,116] In patients without a tumor, or with long-delayed diagnosis and severely symptomatic disease, second-line therapy with rituximab or cyclophosphamide is usually used.[117,118] Approximately 75% of patients recover with minimal sequelae, and the other 25% remain neurologically incapacitated or die. The experience of Dalmau and colleagues[100] in 105 consecutive cases suggests that patients without a diagnosed tumor more frequently require second-line therapy, and second-line therapy may result in substantial improvement in 65% of treated patients.

The association of the LE syndromes with seizures has led Dalmau[24] to propose preliminary clinical criteria for the recognition of antibody associated encephalitides in patients with refractory seizure disorders.[106] In the setting of other psychiatric, autonomic, peripheral nervous system, sleep, or movement disorders, autoantibody-associated encephalitic syndromes should be considered in the differential diagnosis of refractory seizures. Identifying the diagnostic antibodies in serum and CSF would lead to specific immunotherapies and the search for the appropriate associated neoplasms. At present, the antibody testing is performed by a limited number of reliable laboratories, and, for some of these syndromes, the antibody testing is not yet commercially available. In many patients, the decision to institute immunotherapy is based on the clinical, imaging, and CSF abnormalities before definitive diagnosis of the identification of specific autoantibody-associated syndrome.

SUMMARY

Neurologic emergencies are common in patients who have cancer and are associated with significant morbidity and mortality. Timely recognition and treatment may improve symptoms and outcome in some patients. A previously established diagnosis of cancer simplifies diagnostic algorithms and narrows differential diagnosis, but neurologic emergency may be the first clinical manifestation of undiagnosed neoplastic disease with potentially catastrophic outcome. After diagnosis is made, an interdisciplinary team approach including neurology, hematology/oncology, neurosurgery, and radiation oncology team members allows more flexible and effective treatment options.

REFERENCES

1. Schiff D, O'Neill BP, Wang CH, et al. Neuroimaging and treatment implications of patients with multiple epidural spinal metastases. Cancer 1998;83(8):1593–601.
2. Giglio P, Gilbert MR. Neurologic complications of cancer and its treatment. Curr Oncol Rep 2010;12(1):50–9.
3. Barnholtz-Sloan JS, Sloan AE, Davis FG, et al. Incidence proportions of brain metastases in patients diagnosed (1973 to 2001) in the Metropolitan Detroit Cancer Surveillance System. J Clin Oncol 2004;22(14):2865–72.
4. Schouten LJ, Rutten J, Huveneers HA, et al. Incidence of brain metastases in a cohort of patients with carcinoma of the breast, colon, kidney, and lung and melanoma. Cancer 2002;94(10):2698–705.
5. Landis SH, Murray T, Bolden S, et al. Cancer statistics, 1999. CA Cancer J Clin 1999;49(1):8–31, 31.
6. Smedby KE, Brandt L, Backlund ML, et al. Brain metastases admissions in Sweden between 1987 and 2006. Br J Cancer 2009;101(11):1919–24.
7. Eichler AF, Chung E, Kodack DP, et al. The biology of brain metastases-translation to new therapies. Nat Rev Clin Oncol 2011;8(6):344–56.
8. Gabos Z, Sinha R, Hanson J, et al. Prognostic significance of human epidermal growth factor receptor positivity for the development of brain metastasis after newly diagnosed breast cancer. J Clin Oncol 2006;24(36):5658–63.
9. Nguyen TD, DeAngelis LM. Brain metastases. Neurol Clin 2007;25(4):1173–92, x–xi.
10. Schellinger PD, Meinck HM, Thron A. Diagnostic accuracy of MRI compared to CCT in patients with brain metastases. J Neurooncol 1999;44(3):275–81.
11. Patchell RA, Tibbs PA, Walsh JW, et al. A randomized trial of surgery in the treatment of single metastases to the brain. N Engl J Med 1990;322(8):494–500.
12. Chang EL, Hassenbusch SJ 3rd, Shiu AS, et al. The role of tumor size in the radiosurgical management of patients with ambiguous brain metastases. Neurosurgery 2003;53(2):272–80 [discussion: 281–91].
13. Kamar FG, Posner JB. Brain metastases. Semin Neurol 2010;30(3):217–35.
14. Kalkanis SN, Kondziolka D, Gaspar LE, et al. The role of surgical resection in the management of newly diagnosed brain metastases: a systematic review and evidence-based clinical practice guideline. J Neurooncol 2010;96(1):33–43.

15. Mehta MP, Paleologos NA, Mikkelsen T, et al. The role of chemotherapy in the management of newly diagnosed brain metastases: a systematic review and evidence-based clinical practice guideline. J Neurooncol 2010;96(1):71–83.
16. Gerstner ER, Duda DG, di Tomaso E, et al. VEGF inhibitors in the treatment of cerebral edema in patients with brain cancer. Nat Rev Clin Oncol 2009;6(4): 229–36.
17. Ryken TC, McDermott M, Robinson PD, et al. The role of steroids in the management of brain metastases: a systematic review and evidence-based clinical practice guideline. J Neurooncol 2010;96(1):103–14.
18. Vecht CJ, Hovestadt A, Verbiest HB, et al. Dose-effect relationship of dexamethasone on Karnofsky performance in metastatic brain tumors: a randomized study of doses of 4, 8, and 16 mg per day. Neurology 1994;44(4):675–80.
19. Koenig MA, Bryan M, Lewin JL 3rd, et al. Reversal of transtentorial herniation with hypertonic saline. Neurology 2008;70(13):1023–9.
20. Batchelor TT, Duda DG, di Tomaso E, et al. Phase II study of cediranib, an oral pan-vascular endothelial growth factor receptor tyrosine kinase inhibitor, in patients with recurrent glioblastoma. J Clin Oncol 2010;28(17):2817–23.
21. Kreisl TN, Kim L, Moore K, et al. Phase II trial of single-agent bevacizumab followed by bevacizumab plus irinotecan at tumor progression in recurrent glioblastoma. J Clin Oncol 2009;27(5):740–5.
22. Beaumont A, Whittle IR. The pathogenesis of tumour associated epilepsy. Acta Neurochir (Wien) 2000;142(1):1–15.
23. Cocito L, Audenino D, Primavera A. Altered mental state and nonconvulsive status epilepticus in patients with cancer. Arch Neurol 2001;58(8):1310.
24. Dalmau J. Status epilepticus due to paraneoplastic and nonparaneoplastic encephalitides. Epilepsia 2009;50(Suppl 12):58–60.
25. van Breemen MS, Wilms EB, Vecht CJ. Epilepsy in patients with brain tumours: epidemiology, mechanisms, and management. Lancet Neurol 2007;6(5):421–30.
26. Chang EF, Potts MB, Keles GE, et al. Seizure characteristics and control following resection in 332 patients with low-grade gliomas. J Neurosurg 2008; 108(2):227–35.
27. Kirkpatrick PJ, Honavar M, Janota I, et al. Control of temporal lobe epilepsy following en bloc resection of low-grade tumors. J Neurosurg 1993;78(1):19–25.
28. Treiman DM, Walker MC. Treatment of seizure emergencies: convulsive and non-convulsive status epilepticus. Epilepsy Res 2006;68(Suppl 1):S77–82.
29. Jaeckle KA, Ballman K, Furth A, et al. Correlation of enzyme-inducing anticonvulsant use with outcome of patients with glioblastoma. Neurology 2009; 73(15):1207–13.
30. White JR, Walczak TS, Leppik IE, et al. Discontinuation of levetiracetam because of behavioral side effects: a case-control study. Neurology 2003;61(9):1218–21.
31. Helmstaedter C, Fritz NE, Kockelmann E, et al. Positive and negative psychotropic effects of levetiracetam. Epilepsy Behav 2008;13(3):535–41.
32. Forsyth PA, Weaver S, Fulton D, et al. Prophylactic anticonvulsants in patients with brain tumour. Can J Neurol Sci 2003;30(2):106–12.
33. Mikkelsen T, Paleologos NA, Robinson PD, et al. The role of prophylactic anticonvulsants in the management of brain metastases: a systematic review and evidence-based clinical practice guideline. J Neurooncol 2010;96(1):97–102.
34. Aronica E, Gorter JA, Jansen GH, et al. Expression and cellular distribution of multidrug transporter proteins in two major causes of medically intractable epilepsy: focal cortical dysplasia and glioneuronal tumors. Neuroscience 2003;118(2):417–29.

35. Brenner RP. EEG in convulsive and nonconvulsive status epilepticus. J Clin Neurophysiol 2004;21(5):319–31.
36. Drislane FW. Nonconvulsive status epilepticus in patients with cancer. Clin Neurol Neurosurg 1994;96(4):314–8.
37. Blitshteyn S, Jaeckle KA. Nonconvulsive status epilepticus in metastatic CNS disease. Neurology 2006;66(8):1261–3.
38. Sizoo EM, Braam L, Postma TJ, et al. Symptoms and problems in the end-of-life phase of high-grade glioma patients. Neuro Oncol 2010;12(11):1162–6.
39. El Beltagy MA, Kamal HM, Taha H, et al. Endoscopic third ventriculostomy before tumor surgery in children with posterior fossa tumors, CCHE experience. Childs Nerv Syst 2010;26(12):1699–704.
40. Bach F, Larsen BH, Rohde K, et al. Metastatic spinal cord compression. Occurrence, symptoms, clinical presentations and prognosis in 398 patients with spinal cord compression. Acta Neurochir (Wien) 1990;107(1–2):37–43.
41. Schiff D, Batchelor T, Wen PY. Neurologic emergencies in cancer patients. Neurol Clin 1998;16(2):449–83.
42. Aaron AD. The management of cancer metastatic to bone. JAMA 1994;272(15):1206–9.
43. Schiff D, O'Neill BP, Suman VJ. Spinal epidural metastasis as the initial manifestation of malignancy: clinical features and diagnostic approach. Neurology 1997;49(2):452–6.
44. Sun H, Nemecek AN. Optimal management of malignant epidural spinal cord compression. Hematol Oncol Clin North Am 2010;24(3):537–51.
45. Gilbert RW, Kim JH, Posner JB. Epidural spinal cord compression from metastatic tumor: diagnosis and treatment. Ann Neurol 1978;3(1):40–51.
46. Kim JK, Learch TJ, Colletti PM, et al. Diagnosis of vertebral metastasis, epidural metastasis, and malignant spinal cord compression: are T(1)-weighted sagittal images sufficient? Magn Reson Imaging 2000;18(7):819–24.
47. Rose PS, Buchowski JM. Metastatic disease in the thoracic and lumbar spine: evaluation and management. J Am Acad Orthop Surg 2011;19(1):37–48.
48. Witham TF, Khavkin YA, Gallia GL, et al. Surgery insight: current management of epidural spinal cord compression from metastatic spine disease. Nat Clin Pract Neurol 2006;2(2):87–94 [quiz: 116].
49. Sorensen S, Helweg-Larsen S, Mouridsen H, et al. Effect of high-dose dexamethasone in carcinomatous metastatic spinal cord compression treated with radiotherapy: a randomised trial. Eur J Cancer 1994;30A(1):22–7.
50. Patchell RA, Tibbs PA, Regine WF, et al. Direct decompressive surgical resection in the treatment of spinal cord compression caused by metastatic cancer: a randomised trial. Lancet 2005;366(9486):643–8.
51. Fourney DR, Schomer DF, Nader R, et al. Percutaneous vertebroplasty and kyphoplasty for painful vertebral body fractures in cancer patients. J Neurosurg 2003;98(Suppl 1):21–30.
52. Zaidat OO, Ruff RL. Treatment of spinal epidural metastasis improves patient survival and functional state. Neurology 2002;58(9):1360–6.
53. Peters LJ. The ESTRO Regaud lecture. Inherent radiosensitivity of tumor and normal tissue cells as a predictor of human tumor response. Radiother Oncol 1990;17(3):177–90.
54. Maranzano E, Latini P. Effectiveness of radiation therapy without surgery in metastatic spinal cord compression: final results from a prospective trial. Int J Radiat Oncol Biol Phys 1995;32(4):959–67.

55. Abrahm JL, Banffy MB, Harris MB. Spinal cord compression in patients with advanced metastatic cancer: "all I care about is walking and living my life". JAMA 2008;299(8):937–46.
56. Chamberlain MC. Carcinomatous meningitis. Arch Neurol 1997;54(1):16–7.
57. Glass JP, Melamed M, Chernik NL, et al. Malignant cells in cerebrospinal fluid (CSF): the meaning of a positive CSF cytology. Neurology 1979;29(10):1369–75.
58. DeAngelis LM, Boutros D. Leptomeningeal metastasis. Cancer Invest 2005; 23(2):145–54.
59. Chamberlain MC. Neoplastic meningitis. Oncologist 2008;13(9):967–77.
60. Clarke JL, Perez HR, Jacks LM, et al. Leptomeningeal metastases in the MRI era. Neurology 2010;74(18):1449–54.
61. Wasserstrom WR, Glass JP, Posner JB. Diagnosis and treatment of leptomeningeal metastases from solid tumors: experience with 90 patients. Cancer 1982; 49(4):759–72.
62. Graus F, Rogers LR, Posner JB. Cerebrovascular complications in patients with cancer. Medicine (Baltimore) 1985;64(1):16–35.
63. Oberndorfer S, Nussgruber V, Berger O, et al. Stroke in cancer patients: a risk factor analysis. J Neurooncol 2009;94(2):227.
64. Cestari DM, Weine DM, Panageas KS, et al. Stroke in patients with cancer: incidence and etiology. Neurology 2004;62(11):2025–30.
65. Rogers LR. Cerebrovascular complications in patients with cancer. Semin Neurol 2010;30(3):311–9.
66. Zhang YY, Chan DK, Cordato D, et al. Stroke risk factor, pattern and outcome in patients with cancer. Acta Neurol Scand 2006;114(6):378–83.
67. Kim H, Lee JH, Choi SJ, et al. Analysis of fatal intracranial hemorrhage in 792 acute leukemia patients. Haematologica 2004;89(5):622–4.
68. Franchini M, Dario Di Minno MN, Coppola A. Disseminated intravascular coagulation in hematologic malignancies. Semin Thromb Hemost 2010;36(4): 388–403.
69. Seok JM, Kim SG, Kim JW, et al. Coagulopathy and embolic signal in cancer patients with ischemic stroke. Ann Neurol 2010;68(2):213–9.
70. Muzaffar K, Collins SL, Labropoulos N, et al. A prospective study of the effects of irradiation on the carotid artery. Laryngoscope 2000;110(11):1811–4.
71. Cheng SW, Wu LL, Ting AC, et al. Irradiation-induced extracranial carotid stenosis in patients with head and neck malignancies. Am J Surg 1999; 178(4):323–8.
72. Shichita T, Ogata T, Yasaka M, et al. Angiographic characteristics of radiation-induced carotid arterial stenosis. Angiology 2009;60(3):276–82.
73. Kreisl TN, Toothaker T, Karimi S, et al. Ischemic stroke in patients with primary brain tumors. Neurology 2008;70(24):2314–20.
74. Numico G, Garrone O, Dongiovanni V, et al. Prospective evaluation of major vascular events in patients with nonsmall cell lung carcinoma treated with cisplatin and gemcitabine. Cancer 2005;103(5):994–9.
75. Casado-Naranjo I, Calle ML, Falcon A, et al. Intravenous thrombolysis for acute stroke in patients with cancer. J Neurol Neurosurg Psychiatry 2011. [Epub ahead of print].
76. Grimm SA, DeAngelis LM. Intratumoral hemorrhage after thrombolysis in a patient with glioblastoma multiforme. Neurology 2007;69(9):936.
77. Jovin TG, Boosupalli V, Zivkovic SA, et al. High titers of CA-125 may be associated with recurrent ischemic strokes in patients with cancer. Neurology 2005; 64(11):1944–5.

78. Idbaih A, Boukobza M, Crassard I, et al. MRI of clot in cerebral venous thrombosis: high diagnostic value of susceptibility-weighted images. Stroke 2006; 37(4):991–5.
79. Einhaupl KM, Villringer A, Meister W, et al. Heparin treatment in sinus venous thrombosis. Lancet 1991;338(8767):597–600.
80. de Bruijn SF, Stam J. Randomized, placebo-controlled trial of anticoagulant treatment with low-molecular-weight heparin for cerebral sinus thrombosis. Stroke 1999;30(3):484–8.
81. Horowitz M, Purdy P, Unwin H, et al. Treatment of dural sinus thrombosis using selective catheterization and urokinase. Ann Neurol 1995;38(1):58–67.
82. Stam J, De Bruijn SF, DeVeber G. Anticoagulation for cerebral sinus thrombosis. Cochrane Database Syst Rev 2002;4:CD002005.
83. Ferro JM, Bacelar-Nicolau H, Rodrigues T, et al. Risk score to predict the outcome of patients with cerebral vein and dural sinus thrombosis. Cerebrovasc Dis 2009;28(1):39–44.
84. Ferro JM, Canhao P, Stam J, et al. Prognosis of cerebral vein and dural sinus thrombosis: results of the International Study on Cerebral Vein and Dural Sinus Thrombosis (ISCVT). Stroke 2004;35(3):664–70.
85. Pruitt AA. Nervous system infections in patients with cancer. Neurol Clin 2003; 21(1):193–219.
86. Safdieh JE, Mead PA, Sepkowitz KA, et al. Bacterial and fungal meningitis in patients with cancer. Neurology 2008;70(12):943–7.
87. Pruitt AA. Central nervous system infections in cancer patients. Semin Neurol 2010;30(3):296–310.
88. Conen A, Walti LN, Merlo A, et al. Characteristics and treatment outcome of cerebrospinal fluid shunt-associated infections in adults: a retrospective analysis over an 11-year period. Clin Infect Dis 2008;47(1):73–82.
89. Brouwer MC, Heckenberg SG, de Gans J, et al. Nationwide implementation of adjunctive dexamethasone therapy for pneumococcal meningitis. Neurology 2010;75(17):1533–9.
90. Muttaiyah S, Ritchie S, Upton A, et al. Clinical parameters do not predict infection in patients with external ventricular drains: a retrospective observational study of daily cerebrospinal fluid analysis. J Med Microbiol 2008;57(Pt 2):207–9.
91. Tunkel AR, Hartman BJ, Kaplan SL, et al. Practice guidelines for the management of bacterial meningitis. Clin Infect Dis 2004;39(9):1267–84.
92. Rosenfeld MR, Dalmau J. Anti-NMDA-receptor encephalitis and other synaptic autoimmune disorders. Curr Treat Options Neurol 2011;13(3):324–32.
93. Graus F, Keime-Guibert F, Rene R, et al. Anti-Hu-associated paraneoplastic encephalomyelitis: analysis of 200 patients. Brain 2001;124(Pt 6):1138–48.
94. Voltz R, Gultekin SH, Rosenfeld MR, et al. A serologic marker of paraneoplastic limbic and brain-stem encephalitis in patients with testicular cancer. N Engl J Med 1999;340(23):1788–95.
95. Gultekin SH, Rosenfeld MR, Voltz R, et al. Paraneoplastic limbic encephalitis: neurological symptoms, immunological findings and tumour association in 50 patients. Brain 2000;123(Pt 7):1481–94.
96. Bernal F, Shams'ili S, Rojas I, et al. Anti-Tr antibodies as markers of paraneoplastic cerebellar degeneration and Hodgkin's disease. Neurology 2003;60(2): 230–4.
97. Rojas-Marcos I, Rousseau A, Keime-Guibert F, et al. Spectrum of paraneoplastic neurologic disorders in women with breast and gynecologic cancer. Medicine (Baltimore) 2003;82(3):216–23.

98. Deodhare S, O'Connor P, Ghazarian D, et al. Paraneoplastic limbic encephalitis in Hodgkin's disease. Can J Neurol Sci 1996;23(2):138–40.
99. Thuerl C, Muller K, Laubenberger J, et al. MR imaging of autopsy-proved paraneoplastic limbic encephalitis in non-Hodgkin lymphoma. AJNR Am J Neuroradiol 2003;24(3):507–11.
100. Dalmau J, Lancaster E, Martinez-Hernandez E, et al. Clinical experience and laboratory investigations in patients with anti-NMDAR encephalitis. Lancet Neurol 2011;10(1):63–74.
101. Tang T, Tay KY, Chai J, et al. A multimodality approach to reversible paraneoplastic encephalitis associated with ovarian teratomas. Acta Oncol 2009; 48(7):1079–82.
102. Giometto B, Grisold W, Vitaliani R, et al. Paraneoplastic neurologic syndrome in the PNS Euronetwork database: a European study from 20 centers. Arch Neurol 2010;67(3):330–5.
103. Bataller L, Dalmau J. Paraneoplastic neurologic syndromes: approaches to diagnosis and treatment. Semin Neurol 2003;23(2):215–24.
104. Lai M, Hughes EG, Peng X, et al. AMPA receptor antibodies in limbic encephalitis alter synaptic receptor location. Ann Neurol 2009;65(4):424–34.
105. Bataller L, Galiano R, Garcia-Escrig M, et al. Reversible paraneoplastic limbic encephalitis associated with antibodies to the AMPA receptor. Neurology 2010;74(3):265–7.
106. Brashear HR, Caccamo DV, Heck A, et al. Localization of antibody in the central nervous system of a patient with paraneoplastic encephalomyeloneuritis. Neurology 1991;41(10):1583–7.
107. Alamowitch S, Graus F, Uchuya M, et al. Limbic encephalitis and small cell lung cancer. Clinical and immunological features. Brain 1997;120(Pt 6): 923–8.
108. Kayser MS, Kohler CG, Dalmau J. Psychiatric manifestations of paraneoplastic disorders. Am J Psychiatry 2010;167(9):1039–50.
109. Lancaster E, Lai M, Peng X, et al. Antibodies to the GABA(B) receptor in limbic encephalitis with seizures: case series and characterisation of the antigen. Lancet Neurol 2010;9(1):67–76.
110. Lai M, Huijbers MG, Lancaster E, et al. Investigation of LGI1 as the antigen in limbic encephalitis previously attributed to potassium channels: a case series. Lancet Neurol 2010;9(8):776–85.
111. Andrade DM, Tai P, Dalmau J, et al. Tonic seizures: a diagnostic clue of anti-LGI1 encephalitis? Neurology 2011;76(15):1355–7.
112. Kalachikov S, Evgrafov O, Ross B, et al. Mutations in LGI1 cause autosomal-dominant partial epilepsy with auditory features. Nat Genet 2002;30(3): 335–41.
113. Irani SR, Alexander S, Waters P, et al. Antibodies to Kv1 potassium channel-complex proteins leucine-rich, glioma inactivated 1 protein and contactin-associated protein-2 in limbic encephalitis, Morvan's syndrome and acquired neuromyotonia. Brain 2010;133(9):2734–48.
114. Vincent A, Irani SR. Caspr2 antibodies in patients with thymomas. J Thorac Oncol 2010;5(10 Suppl 4):S277–80.
115. Psimaras D, Carpentier AF, Rossi C. Cerebrospinal fluid study in paraneoplastic syndromes. J Neurol Neurosurg Psychiatry 2010;81(1):42–5.
116. Dalmau J, Gleichman AJ, Hughes EG, et al. Anti-NMDA-receptor encephalitis: case series and analysis of the effects of antibodies. Lancet Neurol 2008; 7(12):1091–8.

117. Wong-Kisiel LC, Ji T, Renaud DL, et al. Response to immunotherapy in a 20-month-old boy with anti-NMDA receptor encephalitis. Neurology 2010;74(19):1550–1.
118. Ishiura H, Matsuda S, Higashihara M, et al. Response of anti-NMDA receptor encephalitis without tumor to immunotherapy including rituximab. Neurology 2008;71(23):1921–3.

Neurologic Infectious Disease Emergencies

Amy A. Pruitt, MD

KEYWORDS

- Neurologic infectious diseases
- Central nervous system infections
- Bacterial meningitis • Encephalitis

Nearly 70 years after the discovery of penicillin, neurologic infectious diseases (NIDs) remain an important worldwide source of morbidity and mortality. The ongoing health threat from NIDs stems from several factors: (1) the emergence of large populations of immunocompromised patients, both from the acquired immunodeficiency syndrome (AIDS) and from aggressive treatment regimens with or without solid or hematopoietic cell transplantation (HCT) that have improved survival from many different kinds of malignancies and rheumatologic and neurologic disorders; (2) the increase in international travel allowing rapid global transmission of emerging infectious agents, presenting North American clinicians with illnesses unlikely to be seen with sufficient frequency to maintain diagnostic acumen; (3) the widespread use of antibiotics that have contributed to many clinical successes but that have also driven the emergence of resistant organisms; and (4) the recognition of an increasing number of "infectious mimes," including the immune reconstitution inflammatory syndrome (IRIS) and immune-mediated encephalitides (ADEM and NMDA receptor encephalitis).[1]

The clinician faced with a potential NID must consider 3 sets of data urgently:

1. Patient demographics: is the patient immunocompetent or immunocompromised and, if the latter, by what mechanism are host defenses altered (eg, HIV, corticosteroids, recent penetrating trauma or surgery, recent health care–related exposures)
2. Pace of illness and clinical syndrome (nonspecific altered mental status vs focal findings and associated extraneural infection sites)
3. Laboratory data, including neuroimaging and rapid detection tests to guide initial therapeutic strategy.

In keeping with the topics of this issue, initial emergency diagnosis and management are emphasized with appropriate references to relevant literature for subsequent longer-term interventions.

Department of Neurology, University of Pennsylvania, 3400 Spruce Street, Philadelphia, PA 19104, USA

E-mail address: pruitt@mail.med.upenn.edu

Neurol Clin 30 (2012) 129–159
doi:10.1016/j.ncl.2011.09.011 **neurologic.theclinics.com**

EVALUATING THE PATIENT WITH SUSPECTED CENTRAL NERVOUS SYSTEM INFECTION

Major neurologic infections presenting in urgent care settings, such as emergency rooms or intensive care units, include meningitis, encephalitis, brain abscess, spinal epidural abscess, subdural empyema, and pyomyositis. When patients present with fever, headache, nuchal rigidity, altered mental status, and/or focal signs, emergent evaluation includes physical examination, serologic testing, neuroimaging, and cerebrospinal fluid (CSF) examination.[2] The order of testing depends on a process of triage dictated by the patient's epidemiologic risk factors and physical examination, which will sort the problem into one that best fits meningitis without focal signs, a brain parenchymal localization (focal findings consistent with mass lesion or characteristic infectious pattern), or a spinal cord or a peripheral nerve or muscle problem. **Fig. 1** outlines a broad overview of the urgent evaluation process of a patient with suspected infection.[3–7] The initial triage divides patients into those with minimal alteration in level of alertness and those with more impaired mental status with or without signs of brain parenchymal or specific focal signs. The first obligation is to exclude bacterial processes, most critically bacterial meningitis, and to proceed with imaging studies in those patients whose examination suggests intracranial processes that might preclude lumbar puncture (LP). Computed tomography (CT) of the head (performed as an initial rapid screen, often to be followed by magnetic resonance imaging [MRI]) should be performed before LP if any one of the following is present: depressed level of consciousness (<14 Glasgow Coma Scale), focal or lateralizing examination, new-onset seizures, immunosuppressed state (chronic corticosteroid use, chemotherapy, HIV), or history of central nervous system (CNS) pathology (tumor, stroke, demyelinating disease, previous infection).[8]

A useful strategy is to assume the worst-case, but treatable, scenario, which in most instances is bacterial meningitis, and to ask the following 4 critical questions in designing empiric regimens (**Table 1**):

1. Is *Streptococcus pneumoniae* a possibility (assume penicillin/cephalosporin resistance)?
2. Is coverage for gram negatives necessary?
3. Is *Listeria monocytogenes* a possibility (patients >50 years old, specific exposures)?
4. Is viral encephalitis or tick-borne disease coverage necessary?

BACTERIAL MENINGITIS

Risk Factors and Epidemiology

With the advent of effective vaccination for *Haemophilus influenzae*, community-acquired bacterial meningitis has ceased to be a disease of children and now is one more frequently seen at the extremes of age (elderly, infants and neonates). Other risk factors include crowding (dormitories, military recruits, household contacts), contiguous infection (otitis, sinusitis), bacterial endocarditis (either from intravenous drug abuse or on prosthetic valves), recent neurosurgery or head trauma, ventriculoperitoneal shunts, cochlear implants and other indwelling devices, and immunosuppression (splenectomy, sickle cell disease, thalassemia, malignancy, diabetes, alcoholism, complement and immunoglobulin deficiencies, and immunosuppressive regimens). Prior vaccination status does not preclude infection: patients who have received the 7-valent or 23-valent pneumococcal vaccine can still acquire pneumococcal meningitis, and patients who have received meningococcal vaccine can still be infected with serogroup B meningitis. **Table 1** lists the most common epidemiologic considerations with attendant empiric antibiotic regimen recommendations.

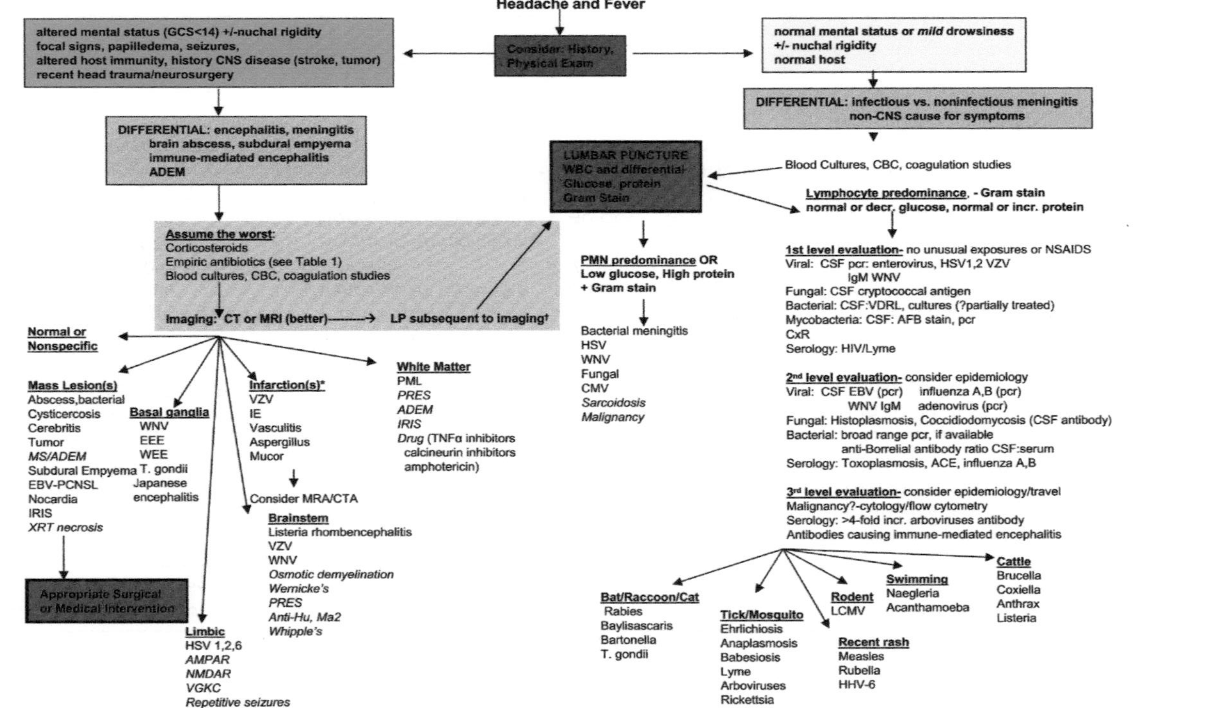

Fig. 1. Urgent evaluation of patient with suspected CNS infection. *Abnormal diffusion-weighted imaging (dwi); dwi also useful in diagnosis of Creutzfeldt-Jakob disease *Italics*, noninfectious processes that may mimic infection. † LP to be done *if* not contraindicated by findings on MRI. ADEM, acute disseminated encephalomyelitis; EBV/PCNSL, Epstein-Barr virus, primary central nervous system lymphoma; EEE/WEE, Eastern/Western equine encephalitis; GCS, Glasgow Coma Scale; IE, infective endocarditis; IRIS, immune reconstitution inflammatory syndrome; NSAIDs, nonsteroidal anti-inflammatory drugs; PCR, polymerase chain reaction; PRES, posterior reversible encephalopathy syndrome; WNV, West Nile Virus; XRT, radiation therapy. (*Data from* Refs.[2–7])

Table 1
Initial empiric coverage for suspected bacterial meningitis or herpes simplex encephalitis by demographic factors

Clinical Setting	Child 1 mo to 17 y	Adults 18–50 y	Adults >50 y	Penetrating Trauma Neurosurgery Shunt, Ventricular Drain	Impaired T-cell Immunity (HIV, Corticosteroids Transplantation)
Potential organisms	*Streptococcus pneumoniae* *Neisseria meningitides*[a] Group B streptococcus *Haemophilus influenzae* (until age 2) *Escherichia coli*	*S pneumoniae* *N meningitidis*[a]	*S pneumoniae* *N meningitidis*[a] *L monocytogenes* Gram-negative bacilli	*Streptococcus aureus* Coagulase-negative staphylococci *Pseudomonas* *S pneumoniae* Streptococci	*S pneumoniae* *N meningitidis*[a] Gram-negative bacilli *Listeria* (consider TB risk by patient origin/ travel)
Empiric antimicrobial regimen[b]	Dexamethasone 0.15 mg/kg q6h for 4 d Ceftriaxone 20–25 mg/kg q6h OR Cefotaxime[c] 75–100 mg/kg q6–8h AND Vancomycin[c] 15 mg/kg q6h Acyclovir[c] 10 mg/kg q8h	Dexamethasone 10 mg q6h for 4 d Ceftriaxone 2 g q12h OR Cefotaxime[c] 2 g IV q6h PLUS Vancomycin[c] 15 mg/kg IV q8h Acyclovir[c] 10 mg/kg q8h Doxycycline PO 100 mg q12h if possibility of tick-borne disease	Dexamethasone 10 mg q6h for 4 d Ceftriaxone 2 g q12h OR Cefotaxime[c] 203 g/d q4–6h PLUS Ampicillin[c] 2 g q4h PLUS Vancomycin[c] 15 mg/k q8h PLUS Acyclovir[c] 10 mg/kg q8h PLUS Doxycycline PO 100 mg q12h if tick-borne disease Possible	Fourth-generation cephalosporin Cefepime[c] 2 g q8h PLUS Vancomycin[c] 15 mg/kg q8h PLUS Gentamicin[c] 1.0–1.3 mg/kg q8h ONLY if high suspicion High-risk MRSA: Vancomycin[c] 15 mg/kg q8h PLUS Rifampin 300 mg–400 mg IV/PO q8h	Ceftazidime[c] 2 g q12h PLUS Vancomycin[c] 15 mg/kg q8h PLUS Ampicillin[c] 2 g q4h High-risk MRSA regimen in previous column *First-Line TB*: Isoniazid 5 mg/kg PO qd; max 300 mg daily Pyridoxine 50 mg PO qd Rifampin 10 mg/kg/d PO; max 600 mg daily Pyrazinamide 15–35 mg/kg/d PO Ethambutol 15–25 mg/kg/d PO

Alternative regimens	Meropenem[c] 40 mg/kg q8h PLUS Vancomycin[c] 15 mg/kg q8h	Meropenem[c] 2 g IV q8h OR chloramphenicol 14–25 mg/kg q6h OR Moxifloxacin 400 mg IV daily PLUS Vancomycin[c] 15 mg/kg IV q8h	Ampicillin[c] 2 g q4h OR TMP 5 mg/kg every 6 h PLUS Vancomycin 15 mg/kg q8h PLUS Meropenem[c] 2 g IV q8h OR Moxifloxacin 400 mg IV daily	Vancomycin[c] 15 mg/kg q8h PLUS Ceftazidime 2 g q8h OR Meropenem[c] 2 g q8h OR Ciprofloxacin 400 mg q8h Metronidazole 400–500 mg q6h MRSA: Linezolid 600 mg IV/PO q12h	Meropenem[c] PLUS Vancomycin[c] PLUS Trimethoprim-sulfamethoxazole 5 mg/kg q6h See high-risk MRSA alternate in previous column TB: moxifloxacin 400 mg IV daily

Abbreviations: h, hour; IV, intravenous; MRSA, methicillin-resistant *Staphylococcus aureus*; PO, oral; q, every.

[a] Ciprofloxacin 500 mg oral one-time dose OR Rifampin 600 mg twice a day for 2 days prophylaxis for contacts.

[b] Doses IV unless otherwise indicated. See text for corticosteroid use. Once specific pathogen identified, local resistance patterns and nosocomial trends should be factored in with infectious disease consultation for definitive, pathogen-specific regimen.

[c] Adjust for renal insufficiency.

Data from Refs.[2–7,22,23,31]

Clinical Presentation

In a Dutch study of 696 episodes of adult community-acquired bacterial meningitis, only 44% of patients had the full triad of fever, altered mental status, and nuchal rigidity, but 85% of episodes had at least 2 of 4 symptoms of headache, fever, neck stiffness, and altered mental status.[9] Roos and Tyler[3] emphasize early vomiting as an important sign, even before headache or altered mental status. Up to one-third of patients with bacterial meningitis had focal signs and 14% were comatose in one study.[10] Immunocompetent patients with *Listeria* meningitis may present with the distinctive rhombencephalitis syndrome with focal cranial nerve and brainstem or other parenchymal deficits (**Fig. 2**).

Elderly patients, patients with partially treated meningitis, and patients on corticosteroids or other immunosuppressive drugs may not have any febrile response, and the clearest emergency distinction between viral and bacterial meningitis appears to be the severity of altered consciousness, seizures, focal neurologic findings, and shock.[11,12] Independent predictors of mortality are seizure activity, depressed level of consciousness (Glasgow Coma Score <13), and CSF white blood cell (WBC) count lower than 1000. Among the elderly with community-acquired meningitis, nearly one-third present in coma, and 16% have seizures. Pneumonia and diabetes are frequent predisposing conditions and additional poor prognostic indicators.[13] In community-acquired meningitis, about 50% of surviving patients have significant sequelae with case-fatality rate highest with *S pneumoniae*.[9]

Microbiology of Acute Bacterial Meningitis

The most common causes of community-acquired bacterial meningitis in adults are *S pneumoniae* and *Neisseria meningitidis* with *L monocytogenes* a consideration in patients older than 50 (see **Table 1**). *H influenzae* is a concern among asplenic or

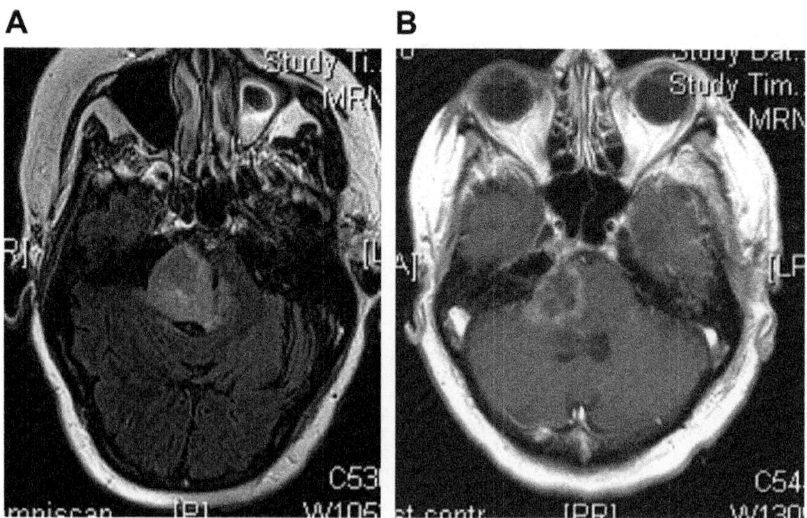

Fig. 2. FLAIR (*A*) and gadolinium-enhanced T1-weighted (*B*) MRI images of a patient with facial numbness, peripheral facial weakness, and rapid obtundation owing to *Listeria monocytogenes* rhombencephalitis. Although diffuse cerebritis predominates in immunocompromised patients, previously healthy patients may have this characteristic focal brainstem parenchymal involvement.

immune-compromised patients. Patients with nosocomially acquired bacterial meningitis occupy a growing number of beds in intensive care units. *Staphylococcus aureus* is a frequent pathogen and gram-negative bacilli (*Klebsiella, Serratia, Pseudomonas, Acinetobacter*) cause up to a third of nosocomial cases.[10,14,15]

Special Considerations in Vulnerable Populations

The risk of patients with HIV/AIDS for NIDs varies with CD4+ count less than 200/mm^3. These patients may present with meningitis caused by conventional bacterial pathogens but also caused by *Toxoplasma gondii*, Epstein-Barr virus (EBV), varicella zoster virus (VZV), *Cryptococcus neoformans,* and, more frequently outside North America, *Mycobacterium tuberculosis*. In such patients, the CSF WBC count and differential may be uninformative depending on the degree of immune suppression.[16] The full spectrum of transplantation-associated infections is beyond the scope of this article and is well covered elsewhere.[17,18] The clinician facing such a patient must cast a broad net to consider bacterial infections but also viral meningitides (VZV, EBV, cytomegalovirus [CMV], toxoplasmosis, and human herpesvirus 6 [HHV6]). For those who require ongoing immunosuppression of graft versus-host-disease, VZV remains a risk, and progressive multifocal leukoencephalopathy (PML) becomes a consideration with duration of immunosuppression.[19]

TREATMENT AND INVESTIGATION OF BACTERIAL MENINGITIS

First Step: Corticosteroids

Current guidelines and several meta-analyses support the use of dexamethasone administered concurrently with antimicrobial agents to abort the dysfunctional release of inflammatory cytokines triggered by bacterial lysis whose consequences include nearby tissue damage and a higher risk of venous infarctions and raised intracranial pressure.[20] A recent meta-analysis subsuming trials in patients who were HIV-positive and HIV-negative from many different parts of the world, suggested that the most solid corticosteroid benefit accrued to adults older than 55 largely in developed countries for whom steroid use decreased incidence of deafness and reduced mortality significantly in *S pneumoniae* cases. It was not clear that dexamethasone harmed any group.[21] Current guidelines recommend use of dexamethasone 10 mg every 6 hours intravenously.[22,23] Brouwer and colleagues[24] looked at 357 episodes of pneumococcal meningitis from 2006 to 2009 when 84% received steroids and compared them with a cohort from 1998 to 2002 when only 3% received steroids. Rates of death and hearing loss were lower in the recent group and, most impressively, mortality fell from 30% to 20%. Dexamethasone should be continued only in patients with cultures positive for pneumococci or with positive Gram stain for diplococci and should not be given to patients who previously received antibiotics. When doses are prescribed as indicated in **Table 1**, intrathecal vancomycin is not required to offset the effect of corticosteroids on CSF penetration.[25]

Other indications for corticosteroids in NID emergencies are control of edema in herpes simplex virus encephalitis[26] and control of initial edema with scolex lysis in cysticerosis.[27] Steroids convincingly reduce mortality in tuberculous meningitis, although the dose and duration of therapy are not fully established.[28–30]

Second Step: Empiric Antibiotics

Table 1 outlines recommendations, emphasizing the resistance of *S pneumoniae* to penicillin, the possibility of methicillin-resistant *S aureus* (MRSA), and the need to cover possible viral encephalitis or tick-borne disease until further microbiologic data emerge.[31]

Third Step: Imaging

Any patient with significant altered mental status needs a CT or MRI before LP. Pyogenic abscesses exhibit several MRI characteristics that suggest infection rather than other etiologies (**Fig. 3**).[32–35]

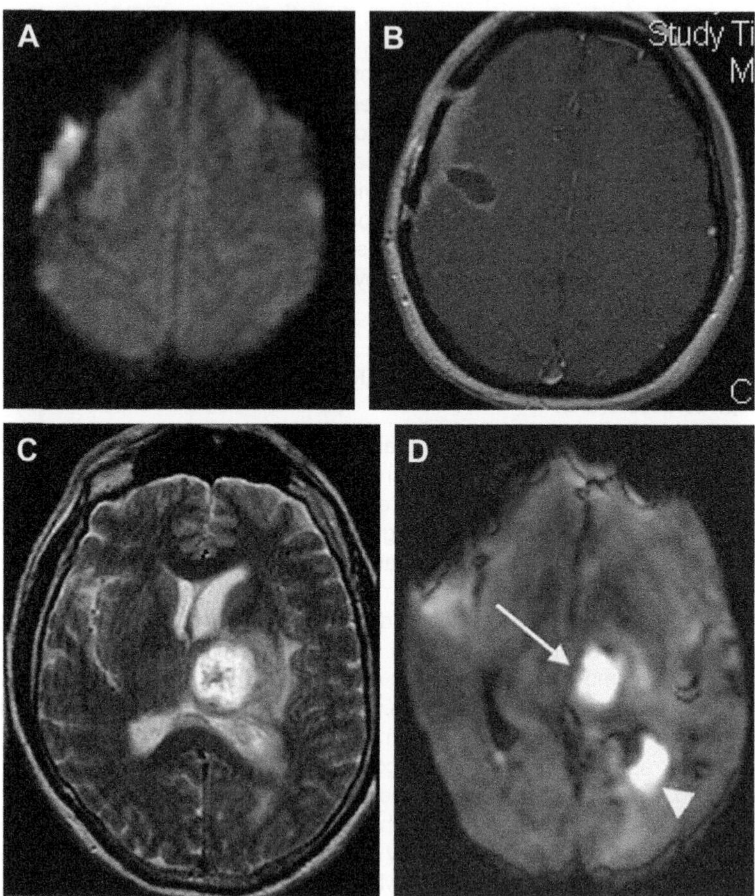

Fig. 3. Suspecting intracranial infection by MRI characteristics. Diffusion-weighted imaging (dwi) MRI (*A*) and gadolinium-enhanced T1-weighted MRI (*B*) in patient presenting with headache and fever 6 weeks after craniotomy for brain tumor. There is evidence of diffusion restriction of viscous purulent material, as well as cerebritis, indicated by parenchymal ring enhancement. Pyogenic abscesses exhibit characteristics suggesting infection rather than other etiologies, including T2 hyperintensity with isointense rim (*C*). (*D*) Another characteristic of purulent material in abscess, namely marked hyperintensity on diffusion-weighted images (*arrow and arrowhead*). Not shown in these figures, other characteristics suggestive of abscesses are increased mean transit time and decreased blood volume on perfusion-weighted images with increased flow in the periphery of the lesion consistent with reactive hyperemia and elevated lactate on proton magnetic resonance spectroscopy. Ventriculitis can be suspected by MRI as well, with decreased apparent diffusion coefficient values and increased signal of dependent intraventricular fluid on dwi. (*Data from* Refs.[32–35])

Fourth Step: Lumbar Puncture and Associated Serologies

Box 1 summarizes the pearls and pitfalls of infection diagnosis by lumbar puncture and serologic studies. A lymphocyte-predominant meningitis is usually seen in viral, tuberculous, fungal, or noninfectious entities, but the presence of lymphocyte predominance does not exclude bacterial meningitis. Decreased CSF glucose level to less than 40 mg/dL is highly suggestive of bacterial meningitis. Although Gram stain and reduced CSF glucose can be helpful in suggesting bacterial meningitis, cultures take several days and a rapid identification of common bacterial pathogens is greatly needed. Several broad-based multiprobe polymerase chain reactions (PCRs) that can detect bacterial DNA within 3 hours have been reported. Target organisms include *Neisseria, H influenzae, S pneumoniae, Streptococcus Agalactiae,* and *Listeria.*[36–38] PCR is not likely to replace culture, as cultures are needed for antimicrobial sensitivity testing; however, molecular methods have been developed to identify antibiotic resistance to penicillin G in *Neisseria meningitidis* strains.[39] Also, surrogate biomarkers, such as galactomannan, have potential as measures of response to antifungal therapy for *Aspergillus*.[40] C-reactive protein (CRP) is an acute-phase reactant that is a nonspecific marker of inflammation in serum or CSF. Although sensitive, it is not very specific for increased risk of bacterial meningitis. Similarly, elevated serum procalcitonin levels can be seen inconsistently in acute bacterial infection, and there is disagreement about their trustworthiness.[3,6]

Fifth Step: Complications of Meningitis

Acute hydrocephalus occurs in up to 8% of meningitis cases, most commonly in cryptococcal meningitis and other fungal infections (**Fig. 4**). *Listeria* is the bacterial pathogen most likely to cause acute hydrocephalus and this complication confers an unfavorable prognosis.[41] Hydrocephalus can be managed with repeated lumbar punctures or with a ventricular drain.

Hyponatremia caused by salt-wasting, syndrome of inappropriate antidiuretic hormone (SIADH), adrenal insufficiency, or iatrogenic overhydration contribute to altered mental status and should be aggressively managed. Seizures occur in 5% of patients with bacterial meningitis before admission and in 15% during hospitalization. Continuous electroencephalogram (EEG) should be considered in selected patients to detect nonconvulsive status epilepticus, as purely electroencephalographic seizures may explain fluctuating level of consciousness in some patients. In one study, periodic epileptiform discharges were frequent in monitored patients, as were seizures, with one or the other occurring in 48% of patients: more than half of these had no clinical correlate.[42] Whether prophylactic antiepileptic drugs would improve outcome is unknown. Survivors of bacterial meningitis remain at risk for more indolent development of communicating hydrocephalus, cognitive impairment, and sensorineural hearing loss.

LYMPHOCYTE-PREDOMINANT MENINGITIS

It is prudent to retain a large differential for the many causes of lymphocyte-predominant meningitis, which is not exclusively caused by viruses. **Fig. 1** outlines a graduated approach to investigate the syndrome at different levels of likelihood given epidemiologic considerations.

Viral Meningitis

Summer and early autumn are the seasons for many viral meningitides, with enteroviral meningitis group (echo, Coxsackie, and enteroviruses types 68–71) and Lyme

Box 1
Cerebrospinal fluid and serologic diagnostic studies

I. Cerebrospinal Fluid (CSF) Standard: White blood cells with differential, glucose, protein, Gram stain, cryptococcal antigen, directed cultures

1. There is no definite cut off for viral versus bacterial meningitis, although >1000 polymorphonuclear leukocytes (PMNs) suggest bacterial etiology; persistent PMN predominance in some West Nile viruses (WNVs)
2. Procalcitonin and C-reactive protein (CRP) are nonspecific; treatment decisions should not be based on these parameters
3. Glucose <50% that of simultaneous serum glucose ominous: bacteria, some fungi (*Aspergillus*), some viruses (herpes simples virus [HSV], WNV), tuberculosis, cancer, neurosarcoidosis
4. Protein elevation reflects blood-brain barrier disruption and is very nonspecific
5. Gram stain may be negative in bacterial infections
6. Polymerase chain reaction (PCR) utility: good for: HSV 1, 2, 6; Epstein-Barr virus (EBV), cytomegalovirus (CMV), rapid enterovirus; untrustworthy for: varicella zoster virus (VZV), HIV, WNV (only very early), *Borrelia*
7. Broad range and specific meningeal pathogen PCR gaining acceptance
8. Tuberculous meningitis: adenosine deaminase (ADA) variably elevated and not reliable; PCR techniques improving
9. Antibody tests and antibody indices:

    Lyme antibody index

    WNV immunoglobulin (Ig) M, VZV IgM, and IgG antibody index

    Coccidioides immitis complement fixation antibody

    HSV serum: CSF antibody ratio <20:1

10. Antigen: *Histoplasma capsulatum, Cryptococcus neoformans*
11. Other special testing: Venereal Disease Research Laboratory: syphilis Galactomannan *Aspergillus*
12. 14-3-3 protein not specific for Creutzfeldt-Jakob disease: elevated in states of rapid neuronal death

II. Serology Standard: complete blood count and differential, retain acute sera for directed antibody testing

1. Viruses

    Measure IgM and IgG antibodies acute and convalescent (fourfold rise in IgG):

    St. Louis, West Nile, Eastern and Western Equine, Japanese encephalitis, Dengue fever

    EBV (antiviral capsid antigen IgM and IgG and EBV nuclear antigen [EBNA])

    VZV, HSV-1(IgM), rabies, HIV (RNA can be checked early when viral load high but enzyme-linked immunosorbent assay [ELISA] weakly positive or negative)

    Borrelia burgdorferi (see #9 in first part of this list)

2. Tick-borne bacterial

    IgG and IgM by indirect immunofluorescence for Rocky Mountain spotted fever (RMSF)

    Lyme ELISA: confirmatory Western blot

    Ehrlichia antibodies by indirect fluorescent antibody

3. Parasites:

Toxoplasma gondii

a. Absence of IgG or IgM antibodies does not exclude *Toxoplasma* encephalitis in patients with AIDS. If positive in a patient with HIV, treat with pyrimethamine/sulfadiazine and folinic acid (incidence reduced among people receiving prophylaxis with sulfadiazine or dapsone and pyrimethamine against *Pneumocystis jiroveci* pneumonia).

b. If toxoplasma serology negative, check CSF EBV PCR and consider brain biopsy of any accessible mass lesion for lymphoma

Taenia solium (cysticercosis)

ELISA, but 50% with solitary lesions will be seronegative

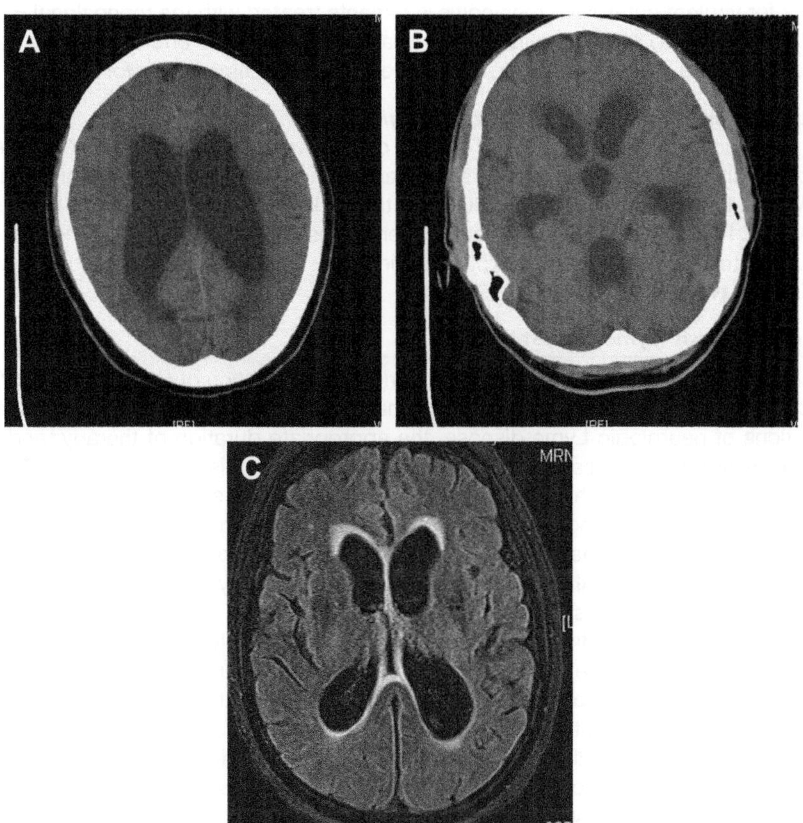

Fig. 4. Acute hydrocephalus complicating meningitis. CT scan of patient with *Coccidiodes immitis* meningitis. Like many such patients with fungal meningitis, this patient required ventriculoperitoneal shunting. The lateral ventricles on the unenhanced CT (*A*) are huge and there is transependymal spread of fluid across the ependymal surface. Lateral third and fourth ventricles are symmetrically enlarged (*B*), demonstrating that circulation of CSF is impeded at the level of the arachnoid villi. (*C*) FLAIR MRI of patient with community-acquired *S pneumoniae* meningitis also with acute hydrocephalus, a poor prognostic sign.

meningitis accounting for many North American cases. HIV seroconversion may be heralded by meningitis with persistent pleocytosis in some patients. Seasonal arthropod-borne viruses, such as West Nile virus (WNV), are concerns in many parts of the United States and the winter season raises the possibility of mumps and lymphocytic choriomeningitis virus (LCMV). Nonseasonal herpesvirus (HSV) type 2 and VZV account for many other cases. Fortunately, HSV type 2 and enteroviral PCRs are quite sensitive and specific and can be used to diagnose this common and usually self-limited illness efficiently.[43] VZV diagnosis is more complex and is summarized both for immunocompetent and immunocompromised patients in **Box 2**. Differential diagnosis includes several noninfectious entities, including sarcoidosis and drug adverse effects (particularly nonsteroidal anti-inflammatory drugs).

Treatment

Treatment of enteroviral meningitis is symptomatic, although in immunocompromised hosts with life-threatening symptoms, pleconaril can be considered.[58] A special group at risk for virulent enteroviral meningitis is patients treated with the monoclonal B-cell antibody rituximab.[59] Herpesviruses are treated with acyclovir 800 mg 5 times daily, famcyclovir 500 mg 3 times daily, or valacyclovir 1 gm 3 times daily for 2 weeks.

Recurring lymphocyte-predominant meningitis

The most common etiology is HSV type 2, often in association with genital herpetic eruption, although many patients are unaware of this infection. Herpes simplex virus (HSV) 2 is treated with acyclovir 100 mg 3 times daily for 5 days if genital herpes is known or 10 days for primary infection Alternatives are famcyclovir 500 mg 3 times daily for 7 to 10 days followed by 250 mg twice daily chronic prophylaxis *or* valacyclovir 500 mg twice daily.

Neuroborreliosis (Lyme Disease)

Neurologic Lyme disease is a potentially serious complication of *Borrelia burgdorferi*. Much confusion exists both in the professional and the lay community about the manifestations of neurologic Lyme disease, the appropriate duration of therapy, and the existence of long-term sequelae of infection. Therefore, this article features **Fig. 6**, a detailed illustration of the appropriate diagnostic process sanctioned by the American Academy of Neurology, to confirm and treat a neurologic syndrome attributable to this organism.[60–66] The most common neurologic sign of Lyme disease is facial palsy, often bilateral. **Table 2**, however, illustrates the myriad of other potentially infection-associated causes of facial palsy.[67,68] Meningitis and radiculitis are other common neurologic syndromes, but brain parenchymal involvement is *rare.* The decision to treat Lyme disease with intravenous (IV) antibiotics versus oral antibiotics is the subject of evolving recommendations, and each institution's infectious disease experts should be consulted for duration of IV treatment.

The current method for diagnosing Lyme neuroborreliosis is demonstration of abnormal CSF with increased leukocyte count, elevated protein, plus intrathecal synthesis of *Borrelia* antibodies. To discriminate between active and past infection can be difficult, as the antibody production can persist for years. Schmidt and colleagues[69] recently showed that measuring CXCL 13, a chemokine that attracts B and T lymphocytes, shows high sensitivity and specificity (100%/90.4%) for acute untreated Lyme disease, a finding that may help mark treatment response and distinguish atypical early cases.

Neurosyphilis

Neurosyphilitic emergencies can present at any time in the course of neurosyphilis. Symptomatic syphilitic meningitis is seen weeks or months to a couple of years

Box 2
Encephalitis and meningoencephalitis

1. Etiology: A significant percentage of cases may remain idiopathic after all appropriate serologic and CSF studies (40%–50%)
2. Radiology: Magnetic resonance imaging (MRI) (fluid-attenuated inversion recovery [FLAIR]) abnormalities in the temporal lobe are found in at least 80% of patients with HSV 1 >48 hours from symptom onset

   VZV may show large/small vessel infarctions but MRI picture also may resemble HSV 1 (**Fig. 5**).

   Flaviviruses (WNV, Eastern Equine Encephalitis, St Louis, Japanese) may show T2 and FLAIR abnormalities in thalami, basal ganglia, and substantia nigra, but, unlike HSV 1, evolution of such abnormalities may be delayed several days
3. PCR Pitfalls:
   a. EBV DNA can be found in peripheral blood mononuclear cells and may be positive in the CNS in many inflammatory disorders; its presence in CSF of immunocompromised hosts *is* significant. EBV acute infection diagnosed by VCA IgM antibodies and absence of antibodies to virus-associated nuclear antigen (EBNA) IgG. In samples collected more than 5 weeks after onset of illness, there should be a decrease in VCA IgG antibody titer and an increase in anti-EBNA IgG.
   b. HSV PCR may be negative in the first 3 days of illness and then remains positive for 2–10 days. CSF antibody becomes positive 8–12 days after illness onset and persists for 30 days. Serum: CSF antibody ratio of less than 20:1 is diagnosis of recent HSV 1 encephalitis.
   c. HIV testing: viral load be very high early on, but PCR IS negative and ELISA weak early on
   d. detection of human herpesvirus 6 (HHV6) in CSF is not definitive evidence that HHV6 is the etiologic organism owing to chromosomal integration
4. Other CSF strategies:
   a. consider repeated cytologies and flow cytometry in suspected malignancy
   b. consider interleukin (IL)-10 in patients with suspected lymphoma (IL-6 elevated in infection and inflammation)
   c. angiotensin-converting enzyme (ACE) level in CSF is of very limited utility
5. Dermatology skin lesions should be biopsied (VZV vs herpes simplex, RMSF, cryptococcus, syphilis, WNV, noninfectious etiologies, such as intravascular lymphoma presenting with fever unknown origin)
6. "New Diseases": consider testing for autoimmune encephalopathies N-methyl-D-aspartate receptor (NMDAR), GluR1/2 alpha-amino3-hydroxy-5-methyl-4-isoxazolepropionic acid receptor (AMPAR), voltage-gated potassium channel (VGKC) antibodies in both children and adults; acute disseminated encephalomyelitis (ADEM) has a different distribution of antecedent infections: measles, group A streptococci, *Mycoplasma pneumoniae*
7. Global Medicine: Read the newspaper and consider travel history for emerging viral infections, often zoonotic pathogens, that cause encephalitis, of which 5 examples follow here:
   a. Toscana virus caused by bites of sand flies: common cause of summer viral meningitis in central Italy
   b. Japanese encephalitis (JE): most common acute viral encephalitis worldwide: half of world population lives where JE can infect; pigs, herons, egrets as amplifying hosts[57]
   c. Paralytic disease can occur with enterovirus 71.[57–59]
   d. Chikungunya virus (togavirus now endemic in India and La Reunion, Zimbabwe, Sri Lanka)

   e. Nipah and Hendra viruses (henipavirus genus of paramyxovirus family: pig farmers, horse workers)

8. Ancillary Studies: Use electroencephalogram (EEG) if fluctuating mental status develops and continue long-term monitoring

9. Empiric Treatment:

   a. Acyclovir 10 mg/kg q8h while investigations under way (**Table 1** for specific therapeutic recommendations).

   b. Consider foscarnet for encephalitis of unknown etiology: 60 mg/kg q8h for 14–21 days.

   c. Consider pleconaril for life-threatening enteroviral meningoencephalitis in immune-compromised patients.

Data from Refs.[44–57]

following primary infection and sometimes causes cranial nerve palsies, including II, IV, VI, VII, and VIII, with acute hearing loss. Skin rash after penile or other genital ulceration and subsequent optic neuritis/neuropathy should raise concern for neurosyphilis, which is included among pathogens presenting with acute infectious visual loss

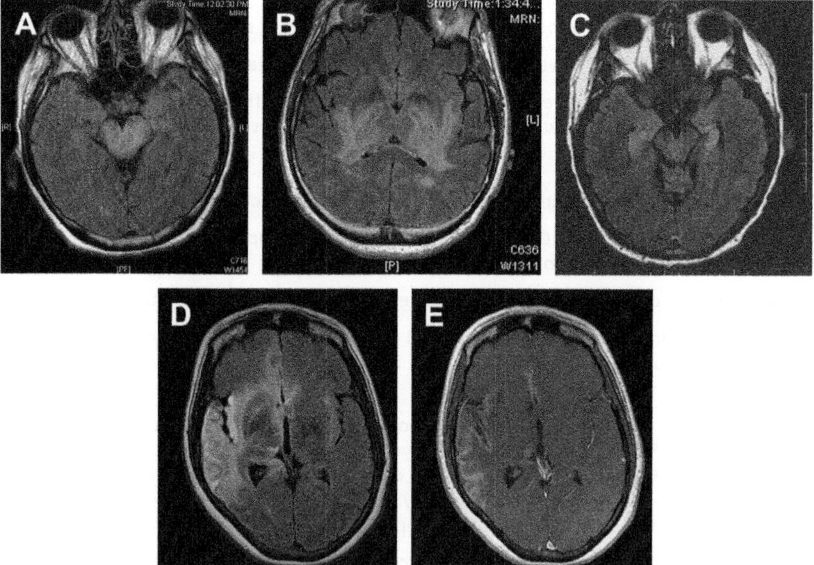

Fig. 5. MRI patterns of viral encephalitis. Although not definitive for specific pathogen and, in fact, as shown in panels *D* and *E*, sometimes misleading, MRI can be helpful. Different characteristic patterns in 3 patients show flavivirus (West Nile virus) or togavirus pattern of brainstem and basal ganglia pathology on FLAIR sequences (*A*, *B*) contrasted with HSV 1 encephalitis with bilateral hippocampal FLAIR abnormality (*C*); and FLAIR (*D*) and gadolinium-enhanced T1 sequences (*E*) of a patient thought to have HSV 1 but who had biopsy-proved varicella zoster virus encephalitis with small vessel vasculitis. There is extensive abnormal FLAIR signal in the right temporal and parietal lobes and genu of corpus callosum, along with sulcal increased FLAIR signal, suggesting proteinaceous fluid (*D*). Compared with the MRI with T1-weighted gadolinium images of *E*, cortical signal looked similar on T1 before gadolinium infusion (not shown), suggesting petechial hemorrhage.

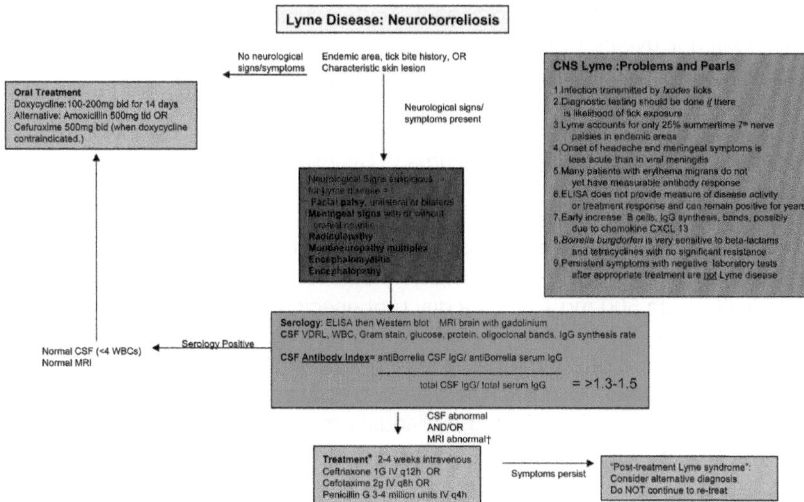

Fig. 6. Diagnosis and treatment of neuroborreliosis. *Some authorities now give 5 to 7 days of IV treatment and followed by change to oral doxycycline for meningitis, cranial neuritis. American Academy of Neurology guidelines recommend 2 weeks of oral or parenteral treatment regimens, but some authorities extend treatment to 4 weeks. †Consider alternative diagnoses if MRI shows only lesions that are nonspecific and CSF negative (see text). (*Data from* Refs.[60–66])

Table 2
Facial nerve palsies: differential diagnosis of infectious processes requiring specific treatment

Most Common Infectious Causes	
Herpes simplex ("Bell palsy"), Borrelia burgdorferi, Varicella zoster virus	
Less Common Infections	**Noninfectious Conditions**
Botulism	Carcinomatous meningitis
Cytomegalovirus[a]	Guillain-Barré syndrome
Epstein-Barr virus	Intranasal influenza vaccine
Diphtheria[b]	Lymphoma meningitis
Guillain-Barré syndrome	Pontine glioma
HIV[a]	Pregnancy
Human herpesvirus 6[a]	Sarcoidosis[b]
Leprosy	Schwannoma
Listeria (rhombencephalitis)	Sjogren
Parotitis/Otitis	
Mucormycosis[a]	
Mycoplasma pneumoniae	
Parotitis	
Syphilis (*Treponema pallidum*)	
Tetanus[b]	
Tuberculosis	

Most common causes are bolded, less common causes listed alphabetically.
[a] Immunocompromised patients.
[b] Often bilateral.

(*Bartonella*, HSV, VZV, CMV, Mucoraceae). Acute ocular manifestations include anterior and posterior uveitis or optic neuritis.[70] Visual deterioration following antibiotic treatment has been ascribed to a Herxheimer reaction, and may require steroids.[71] Among its protean manifestations are convulsive and nonconvulsive status epilepticus; thus, neurosyphilis should be considered in the differential diagnosis of rapidly progressive cognitive change and seizures.[72] Syphilitic meningovasculitis can cause stroke occurring 2 to 5 years after primary infection in patients who do not have HIV.

Diagnosis of neurosyphilis is made by finding a CSF pleocytosis greater than 20, or a reactive CSF-VDRL (Venereal Disease Research Laboratory). Treatment recommendations include penicillin G 3 to 4 μ IV every 4 hours for 2 weeks OR 2.4 procaine intramuscularly (IM) with 500 mg 4 times a day probenecid for 10 to 14 days. Ceftriaxone 2 g IV or IM daily for 10 to 14 days is an alternative. Treatment may be followed with 3 weekly IM injections of 2.4 million units of benzathine penicillin G. CSF should be rechecked at 6 weeks. Outcome is better for patients who are HIV-uninfected, whereas up to 30% of HIV-infected individuals may require retreatment and have residual symptoms.[73]

Cryptococcal Meningitis

Overwhelmingly a disease of the immunocompromised patient (chronic corticosteroids, HIV), immunocompetent individuals also may be at risk for infection with some varieties of the yeast, *Cryptococcus neoformans* var. *gattii*, found in the tropics in decaying heartwood of trees and responsible for recent outbreaks on Vancouver Island in British Columbia and Alberta.[74] Characteristic clinical manifestations in this most common cause of lymphocytic meningitis in patients with HIV are a marked rise in intracranial pressure (ICP) with rapid development of hydrocephalus and visual loss either from invasion of cranial nerves or from sustained elevated pressure. Lung and skin lesions may provide clues.

Repeated lumbar punctures may be necessary to control ICP. Patients are treated with amphotericin 0.7 mg/kg/d or AmBisome (amphotericin B) 5 mg/kg/d with flucytosine 25 mg/kg 4 times daily and 8 to 10 weeks of 400 to 800 mg per day oral fluconazole, followed by 6 months of 200 mg per day in immunocompromised patients.[5,6]

Immune reconstitution inflammatory syndrome

Immune reconstitution inflammatory syndrome (IRIS) refers to the often dramatic and frequently dysfunctional inflammatory response to recent infection after a rapid improvement in the host's immune system, either as a result of withdrawal of immunosuppression or treatment of the underlying immunosuppressive cause, such as AIDS. Thus, it is seen in patients with HIV, in the posttransplant period, or after withdrawal of intense chemotherapy. Neurologists are most likely to encounter IRIS with tuberculous meningitis, cryptococcal meningitis, toxoplasmosis, or PML. Two potentially confusing radiographic pictures should be recognized: (1) diffuse meningeal enhancement with elevated CSF pressure and pleocytosis of several hundred WBCs (**Fig. 7**A)[75] or (2) a mass lesion (see **Fig. 7**B) that can resemble tumor or tumefactive demyelination. Paradoxically, brief courses of corticosteroids can help suppress inflammation and improve outcome.

ENCEPHALITIS: BRAIN PARENCHYMAL DISEASE WITH OR WITHOUT FOCAL SIGNS

More than 100 different agents can cause encephalitis. In the United States, there are about 20,000 reported cases of encephalitis per year, although the actual number is likely larger.[44] The proportion of cases without established etiology in one literature analysis was greater than 50%.[45] Emergency clinical strategy is different from

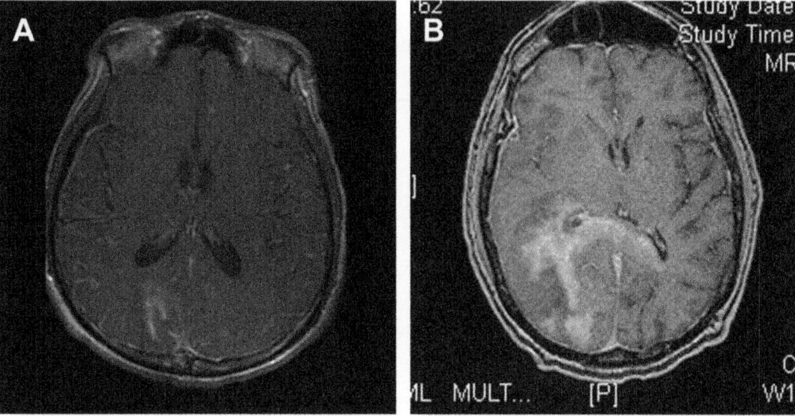

Fig. 7. Two patterns of immune reconstitution inflammatory syndrome (IRIS). (*A*) Gadolinium-enhanced T1-weighted MRI that shows intense leptomeningeal enhancement in a patient recently treated for cryptococcal meningitis who has had rapid rise in CD4 count on antiretroviral therapy and presents with seizures and marked rise in intracranial pressure. (*B*) Gadolinium-enhanced T1-weighted MRI that shows a different HIV-positive patient newly on antiretroviral therapy presenting with hemianopia and a mass lesion resembling high-grade tumor owing to PML with IRIS.

suspected bacterial meningitis, as there are fewer pathogen-specific therapeutic options. In treating a patient with possible encephalitis (defined as 2 or more of the following: fever, CSF pleocytosis, headache, altered mental status, seizures, or focal findings, with or without MRI abnormalities), the short-term goals should be as follows:

1. Treat what is treatable: cover for encephalitis sensitive to acyclovir (HSV, VZV, and possibly EBV) or other antivirals (**Table 3**); consider the possibility that a bacterial cause, such as *Listeria*, *Rickettsia*, or *Borrelia,* requires specific treatment.[46]
2. Provide supportive care with low threshold for continuous EEG monitoring.
3. Use imaging characteristics and epidemiology to dictate specific infectious workup, whereas brain biopsy should be a last resort.
4. Consider autoimmune encephalitis.
5. Save acute serum and CSF for subsequent studies (see **Box 2**).

Unlike bacterial meningitis, viral encephalitis at times can be distinguished by its particular pattern of brain involvement (see **Fig. 5**). Some viruses are likely to produce focal clinical and radiographic signs (John Cunningham [JC] virus, VZV, HSV 1, HHV6), whereas others produce diffuse inflammation. Specific neurotropisms of diagnostic relevance include the following:

1. *Basal ganglia and anterior horn cell infection* with paralytic syndromes and movement disorders are seen with WNV. Other flaviviruses and togaviruses involve preferentially the basal ganglia.
2. *Limbic encephalitis* with memory loss, confusion, and possible seizures or autonomic features is characteristic of HSV types 1 and 6. HSV 1 is the most common nonseasonal encephalitis in North America. HHV6 is associated with the period of engraftment of bone marrow or peripheral blood transplantation.[47] Also targeting mesial temporal structures are some of the antibody-mediated paraneoplastic syndromes such as anti-N-methyl-D-aspartate receptor encephalitis (NMDAR) and antivoltage-gated potassium channel antibody encephalitis

Table 3
Acute infectious encephalitis and possible antiviral treatments

Common	Uncommon
SEASONAL[a] **West Nile virus**	**Eastern equine encephalitis**
Japanese encephalitis[b]	**Western equine encephalitis**
Chikungunya[b]	**Powassan virus**
La Crosse[6]	**Colorado tick virus**
St Louis virus	Naegleria fowleri
Borrelia burgdorferi	Acanthamoeba (Balamuthia mandrillaris)
Rickettsia: Coxiella, Ehrlichia, Babesia	*Leptospirosis*
	LCMV[6]
NONSEASONAL **HSV type 1**[1]	**Rabies**[c]
Varicella zoster[1]	**Cytomegalovirus**[c,2–4]
Epstein-Barr[1,2]	**Mumps**
HIV	**Enteroviruses**[c,5]
Adenoviruses	**HHV6**[c,2+3]
Toxoplasma gondii[c]	*Bartonella henselae*
Cryptococcus neoformans[c]	

[d]*Treatment:* 1 acyclovir, 2 ganciclovir, 3 foscarnet, 4 cidofovir, 5 pleconaril, 6 ribavirin.

No evidence for oral therapy with acyclovir, famciclovir, or valacyclovir, although long-term supplemental oral valacyclovir for HSV encephalitis is in trial.

Bold, viruses; *Italics*, bacteria; Normal font, other (parasites, amoebae, fungi).

Abbreviations: HHV, human herpesvirus; HSV, herpes simplex virus; LCMV, lymphocytic choriomeningitis virus.

[a] Summer/fall except for LCMV in late fall/winter.

[b] Outside North America.

[c] Primarily in HIV or transplant recipient.

[d] Some investigators have recommended Foscarnet 60 mg/kg every 8 hours for 21 days for microbiologically undiagnosed encephalitis.

Data from Refs.[3,5,26,46,54,56,57]

(VGKC).[48] The California Encephalitis Project, as well as other groups, have identified numerous patients with NMDAR antibodies as the likely cause of what was previously deemed infectious encephalitis of unknown cause. Compared with enteroviral, rabies, and HSV 1 encephalitis, these patients were younger, non-white and had lower WBC median CSF cell counts.[49–51] In children, as many as one-third of cases of acute encephalitis are possibly immune-mediated.[52]

CURRENT IMPORTANT ENCEPHALITIC PATHOGENS: NORMAL OR IMMUNOCOMPROMISED HOSTS

West Nile Virus

Most WNV infections are asymptomatic, but 20% of patients develop an acute febrile illness and 1 in 150 develops neuroinvasive disease, including meningitis, encephalitis, and acute flaccid paralysis.[53] These are usually older patients (mean age 60 with vs 46 without neuroinvasive disease) or immunosuppressed patients. A rash may be present, possibly raising diagnostic confusion with Rickettsial diseases.[54] Acute flaccid paralysis, resembling poliomyelitis, is distinctive. Diagnosis is based on serologic testing. Immunoglobulin G (IgG) persists for life, and 18 months after infection, 20% of cases still have detectable IgM. Detection of IgM WNV antibodies in CSF is diagnostic.[55] There is no known specific treatment.[56,76]

Enterovirus 71

Enterovirus 71 is an emerging pathogen with expanding geographic range causing hand-foot-and-mouth disease mostly in children, and neurologic manifestations that include lymphocytic meningitis, encephalitis, and acute flaccid paralysis, as well as transverse myelitis and cerebellitis.[77] Because the geographic range of this RNA virus with a high spontaneous mutation rate is expanding, neurologists and emergency room physicians in North America should be aware of potential cases.[57]

Influenza

Seasonal and nonseasonal influenza is associated with uncommon neurologic complications, including seizures, encephalitis, myositis, and necrotizing encephalopathies. The spectrum and severity of complications of the 2009 H1N1 influenza pandemic are consistent with those of seasonal influenza. Neurologic illness was more frequently reported in children, many of whom had preexisting seizure disorders or other conditions.[78–80]

Varicella Zoster Virus

Varicella zoster virus (VZV) produces a host of neurologic symptoms, both in immunocompromised and in immunocompetent patients (**Box 3**). The most common manifestation is a dermatomal rash but rash is *not* necessary for other complications.[81] Other recognized syndromes include vascular events with a combination of large-vessel and small-vessel strokes and myelopathy. Detection of anti-VZV antibody IgG in the CSF with reduced serum-to-CSF ratio of anti-VZV IgG antibody is the preferred diagnostic test. Alternative tests include anti-VZV IgM in the serum or CSF VZV PCR. CSF IgG antibody is a more sensitive indicator of VZV-related vasculopathy than is PCR.[82,83] Ocular complications can result from trigeminal VZV infection or from retinal necrosis or delayed optic neuropathy.[84,85]

Epstein-Barr Virus

EBV has been associated with a variety of putative neurologic complications in healthy hosts, including meningitis, myelitis, brachial plexitis, and cranial neuritis. A positive EBV PCR in the CSF of healthy hosts does not necessarily represent causal association, although it is significant in immunocompromised patients.[4] Infection usually occurs within weeks of hematopoietic cell transplantation but can present years after transplantation as fulminant lymphoma with multiple contrast-enhancing mass lesions (**Fig. 8**).[86]

An important entity to consider in diffuse or focally abnormal brain MRIs with rapid onset of altered mental status is the posterior reversible encephalopathy syndrome (PRES). Multifocal abnormalities in white matter that resemble encephalitis can occur. The cardinal features include subacute headache, confusion, and seizures, often with cortical visual loss. The MRI picture is consistent with vasogenic edema, primarily in the occipital and parietal lobes, but there are diffuse radiographic presentations, including hemorrhagic lesions and spinal cord involvement. Clinical context dictates evolving diagnostic considerations, as illustrated in **Fig. 8**. The lengthening list of drugs predisposing to PRES includes calcineurin inhibitors, antiangiogenesis agents, and chemotherapeutic drugs.[87]

APPROACH TO THE PATIENT WITH FOCAL CEREBRAL SIGNS OF POSSIBLE INFECTIOUS ORIGIN

Although the bulk of syndromes discussed previously demonstrate presentations dominated by meningeal signs with less prominent focality, much of the differential diagnosis in this section follows from pathogen-suggestive neuroimaging abnormalities outlined on the left-hand side of **Fig. 1**. Of course, many pathogens, notably VZV, assume both patterns.

Box 3
Spectrum of neurologic manifestations of varicella zoster virus

Epidemiology:

- Immunocompetent: usually >60 years
- Immunocompromised: glucocorticoid use, natalizumab, fingolimod, antirejection regimens: calcineurin inhibitors, tumor necrosis factor-α inhibitors

Clinical presentation

- Dermatomal rash or disseminated skin lesions (40% with VZV encephalitis have no history of rash)
- Zoster sine herpete (no rash) occurs in 37% of cases with stroke or meningoencephalitis
- Vasculopathy: transient ischemic attack, ischemic or hemorrhagic stroke
- Segmental motor weakness
- Polyneuritis (cranial nerves [Ramsay Hunt, involving V3 and VII]), lower cranial neuritis (glossopharyngeal, vagus)
- Cerebellar ataxia
- Transverse myelitis
- Necrotizing (acute or progressive outer retinal retinitis, Zoster keratitis)
- Delayed ischemic optic neuropathy after ophthalmic VZV
- Postherpetic neuralgia

Diagnosis:

- Biopsy skin lesions if present
- There may not be CSF pleocytosis
- PCR sensitivity only 30%
- Anti-VZV IgM in serum or CSF, *or*
- VZV DNA by PCR in blood or CSF, *or*
- Anti-VZV IgG in CSF (more often positive in chronic vasculopathy than is PCR) intrathecal synthesis VZV IgG present if: ratio (anti-VZV IgG in CSF/anti-VZV IgG in serum) to (total IgG in CSF/total IgG in serum) ≥1.5

Treatment:

- Acyclovir 10 mg/kg IV q8h × 2 weeks
- Retinal necrosis: ganciclovir and foscarnet
- Postherpetic pain: topical lidocaine, gabapentin, amitriptyline, nortriptyline, desipramine, prega balin, duloxetine; retreatment with IV acyclovir then oral valacyclovir
- Post-VZV encephalitis: check CD4+ count; if <500, consider valacyclovir 500 mg bid chronically

Immunocompetent patients usually have only skin rash in ≤3 dermatomes.

Data from Refs.[81–85]

Progressive Multifocal Leukoencephalopathy

PML, a progressive viral illness caused by papovavirus JC infection, has emerged as an important pathogen. Clinicians should be alert to its varied physical and radiographic manifestations and appropriate workup.[88] Diagnosis is made after suspicious

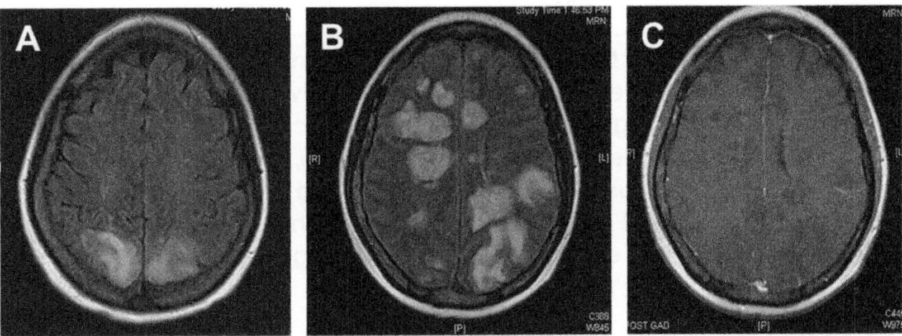

Fig. 8. PRES or infection? Diagnostic confusion illustrated by (*A*), which looks like posterior reversible encephalopathy syndrome (PRES) in a patient 18 days after hematopoietic cell transplantation for acute myelogenous leukemia on cyclosporine. The patient was switched to tacrolimus but continued to worsen over the next month with cytomegalovirus reactivation, graft–versus-host disease, and multifocal FLAIR lesions that enhanced throughout brain ([*B*] FLAIR and [*C*] gadolinium-enhanced T1 sequences) owing to aggressive monoclonal Epstein-Barr virus proliferation producing multicentric lymphoma that was rapidly fatal.

MRI findings lead to CSF PCR for JC virus and brain biopsy is infrequently necessary. Although patients with HIV continue to account for more than 80% of all cases, patients with solid organ and hematopoietic cell transplantation, particularly those taking mycophenolate, and a wide array of patients on immunosuppressives, such as rituximab, natalizumab, and efalizumab for rheumatologic, neurologic, and other conditions, are now recognized as being at risk for PML.[89] Even patients with no discernible prior immunosuppression can develop PML, and the amount of inflammation in such patients may lead to radiographic diagnostic confusion (**Fig. 9**).[90] PML-IRIS further adds to unusual inflammatory lesion development by MRI that can mimic brain tumor (see **Figs. 7** and **9**). Although withdrawal of immune suppression is first-line therapy, emerging strategies include mirtazapine and mefloquine.[85,91]

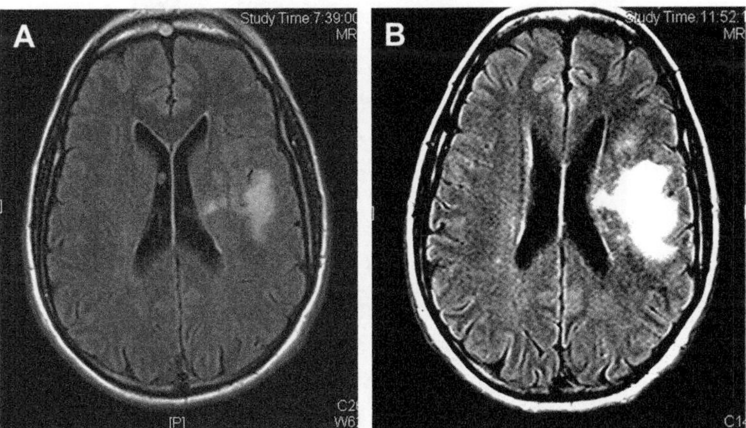

Fig. 9. Rapid progression of progressive multifocal leukoencephalopathy with characteristic white matter abnormality that does not enhance (not shown) in a patient 1 year after HCT for AML. Eighteen days separate (*A*) from (*B*), both FLAIR MRI images. Patient was JC virus positive in CSF.

Brain Abscess

Less common now than in the pre-antibiotic era, brain abscesses are associated, however, with a wider range of organisms than in previous decades. Nonbacterial and uncommon bacterial organisms likely to cause abscess formation in appropriate epidemiologic circumstances include parasites: *T gondii, Taenia solium;* fungi: *Aspergillus*, Mucoraceae, *Histoplasma*, *Candida* species; and bacteria: *Listeria*, *Nocardia*, and *M tuberculosis*. Several of the more common diagnostic and therapeutic emergencies in this category are summarized in the following sections.

Toxoplasma gondii

The most common cause of mass lesions in patients with HIV, this parasitic disease is quite treatable.[16] MRI shows multiple deep microabscesses. Treatment is pyrimethamine 75 to 100 mg/d for 3 to 4 weeks after a 200-mg loading dose, sulfadiazine 1.5 g 4 times a day for 3 to 4 weeks, and folinic acid 10 to 25 mg per day for 3 to 4 weeks. Patients with HIV should continue once-daily trimethoprim/sulfadiazine prophylaxis until the CD4 count exceeds 200.

Neurocysticercosis

Infection of the brain by the larval stage of *T solium* disease is widely prevalent in India, China, and Central and South America, as well as increasingly in the Southwestern United States owing to increasing immigration from seroprevalent areas. MRI is usually suggestive of a scolex (**Fig. 10**). Solitary cysticercus granuloma treatment and steroid use are ongoing areas of therapeutic controversy. The duration of antiseizure treatment may depend on persistence of enhancing lesions and long-term seizure outcome is generally good. If there is residual calcific residue, anti-epileptic drugs likely should be continued.[92] Phenytoin and carbamazepine should be avoided, as they increase metabolism of praziquantel and albendazole.

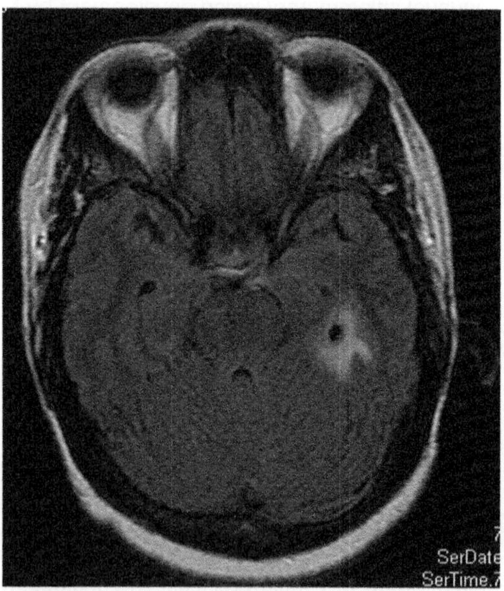

Fig. 10. A 46-year-old patient with new-onset seizure. A Haitian native, the patient was last there more than a decade earlier. Isolated cysticercus scolex seen with small amount of surrounding vasogenic edema on FLAIR MRI image.

Bacterial brain abscess

Postoperative bone infections or paranasal, ear, and pharyngeal infections, as well as pulmonary arteriovenous malformations, dental surgery, endometrial biopsy, and sepsis are all predisposing conditions.[93] Microbiology depends on source: *S aureus* is the most common pathogen postoperatively or after trauma. When the source is hematogenous spread from endocarditis, or urosepsis, *Streptococcus anginosus* (formerly *Streptococcus milleri*), and *Streptococcus viridans* are the culprits, whereas anaerobes (*Bacteroides*, *Peptostreptococcus*, *Actinomyces*, *Fusobacterium*) predominate in lung sources. Enteric gram-negative bacilli often recovered with gastrointestinal or urologic sources. *Pseudomonas* should be considered when ear infections are the source.[4] Empiric coverage should cover gram-positive, gram-negative, and anaerobic organisms (third-generation or fourth-generation cephalosporins and metronidazole). Vancomycin and carbapenems can be used in place of cephalosporins and metronidazole. Surgical intervention is considered in lesions of larger than 2.5 cm, although some abscesses may be drained without open craniotomy.[94] Some authorities believe steroids can be used briefly to control edema.[95] Prophylactic antiepileptic drugs are not recommended.

Subdural empyema, a surgical emergency, is defined as purulent infection between the dura and arachnoid membranes and has risk factors and pathogenesis similar to those of brain abscess.[4] Clinical signs include headache and rapid deterioration in mental status, and CT and/or MRI are often suggestive (**Fig. 11**). Risk factors are similar to those of brain abscess.[96] Lumbar puncture is generally inadvisable because of the risk of raised intracranial pressure.

Infective Endocarditis

Infective endocarditis (IE) in the twenty-first century remains a disease of high morbidity and mortality. In much of the world, IE is no longer a subacute or chronic disease of patients with rheumatic valvular damage, but targets those with degenerative valve disease or prosthetic valves and drug abusers. An important emerging population at risk is patients with health care contact. Current in-hospital mortality

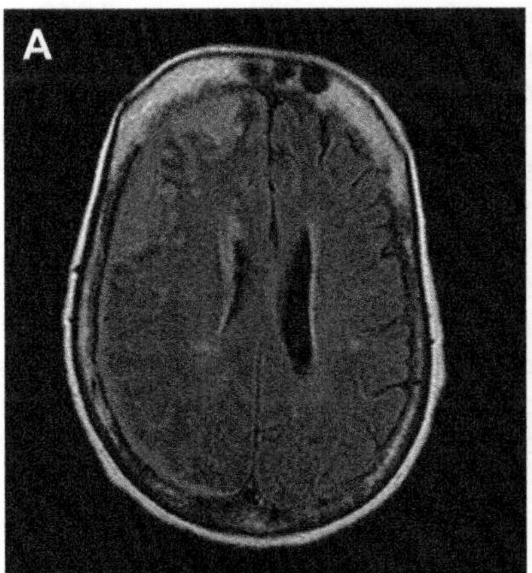

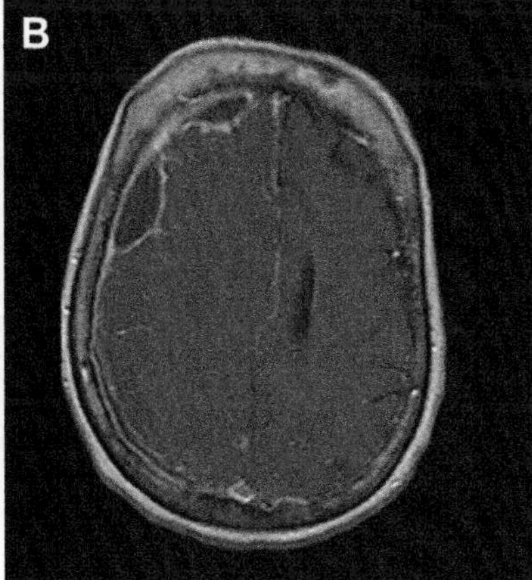

Fig. 11. Patient with long-standing systemic lupus erythematosus on prednisone and azathioprine presented with headache and fever. MRI FLAIR (*A*) shows extradural signal hyperintensity layering along the subdural space. There is intense dural enhancement on the gadolinium image (*B*).

for patients with IE is 14% to 20%.[97] In a recent international survey of 2781 adults with definite IE from 2000 to 2005, the median age was 57.9. Native valve involvement was seen in 72%, recent health care exposure history was elicited in one-quarter of these patients, and *S aureus* was the most common pathogen, whereas culture results were negative in 10%. The most common predisposing conditions were valvular heart disease and about 10% were associated with IV drug abuse. *S aureus* was the causative organism in 68% of drug abusers. *S aureus* and *viridans* streptococci accounted for 28% and 21% of cases respectively in nondrug users.[98]

Neurologic complications continue to contribution to the morbidity and mortality of IE. In the study described above[98], the 16.9% stroke incidence remained stable compared with studies from more than 3 decades ago.[99] We now know, however, that MRI abnormalities are extraordinarily common, as recently demonstrated in a study in which all patients with suspected IE had an admission MRI. Eight-two percent of MRIs done in the first 5 days in hospital were abnormal. MRI helped to diagnose IE by Duke criteria or alter therapeutic decision making in a substantial proportion of patients, although whether this altered the course or outcome of IE remains to be seen.[100] We recommend at least CT or preferably MRI in any patient with suspected IE and altered mental status or focal findings. CT angiography can be done if renal function permits, and MR angiography also may disclose aneurysms. Early surgery decreases mortality.[101]

APPROACH TO THE PATIENT WITH FOCAL FINDINGS SUGGESTIVE OF SPINAL CORD OR PERIPHERAL PROCESSES

Emergency neurologic consultations for rapid onset of dysfunction localizing to the spinal cord raise extensive diagnostic considerations for infection-associated processes with cord tropisms.[102] These include myelitis or postinfectious demyelination with an array of etiologies that can include EBV, *Mycoplasma pneumoniae*, *Treponema pallidum*, and unidentified viruses. Cytomegalovirus can produce a cauda equina inflammatory syndrome. WNV produces an anterior horn syndrome, enterovirus 71 produces a similar picture, and schistosomiasis can invade the cord. Important viral myelitis pathogens include acute VZV and HSV 2, whereas longitudinally extensive intramedullary enhancing lesions of neuromyelitis optica (NMO) and sarcoidosis may mimic infection. Treatment with intravenous acyclovir (see **Table 1**) during workup for causes of myelitis is prudent.

Bacterial spinal epidural abscess is a medical and surgical emergency. Patients present with back pain and point tenderness with or without fever and sometimes in the absence of neurologic abnormalities on initial examination. Patients at risk for spinal epidural abscess often have underlying illnesses, such as diabetes, chronic renal failure, or malignancy. Main routes of infection are hematogenous (prior soft tissue infections or urinary tract or pulmonary infections), contiguous spread from osteomyelitis or muscle abscess, skin punctures through intravenous drug abuse or furuncles, and iatrogenic through invasive procedures on the spine, such as epidural catheters and spinal surgery.[103,104] Common organisms are *S aureus*, gram-negative rods, streptococci, and, *M tuberculosis*.

Management

Lumbar puncture should be avoided because of infection dissemination risk. Four to 6 weeks of antibiotics after immediate decompressive laminectomy are required with vancomycin and antibiotics targeting gram-negative bacilli (piperacillin-tazobactam, cefotaxime, and meropenem). If patients have sensitivity to beta lactam agents, then levofloxacin or aztreonam may be used[83] with subsequent choice of grafting procedure by the neurosurgeon.[105] Prognosis is guarded, with mortality still at 5% to 20%, and complete recovery without neurologic impairments in only 45% of patients.[106] Negative prognostic factors include MRSA infection, motor deficits, elevated CRP, age older than 50, cervical and thoracic as opposed to lumbar area involvement, sepsis, delayed diagnosis and treatment, diabetes, and rheumatoid arthritis, as well as prior spinal surgery.[107]

Pyomyositis

Since the first reports 40 years ago, recognized cases of pyomyositis have increased rapidly and come to neurologists' attention because of pain and weakness. Pyomyositis is heralded by cramping and pain followed by signs of localized tenderness and edema, often in a febrile neutropenic patient and usually without muscle enzyme elevation. Originally described in the tropics, it usually involves transient bacteremia in the setting of preexisting or concurrent muscle injury elicited in more than one-third of the patients. Nearly half have at least one underling disease, such as HIV, diabetes, hematologic malignancies with or without stem cell transplantation, solid cancers, rheumatologic disorders, cirrhosis, or renal insufficiency, it also can be seen in previously healthy patients, often with a history of prior skin infection and in these instances muscle pain in back, buttocks, thighs, or calves can be a critical clue to sepsis.[108] *S aureus* is the most commonly implicated pathogen, and now up to three-fourths of community-acquired strands may be methicillin-resistant (MRSA, strain USA 300), producing an array of new presentations, such as pneumonia with early cavitation, and crops of pustular or vesicular skin lesions.[109] *Escherichia coli*, often fluoroquinolone-resistant, is the most common cause of nosocomial gram-negative bacteremia, both among patients with and those without cancer.[110] This pathogen is emerging as a major myositis culprit in patients with hematologic malignancies.[111] Compared with previously healthy patients, patients with pyomyositis with underling medical conditions have a higher rate of gram-negative infections.[112] MRI shows diffusely abnormal T2 in muscles consistent with edema and aids with rapid diagnosis, leading to prompt debridement and aggressive antimicrobial therapy.

SUMMARY

1. Neurologic infectious diseases remain a significant cause of morbidity and mortality, affecting both healthy hosts and those with HIV and immunosuppression from chemotherapy. There is a growing spectrum of pathogens and their clinical presentations. Timely diagnosis is essential to ensure good-quality survival.
2. Bacterial meningitis etiology differs by age group and site of acquisition. *Streptococcus pneumoniae* remains both the most common community-acquired pathogen in adults and the form with the highest mortality. Dexamethasone reduces mortality in adults with this pathogen.
3. More than half of encephalitis cases remain without definitive etiology and many may be caused by immune-mediated mechanisms, such as NMDAR or VGKC encephalitides.
4. PRES and IRIS are 2 mimes of infection that should be considered in the differential diagnosis of PML, itself a disease now diagnosed in many immune-suppressed patients beyond the HIV population.
5. Indications for neurosurgical intervention for NID treatment include acute hydrocephalus in bacterial or fungal meningitis, brain abscess drainage, subdural

empyema, epidural spinal abscess, and suspected infection of unknown etiology after appropriate serologic and CSF studies.

REFERENCES

1. Tan K, Patel S, Gandhi N, et al. Burden of neuroinfectious diseases on the neurology service in a tertiary care center. Neurology 2008;71:1160–6.
2. Ziai WC, Lewin JJ III. Update in the diagnosis and management of central nervous system infections. Neurol Clin 2008;26:427–68.
3. Roos K, Tyler KL. Meningitis, encephalitis, brain abscess and empyema. In: Hauser SL, Josephson SA, editors. Harrison's neurology in clinical medicine. 2nd edition. New York: McGraw-Hill; 2010. p. 451–83.
4. Honda H, Warren DK. Central nervous system infections: meningitis and brain abscess. Infect Dis Clin North Am 2009;23:609–23.
5. Mace SE. CNS infections as a cause of an altered mental status? What is the pathogen growing in your CNS? Emerg Med Clin North Am 2010;28:535–70.
6. Fitch MT, Abrahamian FM, Moran GJ, et al. Emergency department management of meningitis and encephalitis. Infect Dis Clin North Am 2008;22:33–52.
7. Rincon F, Badjatia N. CNS infections in the neurointensive care unit. Curr Treat Options Neurol 2006;8:135–44.
8. Hasbun R, Abrahams J, Jekel J, et al. Computed tomography of the head before lumbar puncture in adults with suspected meningitis. N Engl J Med 2001;345: 1727–33.
9. Van de Beek D, de Gans J, Spanjaard L, et al. Clinical features and prognostic factors in adults with bacterial meningitis. N Engl J Med 2004;351:1849–59.
10. Durand ML, Calderwood SB, Weber DJ, et al. Acute bacterial meningitis in adults. A review of 493 episodes. N Engl J Med 1993;328:21–8.
11. Brivet FG, Ducuing S, Jacobs F, et al. Accuracy of clinical presentation for differentiating bacterial from viral meningitis in adults: a multivariate approach. Intensive Care Med 2005;31:1654–60.
12. Safdieh JE, Mead PA, Sepkowitz A, et al. Bacterial and fungal meningitis in patients with cancer. Neurology 2008;70:943–7.
13. Cabellos C, Verdquer R, Olmo M, et al. Community-acquired bacterial meningitis in elderly patients: experience over 30 years. Medicine 2009;88:115–9.
14. Kourbeti IS, Jacobs AV, Koslow M, et al. Risk factors associated with postcraniotomy meningitis. Neurosurgery 2007;60:317–25.
15. Pizon AF, Bonner MR, Want HE, et al. Ten years of clinical experience with adult meningitis at an urban academic medical center. J Emerg Med 2006;30:367–70.
16. Walker M, Zunt JR. Parasitic CNS infections in immunocompromised hosts. Clin Infect Dis 2005;40:1005–15.
17. Saiz A, Graus F. Neurologic complications of hematopoietic cell transplantation. Semin Neurol 2010;30:287–95.
18. Rosenfeld MR, Pruitt AA. Neurologic complications of bone marrow, stem cell, and organ transplantation in patients with cancer. Semin Oncol 2006;33:352–61.
19. Pruitt AA. Central nervous system infections in cancer patients. Semin Neurol 2010;30:296–310.
20. Van de Beek D, de Gans J, McIntyre P, et al. Corticosteroids for acute bacterial meningitis. Cochrane Database Syst Rev 2007;1:CD004405.
21. Van de Beek D, Farrar JJ, de Gans J, et al. Adjunctive dexamethasone in bacterial meningitis: a meta-analysis of individual patient data. Lancet Neurol 2010;9: 254–63.

22. Tunkel AR, Hartman BJ, Kaplan SL, et al. Practice guidelines for the management of bacterial meningitis. Clin Infect Dis 2004;39:1267–84.
23. Nudelman Y, Tunkel AR. Bacterial meningitis: epidemiology, pathogenesis and management update. Drugs 2009;69:2577–96.
24. Brouwer MC, Heckenberg SG, de Gans J, et al. Nationwide implementation of adjunctive dexamethasone therapy for pneumococccal meningitis. Neurology 2010;75:1533–9.
25. Ricard JD, Wolff M, Lacherade JC, et al. Levels of vancomycin in CSF of adult patients receiving adjunctive corticosteroids to treat pneumococcal meningitis: a prospective multicenter observational study. Clin Infect Dis 2007;44:250–5.
26. Kamei S, Seikizawa T, Shiota H, et al. Evaluation of combination therapy using acyclovir and corticosteroids in adult patients with HSV encephalitis. J Neurol Neurosurg Psychiatry 2005;76:1544–9.
27. Abba K, Ramaratnam S, Ranganathan LN. Antihelmintics for people with neurocysticercosis. Cochrane Database Syst Rev 2010;3:CD000215.
28. Thwaites GE, Nguyen DB, Nguyen HD, et al. Dexamethasone for the treatment of tuberculous meningitis in adolescents and adults. N Engl J Med 2004;351: 1741–51.
29. Sinner SW. Approach to the diagnosis and management of tuberculous meningitis. Curr Infect Dis Rep 2010;12:291–8.
30. Prasad K, Singh MB. Corticosteroids for managing tuberculous meningitis. Cochrane Database Syst Rev 2008;1:CD002244.
31. Chapman AS, Bakken JS, Folk SM, et al. Diagnosis and management of tickborne rickettsial diseases: rocky mountain spotted fever, ehrlichioses, and anaplasmosis—United States: a practical guide for physicians and other health-care and public health professionals. MMWR Recomm Rep 2006; 55(RR-4):1–27.
32. Cahill DP, Barker FG, Davis KR, et al. Case 10-2010: a 37-year-old woman with weakness and a mass in the brain. Case records MGH. N Engl J Med 2010;362: 1326–33.
33. Kastrup O, Wanke I, Maschke M. Neuroimaging of infections of the central nervous system. Semin Neurol 2008;28:511–22.
34. Ben Salem D, Peruse de Montclos E, Couaillier JF, et al. Urgences neuroradiologiques en pathologie infectieuse. J Neuroradiol 2004;31:301–12.
35. Hong JT, Son BC, Sun JH, et al. Significance of diffusion-weighted imaging and apparent diffusion coefficient maps for the evaluation of pyogenic ventriculitis. Clin Neurol Neurosurg 2008;110:137–44.
36. Van Gastel E, Bruynseels P, Verstrepen W, et al. Evaluation of a real-time PCR assay for the diagnosis of pneumococcal and meningococcal meningitis in a tertiary care hospital. Eur J Clin Microbiol Infect Dis 2007;26:651–3.
37. Rothman R, Ramachandran P, Yang S, et al. Use of quantitative broad-based polymerase chain reaction for detection and identification of common bacterial pathogens in cerebrospinal fluid. Acad Emerg Med 2010;17:741–7.
38. Hedberg ST, Olcen P, Fredlung H, et al. Real-time PCR detection of five prevalent bacteria causing acute meningitis. APMIS 2009;117:856–60.
39. Taha MK, Vazquez JA, Hong E, et al. Target gene sequencing to characterize the penicillin G susceptibility of *Neisseria meningitides*. Antimicrobial Agents Chemother 2007;51:2784–92.
40. Chen SC, Kontoyiannis DP. New molecular and surrogate biomarker-based tests in the diagnosis of bacterial and fungal infection in febrile neutropenic patients. Curr Opin Infect Dis 2010;23:567–77.

41. Kasanmoentalib ES, Brouwer MC, Van der Ende A, et al. Hydrocephalus in adults with community acquired bacterial meningitis. Neurology 2010;75:918–23.
42. Carrera E, Claassen J, Oddo ML, et al. Continuous electroencephalographic monitoring of critically ill patients with CNS infections. Arch Neurol 2008;65: 1612–8.
43. Kost CB, Rogers B, Oberste S, et al. Multicenter beta trial of the GeneXpert enterovirus assay. J Clin Microbiol 2007;45:1081–6.
44. Granerod J, Cunningham R, Zuckerman M, et al. Causality in acute encephalitis: defining aetiologies. Epidemiol Infect 2010;138:783–800.
45. Granerod J, Tam CC, Crowcroft NS, et al. Challenge of the unknown: a systematic review of acute encephalitis in non-outbreak situations. Neurology 2010;75: 924–32.
46. Tunkel AR, Glaser CA, Bloch KC, et al, Infectious Diseases Society of America. The management of encephalitis: clinical practice guidelines by the Infectious Diseases Society of America. Clin Infect Dis 2008;47:303–27.
47. Seeley WW, Marth FM, Holmes TM, et al. Post-transplant acute limbic encephalitis. Neurology 2007;69:156–65.
48. Vincent A, Buckley C, Schott JM, et al. Potassium channel antibody-associated encephalopathy: a potentially immunotherapy-responsive form of limbic encephalitis. Brain 2004;127(pt 3):701–12.
49. Prüss H, Dalmau J, Harms L, et al. Retrospective analysis of NMDA receptor antibodies in encephalitis of unknown origin. Neurology 2010;75:1735–9.
50. Gable MS, Gaval S, Radner A, et al. Anti-NMDA receptor encephalitis: report of ten cases and comparison with viral encephalitis. Eur J Clin Microbiol Infect Dis 2009;28:1421–9.
51. Glaser CA, Honarmand S, Anderson L, et al. Beyond viruses: clinical profiles and etiologies associated with encephalitis. Clin Infect Dis 2006;43:1565–77.
52. Florance NR, Davis RL, Lam C, et al. Anti-N-methyl-D-aspartate receptor (NMDAR) encephalitis in children and adolescents. Ann Neurol 2009;66:11–8.
53. Petersen LR, Hayes EB. West Nile virus in the Americas. Med Clin North Am 2008;92:1307–22.
54. Reznicek JE, Mason WJ, Kaul DR, et al. Avoiding a rash diagnosis. N Engl J Med 2011;364:466–71.
55. Davis LE, DeBiasi R, Goade DE, et al. West Nile virus neuroinvasive disease. Ann Neurol 2006;60:286–300.
56. Solomon T, Hart IJ, Beeching NJ. Viral encephalitis: a clinician's guide. Pract Neurol 2007;7:288–305.
57. Tyler KL. Emerging viral infections of the CNS parts I and II. Arch Neurol 2009; 66:939–48, 1065–74.
58. Desmond RA, Accortt NA, Talley L, et al. Enteroviral meningitis: natural history and outcome of pleconaril therapy. Antimicrobial Agents Chemother 2006;50: 2409–14.
59. Ganjoo KN, Raman R, Sobel RA, et al. Opportunistic enteroviral meningoencephalitis: an unusual treatable complication of rituximab therapy. Leuk Lymphoma 2009;50:673–5.
60. Halperin JJ, Shapiro ED, Logigian EL, et al. Practice parameter: treatment of nervous system Lyme disease. Neurology 2007;69:91–102.
61. Halperin JJ. Nervous system Lyme disease. J R Coll Physicians Edinb 2010; 40(3):248–55.
62. Blanc F, Jaulhac B, Fleury M, et al. Relevance of the antibody index to diagnose Lyme neuroborreliosis among seropositive patients. Neurology 2007;69:953–8.

63. Lantos PM, Charini WA, Medoff G, et al. Final report of the Lyme disease review panel of the Infectious Diseases Society of America. Clin Infect Dis 2010;51:1–5.
64. Wormser GP, Dattwyler RJ, Shapiro ED, et al. The clinical assessment, treatment, and prevention of Lyme disease, human granulocytic anaplasmosis, and babesiosis: clinical practice guidelines by the Infectious Diseases Society of America. Clin Infect Dis 2006;41:1089–134.
65. Fallon BA, Keilp JG, Corbera KM, et al. A randomized, placebo-controlled trial of repeated IV antibiotic therapy for Lyme encephalopathy. Neurology 2008;70: 992–1003.
66. Feder HM, Johnson BJ, O'Connell S, et al. A critical appraisal of chronic Lyme disease. N Engl J Med 2007;357:422–30.
67. Gleeson T, Etienne M. Cranial nerve VII palsy as the first sign of cephalic tetanus after an earthquake. Arch Neurol 2011;68:536–7.
68. Yis U, Kurul SH, Cakmakci H, et al. *Mycoplasma pneumoniae*: nervous system complications in childhood and review of the literature. Eur J Pediatr 2008;167: 973–8.
69. Schmidt C, Plate A, Angele B, et al. A prospective study on the role of CXCL13 in Lyme neuroborreliosis. Neurology 2011;76:1051–8. Accompanying editorial: Tuman H, David D. Are high CSF levels of CXCL 13 helpful for diagnosis of Lyme neuroborreliosis? Neurology 2011;76:1036–7.
70. Pless ML, Korshinsky D, LaRocque RC, et al. Case records of the MGH. Case 26-2010: a 54-year-old man with loss of vision and a rash. N Engl J Med 2010;363:865–74.
71. Kiss S, Damico FM, Young LH. Ocular manifestations and treatment of syphilis. Semin Ophthalmol 2005;20:161–7.
72. Marra CM. Update on neurosyphilis. Curr Infect Dis Rep 2009;11:127–34.
73. Ghanem KG, Moore RD, Rompalo AM, et al. Neurosyphilis in a clinical cohort of HIV-1-infected patients. AIDS 2008;22:1145–51.
74. Bestard J, Siddiqi ZA. Cryptococcal meningoencephalitis in immunocompetent patients: changing trends in Canada. Neurology 2010;74:1233–4.
75. Airas L, Paivarinta M, Roytta M, et al. Central nervous system immune reconstitution inflammatory syndrome (IRIS) after hematopoietic stem cell transplantation. Bone Marrow Transplant 2009;34:1–4.
76. Granwehr BP, Lillibridge KM, Higgs S, et al. West nile virus: where are we now? Lancet Infect Dis 2004;4:547–56.
77. Ooi MH, Wong SC, Pidin Y, et al. Human enterovirus 71 disease in Sarawak, Malaysia: a prospective clinical, virological and molecular epidemiological study. Clin Infect Dis 2007;44:646–56.
78. Ekstrand JJ, Herener A, Rawlings J, et al. Heightened neurologic complications in children with pandemic H1N1 influenza. Ann Neurol 2010;68:762–6.
79. Kedia S, Stroud B, Parsons J, et al. Pediatric neurological complications of 2009 pandemic influenza A (H1N1). Arch Neurol 2011;68:455–62.
80. Augarten A, Aderka D. Alice in wonderland syndrome in H1N1 influenza. Pediatr Emerg Care 2011;27:120.
81. Nagel MA, Gilden DH. The protean neurologic manifestations of varicella-zoster virus infection. Cleve Clin J Med 2007;74:489–94.
82. Nagel MA, Cohrs RJ, Mahalingam R, et al. The varicella zoster virus vasculopathies: clinical, CSF, imaging and virologic features. Neurology 2008;70:853–60.
83. Gilden D, Cohrs RJ, Mahalingam R, et al. Varicella zoster virus vasculopathies: diverse clinical manifestations, laboratory features, pathogenesis, and treatment. Lancet Neurol 2009;8:731–40.

84. Nakamoto BK, Dorotheo EU, Biousse V, et al. Progressive outer retinal necrosis presenting with isolated optic neuropathy. Neurology 2004;63:2423–5.
85. Salazar R, Russman AN, Nagel MA, et al. Varicella zoster virus ischemic optic neuropathy and subclinical temporal artery involvement. Arch Neurol 2011;68: 517–20.
86. Ahmad I, Cau NV, Kwan J, et al. Preemptive management of Epstein-Barr virus reactivation after hematopoietic stem-cell transplantation. Transplantation 2009; 8:140–5.
87. Fugate JF, Claasen DO, Cloft HJ. Posterior reversible encephalopathy syndrome: associated clinical and radiologic findings. Mayo Clin Proc 2010;85:427–32.
88. Aksamit AJ. Progressive multifocal leukoencephalopathy. Curr Treat Options Neurol 2008;10:178–85.
89. Carson KB, Evens AM, Richey EA, et al. Progressive multifocal leukoencephalopathy after rituximab therapy in HIV-negative patients: a report of 57 cases from the Research on Adverse Drug Events and Reports project. Blood 2009; 113:4834–40.
90. Gheuens S, Pierone G, Peeters P, et al. Progressive multifocal leukoencephalopathy in individuals with minimal or occult immunosuppression. J Neurol Neurosurg Psychiatr 2010;81:247–54.
91. Brickelmaiaer M, Lugovskoy A, Kartikeyan R, et al. Identification and characterization of mefloquine efficacy against JC virus in vitro. Antimicrobial Agents Chemother 2009;53:1840–9.
92. Singh G, Rajshekhar V, Murthy JM, et al. A diagnostic and therapeutic scheme for a solitary cysticercus granuloma. Neurology 2010;75:2236–45.
93. Bernardini GL. Diagnosis and management of brain abscess and subdural empyema. Curr Neurol Neurosci Rep 2004;4:448–56.
94. Tseng JH, Tseng MY. Brain abscess in 142 patients: factors influencing outcome and mortality. Surg Neurol 2006;65:557–62.
95. Hakan T, Cerana N, Erdem I, et al. Bacterial brain abscesses: an evaluation of 96 cases. J Infect 2006;52:359–66.
96. Osborn MK, Steinberg JP. Subdural empyema and other suppurative complications of paranasal sinusitis. Lancet Infect Dis 2007;7:662–7.
97. Cabell CH, Jollis JG, Peterson GE, et al. Changing patient characteristics and the effect on mortality in endocarditis. Arch Intern Med 2002;162:90–4.
98. Murdoch DR, Corey GR, Hoen B, et al. Clinical presentation, etiology and outcome of infective endocarditis in the 21st century. Arch Intern Med 2009; 169:463–73.
99. Pruitt AA, Rubin RH, Karchmer AW, et al. Neurological complications of bacterial endocarditis. Medicine (Baltimore) 1978;57:329–43.
100. Duval X, Lung B, Kelin I, et al. Effect of early clinical MR imaging on clinical decisions in infective endocarditis. Ann Intern Med 2010;152:497–504.
101. Vikram HR, Buencosejo J, Hasbun R, et al. Impact of valve surgery on 6-month mortality in adults with complicated, left-sided native valve endocarditis: a propensity analysis. JAMA 2003;290:3207–14.
102. Jacob A, Weinshenker BG. An approach to the diagnosis of acute transverse myelitis. Semin Neurol 2008;28:105–20.
103. Darouiche RO. Spinal epidural abscess. N Engl J Med 2006;355:2012–20.
104. Pradilla G, Nagahama Y, Spivak AM, et al. Spinal epidural abscess: current diagnosis and management. Curr Infect Dis Rep 2010;12:484–91.
105. Sendi P, Bregenzer T, Zimmerli W. Spinal epidural abscess in clinical practice. QJM 2008;101:1–12.

106. Reihsaus E, Waldbaur H, Seeling W. Spinal epidural abscess: a meta-analysis of 915 patients. Neurosurg Rev 2000;23:175–204.
107. Pradilla G, Ardila GP, Hsu W, et al. Epidural abscesses of the CNS. Lancet Neurol 2009;8:292–300.
108. Moellering RC Jr, Abbott GF, Ferraro MJ. Case Records of the MGH. Case 2-2011: a 30-year-old woman with shock after treatment of a furuncle. N Engl J Med 2011;364:266–75.
109. Moellering RC Jr. The growing menace of community-acquired methicillin-resistant *Staphylococcus aureus*. Ann Intern Med 2006;144:368–70.
110. Wisplinghoff H, Bischoff T, Tallent SM, et al. Nosocomial bloodstream infections in US hospitals: analysis of 24,179 cases from a prospective nationwide surveillance study. Clin Infect Dis 2004;39:309–17.
111. Vigil KJ, Johnson JR, Johnston BD, et al. *E coli* pyomyositis: an emerging infectious disease among patients with hematologic malignancies. Clin Infect Dis 2010;50:374–80.
112. Crum NF. Bacterial pyomyositis in the United States. Am J Med 2004;117:420–8.

Neuromuscular Disorders and Acute Respiratory Failure: Diagnosis and Management

Kourosh Rezania, MD[a,*], Fernando D. Goldenberg, MD[a], Steven White, MD[b]

KEYWORDS

• Neuromuscular • Respiratory failure • ALS • Myasthenia gravis • Guillain-Barré • CIDP • Critical illness myopathy

The diagnostic approach to a patient with respiratory failure starts with the determination of whether the respiratory failure is the result of a cardiopulmonary disease versus a primary neurologic disorder. The latter can occur in the setting of either a central nervous system (CNS) disease such as cervical myelopathy, lower brainstem injury, or diffuse bihemispheric involvement, or a neuromuscular disease (NMD). This review focuses on NMDs that result in respiratory impairment because of weakness of the respiratory muscles.

An NMD may result in respiratory weakness when there is impaired function of a large proportion of the motor units that innervate the respiratory muscles. A motor unit is referred to a motor neuron (located in the anterior horn cells of the spinal cord or the motor nuclei of the cranial nerves in the medulla and pons), its axon, and all the myofibers that it innervates (**Fig. 1**). Neuromuscular weakness may also result from diseases that primarily affect the myofiber plasma membrane or its contractile apparatus.[1]

PATHOPHYSIOLOGY

NMDs often present with acute or subacute respiratory weakness and a rapidly evolving respiratory failure. On the other hand, the more indolent NMDs may also

This work has not been supported by a grant.
The authors have nothing to disclose.

[a] Department of Neurology, The University of Chicago Medical Center, 5841 South Maryland Avenue, MC 2030, Chicago, IL 60637, USA
[b] Department of Medicine, The University of Chicago Medical Center, 5841 South Maryland Avenue, MC 6076, Chicago, IL 60637, USA
* Corresponding author.
E-mail address: krezania@neurology.bsd.uchicago.edu

Neurol Clin 30 (2012) 161–185
doi:10.1016/j.ncl.2011.09.010 **neurologic.theclinics.com**
0733-8619/12/$ – see front matter

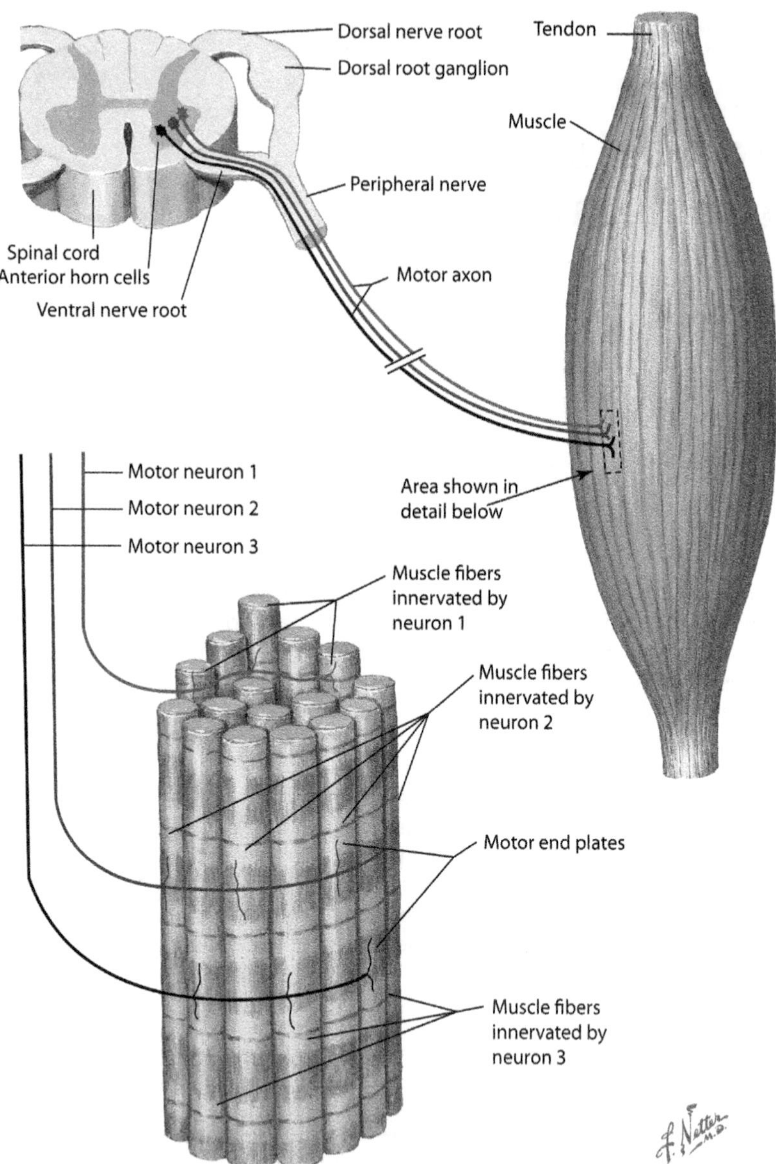

Fig. 1. A motor unit. (*Courtesy of* Netter Images; with permission.)

present with an acute respiratory failure, which could be the result of disease progression to a point that the compensatory mechanisms are overwhelmed, or emergence of a superimposed respiratory disease such as atelectasis, pneumonia (bacterial, viral or aspiration), or pulmonary embolism.

NMDs may result in respiratory insufficiency with 3 potential mechanisms.[2,3] A combination of these mechanisms is often implicated in an individual patient:

1. Weakness of the upper airway muscles. Weakness of the oropharyngeal muscles and tongue may result in impaired swallowing, which predisposes to aspiration of the food or respiratory secretions. Aspiration then results in atelectasis and pneumonia. Paralysis of the vocal cords and significant weakness of the tongue and pharyngeal muscles may also result in partial upper airway obstruction.[2,4]
2. Weakness of the inspiratory and expiratory muscles. The diaphragm, intercostal muscles, and accessory muscles are the main muscles of inspiration (**Fig. 2**). Weakness of these muscles may result in abnormal sigh mechanism, atelectasis caused by decreased lung expansion, and subsequent ventilation/perfusion (V/Q) mismatch. Hypoxemia may be the result of V/Q mismatch early in the course of the respiratory failure. The relative contribution of different inspiratory muscles changes in different positions. The diaphragm is the most important contributor in the supine position; therefore, diaphragmatic weakness is often associated with orthopnea. Progressive weakness of the inspiratory muscles leads to a decreased tidal volume. Compensatory tachypnea develops to maintain normal minute ventilation. This persistent tachypnea and increased work of breathing of the already weakened respiratory musculature may eventually lead to muscle exhaustion, with the evolving inability to maintain a normal minute ventilation,

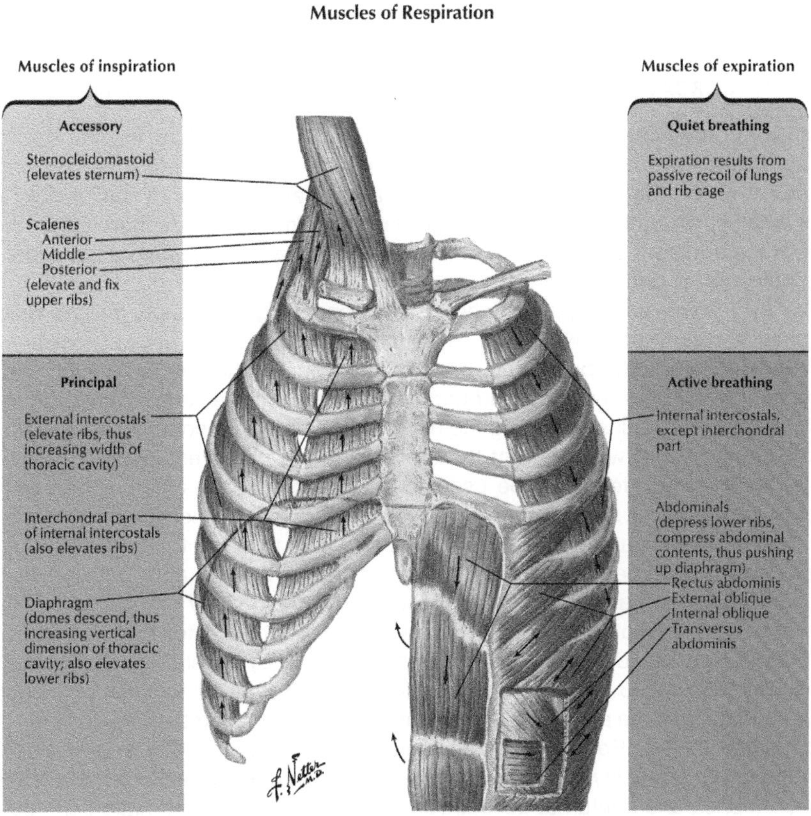

Fig. 2. Inspiratory and expiratory muscles. (*Courtesy of* Netter Images; with permission.)

resulting in progressive hypercapnia and respiratory acidosis. Hypoxemia develops in an earlier stage of the respiratory failure than CO_2 retention (hypercapnia). The latter is usually present later in the course, and is associated with significant weakness and fatigue.[5,6] Weakness of the expiratory muscles (ie, internal intercostals and abdominal muscles [see **Fig. 2**]), results in impaired coughing and clearance of respiratory secretions, which leads to mucous plugging, atelectasis, and pneumonia. Adequate strength of the inspiratory and expiratory muscles is essential for an effective cough. There should also be coordination between the muscles of the upper airways and the expiratory muscles so that the glottis opens during a forceful contraction of the expiratory muscles.

3. Concomitant cardiopulmonary disease. Patients with NMD often have a concomitant cardiomyopathy and congestive heart failure. They may also develop aspiration pneumonia and atelectasis, as mentioned earlier. The latter further decreases the lung compliance and increases the workload on the already weak muscles. Immobility may result in deep vein thrombosis and subsequent pulmonary embolization.

Sleep exacerbates the hypoventilation associated with respiratory muscle weakness. The rapid eye movement (REM) stage is associated with hypotonia and flaccidity of the accessory muscles. Therefore, patients with diaphragmatic weakness may develop hypoxia and hypercapnia during the REM stage, if they sleep in the supine position. As the respiratory muscle weakness deteriorates, hypoventilation develops during the other stages of sleep, followed by wakefulness.[7]

GENERAL APPROACH TO A PATIENT WITH IMPENDING RESPIRATORY FAILURE

When confronted with a patient with symptoms of respiratory failure, the first step is to secure the airways, provide adequate oxygenation and stabilize the hemodynamic status.[1] It should be decided whether the patient has respiratory insufficiency, and if so, whether intubation and mechanical ventilation are needed. A short history often reveals the apparent cause (ie, a cardiopulmonary disease, a neurologic disorder, or a combination of both).

The symptoms and signs that herald an impending respiratory failure include dysphagia, cough after swallowing, dysphonia, shortness of breath at rest or with minimal exertion, orthopnea, tachycardia, tachypnea, shallow breathing, use of accessory respiratory muscles, and paradoxic breathing. Weakness of the trapezius and the truncal muscles (including the neck flexors and extensors) is usually associated with significant weakness of the diaphragm and other respiratory muscles. A single breath count test may be used to assess for poor respiratory reserve.[2,3,6] Counting out loud in a single breath after a deep inspiration, an individual with a normal respiratory reserve can count to about 50. Being able to count to 25 and 10 roughly correlates with a forced vital capacity (FVC) of greater than 2L and 1L, respectively. Counts less than 15 are associated with substantial respiratory compromise.[6] Staccato speech (interrupted talking) is another clinical evidence for low and impaired respiratory reserves. Dysphagia can be tested clinically by observing the patient after swallowing 88.7 mL (3 oz) of water. Coughing implicates the dysfunction of the upper airways, leading to the aspiration of oropharyngeal content, and the necessity of withholding oral intake. Because FVC decreases about 10% in the supine position compared with sitting in nonobese individuals,[8] diaphragmatic weakness may present with orthopnea and nocturnal desaturation, because the diaphragmatic contribution diminishes during sleep.[2]

Patients should undergo immediate endotracheal intubation and mechanical ventilation if they present with respiratory or cardiac arrest, shock, impaired consciousness, respiratory distress, or evidence of active aspiration caused by the weakness of the upper airways. Patients with the weakness of the bulbar or respiratory muscles who do not have these criteria for intubation should be closely monitored, both by clinical measures and when practical and possible in the clinical setting, by spirometry and measurements of respiratory muscle strength. Intubation may then become necessary if the respiratory status continues to deteriorate.

When practical in the clinical situation, the pulmonary function tests (PFTs) to be monitored at regular intervals are the FVC, negative inspiratory force (NIF, also known as maximal inspiratory pressure [Pi max]) and positive expiratory force (PEF, or maximal expiratory pressure [Pe max]), obtained by respiratory muscle strength testing. NIF predicts the ability to maintain adequate alveolar ventilation and the PEF predicts the ability to cough and clear the airways. These tests may be performed in a pulmonary function laboratory or at the bedside with suitable equipment. NIF can be measured in the intubated patients in a critical care unit by qualified respiratory therapists. It has been suggested that PEF is the most sensitive parameter to assess for respiratory weakness in chronic NMD.[9] However, FVC and NIF are simpler to use in critically ill patients, and assess the diaphragmatic function.[6]

FVC is normally about 60 to 70 mL/kg; specific values for a given patient are dependent on age, race, and height and should be expressed as a percentage of predicted for a given patient.[10] FVC of 30 mL/kg (50%–60% of predicted) is associated with a weak cough. Subjective dyspnea also occurs when FVC is less than 30 mL/kg, but there is variability between the patients based on the age and the presence of underlying cardiopulmonary disease.[5,6] FVC less than 25 mL/kg is associated with a weak sigh (and development of atelectasis and hypoxemia) and FVC of 15 mL/kg or 1L (<30%–35% of predicted) is considered an indication for mechanical ventilation[2,6] in the appropriate clinical setting. FVC and NIF may be spuriously low if there is significant weakness of the facial and bulbar muscles or if there is significant air leak around the device mouthpiece during testing. Tidal volume changes only slightly in the early stages of respiratory failure but may decrease significantly with advanced neuromuscular weakness. Other less commonly used PFTs include peak cough flow rate (PCFR) and sniff nasal inspiratory pressure (SNIP).

DIAGNOSTIC APPROACH TO THE UNDERLYING NMD

History

A focused history should be obtained from the patient or family or by reviewing the medical records.[1] The following aspects are especially important:

1. A known underlying NMD: patients with amyotrophic lateral sclerosis (ALS) inexorably develop respiratory failure as a result of disease progression or aspiration. Patients with dystrophinopathy predictably become ventilator dependent later in the course, and myotonic dystrophy is associated with respiratory muscle weakness, as well as sleep-related breathing disorder and central hypoventilation.[11] Previous episodes of generalized weakness may suggest hypokalemic periodic paralysis or myasthenia gravis (MG) crisis, and previous episodes of rhabdomyolysis may denote an underlying metabolic myopathy affecting the glycogen or lipid pathways, such as carnitine palmitoyl transferase type II (CPT-II) deficiency.
2. A preexisting medical disease: an underlying cancer may suggest a paraneoplastic syndrome such as Lambert-Eaton myasthenic syndrome (LEMS), MG, or rarely, paraneoplastic motor neuronopathy. On the other hand, neoplastic infiltration of

the nerve roots and the peripheral nerves often occurs with lymphoid malignancies and metastatic carcinoma. History of monoclonal gammopathy may be present in patients in chronic inflammatory demyelinating polyneuropathy (CIDP) and POEMS (polyneuropathy, organomegaly, endocrinopathy, M spike, skin changes). Patients with bone marrow transplantation are predisposed to autoimmune disease like MG and Guillain-Barré syndrome (GBS). Human immunodeficiency virus (HIV) infection may be associated with GBS, CIDP, myositis, HIV myopathy, and polyradiculopathy. Polyradiculopathy may be infectious (eg, cytomegalovirus) or malignant (eg, lymphoma). Critical illness neuropathy and myopathy (CIN/M) are the most common causes of weakness in critically ill patients in the intensive care unit (ICU) (see later discussion).

3. Illicit substance use and alcoholism could be associated with rhabdomyolysis.
4. Recent respiratory or gastrointestinal infections could be present in patients with GBS or MG exacerbation. Gastrointestinal symptoms are also seen in botulism, and abdominal pain often precedes the onset of respiratory weakness in acute intermittent porphyria.
5. History of recent major surgery may suggest GBS and CIN/M.[12]
6. Medications: a large proportion of patients with cancer or history of transplantation who are admitted to the ICU have been treated with neurotoxic medications (**Box 1**). However, toxic neuropathy is generally not a common cause of respiratory failure. Furthermore, several medications are implicated in precipitation of MG

Box 1
Some of the drugs and toxins that may be associated with weakness as a result of polyneuropathy

Vinca alkaloids (vincristine, vinblastine)

Taxanes (taxol)

Platinum compounds (cisplatin, oxaliplatin)

Suramin

Tacrolimus, sirolimus

Thalidomide

Bortezomib

Amiodarone

Metronidazole

Nitrofurantoin

Tumor necrosis factor α blockers

Gold

Metals (arsenic, lead, inorganic mercury, thallium)

Hydrocarbons (n-hexane)

Buckthorn

Diphtheria

Saxitoxin

Tetrodotoxin

Tick paralysis (North American type)

crisis (**Box 2**). Barbiturates and several other antiepileptics, sulfonamides and other antibiotics, and a large number of other medications have been associated with precipitation of porphyria attack.

7. Diet: fasting and low carbohydrate intake may precipitate a porphyria attack, as well as weakness and rhabdomyolysis in patients with a variety of metabolic muscle diseases such as CPT-II. Recent intake of a high-carbohydrate diet is often encountered before an episode of paralysis in hypokalemic periodic paralysis. Intake of canned food and seafood may precede botulism and saxitoxin poisoning, respectively. Intake of the buckthorn fruit has rarely been implicated in acute neuropathy.

Examination

The accurate assessment of the muscle weakness in patients who are critically ill is often limited by the lack of cooperation. In these patients, inspection may reveal lack of spontaneous movements, muscle involuntary activity (fasciculations, myokymia), and muscle atrophy.[13] Generalized areflexia and hypotonia suggest demyelinating neuropathy (ie, GBS) or polyradiculopathy. Myalgia and muscle tenderness may represent myositis or rhabdomyolysis. **Table 1** summarizes the patterns of muscle weakness in different classes of NMD.

Electromyography and Nerve Conduction Study

Electromyography (EMG) is a valuable tool in the diagnosis of NMDs. It should preferably be conducted in the neurophysiology laboratory, where the electrical interference is minimal. On the other hand, EMG is commonly conducted in critically ill patients in the ICU. **Table 2** summarizes the EMG characteristics of different categories of NMD.

Other Workup

Other laboratory testing, including a nerve and muscle biopsy, is often needed to establish the diagnosis of an NMD. Such a laboratory workup should be tailored to

Box 2
Drugs associated with neuromuscular junction impairment or worsening of MG symptoms

Antibiotics: aminoglycosides, colistin, polymyxin, macrolides, quinolones, imipenem, ciprofloxacin, tetracyclines

Antiarrhythmics: procainamide, quinidine, lidocaine, trimethaphan

Neuromuscular junction blockers (succinylcholine, vecuronium)

Quinine

Phenytoin

Immunosuppressants: steroids, cyclosporine

Antirheumatics: chloroquine, D-penicillamine

Psychotropics: lithium, chlorpromazine

Calcium channel blockers

β-Blockers

Magnesium

Iodinated contrast

Table 1
Clinical characteristics of different categories of NMD, based on the localization of the lesion in a motor unit

Disease Category	Clinical Characteristics
Motor neuronopathy	Muscle atrophy Fasciculations Frequent involvement of bulbar muscles Lack of sensory signs and symptoms DTRs: decreased or increased ± pathologic reflexes Lack of ocular motor involvement until late in the course
Polyradiculopathy and neuropathy	Loss of deep tendon reflexes Motor and sensory impairment ± Ocular motor involvement ± Autonomic involvement
Neuromuscular junction disorder	Significant ocular motor involvement Frequent involvement of bulbar muscles Proximal → distal limb weakness Muscle atrophy usually not present DTRs: normal or decreased
Myopathy	Proximal → distal limb weakness DTRs: normal or decreased ± Myalgia ± Rhabdomyolysis

Abbreviation: DTR, deep tendon reflex.

an individual patient, based on the clinical and EMG findings. The clinical and laboratory features of different NMDs are described in **Tables 3–6**.

GBS

GBS is an acute polyradiculoneuropathy caused by autoimmunity against the structural components of the peripheral nerves.[28] Acquired inflammatory demyelinating polyneuropathy (AIDP) is the most common subtype of GBS in the United States and Europe. Axonal subtypes, acute motor axonal neuropathy (AMAN), and acute motor and sensory axonal neuropathy occur in less than 10% of cases in North America and Europe.[28,29] AMAN is particularly common in China, and another variant, Miller Fisher syndrome (MFS), is more prevalent in Japan.[28,29] AIDP is characterized by progressive weakness, with maximal weakness present within 4 weeks, but usually within 2 weeks after the onset.[30,31] The weakness typically affects both proximal and distal limb muscles and frequently the truncal and respiratory muscles. Reflexes are typically absent early in the course. Facial diplegia is seen in 70% of patients.[29] Ocular motor involvement is less common, except in patients who are positive for the GQ1b antibody, including those with MFS. Sensory symptoms are commonly present, including severe pain in some patients.[29] Dysautonomia, resulting from hypoactivity or hyperactivity of the sympathetic and parasympathetic systems, occurs in about two-thirds of patients. Although mild in most patients, dysautonomia can be severe and even fatal. The symptoms may include severe fluctuations in blood pressure, heart arrhythmia, abnormal pupillary response, bladder atonia, and ileus.[29,32]

A history of a respiratory or gastrointestinal tract infection 3 weeks or less before the onset is present in about two-thirds of patients with AIDP.[29] *Campylobacter jejuni* is the most commonly encountered pathogen, and is associated with seropositivity to IgG GM1, an axonal form, and less favorable prognosis.[33–36] Cytomegalovirus is the

Table 2
EMG characteristics in different categories of NMD

Disease Category	EMG-NCS Features
Motor neuronopathy	Reduced CMAP amplitudes Normal or mildly reduced motor CV Normal SNAPs Fibrillations, positive waves, and fasciculations in multiple myotomes Reduced recruitment, neurogenic MUs
Polyradiculopathy and neuropathy	*Demyelinating:* Significant slowing of CV Marked prolongation of distal latencies Conduction block, temporal dispersion SNAPs abnormal Fibrillations and positive waves if there is concomitant axonal loss *Axonal:* Reduced CMAP amplitudes Normal or mildly reduced motor CV SNAPs abnormal (except for AMAN) Fibrillations and positive waves in multiple myotomes Reduced recruitment, neurogenic MUs
Neuromuscular junction disorder	*Postsynaptic:* Normal baseline CMAP amplitude Normal SNAPs Decrement of CMAP amplitude with low frequency (2–5 Hz) repetitive stimulation Needle EMG normal, or may show neurogenic or myopathic units *Presynaptic:* Low baseline CMAP amplitude Facilitation of CMAP amplitude after brief (ie, 10 s) exertion Facilitation of the CMAP amplitude with high-frequency (20–50 Hz) repetitive stimulation Decrement of the CMAP amplitude with low-frequency (2–5 Hz) repetitive stimulation
Myopathy	CMAP amplitude reduced or normal SNAPs normal ± Fibrillations and positive waves Myopathic (short duration ± polyphasic) units Early recruitment

Abbreviations: CMAP, compound muscle action potential; CV, conduction velocity; MU, motor unit; SNAP, sensory nerve action potential.

second most common infection associated with GBS.[33,36] Other more commonly encountered pathogens are Epstein-Barr virus, *Mycoplasma pneumoniae*, HIV, and *Haemophilus influenzae*.[29]

Respiratory failure is one of the most serious short-term complications of GBS, and occurs in about 30% of patients.[37] A large proportion of patients with GBS develop phrenic neuropathy, although the accessory nerve is spared except in the more severe cases.[6] About 25% of patients with GBS who are unable to walk need mechanical ventilation[29]; and intubation and mechanical ventilation are required in 30% to 50% of patients admitted to the ICU.[37–40]

It is recommended to assess FVC every 2 to 4 hours during the day and every 4 to 6 hours at night in a patient with declining respiratory function.[6] NIF should be measured

Table 3
Clinical and laboratory features and suggested treatments of neuropathies that may cause respiratory failure

Type of Neuropathy	Clinical Features	EMG and Laboratory Findings	Treatment in the Acute Stage (Besides Supportive Care)
CIDP	Proximal and distal weakness Proximal and distal sensory impairment Progressive course >2 mo Hypertrophic polyradiculopathy (uncommon) Cranial neuropathy (uncommon)	EMG: demyelinating features High CSF protein (always >45 mg/dL) Albuminocytologic dissociation	Steroids IVIG Consider steroid sparing agents and tapering steroids
POEMS[14,15]	Polyneuropathy Organomegaly (hepatomegaly, splenomegaly, lymphadenopathy) Endocrinopathy (diabetes, hypothyroidism, gynecomastia) Skin lesions (edema, clubbing, hypertrichosis, hyperpigmentation)	EMG: severe, primarily demyelinating neuropathy, but axonal loss always present M spike (usually IgG or IgA paraprotein, λ chain in >95%). $\pm$ Sclerotic plasmacytoma ↑ serum VEGF Multiorgan failure, ascites, pleural effusion,	Irradiation or resection of plasmacytoma Melphalan, dexamethasone, IVIG Consider autologous stem cell transplantation, thalidomide or bevacizumab
Vasculitis and collagen vascular disease	Underlying systemic vasculitis (eg, polyarteritis nodosa) may be present Multifocal neuropathy which becomes confluent Sensory and motor involvement Neuropathic pain	EMG: axonal polyneuropathy or mononeuropathy multiplex Positive serology (ANCA, ANA, SSA, SSB, others) Nerve and muscle biopsy	Steroids Immunosuppressants
Saxitoxin, tetrodotoxin[16–18]	Onset within hours after intake of contaminated mussels, oysters, or clam (saxitoxin), and fish (tetrodotoxin) Limb, bulbar, and respiratory weakness Headaches, encephalopathy, ataxia, nausea, vomiting Cardiac arrhythmias Mechanism: blockage of Na channels	EMG: conduction block and small amplitude CMAP and SNAP Toxin detection in urine	Induced emesis to remove unabsorbed toxin

Tick paralysis North American types[19]	*Dermacentor variabilis* (dog tick), *Dermacentor andersoni* (wood tick) Children predominantly affected Ascending paralysis, areflexia, ataxia, truncal, bulbar weakness, and respiratory failure Progression over hours to few days	EMG: prolonged latency, slow CV (axonal range), low CMAP and SNAP amplitudes CSF protein normal Potential mechanism: impaired saltatory conduction at the terminal axons	ICU admission and close observation Tick removal results in rapid and complete recovery
Hypophosphatemia	Risk factors: hyperalimentation without adding inorganic phosphate,[20,21] anorexia/bulimia,[22] treatment of diabetic ketoacidosis,[23] hemodialysis[24] Generalized weakness, respiratory muscle weakness, rhabdomyolysis, polyneuropathy, encephalopathy	EMG: ± polyneuropathy with either axonal or demyelinating features[20,21]	Rapid improvement with parenteral phosphate supplementation, suggests a reversible metabolic impairment of the myofiber function in most cases
Acute intermittent and variegate porphyria[25]	Abdominal pain, followed by progressive weakness Motor → sensory, ± respiratory failure, bulbar and facial muscle weakness CNS demyelination Psychiatric features Dysautonomia Recent use of specific medications and hormones	EMG: axonal, predominantly motor neuropathy ↑ Urinary porphobilinogen and σ aminolevulinic acid Porphobilinogen deaminase assay	Intravenous glucose and heme arginate Symptomatic treatment of pain (eg, meperidine), Gastrointestinal symptoms
Diphtheria[26,27]	Polyneuropathy occurs in at least 15%, 20% of which develop respiratory failure Onset of neuropathy weeks after the onset of infection Bulbar weakness universal ± Ocular motor weakness Sensory and autonomic impairment in all of the patients Cardiomyopathy (often fatal)	EMG: prolonged distal motor latencies, ± slow motor conduction velocities CSF: high protein, mildly increased cell count ± albuminocytological dissociation Positive throat culture for *Corynebacterium diphtheriae*	Diphtheria antitoxin within the first 2 d of onset

Abbreviations: ANA, antinuclear antibodies; ANCA, antineutrophil cytoplasmic antibodies; CMAP, compound muscle action potential; CSF, cerebrospinal fluid; CV, conduction velocity; VEGF, vascular endothelial growth factor; SSA and SSB, Sjogren syndrome associated antibodies.

Table 4
Clinical and laboratory features and suggested treatments of neuromuscular junction disorders that may cause respiratory failure

Neuromuscular Junction Disorder	Clinical Features	Treatments (Other than Close Monitoring and Respiratory Care)
LEMS[75,76]	Muscle weakness (especially proximal lower extremity weakness) Ptosis (ophthalmoparesis uncommon) Hyporeflexia Dysautonomia Muscle pain Association with small cell lung cancer in two-thirds of patients Antibodies to P/Q voltage gated calcium channels in 90% of patients	Treatment of small cell lung cancer 3,4-DAP PE or IVIG Avoid calcium channel blockers
Botulism[77–79]	Abdominal pain, nausea, or vomiting, diarrhea preceding weakness Bulbar and ocular motor involvement Respiratory failure in 20%–30% of patients Autonomic impairment (unreactive pupils, urinary retention, fluctuations in pulse and blood pressure) Recent intake of canned food, soft tissue trauma, and infected wounds	Close monitoring in ICU Administration of botulinum antitoxin
Hypermagnesemia[80,81]	Underlying renal failure, laxative abuse, magnesium-containing antiacids, tocolysis Respiratory depression Quadriparesis	Rapid improvement with calcium gluconate intravenously
Organophosphate poisoning[82,83]	Suicidal attempt or accidental exposure. Respiratory failure common, bulbar weakness, quadriparesis, fasciculations, cramps, miosis	Intravenous atropine and pralidoxime
Snake venom[84–86]	Progressive bulbar paralysis and respiratory failure, ptosis, and ophthalmoparesis Pathogenesis: *Bungarus* sp: presynaptic (β-BTX), postsynaptic: nicotinic AChR (α-BTX and γ-BTX); Cobra: nicotinic AChR (α-cobra toxin)	Appropriate snake antitoxin Supportive care of respiratory failure and rhabdomyolysis (if present)

(*continued on next page*)

Table 4
(*continued*)

Neuromuscular Junction Disorder	Clinical Features	Treatments (Other than Close Monitoring and Respiratory Care)
Tick paralysis Australian type[87]	*Ixodes holocyclus* (marsupial tick) Rapidly progressive ascending paralysis, with early cranial nerve involvement Respiratory failure common and potentially fatal EMG: low motor amplitudes, normal sensory responses; normal repetitive stimulation Possible mechanism: interference by neurotoxin with ACh release an NMJ (similar to botulinum toxin)	Antitoxin to be injected before tick removal More severe, and longer time to recovery than the North American type ICU admission and respiratory support in the acute stage
Prolonged neuromuscular block[88]	Underlying kidney or liver failure, hypermagnesemia, medication interaction (eg, sevoflurane), cholinesterase or pseudocholinesterase deficiency Use of a neuromuscular blocker (eg, mivacurium, rapacuronium) Generalized weakness, ophthalmoparesis, ptosis, failure to wean	Avoidance of use of neuromuscular blocker

Abbreviations: ACh, acetylcholine; BTX, bungarotoxin; DAP, diaminopyridine; NMJ, neuromuscular junction.

at the same time if possible, because it may be more sensitive to declines in respiratory function.

The patients with significant respiratory muscle weakness may deteriorate clinically, as shown by distress, fatigue, accessory muscle use, and thoracoabdominal dyssynchrony, before such deterioration is reflected in either arterial blood gas (ABG) or pulmonary function measurements. Therefore, intubation, either elective or emergent, is a bedside clinical judgment.

Because emergency intubation substantially increases the risk of complications such as aspiration and hypoxemia, it is essential to anticipate the need for intubation and mechanical ventilation and proceed with elective intubation in selected patients. Criteria proposed for elective intubation and MV in patients with GBS include significant respiratory distress, fatigue, sweating, tachycardia, active aspiration, and FVC of 10 to 12 mL/kg (<30%–35% of predicted), and Pa_{CO_2} greater than 50 mm Hg. Elective intubation should be considered in the presence of a higher FVC if the condition is rapidly deteriorating, if there is inefficient cough, inability to clear bronchial secretions despite vigorous chest physiotherapy,[38,39,41] or if the patient has a significant concomitant morbidity such as active cardiac ischemia or heart failure.

Predictive parameters for mechanical ventilation in GBS include rapidly progressive course as manifested by time to peak disability less than 7 days, time from the onset of symptoms to hospitalization less than 7 days, and more than 30% reduction of vital capacity, NIF, and PEF.[40,42] Significant bulbar dysfunction, facial weakness, impaired cough, dysautonomia, and inability to lift the elbow or head off the bed are other suggested predictors of need for mechanical ventilation. On the other hand, an FVC less

Table 5
Clinical and laboratory features and suggested treatments of diseases of the motor neuron that may cause respiratory failure

Disease of the Motor Neuron	Clinical Features and Pertinent Paraclinical Findings	Treatment in the Acute Phase
Poliomyelitis	Myalgia and meningoencephalitis, followed by asymmetrical paralysis ± bulbar and respiratory muscle weakness ± dysautonomia EMG: ↓ CMAP amplitudes, denervation in multiple myotomes, CSF: ↑ WBC (neutrophils early on), ↑ protein, normal glucose Serology: ↑ IgM titer in CSF	Supportive treatment
West Nile meningoencephalitis[89]	Motor neuronopathy (similar to poliomyelitis) Asymmetrical weakness, ± diaphragm weakness, facial weakness common Meningoencephalitis (headaches, ataxia, seizures) EMG: CSF: similar to polio + ↑ IgM titer in serum and CSF	Supportive treatment Mortality higher in age >75 y
Tetanus[90]	Risk factors: lack of adequate vaccination, puncture wounds, tongue piercing, poor hygiene childbirth (for the neonatal form) Severe, painful muscle spasms that may last seconds to minutes Generalized form: opisthotonus, generalized spasms, respiratory failure, dysautonomia, ± rhabdomyolysis and renal failure Milder, local forms: trismus, face muscle spasms (risus sardonicus), dysphagia, neck stiffness, and local limb spasms EMG: continuous high-frequency motor unit discharges during periods of spasms Wound culture positive in 30%–50% Mechanism: tetanospasmin induces sustained firing of motor neurons as a result of impaired release of inhibitory neurotransmitters (GABA and glycine)	Human tetanus immunoglobulin administration Treatment of respiratory failure, rhabdomyolysis, cardiac arrhythmias and dysautonomia Antispasmodics: diazepam, baclofen, magnesium sulfate Antibiotic and surgical treatment of wound

than 20 mL/kg, NIF less than negative 30 cm H_2O and PEF less than 40 cm H_2O (20/30/40 rule) during the course of hospitalization are other PFT parameters that have been suggested to predict intubation and mechanical ventilation.[42,43]

Noninvasive, positive pressure ventilation (NIV or NIPPV) is not a good choice in patients with respiratory failure and significant bulbar muscle weakness, because there is increased risk of aspiration or collapse of the upper airways.[2] NIV should also be avoided in patients who are likely to need a long duration of respiratory support. Other important supportive management issues include deep vein thrombosis and peptic ulcer disease prophylaxis, and appropriate treatment of the cardiac arrhythmias, fluctuations in the blood pressure, ileus, and urinary retention.

Plasma exchange (PE) and intravenous immunoglobulins (IVIG) are both proved to be effective in the treatment of GBS.[28,44] PE is more effective when it is given early in the course, and the usual regimen is a total exchange of about 5 plasma volumes of 50 mL/kg during 1 to 2 weeks.[28,45] IVIG has replaced PE as the preferred method of treatment in many hospitals, after a large randomized clinical trial showed its equal efficacy to PE.[46] The usual dose is 2 g/kg over a 3 to 5-day period.[45] The mortality of GBS is estimated at 3% to 10%; the most common causes of death are the complications of dysautonomia and respiratory failure.[29,32] **Table 3** summarizes the clinical and paraclinical features of some of the other neuropathies that could be associated with respiratory failure.

GENERALIZED MG

Generalized MG is a commonly encountered neuromuscular cause of respiratory failure. Involvement of the facial and oropharyngeal muscles happens during the course of the disease in most patients, causing facial weakness, dysphagia, and dysarthria (nasal speech). MG crisis is referred to exacerbation of the generalized weakness, with associated respiratory insufficiency and the need for mechanical ventilation. MG rarely presents with isolated stridor or respiratory failure.[47–49] The course of MG is unpredictable, especially in the first 2 years of diagnosis. MG crisis occurs in approximately 15% to 20% of patients some time during the course, but most often during the first year after the onset of symptoms.[50] MG crisis may be precipitated by the disease progression, treatment with high-dose steroids, anticholinesterases, and other medications that affect the neuromuscular transmission (see **Table 3**).[3,50,51] Intercurrent infections, pregnancy, surgery, and other sorts of stress (including emotional) are other causes of MG crisis.

MG diagnosis is usually made based on the clinical grounds and seropositivity to the acetylcholine receptors (AChR) autoantibodies, present in about 85% of the generalized cases.[52] Antibodies to the muscle specific kinase are found in about 40% of the seronegative patients.[53] EMG is useful to differentiate MG from neuropathies such as GBS, myopathies, motor neuron diseases (MNDs), and other neuromuscular transmission diseases such as LEMS and prolonged effect of the neuromuscular blockers (see **Table 1**). The edrophonium (Tensilon) test can be used at the bedside to diagnose MG.[52,54] Edrophonium is given intravenously, and the patient is watched for immediate improvement of the MG symptoms, usually ptosis or ocular movements. If the appropriate target symptoms are present, the sensitivity is 71% to 95%.[54] Cardiac monitoring is strongly recommended, because there is a low risk of serious side effects like bradycardia and asystole. It has been suggested that because of its maximum effect at 15 to 30 minutes, 2 mg of intramuscular neostigmine could provide better diagnostic results in patients with respiratory weakness, because the PFT data can be repeated during that interval.[6]

Table 6
Clinical and laboratory features and suggested treatments of some of the muscle diseases that could cause acute respiratory failure

Type of Myopathy	Clinical Features	EMG and Laboratory Findings	Treatment in the Acute Stage (Besides Supportive Care)
Polymyositis, dermatomyositis[91–93]	Proximal → distal limb weakness usually present Respiratory failure caused by diaphragm and intercostal weakness can rarely be the predominant symptom Skin rash in dermatomyositis Cardiomyopathy, interstitial lung disease	EMG: myopathies, with spontaneous activity ↑ CPK Muscle biopsy Underlying malignancy should be excluded in polymyositis >50	Steroids IVIG
Rhabdomyolysis[84,94,95]	Proximal → distal weakness, and myalgia ± respiratory failure Causes: Drugs: statins, colchicine, clofibrate, others Cocaine, heroin, alcohol Neuroleptic malignant syndrome, serotonin syndrome Snake venom (*Bungarus candidus* and *multicinctus*), cobra, coral, rattlesnake Wild mushroom Tetanus	Markedly ↑ CPK Myoglobinuria, kidney dysfunction	Monitor renal function, IV hydration, alkalinize urine Specific antivenom immunoglobulin in the case of envenomation
Acid maltase deficiency[96,97]	Diaphragmatic weakness and respiratory failure common in the adult form ± proximal → distal weakness, paraspinal atrophy, winging scapula Sleep-disordered breathing common	EMG: myopathic units, fibrillations, myotonic discharges, especially in the paraspinal muscles CPK: normal to markedly ↑, urine hexose tetrasaccharide ↑ Muscle biopsy or assessment of α glucosidase activity in blood or skin fibroblasts	BIPAP Long-term IV enzyme replacement

Mitochondrial myopathy[98–100]	Respiratory failure could be central (↓ respiratory drive) or as a result of respiratory muscle weakness Symmetric ophthalmoparesis and ptosis Proximal → distal weakness ± Cardiomyopathy, diabetes, seizures, neuropathy	EMG: ± myopathic units CPK: normal or mild ↑ ± ↑ lactate Diagnosis by muscle biopsy	Supportive care (mechanical ventilation vs BIPAP)
Deficiency of β oxidation or fatty acid transport enzymes[101–104]	Respiratory failure rare in very long chain acyl-CoA, CPT-II Recurrent rhabdomyolysis ± muscle weakness Precipitating factors: fasting, infections, endurance exercise	↑ urinary dicarboxylic acids Assessment of blood acylcarnitines Enzyme activity in the muscle	Monitor renal function, IV hydration, alkalinize urine
Hypokalemic periodic paralysis[105,106]	Proximal → distal weakness, ↓ reflexes Cranial nerves not affected Respiratory failure rare Precipitated by high-carbohydrate diet, rest after exercise, and medications such as insulin and β agonists	↓ K during attack Thyrotoxicosis often present CPK: normal or mildly ↑ EMG: CMAP amplitude diminished during attack and insertional activity decreased during attack, ± fibrillations and myopathic units	KCl supplementation during attack Prophylaxis: acetazolamide and dichlorphenamide Secondary causes of hypokalemia to be excluded

Abbreviations: CMAP, compound muscle action potential; CPK, creatine phosphokinase; IV, intravenous.

Respiratory failure in MG may present with tachycardia, anxiety, restlessness, and tachypnea in the early stage. Later in the course and with worsening hypoxemia and the emergence of hypercapnia, patients develop cyanosis, encephalopathy, and headaches. MG patients with questionable status should be closely monitored in the ICU with repeated clinical evaluation as well as bedside FVC and NIF.[5] However, given the fluctuating nature of the weakness, it is often difficult to predict the need for mechanical ventilation in MG, even with close monitoring.[2,55] An ABG measurement should be obtained if there is suspicion of evolving respiratory failure. Intubation is recommended with marginal and declining respiratory status, FVC less than 15 mL/kg, Pa_{O_2} less than 60 mm Hg and Pa_{CO_2} greater than 50 mm Hg.[6] Oral intake should be stopped, and intubation should also be considered in patients with aspiration or significant weakness of the oropharyngeal muscles. In a retrospective study, the mortality of MG crisis was 4% and the parameters that predicted prolonged intubation included a preintubation bicarbonate level greater than 30 mg/dL,peak vital capacity less than 25 mL/kg on day 1 to 6 after intubation, and age older than 50 years.[50]

The use of NIV (intermittent bilevel positive airway pressure [BIPAP]) early in the course of the MG crisis may prevent the development of atelectasis and lead to a lesser need for intubation and mechanical ventilation. In 2 retrospective studies on respiratory failure in MG, BIPAP prevented intubation and mechanical ventilation in 60% to 70% of the trials.[56,57] Hypercapnia (a P_{CO_2} >45 mm Hg) was a strong predictor of the failure of BIPAP in one of those studies.[57]

PE and IVIG with the same dose mentioned under GBS have been shown to be effective in myasthenic crisis.[58] Although PE was more effective for improving the respiratory status than IVIG in a study, it was also associated with more side effects and increased length of ICU stay.[59] Starting a high dose of corticosteroids is a potential cause of MG crisis, and should be avoided unless the patient is already on mechanical ventilation. If the patient is on a low dose of prednisone, the dose should be increased, preferably after the respiratory function has started to improve with either PE or IVIG. Anticholinesterase inhibitors such as pyridostigmine should be withheld in patients on mechanical ventilation for the potential cardiovascular side effects such as arrhythmias, increasing bronchial secretions, and increased airway resistance.[58] Pyridostigmine, which is also available in the intravenous form, may be restarted when the patient is being weaned off. It can be started at 30 mg orally every 3 to 4 hours, and increased to 60 mg every 3 to 4 hours. Higher doses (up to 120 mg every 3–4 hours) are sometimes used; however, higher doses often do not improve the symptoms, and the weakness may paradoxically deteriorate.[58] **Table 4** summarizes the clinical and laboratory characteristics of other more commonly encountered neuromuscular junction transmission diseases.

ALS

MND is characterized by progressive degeneration of the motor neurons. The less common variants of MND (spinal muscular atrophy and spinobulbar muscular atrophy) are diseases of the lower motor neurons (which are located in the motor brainstem nuclei and the anterior horns of the spinal cord). On the other hand, ALS is characterized by the progressive degeneration of the lower and upper motor neurons. Respiratory failure emerges in almost all patients with ALS, and is the cause of death in most of these patients.[60,61] Respiratory muscle weakness is predominantly secondary to diffuse denervation (lower MND); however, upper motor neuron impairment is also implicated in the respiratory symptoms in ALS.[62,63] Bulbar muscle dysfunction caused by lower motor neuron (bulbar palsy) or upper motor neuron (pseudobulbar palsy) disease, also invariably complicates the clinical course of ALS.[64] Bulbar-onset ALS is more common in older patients; 43% of patients with ALS older than 70 years presented with bulbar symptoms in a study.[65] Bulbar weakness results in aspiration and impaired cough, as well as malnutrition, which leads to further weakness and atrophy of the respiratory muscles.[64] Early symptoms of respiratory failure in ALS include exertional dyspnea, orthopnea, frequent nocturnal arousals, daytime somnolence, morning headaches, and impaired memory and concentration.[63]

Because respiratory failure may even occur early in the course of ALS, the treatment plan and the patient's wish for intubation and mechanical ventilation should be discussed before an emergency situation arises.[7] Patients with ALS should be closely monitored with PFTs such as supine and upright FVC, PEF, NIF, and PCFR.[7] The efficacy of the airway mucous clearance is largely determined by the strength of the cough as assessed by the PCFR.[64,66] These tests may be spuriously low when bulbar and facial weakness is present, and when there is inadequate control of the voluntary respiratory muscles because of upper motor neuron involvement. SNIP is another method that can be effectively used in patients with significant bulbar weakness, because it does not require a tight seal around a mouthpiece.[63] SNIP has been shown to correlate with the transdiaphragmatic pressure, and SNIP less than 40 cm H_2O correlates with nocturnal hypoxemia.[67] Nighttime pulse oximetry may also provide evidence for intermittent nocturnal hypoventilation, because the hypoventilation generally deteriorates during sleep.

The timely institution of adequate nutrition through percutaneous endoscopic gastrostomy has been shown to improve the survival and the quality of life in patients with ALS.[61] The procedure-related morbidity is substantially lower when percutaneous endoscopic gastrostomy is performed with FVC greater than 50% predicted and SNIP greater than 40 cm H_2O; and the rate of procedure-associated complications (including intubation and mechanical ventilation) substantially increases in patients with more advanced respiratory failure.[61,67] The use of NIV has been recommended with the presence of signs and symptoms of respiratory failure, greater than 1 minute of nocturnal O_2 desaturation of less than 90%, FVC less than 50%, SNIP less than 40 cm H_2O, and PCFR less than 270 L/min.[63,68] Aspiration and increased secretions as a result of bulbar weakness may result in difficulties in the use of NIV in patients with ALS. Because mucous plugging could result in serious complications such as atelectasis and pneumonia, frequent chest physiotherapy, frequent suctioning, and use of assistive cough devices are recommended in patients with a weak cough.[63]

Because continuous positive airway pressure causes increased workload on the already weak respiratory muscles, it is better avoided in patients with ALS.[7] Caution should also be exercised in the use of medications that suppress the respiratory drive (such as benzodiazepines and narcotics). The use of nocturnal supplemental oxygen in patients with significant respiratory muscle weakness (including ALS) has also been shown to suppress the respiratory drive and cause hypercapnia.[63,69]

RESPIRATORY WEAKNESS IN THE ICU

In patients with respiratory muscle weakness in the ICU, it should first be determined whether the weakness preceded (and led to) the ICU admission. GBS and MG crisis are the most commonly encountered acute NMDs that result in ICU admission. On the other hand, Critical Illness Myopathy and Polyneuropathy (CIM and P) account for most patients who develop weakness (or cannot be weaned from the ventilator) after being admitted to the ICU for another reason.

In a retrospective study on 92 ICU patients who underwent EMG, 28% had a primary NMD (GBS, MG, and MND) that resulted in the ICU admission. CIM and P accounted for 42% and 13% of the cases, respectively.[70] Electrophysiologic evidence for CIM and P was present in 50% of ICU patients with a stay of more than 3 days in another study.[71] Of patients with ICU stay of more than 1 week, 50% to 70% develop clinical CIM and P; this figure may reach 100% in patients with a long ICU stay with sepsis and end-organ damage.[71] CIM and P often emerges in the setting of treatment with high-dose corticosteroids and neuromuscular blockers. Other risk factors include sepsis, long ICU stay, encephalopathy, and need for vasopressor support.[71,72] The clinical picture consists of generalized weakness, lack of tolerance of weaning from the ventilator when the patient is off sedation, and lack of cardiopulmonary explanation. Examination reveals flaccidity and hyporeflexia, and muscle atrophy can be prominent in chronic cases. Muscle atrophy results in the prominence of the hand tendons and the tibia in patients with severe critical illness polyneuropathy (CIP).[13] Facial weakness and ophthalmoparesis are rare and these features point to other differential diagnoses (ie, MG, prolonged neuromuscular blockade, GBS).[71] Examination of the sensation is usually complicated by encephalopathy and sedation, but there is a stocking-gloves decrease of sensation when CIP is present.[13] Creatine phosphokinase (CPK) level was markedly increased in a retrospective study in about 50% during the first 5 days after the onset of the weakness, with subsequent gradual normalization.[73] The nerve conduction study may be normal, or shows abnormally low compound muscle action potential amplitudes in CIM. It reveals an axonal sensorimotor neuropathy in CIP. Abnormal spontaneous activity is seen in some cases of myopathy, and is uniformly present in the more distal muscles in CIP.[71] Direct muscle stimulation has been used to distinguish CIP and CIM (muscle is inexcitable in CIM).[74] If a muscle biopsy is performed, it may show myosin loss, myofiber atrophy, or a necrotizing myopathy (myofiber necrosis, vacuolization, and phagocytosis).[71] Minimizing the use of high doses of steroids and neuromuscular blocking agents and aggressive insulin treatment (keeping the blood sugar at 80 to 110 mg/dL) have been suggested to reduce the incidence of CIM and CIP.

REFERENCES

1. Bella I, Chad DA. Neuromuscular disorders and acute respiratory failure. Neurol Clin 1998;16:391.
2. Mehta S. Neuromuscular disease causing acute respiratory failure. Respir Care 2006;51:1016.
3. Yavagal DR, Mayer SA. Respiratory complications of rapidly progressive neuromuscular syndromes: Guillain-Barré syndrome and myasthenia gravis. Semin Respir Crit Care Med 2002;23:221.
4. Teramoto K, Kuwabara M, Matsubara Y. Respiratory failure due to vocal cord paresis in myasthenia gravis. Respiration 2002;69:280.
5. Green DM. Weakness in the ICU: Guillain-Barré syndrome, myasthenia gravis, and critical illness polyneuropathy/myopathy. Neurologist 2005;11:338.
6. Ropper AH, Gress DR, Diringer MN, et al. Neurological and neurosurgical intensive care. 4th edition. Philadelphia: Lippincott Williams & Wilkins; 2004.
7. Oppenheimer EA. Treating respiratory failure in ALS: the details are becoming clearer. J Neurol Sci 2003;209:1.
8. Vilke GM, Chan TC, Neuman T, et al. Spirometry in normal subjects in sitting, prone, and supine positions. Respir Care 2000;45:407.
9. Griggs RC, Donohoe KM, Utell MJ, et al. Evaluation of pulmonary function in neuromuscular disease. Arch Neurol 1981;38:9.
10. Stanojevic S, Wade A, Stocks J, et al. Reference ranges for spirometry across all ages: a new approach. Am J Respir Crit Care Med 2008;177:253.

11. Kumar SP, Sword D, Petty RK, et al. Assessment of sleep studies in myotonic dystrophy. Chron Respir Dis 2007;4:15.
12. Arnason BG, Asbury AK. Idiopathic polyneuritis after surgery. Arch Neurol 1968; 18:500.
13. Wijdicks EF. Generalized weakness in the intensive care unit. In: Wijdicks EF, editor. Neurological complications of critical illness. Oxford University Press; 2009.
14. Allam JS, Kennedy CC, Aksamit TR, et al. Pulmonary manifestations in patients with POEMS syndrome: a retrospective review of 137 patients. Chest 2008;133: 969.
15. Mokhlesi B, Jain M. Pulmonary manifestations of POEMS syndrome: case report and literature review. Chest 1999;115:1740.
16. Garcia C, del Carmen Bravo M, Lagos M, et al. Paralytic shellfish poisoning: post-mortem analysis of tissue and body fluid samples from human victims in the Patagonia fjords. Toxicon 2004;43:149.
17. Jen HC, Lin SJ, Lin SY, et al. Occurrence of tetrodotoxin and paralytic shellfish poisons in a gastropod implicated in food poisoning in southern Taiwan. Food Addit Contam 2007;24:902.
18. Lehane L. Paralytic shellfish poisoning: a potential public health problem. Med J Aust 2001;175:29.
19. Felz MW, Smith CD, Swift TR. A six-year-old girl with tick paralysis. N Engl J Med 2000;342:90.
20. Iguchi Y, Mori K, Koike H, et al. Hypophosphataemic neuropathy in a patient who received intravenous hyperalimentation. J Neurol Neurosurg Psychiatry 2007;78:1159.
21. Siddiqui MF, Bertorini TE. Hypophosphatemia-induced neuropathy: clinical and electrophysiologic findings. Muscle Nerve 1998;21:650.
22. Oud L. Transient hypoxic respiratory failure in a patient with severe hypophosphatemia. Med Sci Monit 2009;15:CS49.
23. Liu PY, Jeng CY. Severe hypophosphatemia in a patient with diabetic ketoacidosis and acute respiratory failure. J Chin Med Assoc 2004;67:355.
24. Demirjian S, Teo BW, Guzman JA, et al. Hypophosphatemia during continuous hemodialysis is associated with prolonged respiratory failure in patients with acute kidney injury. Nephrol Dial Transplant 2011. [Epub ahead of print].
25. Hift RJ, Meissner PN. An analysis of 112 acute porphyric attacks in Cape Town, South Africa: evidence that acute intermittent porphyria and variegate porphyria differ in susceptibility and severity. Medicine (Baltimore) 2005;84:48.
26. Logina I, Donaghy M. Diphtheritic polyneuropathy: a clinical study and comparison with Guillain-Barré syndrome. J Neurol Neurosurg Psychiatry 1999;67:433.
27. Piradov MA, Pirogov VN, Popova LM, et al. Diphtheritic polyneuropathy: clinical analysis of severe forms. Arch Neurol 2001;58:1438.
28. Hughes RA, Cornblath DR. Guillain-Barré syndrome. Lancet 2005;366:1653.
29. van Doorn PA, Ruts L, Jacobs BC. Clinical features, pathogenesis, and treatment of Guillain-Barré syndrome. Lancet Neurol 2008;7:939.
30. Asbury AK, Cornblath DR. Assessment of current diagnostic criteria for Guillain-Barré syndrome. Ann Neurol 1990;27(Suppl):S21.
31. Van der Meche FG, Van Doorn PA, Meulstee J, et al. Diagnostic and classification criteria for the Guillain-Barré syndrome. Eur Neurol 2001;45:133.
32. Winer JB, Hughes RA, Osmond C. A prospective study of acute idiopathic neuropathy. I. Clinical features and their prognostic value. J Neurol Neurosurg Psychiatry 1988;51:605.

33. Hadden RD, Karch H, Hartung HP, et al. Preceding infections, immune factors, and outcome in Guillain-Barré syndrome. Neurology 2001;56:758.
34. Hughes RA, Rees JH. Guillain-Barré syndrome. Curr Opin Neurol 1994;7:386.
35. Rees JH, Soudain SE, Gregson NA, et al. *Campylobacter jejuni* infection and Guillain-Barré syndrome. N Engl J Med 1995;333:1374.
36. Van Koningsveld R, Van Doorn PA, Schmitz PI, et al. Mild forms of Guillain-Barré syndrome in an epidemiologic survey in The Netherlands. Neurology 2000;54:620.
37. Orlikowski D, Prigent H, Sharshar T, et al. Respiratory dysfunction in Guillain-Barré syndrome. Neurocrit Care 2004;1:415.
38. Chevrolet JC, Deleamont P. Repeated vital capacity measurements as predictive parameters for mechanical ventilation need and weaning success in the Guillain-Barré syndrome. Am Rev Respir Dis 1991;144:814.
39. Ropper AH, Kehne SM. Guillain-Barré syndrome: management of respiratory failure. Neurology 1985;35:1662.
40. Sharshar T, Chevret S, Bourdain F, et al. Early predictors of mechanical ventilation in Guillain-Barré syndrome. Crit Care Med 2003;31:278.
41. Wijdicks EF, Borel CO. Respiratory management in acute neurologic illness. Neurology 1998;50:11.
42. Lawn ND, Fletcher DD, Henderson RD, et al. Anticipating mechanical ventilation in Guillain-Barré syndrome. Arch Neurol 2001;58:893.
43. Hughes RA. Management of acute neuromuscular paralysis. J R Coll Physicians Lond 1998;32:254.
44. Elovaara I, Apostolski S, van Doorn P, et al. EFNS guidelines for the use of intravenous immunoglobulin in treatment of neurological diseases: EFNS task force on the use of intravenous immunoglobulin in treatment of neurological diseases. Eur J Neurol 2008;15:893.
45. Randomised trial of plasma exchange, intravenous immunoglobulin, and combined treatments in Guillain-Barré syndrome. Plasma Exchange/Sandoglobulin Guillain-Barré Syndrome Trial Group. Lancet 1997;349:225.
46. van der Meche FG, Schmitz PI. A randomized trial comparing intravenous immune globulin and plasma exchange in Guillain-Barré syndrome. Dutch Guillain-Barré Study Group. N Engl J Med 1992;326:1123.
47. Hanson JA, Lueck CJ, Thomas DJ. Myasthenia gravis presenting with stridor. Thorax 1996;51:108.
48. Kim WH, Kim JH, Kim EK, et al. Myasthenia gravis presenting as isolated respiratory failure: a case report. Korean J Intern Med 2010;25:101.
49. Vaidya H. Case of the month: unusual presentation of myasthenia gravis with acute respiratory failure in the emergency room. Emerg Med J 2006;23:410.
50. Thomas CE, Mayer SA, Gungor Y, et al. Myasthenic crisis: clinical features, mortality, complications, and risk factors for prolonged intubation. Neurology 1997;48:1253.
51. Argov Z, Mastaglia FL. Drug therapy: disorders of neuromuscular transmission caused by drugs. N Engl J Med 1979;301:409.
52. Meriggioli MN, Sanders DB. Autoimmune myasthenia gravis: emerging clinical and biological heterogeneity. Lancet Neurol 2009;8:475.
53. McConville J, Farrugia ME, Beeson D, et al. Detection and characterization of MuSK antibodies in seronegative myasthenia gravis. Ann Neurol 2004;55:580.
54. Pascuzzi RM. The edrophonium test. Semin Neurol 2003;23:83.

55. Rieder P, Louis M, Jolliet P, et al. The repeated measurement of vital capacity is a poor predictor of the need for mechanical ventilation in myasthenia gravis. Intensive Care Med 1995;21:663.
56. Rabinstein A, Wijdicks EF. BiPAP in acute respiratory failure due to myasthenic crisis may prevent intubation. Neurology 2002;59:1647.
57. Seneviratne J, Mandrekar J, Wijdicks EF, et al. Noninvasive ventilation in myasthenic crisis. Arch Neurol 2008;65:54.
58. Lacomis D. Myasthenic crisis. Neurocrit Care 2005;3:189.
59. Qureshi AI, Choudhry MA, Akbar MS, et al. Plasma exchange versus intravenous immunoglobulin treatment in myasthenic crisis. Neurology 1999;52:629.
60. Corcia P, Pradat PF, Salachas F, et al. Causes of death in a post-mortem series of ALS patients. Amyotroph Lateral Scler 2008;9:59.
61. Miller RG, Jackson CE, Kasarskis EJ, et al. Practice parameter update: the care of the patient with amyotrophic lateral sclerosis: multidisciplinary care, symptom management, and cognitive/behavioral impairment (an evidence-based review): report of the Quality Standards Subcommittee of the American Academy of Neurology. Neurology 2009;73:1227.
62. de Carvalho M, Pinto S, Swash M. Association of paraspinal and diaphragm denervation in ALS. Amyotroph Lateral Scler 2010;11:63.
63. Hardiman O. Management of respiratory symptoms in ALS. J Neurol 2011; 258:359.
64. Hadjikoutis S, Wiles CM. Respiratory complications related to bulbar dysfunction in motor neuron disease. Acta Neurol Scand 2001;103:207.
65. Haverkamp LJ, Appel V, Appel SH. Natural history of amyotrophic lateral sclerosis in a database population. Validation of a scoring system and a model for survival prediction. Brain 1995;118(Pt 3):707.
66. Leiner GC, Abramowitz S, Small MJ, et al. Expiratory peak flow rate. Standard values for normal subjects. Use as a clinical test of ventilatory function. Am Rev Respir Dis 1963;88:644.
67. Morgan RK, McNally S, Alexander M, et al. Use of Sniff nasal-inspiratory force to predict survival in amyotrophic lateral sclerosis. Am J Respir Crit Care Med 2005;171:269.
68. Bach JR. Amyotrophic lateral sclerosis: prolongation of life by noninvasive respiratory AIDS. Chest 2002;122:92.
69. Gay PC, Edmonds LC. Severe hypercapnia after low-flow oxygen therapy in patients with neuromuscular disease and diaphragmatic dysfunction. Mayo Clin Proc 1995;70:327.
70. Lacomis D, Petrella JT, Giuliani MJ. Causes of neuromuscular weakness in the intensive care unit: a study of ninety-two patients. Muscle Nerve 1998; 21:610.
71. Zink W, Kollmar R, Schwab S. Critical illness polyneuropathy and myopathy in the intensive care unit. Nat Rev Neurol 2009;5:372.
72. Lacomis D, Zochodne DW, Bird SJ. Critical illness myopathy. Muscle Nerve 2000;23:1785.
73. Douglass JA, Tuxen DV, Horne M, et al. Myopathy in severe asthma. Am Rev Respir Dis 1992;146:517.
74. Rich MM, Bird SJ, Raps EC, et al. Direct muscle stimulation in acute quadriplegic myopathy. Muscle Nerve 1997;20:665.
75. Jiang JR, Shih JY, Wang HC, et al. Small-cell lung cancer presenting with Lambert-Eaton myasthenic syndrome and respiratory failure. J Formos Med Assoc 2002;101:871.

76. Tseng A, Claussen GC, Oh SJ. Respiratory failure in Lambert-Eaton myasthenic syndrome precipitated by calcium-channel blockers: report of a case and literature review. J Clin Neuromuscul Dis 2002;4:60.
77. Kongsaengdao S, Samintarapanya K, Rusmeechan S, et al. An outbreak of botulism in Thailand: clinical manifestations and management of severe respiratory failure. Clin Infect Dis 2006;43:1247.
78. Lewis SW, Pierson DJ, Cary JM, et al. Prolonged respiratory paralysis in wound botulism. Chest 1979;75:59.
79. Wongtanate M, Sucharitchan N, Tantisiriwit K, et al. Signs and symptoms predictive of respiratory failure in patients with foodborne botulism in Thailand. Am J Trop Med Hyg 2007;77:386.
80. Castelbaum AR, Donofrio PD, Walker FO, et al. Laxative abuse causing hypermagnesemia, quadriparesis, and neuromuscular junction defect. Neurology 1989;39:746.
81. Ferdinandus J, Pederson JA, Whang R. Hypermagnesemia as a cause of refractory hypotension, respiratory depression, and coma. Arch Intern Med 1981;141:669.
82. Goswamy R, Chaudhuri A, Mahashur AA. Study of respiratory failure in organophosphate and carbamate poisoning. Heart Lung 1994;23:466.
83. Noshad H, Ansarin K, Ardalan MR, et al. Respiratory failure in organophosphate insecticide poisoning. Saudi Med J 2007;28:405.
84. Faiz A, Ghose A, Ahsan F, et al. The greater black krait (*Bungarus niger*), a newly recognized cause of neuro-myotoxic snake bite envenoming in Bangladesh. Brain 2010;133:3181.
85. Nirthanan S, Gwee MC. Three-finger alpha-neurotoxins and the nicotinic acetylcholine receptor, forty years on. J Pharmacol Sci 2004;94:1.
86. Rowan EG. What does beta-bungarotoxin do at the neuromuscular junction? Toxicon 2001;39:107.
87. Grattan-Smith PJ, Morris JG, Johnston HM, et al. Clinical and neurophysiological features of tick paralysis. Brain 1997;120(Pt 11):1975.
88. Imerman B, Caruso LJ, Zori RT. Prolonged neuromuscular block in a patient undergoing renal transplantation. J Clin Anesth 2001;13:540.
89. Betensley AD, Jaffery SH, Collins H, et al. Bilateral diaphragmatic paralysis and related respiratory complications in a patient with West Nile virus infection. Thorax 2004;59:268.
90. Poudel P, Budhathoki S, Manandhar S. Tetanus. Kathmandu Univ Med J (KUMJ) 2009;7:315.
91. Blumbergs PC, Byrne E, Kakulas BA. Polymyositis presenting with respiratory failure. J Neurol Sci 1984;65:221.
92. Dauriat G, Stern JB, Similowski T, et al. Acute respiratory failure due to diaphragmatic weakness revealing a polymyositis. Eur J Intern Med 2002;13:203.
93. Sano M, Suzuki M, Sato M, et al. Fatal respiratory failure due to polymyositis. Intern Med 1994;33:185.
94. Bedry R, Baudrimont I, Deffieux G, et al. Wild-mushroom intoxication as a cause of rhabdomyolysis. N Engl J Med 2001;345:798.
95. Francis L, Bonilla E, Soforo E, et al. Fatal toxic myopathy attributed to propofol, methylprednisolone, and cyclosporine after prior exposure to colchicine and simvastatin. Clin Rheumatol 2008;27:129.
96. Mellies U, Ragette R, Schwake C, et al. Sleep-disordered breathing and respiratory failure in acid maltase deficiency. Neurology 2001;57:1290.
97. Rosenow EC 3rd, Engel AG. Acid maltase deficiency in adults presenting as respiratory failure. Am J Med 1978;64:485.

98. Barohn RJ, Clanton T, Sahenk Z, et al. Recurrent respiratory insufficiency and depressed ventilatory drive complicating mitochondrial myopathies. Neurology 1990;40:103.
99. Cros D, Palliyath S, DiMauro S, et al. Respiratory failure revealing mitochondrial myopathy in adults. Chest 1992;101:824.
100. Kim GW, Kim SM, Sunwoo IN, et al. Two cases of mitochondrial myopathy with predominant respiratory dysfunction. Yonsei Med J 1991;32:184.
101. Gentili A, Iannella E, Masciopinto F, et al. Rhabdomyolysis and respiratory failure: rare presentation of carnitine palmityl-transferase II deficiency. Minerva Anestesiol 2008;74:205.
102. Joutel A, Moulonguet A, Demaugre F, et al. Type II carnitine palmitoyl transferase deficiency complicated by acute respiratory failure. Rev Neurol (Paris) 1993;149:797 [in French].
103. Smolle KH, Kaufmann P, Gasser R. Recurrent rhabdomyolysis and acute respiratory failure due to carnitine palmityltransferase deficiency. Intensive Care Med 2001;27:1235.
104. Tong MK, Lam CS, Mak TW, et al. Very long-chain acyl-CoA dehydrogenase deficiency presenting as acute hypercapnic respiratory failure. Eur Respir J 2006;28:447.
105. Abbasi B, Sharif Z, Sprabery LR. Hypokalemic thyrotoxic periodic paralysis with thyrotoxic psychosis and hypercapnic respiratory failure. Am J Med Sci 2010; 340:147.
106. Ryan AM, Matthews E, Hanna MG. Skeletal-muscle channelopathies: periodic paralysis and nondystrophic myotonias. Curr Opin Neurol 2007;20:558.

Ischemic Stroke: Emergencies and Management

Roger E. Kelley, MD*, Sheryl Martin-Schild, MD, PhD

KEYWORDS

- Acute ischemic stroke • Thrombolytic therapy
- Cerebral angioplasty • Cerebral edema • Vascular dissection

It is now increasingly recognized that acute ischemic stroke is an emergent issue that is potentially amenable to interventions that may have a significant effect on outcome. Naturally, when one is talking about interventional therapy for acute ischemic stroke, outside of aspirin, there is a trade-off between risks versus benefits. The major issue is what to do about clots. The development and propagation of thrombus, as well as thromboembolic mechanism, is at the center of interventional therapy. For years, it was theorized that antithrombotic therapy with unfractionated heparin, an agent that binds with antithrombin III and interferes with the intrinsic coagulation pathway, would block thrombin formation and protect against the propagation of thrombus with a salutatory effect on ischemic stroke. Anecdotally, there was some support for efficacy, but scientific support was lacking.

One of the major challenges is to effectively determine whether or not an intervention is having an effect on outcome. The natural history of stroke is quite variable. Several neuroprotective trials demonstrated that a relatively minor stroke tends to have a good outcome, within a finite period of time, as part of the natural history. This finding can make it difficult to detect a positive effect of an intervention unless the effect is substantial. A major question is what constitutes a certifiable significant effect that potentially justifies approval by the Food and Drug Administration (FDA). Will a 20% difference between study intervention versus placebo suffice? The magnitude will impact the choice of the patient population in terms of how the potential agent is being assessed. A higher-risk population is easier for the detection of an effect than a lower-risk population. Furthermore, the potential efficacy will very much impact on how the study will need to be powered to determine a possible effect. In other words, an agent that limits infarct size by 50% or greater, within a certain therapeutic time

Department of Neurology, Tulane University School of Medicine, 1430 Tulane Avenue 8065, New Orleans, LA 70112, USA
* Corresponding author.
E-mail address: rkelley2@tulane.edu

Neurol Clin 30 (2012) 187–210
doi:10.1016/j.ncl.2011.09.014 **neurologic.theclinics.com**
0733-8619/12/$ – see front matter

window, will need less study patients to demonstrate a positive effect on outcome than a drug that limits infarct size by 30%.

The concept of therapeutic window for efficacy versus detriment is extremely important in clinical decision making. There is a limited time for correction of circulatory compromise before the ischemic cascade[1] evolves into a danger zone for potential hemorrhagic conversion of the evolving infarct (**Fig. 1**). Furthermore, the concept of reperfusion injury[2] is very real because the restoration of the circulation to irreversibly infarcted tissue can promote expanded brain tissue injury as excitatory neurotoxins, including free oxygen radicals, have enhanced access to the infarct with subsequently enhanced infarction size.

Four major targets of therapeutic intervention in acute ischemic stroke are the (1) restoration of the circulation with a timeframe in which the restored perfusion has more of a salutatory effect than a detrimental effect; (2) interference of the ischemic cascade pathways, which is predicated on reversible versus irreversible interference; (3) lowering cerebral metabolic demand so that the susceptible brain tissue is protected against impaired perfusion; and (4) protection against recurrent ischemic events. Examples of reperfusion of an occlusive cerebrovascular event include thrombolytic therapy,[3] the potential for ultrasound to enhance thrombolysis[4] and angioplasty with stenting,[5] and mechanical embolectomy with devices, such as the Merci clot retrieval device[6] (Concentric Medical of Mountain View, CA, USA) and the Penumbra clot retrieval device[7] (Penumbra, Inc, Alameda, CA, USA). Several efforts have been made with neuroprotective agents to interfere with the generation of cerebral infarcted tissue.[8] However, to date, even with various near misses,[9] no agent has been found to improve outcome in a statistically significant fashion that would justify its release by the FDA.[10] Certain neuroprotective approaches are designed to reduce the metabolic need of brain tissue that is underperfused. The prototypical approach is hypothermia, which is well established as having potential in protecting the brain against anoxic/ischemic insults, such as during cardiac arrest.[11] However, there

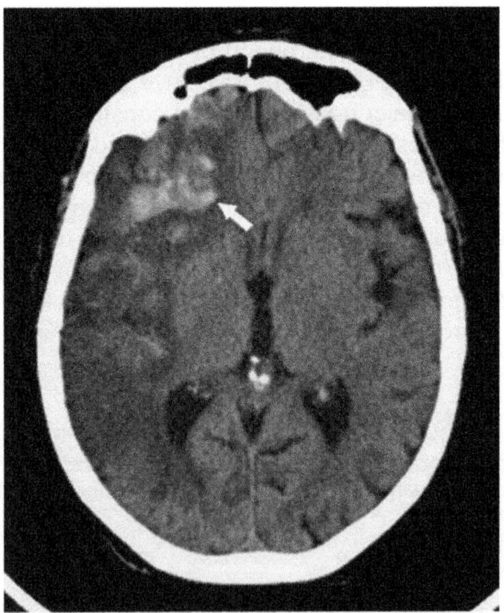

Fig. 1. Hemorrhagic conversion of an acute middle artery distribution cerebral infarct on noncontrast CT brain scan with arrow identifying the associated hemorrhagic transformation.

have been various potential clinical barriers with hypothermia, and it is not yet ready for prime time in our present armamentarium for acute ischemic stroke.[12]

MECHANISM OF ISCHEMIC INSULT

A major issue in stroke management is the determination of the presumptive mechanism of the cerebral ischemic insult. Naturally, vessel occlusion would be expected to be more amenable to thrombolytic therapy than a nonobstructed vessel. Cardio-embolic stroke implies clot formation in the heart that traverses into the cerebral circulation. Embolic occlusion of a cerebral artery would be expected to be especially responsive to therapy designed to break up a clot. On the other hand, in situ small vessel thrombosis, the most commonly cited mechanism of lacunar-type stroke, may be less amenable to thrombolysis. Artery-to-artery embolism is a commonly cited mechanism for ischemic stroke and can be related to carotid or aortic arch plaque formation. There is also the potential for hemodynamic compromise with vessel stenosis and this might be more relevant in vertebrobasilar ischemia.[13] This concept is important because carotid intervention, despite significant stenosis, is not necessarily going to be beneficial for patients with symptoms referable to the vertebrobasilar system.

Potential mechanisms of ischemic stroke are summarized in **Box 1**. It is important to recognize that a significant percentage of patients with ischemic stroke have a mechanism that cannot be readily determined.[14] This point is perhaps of greater importance for the so-called stroke in the young, which is attributed to stroke in patients who are 45 years of age or younger and have no ongoing, well-recognized risk factors for ischemic stroke. In such patients, more esoteric causes of stroke are often brought

Box 1
Potential mechanisms of ischemic stroke

1. Large-artery thrombotic
2. Small-artery thrombotic (lacunar-type)
3. Artery-to-artery embolism
4. Cardio-embolic
5. Cerebrovascular dissection
6. Cerebral vasculitis
7. Cerebral sinovenous thrombosis
8. Hematological occlusive process (eg, sickle cell disease, thrombocytosis, polycythemia)
9. Iatrogenic (eg, ENT procedures affecting the extracranial vasculature)
10. Septic embolism from infectious endocarditis
11. Sympathomimetic agent–induced vasospasm
12. Hypotensive with cerebral hypoperfusion (eg, watershed infarction)
13. Secondary cerebral ischemia following aneurysmal rupture
14. Noninflammatory cerebral vasculopathy (eg, moyamoya disease)
15. Hypercoagulability (eg, antiphospholipid syndrome; antithrombin III, protein S, or protein C deficiency; malignancy related)
16. Nonseptic embolism from marantic endocarditis

into the differential diagnosis (**Box 2**), such as vascular dissection, migraine, hypercoagulable state, vasculitis, oral contraceptive use in women, and paradoxic cerebral embolism.[15]

The determination of the stroke mechanism helps in terms of diagnostic yield for investigational studies. Naturally, the history of standard cardiac disease–related risk factors, including advanced age, hypertension, hyperlipidemia, and diabetes mellitus, will more likely identify a cardiogenic mechanism than in an individual aged 45 years or younger without these risk factors. In such a circumstance, mechanisms, such as paradoxic cerebral embolism, through a patent foramen ovale, atrial myxoma, and endocarditis will be of potentially higher yield diagnostically than in a 70-year-old patient with long-standing hypertension and hyperlipidemia with a history of myocardial infarction. In our evolving health care system, whereby diagnostic study choice might be dictated by the expected yield frequency, we may be faced with paradigms that mandate risk stratification from the start. Presently, we have available a virtual cornucopia of diagnostic studies in acute ischemic stroke that seems to increasingly expand, especially when we start to factor in genetic studies. However, cost issues raise the important question of how such studies will impact patient management to justify cost.

GENERAL PRINCIPLES OF ISCHEMIC STROKE MANAGEMENT

The ABCs of resuscitation for acute ischemic stroke must be attended to, especially in patients with moderate to severe infarction of the cerebral hemispheres, the brainstem, or the cerebellum. The airway may be compromised by pharyngeal muscle dysfunction, and loss of control of the oropharyngeal secretions increases the risk for aspiration. Most patients do not require supplemental oxygen to keep normal oxygen saturations. Respiratory compromise will mandate ventilator support. Noninvasive positive-pressure ventilator support may suffice but, if patients are at a high risk for aspiration, this option is contraindicated. Unfortunately, the requirement for

Box 2
Differential diagnosis of ischemic stroke in the young

1. Paradoxical cerebral embolism via patent foramen ovale
2. Migrainous infarction
3. Oral contraceptive with resultant hypercoagulopathy
4. Infectious endocarditis
5. Connective tissue disorder
6. Cerebrovascular dissection
7. Moyamoya disease
8. Cocaine-induced vasculitis
9. Anticlotting deficiency
10. Sinovenous thrombosis
11. Sickle cell disease
12. Polycythemia vera
13. Thrombocytosis
14. Meningovascular syphilis

endotracheal intubation is associated with a high 30-day mortality rate after ischemic stroke.

Neurological checks and vital signs are typically ordered every 4 hours in patients with moderate to large infarcts, with closer monitoring after thrombolytic therapy in an intensive care unit as well as for those patients who are neurologically unstable. For patients receiving recombinant tissue plasminogen activator (rt-PA), the blood pressure should be measured every 15 minutes for 2 hours after the initiation of the infusion, then every 30 minutes for 6 hours, and then every 60 minutes until 24 hours after the initiation of treatment.

Patients seen on an emergency basis with symptoms of stroke need an immediate complete blood count (CBC), platelet count, prothrombin time/international normalization ratio (INR), partial thromboplastin time, and metabolic studies to assess for significant hypoglycemia or hyperglycemia, as well as a noncontrast computed tomography (CT) brain scan and electrocardiogram (EKG). In certain medical centers, the magnetic resonance imaging (MRI) brain scan will be substituted for the CT brain scan as long as imaging sequences are available that can reliably distinguish an ischemic insult from a hemorrhagic one. It is common to see an imaging protocol, at certain centers, that attempts to compare perfusion with diffusion imaging, looking for the so-called mismatch between perfusion and diffusion lesion supportive of reversibly impaired tissue often termed the ischemic penumbra.[16] Such imaging assessment of salvageable brain tissue has been reported to be of value with both MR[17] as well as perfusion CT scan techniques.[18] In addition, incorporation of such potential mismatch assessment, with either MR or CT techniques, along with vessel imaging which can include, respectively, magnetic resonance angiography (MRA) or CT angiography (CTA) (**Fig. 2**). Alternatively, transcranial Doppler ultrasonography (TCD) can be used in the emergency department setting to assess for vessel patency

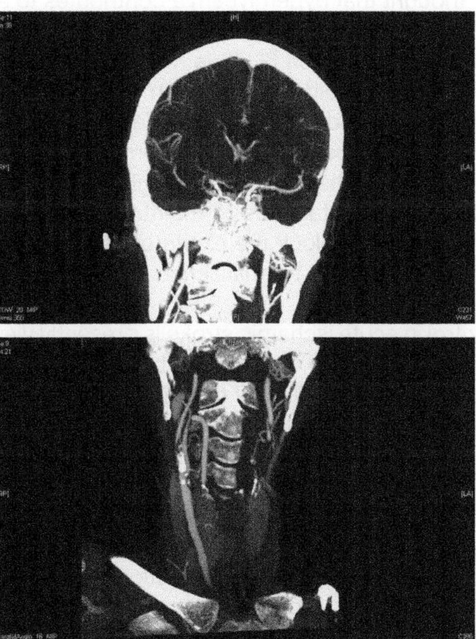

Fig. 2. CT angiogram that demonstrates (*top*) total middle cerebral artery occlusion ipsilateral to (*bottom*) high-grade internal carotid artery origin stenosis.

in a noninvasive fashion.[19] However, studies that delay the administration of thrombolytic therapy are counterproductive. Certain readily available imaging findings, such as the hyperdense middle cerebral artery on CT brain scan, reflective of a presence of a clot may have an impact on the response to therapy.[20]

Appropriate monitoring is important in terms of protection of the airway, and protection against aspiration, as well as the monitoring of effective breathing, with pulse oximetry and adequate circulation with the assessment of an adequate mean arterial pressure, for the clinical situation. Respiratory compromise will mandate ventilator support, if necessary, although noninvasive respiratory support has its potential advantages as long as aspiration risk does not contraindicate this option. In this regard, a swallowing study becomes mandatory for any patient with clinically significant neurologic deficits in acute ischemic stroke. Cardiac monitoring can be of particular value if there is evidence of cardiac ischemia associated with the stroke or risk of cardiac arrhythmia that may impact management, such as paroxysmal atrial fibrillation. This arrhythmia is reported to be present in up to 9.2% of patients with definite ischemic stroke or transient ischemic attack.[21] The yield of finding this potential cardio-embolic source correlates with the diligence with which it is sought and might well require Holter monitoring up to day 7 of the time of presentation of the arrhythmia.[22] Stroke units are particularly well suited for such monitoring of patients with acute ischemic stroke and are clearly established to improve outcome. Blood pressure monitoring, mentioned previously, is important not only from the standpoint of protection against unacceptable elevation following thrombolytic therapy but also in terms of avoiding relative hypotension, which can, at least theoretically, lead to extension of the infarction. Stroke units are particularly well suited for such monitoring of the patients' neurologic and hemodynamic status and have clearly been demonstrated to have a positive impact on outcome.

Optimal blood sugar management is still under investigation in acute ischemic stroke. It is generally thought that hyperglycemia contributes to adverse outcomes.[23] However, use of an insulin sliding scale, as opposed to continuous insulin infusion, may not be the optimal approach.[24] It is generally accepted that dextrose-containing intravenous fluids should be avoided in the acute stroke setting. There is also evidence that persistent body temperature elevation has an adverse effect on stroke outcome and this should be avoided.[25] Patients with ischemic stroke are often volume depleted. In such circumstances, the administration of intravenous normal saline at 1 to 2 mL/kg/h is advantageous to maintain fluid balance. In addition, the electrolyte magnesium serves to block the excitatory glutamate receptor, which has led to a recommendation for the normalization of the serum magnesium when deficient.

Blood pressure control in acute ischemic stroke is presently viewed as permissive in terms of acceptable ballpark values of a systolic blood pressure of 180 ± 20 mm Hg and a diastolic blood pressure of 110 ± 10 mm Hg. This approach is primarily based on the theoretical concerns over too aggressive blood pressure control promoting hypoperfusion in the setting of the disruption of cerebral autoregulation.[26] Such hypoperfusion, in turn, promote the extension of the infarct and worsen outcomes. The natural corollary of this is that hypertensive therapy might have a potential benefit in protecting susceptible brain tissue in the region of the infarct (ie, the penumbra). However, such an approach, despite the theoretical attractiveness, has not been clearly established as beneficial.[27] From a practical standpoint, it is advisable to avoid antihypertensive agents, with markedly elevated blood pressure, that can cause a precipitous drop in blood pressure with the potential for cerebral hypoperfusion. Agents that have been specifically cited for such blood pressure management include labetalol and nicardipine. Labetalol boluses result in mild and fairly predictable decreases in blood pressure, and nicardipine can be rapidly titrated for a target blood pressure with little effect on heart rate or cerebral vasoreactivity. On the other hand, agents, such as nifedipine or clonidine, are best avoided. In the malignant intractable elevation of the blood pressure, the agent sodium nitroprusside may still have a place in management as long as an arterial line is available for accurate monitoring of the antihypertensive effect and intracranial hypertension is not suspected. It is important to keep in mind that blood pressure guidelines with the use of an agent, such as rt-PA, are systolic blood pressure less than or equal to 185 mm Hg and diastolic blood pressure less than or equal to 110 mm Hg. Therefore, with the use of such a thrombolytic agent, labetalol, nicardipine, or the nitroglycerin patch are attractive choices.

As long as there are not concerns about aspiration, enteral nutrition is preferred over parenteral alimentation. Over the longer term, if aspiration remains a concern, then the percutaneous enteral gastrostomy tube becomes indicated. Elevation of the head to roughly 30° can protect against aspiration, although flat positioning of the head may improve blood flow velocity in the acute setting.[28] Proper nutrition is an important means to promote recovery after stroke and needs to be instituted as soon as feasible.

Prevention of deep venous thrombosis (DVT), and the subsequent concern about pulmonary embolism, is of the utmost importance in acute ischemic stroke. It is well established that subcutaneous heparin or heparinoid is indicated for DVT prophylaxis in acute ischemic stroke and is part of the guidelines of both the American Academy of Neurology and the American Stroke Association[29] for acute ischemic stroke management. Naturally, the risk of DVT is reflective of immobility and the longer patients are immobile, the greater the likelihood of complications of immobility, such as DVT, pressure sores of the skin, and infections related to a prolonged recumbent posture. Unfractionated heparin, with a dosage of 5000 units subcutaneous twice a day, is the most cost-effective but may not have the efficacy of low-molecular-weight heparins, such as enoxaparin.[30] Intermittent pressure stockings can also be advantageous in such a clinical setting, especially if the use of heparin or heparinoid is contraindicated for reasons, such as heparin-induced thrombocytopenia.[31] Every effort should be made to mobilize patients with acute stroke as early as possible in an enhanced effort to protect against such potential problems with prolonged immobility.

It is well recognized that part of the early mobilization effort includes rehabilitative specialists to assess various functional limitations and determine how best to address these limitations when they are present. The assessment of swallowing function, often with the input of a speech pathologist, is vitally important to protect against aspiration pneumonia in patients who have had a stroke who are susceptible to such aspiration. This risk is usually associated with either larger hemispheric infarcts, which impact on the level of alertness, or infarcts involving the brainstem or cerebellum, which impair bulbar function with secondary dysphagia. Speech therapists also help in assessing and promoting the recovery of associated communication deficits both in terms of aphasia and dysarthria. Occupational and physical therapists work in tandem in the assessment and therapeutic intervention for motor, coordination, and gait deficits that may be associated with the acute ischemic stroke. Multidisciplinary rounds in stroke units can be beneficial for the coordination of various services in an effort to promote optimal recovery for the stroke victim. This includes the potential neuropsychological assessment when cognitive deficits interfere with the neurorehabilitative process. Denial, neglect, and resistance to the rehabilitative specialists, not uncommonly seen with nondominant hemispheric infarcts, can be quite counterproductive to the therapists' efforts. It is also important to screen for depression, which is commonly encountered in patients who have had a stroke. Significant depression, with the tendency toward social withdrawal associated with it, can impede the level of cooperation expected of patients in the neurorehabilitative process. Selective serotonin reuptake inhibitors, such as fluoxetine, have been reported to improved depressed mood in acute stroke[32] and may also help in the recovery of motor function.[33] **Box 3** summarizes general principles in the assessment and management of acute ischemic stroke.

THROMBOLYTIC THERAPY

A major advance in improving acute ischemic stroke outcome has been the demonstration that certain agents have the potential to disrupt a clot obstructing a cerebral vessel. It clearly makes theoretical sense that the restoration of impaired cerebral blood flow should help ischemic stroke outcomes *if* it can be done in a timely fashion. Demonstration of efficacy in thrombolytic therapy was not an overnight event, however. Initial attempts at clot lysis, with an agent such as streptokinase,[34] were not only not helpful but potentially harmful. However, there was scientific support for such an approach with various laboratory models of ischemic stroke as well as the obvious impetus from several cardiac interventional trials.

Box 3
Basic assessment and management measures in acute ischemic stroke

1. Assess vital signs to ensure adequate breathing, regularity of pulse, presence or absence of fever, and blood pressure range that is appropriate for the clinical presentation
2. Protection against elevated body temperature with an agent, such as acetaminophen
3. Avoidance of hyperglycemia and hypoglycemia; generally, dextrose-containing intravenous fluids are avoided
4. Stat (immediate) noncontrast CT brain scan with option of diffusion/perfusion–weighted MRI with gradient echo at certain centers; protocols at certain centers may include perfusion CT brain scan with CTA or MRA
5. Stat blood work, including CBC, prothrombin time/INR, partial thromboplastin time and metabolic profile
6. EKG to assess for cardiac arrhythmia, such as atrial fibrillation, as well as for acute myocardial ischemia
7. Determination of the appropriateness of possible interventional therapy, such as thrombolytic therapy, clot retrieval, mechanical disruption, or angioplasty with stenting
8. Assessment of swallowing capacity in an effort to avoid aspiration
9. DVT prophylaxis
10. Early mobilization to protect against potential complications of immobility, such as skin breakdown, DVT, and infections
11. Heart rhythm monitoring
12. Further assessment of stroke mechanism, which might include carotid/vertebral duplex scan, cerebral angiography, transcranial Doppler ultrasound, lipid profile, platelet function studies, assessment for a hypercoagulable state, 2-dimensional or transesophageal echocardiography, evaluation for a connective tissue disorder, sickle cell preparation, blood cultures, syphilis serology
13. Initiation of aspirin at 160 to 325 mg/d if no contraindication
14. Rehabilitation services consultation, which can include speech therapy, occupational therapy, and physical therapy as appropriate

Rt-PA was released by the FDA in the United States for the treatment of acute ischemic stroke in 1996. This release was based on the National Institutes of Neurologic Diseases and Stroke (NINDS) trial,[35] which demonstrated roughly a 30% improvement in the rate of essentially full recovery from stroke at 3 months compared with placebo. The 6.4% risk of symptomatic brain hemorrhage associated with rt-PA has tempered enthusiasm along with the indications for its use (**Box 4**) and the contraindications for its use (**Box 5**). Despite initial concerns about just how effective thrombolytic therapy is as opposed to concerns about bleeding risk, cumulative information from ongoing studies has convincingly demonstrated its efficacy and justified its use.[36] Concern about the risk of brain hemorrhage remains with rt-PA, and this risk tends to be enhanced in patients with larger infarcts with a National Institutes of Health (NIH) Stroke Scale greater than 22, those with an early infarction pattern on CT brain scan that involves more than one-third of the middle cerebral artery territory and those of advanced age with an increased risk of underlying cerebral amyloid angiopathy.

Challenges related to the 3-hour time window for the availability of intravenous infusion has led to no more than 5% of patients with acute ischemic stroke receiving this agent.[37] However, this percentage can clearly be improved in sophisticated centers that are geared to reduction in the door-to-needle time for the administration of this agent.

The dose of rt-PA is 0.9 mg/kg up to a maximum of 90 mg, with 10% given by intravenous bolus over 1 minute and the remainder infused over 1 hour. The patient is generally carefully monitored in an intensive-care-unit setting for at least the first 48 hours, and a follow-up CT brain scan is obtained at 24 hours to assess for possible subclinical hemorrhagic transformation of the infarct and to allow guidance in terms of initiation of antiplatelet or anticoagulant therapy, which needs to be held for at least 24 hours after the rt-PA infusion. Naturally, clinical evidence of intracerebral hemorrhage, based on neurologic worsening, mandates an immediate CT brain scan. The demonstration of intracerebral hemorrhage leads to efforts to limit the amount of bleeding with 6 to 8 units of cryoprecipitate or fresh frozen plasma and 10 units of single-donor platelets. Neurosurgical consultation is also recommended in case there is a potential benefit from hematoma evacuation. An additional concern with rt-PA is the risk of orolingual angioedema, which is enhanced in patients receiving angiotensin-converting enzyme inhibitors. This condition has the potential to

Box 4
Indications for the use of recombinant intravenous tissue plasminogen activator in acute ischemic stroke

1. Presentation, evaluation, and treatment within 3.0 to 4.5 hours
2. Finite neurologic deficit on neurologic examination as assessed by the NIH Stroke Scale with the absence of spontaneous significant resolution during initial evaluation
3. Noncontrast CT brain scan, or alternative MRI at certain centers, that is compatible with an acute ischemic stroke
4. Lack of an alternative explanation for the neurologic presentation, such as severe hypoglycemia or hyperglycemia or the residua of a focal seizure (ie, Todd paralysis)
5. Effort to address potential risks versus benefits of this agent with patients and close family members, which is documented in the records and with some centers requesting an effort at an informed consent form; informed consent is presumably most appropriate, at this time, for use of this agent beyond the standard 3-hour therapeutic window
6. Persistent neurologic deficit that is not rapidly resolving during the evaluation process

Box 5
Contraindications to the use of intravenous rt-PA in acute ischemic stroke

1. Clinical or imaging evidence of intracerebral or subarachnoid hemorrhage
2. Intracranial or intraspinal surgery within 3 months of presentation
3. Prior ischemic stroke within 3 months of presentation
4. Serious head trauma within 3 months of presentation
5. History of intracranial hemorrhage
6. Persistently uncontrolled high blood pressure at the time of presentation with systolic blood pressure greater than 185 mm Hg or diastolic blood pressure greater than 110 mm Hg; agents, such as intravenous labetalol or nicardipine and nitroglycerin paste, may be considered for the maintenance of adequately controlled blood pressure, with recognition that the blood pressure may fluctuate to a significant degree in the acute stroke setting
7. Seizure at the onset of the stroke that is thought to likely explain the deficit at the time of presentation
8. Active internal bleeding
9. Evidence of intracranial neoplasm, arteriovenous malformation, or cerebral aneurysm
10. Acute myocardial infarction within the previous 3 months[a]
11. Bleeding abnormality, which can include warfarin therapy with an INR greater than 1.7 or a prothrombin time greater than 15 seconds, use of heparin within 48 hours of presentation with a significantly prolonged activated partial thromboplastin time at the time of presentation, or a platelet count less than 100,000/mm[3b]
12. For the 3.0- to 4.5-hour window: aged 80 years or older, prior ischemic stroke with diabetes mellitus, and any recent use of an oral anticoagulant

[a] Initially viewed as an absolute contraindication, but now viewed, at least by some, as a relative contraindication dependent on the risk of transmural rupture.
[b] The release of the agent dabigatran for stroke prevention in atrial fibrillation has necessitated avoiding within 48 hours of dosing, with a normal activated partial thromboplastin time (aPTT), as a guideline.

compromise the airway, and there have been reports of response to antihistamine agents along with steroid therapy.

The sooner patients receive the rt-TPA, the greater the likelihood of a positive response. In a report of cumulative experience with this agent,[38] the odds ratio (OR) of an excellent outcome, compared with placebo, is 2.8 for patients treated within 90 minutes, 1.6 for patients treated within 91 to 180 minutes, 1.4 for patients treated at 181 to 270 minutes, and 1.2 for patients treated within 271 to 360 minutes. Patients most likely to benefit are reported to be those with milder neurologic deficit, absence of diabetes mellitus and normal blood glucose, normal CT brain scan, and normal blood pressure.[39] Despite this, it seems that the quicker recanalization is effectively achieved, the more likely is one to see an improved outcome with revascularization procedures.[40]

The Alteplase Thrombolysis for Acute Noninterventional Therapy in Ischemic Stroke (ATLANTIS) trial[41] did not find that potential benefits of extending the administration of rt-PA to a 3- to 5-hour window was associated with improvement that would justify the increased risk of cerebral hemorrhage. It was speculated that a mismatch between clinical deficit and diffusion-weighted imaging (DWI) MRI might identify patients more likely to benefit from rt-PA in the 3- to 6-hour therapeutic window. However, such a therapeutic approach did not translate into improved outcomes or enhanced reperfusion.[42] Despite these discouraging results for the extension of the therapeutic window for rt-PA, Hacke and colleagues,[43] for the European Cooperative Acute Stroke Study (ECASS) investigators, reported a 52.4% favorable outcome with rt-PA compared with 45.2% with placebo (OR = 1.34, *P* = .04). It is important to note that this study excluded patients aged more than 80 years, those with a combination of previous stroke and diabetes mellitus, and those on oral anticoagulant therapy even if the INR was in the nontherapeutic range. The risk of cerebral hemorrhage was 27.0% with rt-PA compared with 17.6% for placebo, but symptomatic hemorrhage, respectively, was 2.4% vs 0.2%, *P* = .008). Furthermore, the mortality rate was not statistically significantly different (7.7% vs 8.4%).

In the scientific advisory from the American Heart Association/American Stroke Association,[44] which recommended an extended window of rt-PA to 4.5 hours based on this ECASS study, symptomatic cerebral hemorrhage was interpreted as being 7.9%, by NINDS study criteria, with rt-PA compared with 3.5% with placebo (OR = 2.38, *P* = .0008). To date, the FDA has not approved the extension of the window to 4.5 hours, which creates a dilemma for the clinician treating acute ischemic stroke. In such a circumstance, if one is convinced that intravenous rt-PA is a legitimate option with a 3.0- to 4.5-hour window, then an informed consent should probably be developed and approved by the medical center administration whereby patients and family members are made aware that there is scientific support for the use of such an agent with an extended window, but that the evidence, to date, has not resulted in approval by the FDA.

Intra-arterial thrombolytic therapy is an exciting option for acute ischemic stroke for patients who are beyond the therapeutic window for intravenous rt-PA and at centers that have special expertise in the use of such therapy. However, the time window for therapeutic benefit versus enhanced risk of hemorrhagic complication is still being worked out. Efforts have been made to combine intravenous rt-PA with intra-arterial rt-PA, the so-called bridging therapy.[45]

This therapy theoretically allows immediate access to intravenous therapy but is in recognition that the recanalization success with this approach can be improved on. A recent study reported an acute recanalization rate with intravenous rt-PA of only 21.25%.[46] The use of intra-arterial thrombolysis has been reported to have a recanalization rate substantially greater than intravenous therapy.[47] Unfortunately, the bridging trial reported by Lewandowski and colleagues,[48] consisting of 0.6 mg/kg intravenous rt-PA with 10% by bolus and the remainder over 30 minutes, at a maximum dose of 60 mg, followed by intra-arterial rt-PA administered to the clot within 2 hours of the intravenous dose, with a maximum dose of 20 mg, reported a treatment mortality of 29%. This finding was in distinction from 5.5% in the comparison group that only received the intra-arterial rt-PA (*P* = .06). Despite this sobering endpoint, the researchers made note of the 54% successful recanalization rate versus 10% (*P* = .03) as well as the improved NIHSS scores in survivors at 3 months out. This finding has led to the Interventional Management of Stroke (IMS) trial, which has progressed to a pivotal IMS-III study in progress.[47] Preliminary data suggests an acceptable safety profile and improved outcomes compared with historical controls from the NINDS trial.[34] An example of successful recanalization is demonstrated in **Fig. 3**.

Most patients with acute ischemic stroke are not eligible for intravenous rt-PA because of the time-window limitations. However, imaging studies have suggested that perfusion-diffusion mismatch[17] (ie, relative sparing of perfusion adjacent to the area of completed infarction demonstrating tissue at risk) (**Fig. 4**) may allow the identification of patients beyond the 3-hour, or 4.5-hour, window of opportunity who still may benefit from thrombolytic therapy. Such potential efficacy beyond the standard time window, with the use of intra-arterial thrombolytic therapy alone, was supported

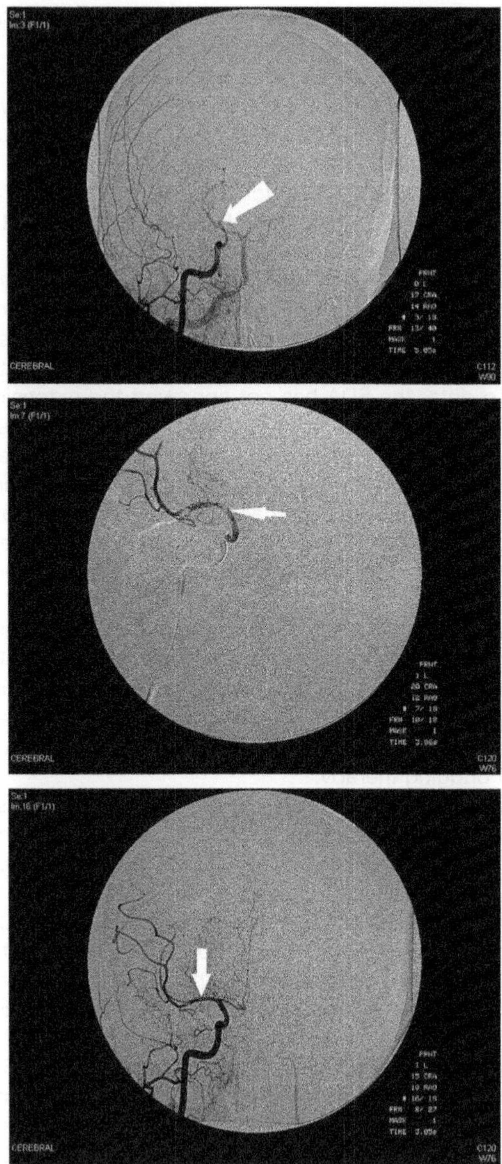

Fig. 3. Distal right internal carotid artery near occlusion (*top*) with successful reconstitution of right middle cerebral artery flow (*middle*) along with anterior cerebral artery flow (*bottom*) with intra-arterial thrombolytic therapy (*arrows*).

by the Prolyse in Acute Cerebral Thromboembolism (PROACT) study.[49,50] These studies (PROACT-I and -II) looked at the recanalization rate of intra-arterial recombinant prourokinase as a function of safety and outcome in acute ischemic stroke with a 6-hour therapeutic window. Both groups received intravenous heparin as part of the study protocol, with the control group receiving heparin alone. The recanalization rate was 66% in the study group compared with 18% in the control group

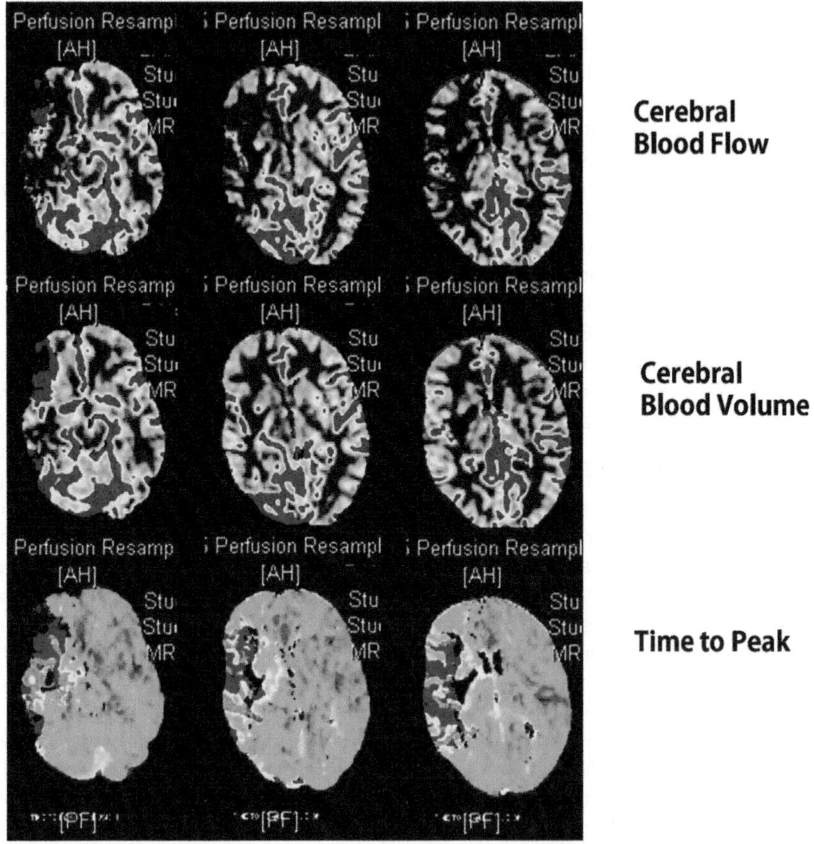

Fig. 4. CT cerebral blood flow versus blood volume perfusion imaging, which demonstrates a large mismatch that reflects susceptible versus infarcted tissue as demonstrated in the time-to-peak image.

($P<.001$), and with good outcome at 90 days, 40% in the study group compared with 25% in the control group (OR = 2.13, $P = .04$). However, the 10% risk of intracerebral hemorrhage in the study group, compared with 2% in the control group ($P = .06$), translated into this thrombolytic agent never being approved by the FDA for such an indication. Despite this, the most recent Guidelines for the Management of Adults with Ischemic Stroke from the American Stroke Association Stroke Council[26] list intra-arterial thrombolysis as a therapeutic option for patients treated within 6 hours of a major stroke associated with middle cerebral artery occlusion and who have access to a facility with acceptable expertise in the interventional realm for such a procedure.

The challenge of the consequences of symptomatic severe occlusive vertebrobasilar disease has led several qualified centers to extend the therapeutic window for intra-arterial thrombolytic therapy to up to 24 hours. This extension is based on the natural history of severe brainstem stroke in terms of the cumulative severe morbidity and mortality, which is 90% or greater, whereas successful revascularization has the potential to make a significant improvement in outcome.[51] There are several presentations and anecdotal reports of great saves in terms of patients who seemed to be headed toward an irretrievable locked-in state who recovered remarkably well with such therapy. Generally, these are patients who are beyond the 3-hour window for intravenous rt-PA based on the time involved in determining the degree of vascular involvement with neurovascular imaging. However, faster determination of the occlusive process with noninvasive imaging techniques, such as CTA, may expedite the detection and potential for intervention in severe vertebrobasilar occlusive disease.[52] However, a recent study reported that contrast-enhanced MRA was the most sensitive noninvasive test for vertebral artery stenosis when compared with CTA and ultrasound.[53]

Montavont and colleagues[54] looked at 18 consecutive patients with vertebrobasilar ischemia who were treated with intravenous rt-PA within 7 hours of presentation. At 3 months, they reported that 10 patients were independent, with a modified Rankin Scale of 0 to 2, whereas 8 had a poor outcome with a modified Rankin Scale of 3 to 6. In a systematic analysis of intra-arterial versus intravenous thrombolytic therapy for basilar artery occlusion,[55] Lindsberg and Mattle reported that recanalization was more frequent with intra-arterial versus intravenous therapy (65% vs 53%, P =.05), with similar frequency of good outcomes in both groups (24% vs 22%). However, only 2% of those patients who failed to recanalize had a good outcome. The Basilar Artery International Cooperation Study (BASICS) looked at the treatment and outcomes in acute basilar artery occlusion.[56] There were 619 patients in this registry and 27 were excluded because they did not receive either antithrombotic therapy alone, intravenous therapy, or intra-arterial thrombolysis, and all had a poor outcome. For those who received some form of therapy, 68% had a poor outcome, and no statistically significant superiority was found for any of the 3 treatment arms. This finding underscores the expected poor prognosis in acute basilar artery thrombosis even with thrombolytic therapy.

In summary, there is now an established 3-hour window for the use of intravenous rt-PA for patients who fulfill the criteria, assuming that they and their loved ones are in agreement with receiving this agent with the recognition of its relatively small, but real, risk of serious hemorrhagic complications. This established window is viewed as a standard of care, and there are potential medicolegal ramifications for its use, or nonuse, with most of these ramifications related to failure to use this agent for patients who were eligible to receive it. The extension of the therapeutic window for rt-PA to up to 4.5 hours is potentially exciting, with an endorsement by the Stroke Council of the American Stroke Association, but there is also a lack of approval for this extended window by the FDA. It is advisable, at this time, to seriously consider it as an option for a person who qualifies for the extended window, with the availability of an informed consent to clearly spell what seem to be less of a benefit/risk ratio compared with the 3-hour window. The availability of extended windows for thrombolytic therapy, particularly in reference to intra-arterial rt-PA, should be predicated on the experience and critical mass of the particular stroke center to avoid what could be interpreted as a haphazard window of availability depending on the coverage at the particular center at any one time. Because of the lack of definitive controlled trials of the extended window with either intravenous/intra-arterial rt-PA bridging or intra-arterial rt-PA alone, and without FDA approval for such an indication, it is expected that a protocol will be in place for a particular medical center that is approved by that institution's human subjects committee along with an informed consent.

CLOT-RETRIEVAL/ANGIOPLASTIC DEVICES

There are now 2 FDA-approved clot-retrieval devices available for patients with acute ischemic stroke: the Merci clot-retrieval device[6,57–59] and the Penumbra clot-retrieval device.[7,60] Their release by the FDA was based on their demonstrated ability to extract a clot within the intracerebral circulation and restore blood flow through that particular involved vessel. Their impact on outcome in acute ischemic stroke has been favorable, with the caveat that such an interventional procedure is operator dependent and reflects the skill and experience of a particular interventionalist. The therapeutic window is generally viewed within 3 to 8 hours of presentation, taking into account the accepted first choice of intravenous rt-PA for patients presenting within the 3-hour window who do not have contraindications to its use.

In the Mechanical Embolus Removal in Cerebral Ischemia (MERCI) trial,[6] with a mean procedural time of 2.1 hours, with a 3- to 8-hour therapeutic window, the recanalization rate was 48% for patients with documented occlusions of either the middle cerebral artery, terminal internal carotid artery, or the basilar artery. This finding was compared with the reported 18% in the PROACT-II historical control arm ($P<.0001$).[50] For patients in the MERCI trial who did not have good recanalization, adjuvant intra-arterial rt-PA was available with or without angioplastic intervention. The significant periprocedural complication rate was 7.1%, and intracerebral hemorrhage was observed in 7.8%. Of particular note, from an outcome standpoint, good neurologic recovery was seen in 46% of those patients who were successfully recanalized but in only 10% of those who did not recanalize ($P<.0001$).

In the Multi MERCI trial, the newer-generation embolus-retrieval device was tested in patients with persistent large vessel clot despite intravenous rt-PA.[57] This test was compared with a recanalization rate of approximately 48% and an enhanced rate of up to 60% when combined with intra-arterial thrombolytic agents. The results provide caution about the potential benefits versus risks of such intervention, however. Despite a recanalization rate of 57.3% with this device, along with 69.5% when combined with thrombolytic therapy, favorable outcome was 36% clinically and the mortality rate was a worrisome 34%, whereas the symptomatic intracerebral hemorrhage rate was 9.8%. The investigators noted that clinical outcome was reflective of the recanalization rate, which was also emphasized in the pooled analysis of the MERCI and Multi MERCI trials,[58] and this pooled analysis also reported greater success with second-division middle cerebral artery occlusions than with trunk occlusions.[59]

The Penumbra device, consisting of a reperfusion catheter and separator with or without a thrombus removal ring, was reported to have a recanalization rate of 100% in one international study of 20.[60] Kulcsar and colleagues[61] reported their experience with this device in 27 consecutive patients. They observed a recanalization rate of 93%, no symptomatic intracerebral hemorrhages, significant clinical improvement in roughly 50%, and an all-cause 3-month mortality of 11%. The mean time to initial angiographic imaging was 4 hours and 26 minutes in this study, and the mean time to attain revascularization was an additional 97 minutes in a patient population who had presented within 3 hours of their stroke onset.

In addition to the Multi MERCI and Penumbra, there are various alternatives involving either microwire or microcatheter clot disruption, which may also include the incorporation of angioplasty once the reestablishment of vessel patency has been achieved. In a study by Noser and colleagues,[62] clot maceration with microcatheter/microwire was followed by either angioplasty, stent, or snare in 32 patients who also received adjuvant thrombolytic therapy. They reported a favorable outcome in 59% and a mortality rate of 12.5%. Somewhat more sobering was a report of balloon angioplasty with or without snare, in addition to either intravenous or intra-arterial thrombolytic therapy.[63] Although the recanalization rate was impressive at 86%, the mortality rate was 53%.

In summary, clot-retrieval devices are now available at up to an 8-hour therapeutic window of intervention and addition to refinements in microwire/microcatheter clot maceration as well as angioplasty with or without snare endovascular interventions. This evolution of what has been termed aggressive mechanical clot disruption requires special expertise in terms of the application of such procedures in the acute ischemic stroke setting. Various devices have been FDA approved, based on their potential success in recanalization, which is clearly correlated with improved outcome, although the review process for such device approval has caused some consternation among stroke specialists.[64] As of the present time, one can draw their own conclusions about the choice of procedure based on the data at hand. However, one must also factor in the delicacy of such intervention, with reported results most assuredly reflective of procedural skills and experience.

ASPIRIN IN ACUTE ISCHEMIC STROKE

Two studies have demonstrated modest improvement in outcome with aspirin therapy in acute ischemic stroke. Naturally, this assumes that patients are tolerant of aspirin and that there is no contraindication, such as the withholding of both antiplatelet and anticoagulant therapy for at least 24 hours after the administration of rt-PA. The International Stroke Trial (IST) Collaborative Group looked at 330 mg of aspirin administered within the first 48 hours of an acute ischemic stroke,[65] whereas the Chinese Acute Stroke Trial (CAST) looked at a dose of 160 mg of aspirin.[66] Pooled data of the 40,000 patients entered in the 2 trials reported a 1.6% versus 2.3% reduced risk of recurrent stroke with aspirin, although the risk of hemorrhagic stroke was a bit higher at 1.0% versus 0.8%.[67]

There has been some interest in clopidogrel loading in acute ischemic stroke in an effort to protect against the extension of the infarction and progression of the neurologic deficit. This approach has been extrapolated from cardiac studies, which have suggested that higher-dose clopidogrel (600 mg vs 300 mg) in acute ST-segment elevation myocardial infarction is beneficial.[68] However, as with many antiplatelet studies, there are conflicting reports; the Clopidogrel Optimal Loading Dose Usage to Reduce Recurrent Events/Optimal Antiplatelet Strategy for Interventions (CURRENT-OASIS 7) investigators[69] reported no difference between double-dose versus standard-dose clopidogrel or aspirin in acute coronary syndromes.

ANTICOAGULANT THERAPY IN ACUTE ISCHEMIC STROKE

Anticoagulant therapy in acute ischemic stroke was, for years, a commonly used therapeutic regimen in an effort to promote dissolution of thrombus formation or propagation of the thrombus, which was viewed as a common mechanism of stroke-in-evolution. However, the IST report[65] was one of several studies that have led to the recommendation that the only clear indication for anticoagulant therapy in the acute ischemic stroke setting is for DVT prophylaxis.[26] In IST, for example, subcutaneous heparin, at 5000 or 12,500 IU twice a day, was not found to be beneficial in acute ischemic stroke, although most clinicians recognize the value of lower-dose anticoagulant therapy in patients who have had a stroke with limited mobility for the protection against DVT and risk of pulmonary embolism. A pivotal trial that led to a rethinking of full-dose anticoagulants in acute ischemic stroke was the Trial of ORG 10,172 in Acute Stroke Treatment (TOAST).[70] This study of the low-molecular-weight heparinoid danaparoid reported no significant improvement in acute ischemic stroke outcome at 3 months, although there was an apparent positive response at 7 days.

Bath and colleagues[71] published a meta-analysis of randomized controlled trials of low-molecular-weight heparins and heparinoids in acute ischemic stroke and concluded that any potential benefit in the reduction of venous thromboembolic events was negated by an increased risk of extracranial bleeding. Perhaps even more sobering was the report that low-molecular-weight heparin was not superior to aspirin in patients with acute ischemic stroke in terms of functional outcome at 2 weeks or 3 months.[72] The investigators could not exclude some potential benefit. However, agents, such as activated factor X inhibitor idraparinux, apparently may produce more harm than any potential good.[73] On the other hand, there is clearly support for the efficacy of anticoagulant therapy in the protection against ischemic stroke in patients with significant risk of cardio-embolism, such as higher-risk nonvalvular atrial fibrillation,[74] let alone valvular atrial fibrillation.

The use of anticoagulant therapy in acute ischemic stroke has not been completely abandoned by some. Camerlingo and colleagues[75] reported some benefit with intravenous heparin administered within 3 hours of a nonlacunar stroke, although the increased risk of symptomatic intracerebral hemorrhage tended to negate this benefit. This benefit was also suggested by the TOAST study,[69] which reported some potential benefit from danaparoid in large-artery occlusive disease. Moonis and Fisher[76] have addressed the potential benefit of unfractionated heparin and low-molecular-weight heparin in such circumstances whereby the risk of early recurrent stroke, on an embolic mechanism, is quite substantial. In reference to this, Hallevi and colleagues[77] reported that warfarin could generally be safely started shortly after cardioembolic stroke, whereas heparin and enoxaparin bridging enhances the risk of serious bleeding. Other than for the protection against recurrent cardioembolic stroke, anticoagulant therapy is often initiated sooner rather than later in patients with ischemic strokes who have either cerebrovascular dissection,[78] cerebral sinovenous thrombosis,[79] or a well-documented hypercoagulable state[80] whereby it is thought that the potential benefit outweighs the risk of hemorrhagic complications. However, many of these reports of the potential salutary effect on outcome have been somewhat conflicting, although the benefits of anticoagulation in venous thrombosis are generally supportive both on theoretical grounds as well as clinically.[81]

ULTRASOUND-ENHANCED THROMBOLYSIS

It has been observed experimentally that ultrasound exposure can promote the disruption of fibrin deposition within thrombus formation, which can theoretically promote greater penetration of thrombolytic material into the clot.[4,82] This finding has led to the use of a low MHz-KHz–frequency ultrasound exposure in the clinical setting of acute ischemic stroke treatment, and it has been reported that the administration of microbubbles, in combination with ultrasound, can enhance the clot lysis.[4] Alexandrov and colleagues[83] compared the application of continuous 2-MHz transcranial Doppler ultrasonography with placebo in 126 patients being treated with intravenous rt-PA for acute ischemic stroke. Complete recanalization or dramatic clinical recovery within 2 hours of the administration of the thrombolytic agent was seen in 49% of study patients versus 30% of controls ($P = .03$). However, there has been concern that such therapy can also increase the risk of hemorrhagic transformation of the infarct,[84] and this has been the major limitation in wider applications of this modality. According to one recent study,[85] the combination of 3 doses of 2.5 g of microbubbles with continuous TCD monitoring for 2 hours was reported to enhance reperfusion, but also hemorrhagic transformation of the infarct, but not necessarily the risk of symptomatic intracranial hemorrhage.

EVALUATION AND TREATMENT OF CEREBRAL EDEMA ASSOCIATED WITH ISCHEMIC STROKE

There are several potential explanations for deteriorating stroke manifestations in patients who present with a mild to moderate deficit.[86] Naturally, clinical worsening associated with recurrent stroke can be seen with a high-risk source of cerebral embolism or an ongoing malicious hypercoagulable state, along with aggressive cerebral vasculitis or propagation of the thrombus that can be seen as part of the pathogenesis of vascular dissection. However, the most common mechanism is probably the evolution of the infarction as part of the ischemic cascade, with development of cytotoxic edema in the area of infarction. The swelling of the infarct tends to peak over 3 to 5 days and can lead to rapid deterioration in death especially in clinical scenarios, such as the malignant middle cerebral artery syndrome.[87]

General measures to address increased intracranial pressure, such as hyperventilation, mannitol,[88] hypertonic (10%) saline,[89] high-dose barbiturates,[90] and steroids, are not necessarily beneficial in such a setting, although they are not infrequently used to buy time against this irreversible process.[90] Hypothermia may have at least a temporary benefit for severe brain swelling associated with massive cerebral infarction (**Fig. 5**).[91]

Hemicraniectomy is now accepted as a means to improve both mortality and outcome in massive middle cerebral artery infarcts based on the pooled analysis of 3 randomized trials.[92] This compilation, looking at 93 patients aged 60 years or younger, with surgical decompression within 48 hours of stroke onset versus no intervention, found a mortality rate of 22% compared with 71% favoring decompression. Furthermore, moderate to severe disability or death was also in favor of decompression

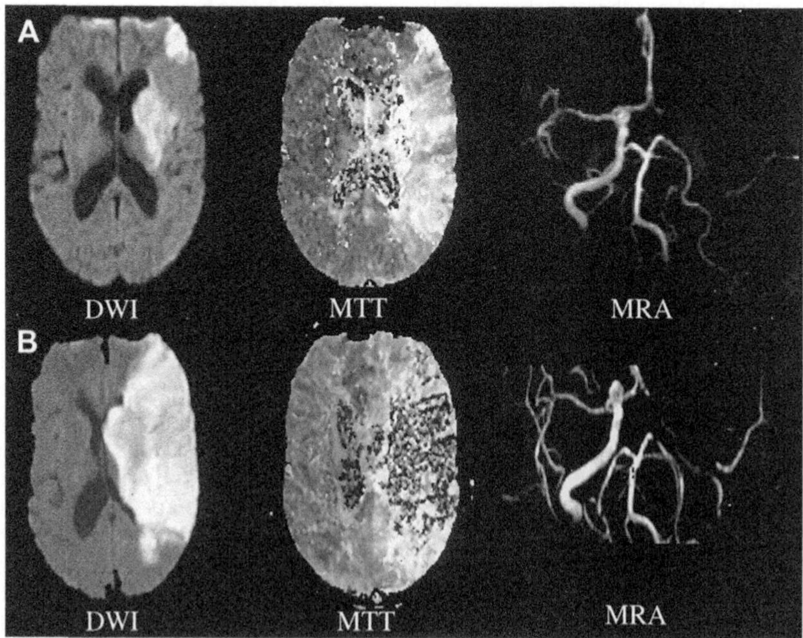

Fig. 5. Evolution from time of presentation (*A*) and 24 hours later (*B*) of a massive cerebral hemispheric infarction as demonstrated by diffusion-weighted (MR) imaging and mean transit time (MTT) related to ipsilateral internal carotid artery occlusion by magnetic resonance angiography (MRA).

(57% vs 79%). In addition, suboccipital decompressive craniectomy can be a lifesaving measure with malignant cerebellar infarction.[93] Naturally, one has to keep in perspective the expectations of patients and their families in terms of the potential for the promotion of severe, longstanding functional morbidity with such interventions.

SUMMARY

The past 40 years have seen the evolution of acute ischemic stroke management from the unproven therapies du jour, such as steroids, heparin for stroke in evolution, and hypervolemic-hemodilution, to more of a scientific basis for our decision-making process.[8] This evolution has been directly related to the advancements in imaging of stroke from the early days of CT brain scan to the presently available MR and CT techniques that allow for both assessment of tissue viability and for circulatory compromise in a matter of minutes. In addition, it has been related to carefully designed, controlled clinical trials of potential therapies, which have led to the recognition of the benefits of thrombolytic therapy in the acute setting but have also left us bemused and frustrated over the lack of benefit for several potential neuroprotective agents that have been studied that seemed to have significant promise at one time.

The art and science of stroke therapy is still in evidence with the newer interventional tools that have become available. We know, by studies and by commonsense, that the effective reestablishment of blood flow with various endovascular techniques should improve outcomes in stroke if the restoration of flow can be achieved while there is ample viable tissue to salvage. It is not out of the realm of possibility that we may soon develop combined approaches that reestablish blood flow and protect the brain from possible adverse consequences of reperfusion, and this remains a very exciting aspect of acute ischemic stroke management. However, it is always important to keep things in perspective in view of the recent NINDS Clinical Alert for angioplasty combined with stenting in the recently halted Stenting versus Aggressive Medical Management for Preventing Recurrent Stroke in Intracranial Stenosis (SAMMPRIS), which reflected an unacceptably high mortality rate when compared with aggressive medical therapy for symptomatic high-grade intracranial stenosis.

REFERENCES

1. Ginsberg MD. Advances in the pathophysiology of brain ischemia: penumbra, gene expression, neuroprotection: the 2002 Thomas Willis lecture. Stroke 2003; 34:214–23.
2. D'Ambrosia AL, Pinksy DJ, Connolly ES. The role of the complement cascade in ischemic/reperfusion injury: implications for neuroprotection. Mol Med 2001;7: 367–82.
3. Bourekas EC, Slivka A, Shah R, et al. Intra-arterial thrombolysis within three hours of stroke onset in middle cerebral artery strokes. Neurocrit Care 2009;11:217–22.
4. Molina CA, Barreto AD, Tsivgoulis G, et al. Transcranial ultrasound in clinical thrombolysis (TUSCON) trial. Ann Neurol 2009;66:28–38.
5. Liebeskind DS. Reperfusion for acute ischemic stroke: arterial revascularization and collateral therapeutics. Curr Opin Neurol 2010;23:36–45.
6. Smith WS, Sung G, Starkman S, et al. Safety and efficacy of mechanical embolectomy in acute ischemic stroke: results of the MERCI trial. Stroke 2005;36: 1432–8.
7. Penumbra Pivotal Stroke Trial Investigators. The penumbra pivotal stroke trial: safety and effectiveness of a new generation of mechanical devices for clot removal in intracranial large vessel occlusive disease. Stroke 2009;40:2761–8.

8. van der Worp HB, van Gijn J. Acute ischemic stroke. N Engl J Med 2007;357:572–9.
9. O'Collins VE, Macleod MR, Donnan GA, et al. 1,026 experimental treatments in acute stroke. Ann Neurol 2006;59:467–77.
10. Fisher M. New approaches to neuroprotective drug development. Stroke 2011;42(Suppl 1):S24–7.
11. Bernard SA, Gray TW, Buist MD, et al. Treatment of comatose survivors of out-of-hospital cardiac arrest with induced hypothermia. N Engl J Med 2002;346:557–63.
12. Hacke W, Kaste M, Bogousslavsky J, et al. European Stroke Initiative recommendations for stroke management-update 2003. Cerebrovasc Dis 2003;16:311–37.
13. Savitz SI, Caplan LR. Vertebrobasilar disease. N Engl J Med 2005;352:2618–26.
14. Ay H, Furie KL, Singhal A, et al. An evidence-based causative classification system for acute ischemic stroke. Ann Neurol 2005;58:688–97.
15. Ferro JM, Massaro AR, Mas JL. Aetiological diagnosis of ischaemic stroke in young adults. Lancet Neurol 2010;9:1085–96.
16. Schaller B, Graf R. Cerebral ischemia and reperfusion: the pathophysiologic concept as a basis for clinical therapy. J Cereb Blood Flow Metab 2004;24:352–71.
17. Albers GW, Thijs VN, Wechsler LR, et al. Magnetic resonance imaging profiles predict clinical response to early reperfusion: the diffusion and perfusion imaging evaluation for understanding stroke evolution (DEFUSE) study. Ann Neurol 2006;60:508–17.
18. Wintermark M, Flanders AE, Velthuis B, et al. Perfusion-CT assessment of infarct core and penumbra. Stroke 2006;37:979–85.
19. Alexandrov AV, Felberg RA, Demchuk AM, et al. Deterioration following spontaneous improvement: sonographic findings in patients with acute resolving symptoms of cerebral ischemia. Stroke 2000;31:915–9.
20. Aries MJ, Uyttenboogaart M, Koopman K, et al. Hyperdense middle cerebral artery sign and outcome after intravenous thrombolysis for acute ischemic stroke. J Neurol Sci 2009;285:114–7.
21. Alhadramy O, Jeerakathil TJ, Majumdar SR, et al. Prevalence and predictors of paroxysmal atrial fibrillation on Holter monitor in patients with acute stroke and transient ischemic attack. Stroke 2010;41:2596–600.
22. Stahrenberg R, Weber-Kruger M, Seegers J, et al. Enhanced detection of paroxysmal atrial fibrillation by early and prolonged continuous Holter monitoring in patients with cerebral ischemia presenting in sinus rhythm. Stroke 2010;41:2884–8.
23. Capes SE, Hunt D, Malmberg K, et al. Stress hyperglycemia and prognosis of stroke in non-diabetic and diabetic patients: a systemic overview. Stroke 2001;32:2426–32.
24. Cheung NW, Chipps DR. Sliding scale insulin: will the false idol finally fall? Intern Med J 2010;40:662–4.
25. Reith J, Jorgensen S, Pedersen PM, et al. Body temperature in acute stroke: relation to stroke severity, infarct size, mortality and outcome. Lancet 1996;347:422–5.
26. Willmot M, Leonardi-Bee J, Bath PM. High blood pressure in acute stroke and subsequent outcome: a systematic review. Hypertension 2004;43:18–24.
27. Mistri AK, Robinson TG, Potter JF. Pressor therapy in acute ischemic stroke: systematic review. Stroke 2006;37:1565–71.
28. Wojner-Alexander AW, Garami Z, Chemyshev OY, et al. Heads down: flat positioning improves blood flow velocity in acute ischemic stroke. Neurology 2005;64:1354–7.

29. Adams HP Jr, del Zoppo G, Alberts MJ, et al. Guidelines for the early management of adults with ischemic stroke. Circulation 2007;115:478–534.
30. Lassen MR, Gallus A, Raskob GE, et al. Apixaban or enoxaparin for thromboprophylaxis after knee replacement. N Engl J Med 2009;361:594–604.
31. Butt A, Aronow WS, Chandy D. Heparin-induced thrombocytopenia and thrombosis. Compr Ther 2010;36:23–7.
32. Starkstein SE, Mizrahi R, Power BD. Antidepressant therapy in post-stroke depression. Expert Opin Pharmacother 2008;9:1291–8.
33. Chollet F, Tardy J, Albucher JF, et al. Fluoxetine for motor recovery after acute ischaemic stroke (FLAME): a randomized placebo-controlled trial. Lancet Neurol 2011;10:47–54.
34. The Multicenter Acute Stroke Trial-Europe Study Group. Thrombolytic therapy with streptokinase in acute ischemic stroke. N Engl J Med 1996;335:145–50.
35. The National Institute of Neurological Disorders and Stroke rt-PA Stroke Study Group. Tissue plasminogen activator for acute ischemic stroke. N Engl J Med 1995;333:1581–7.
36. The ATLANTIS, ECASS and NINDS rt-PA Study Group Investigators. Association of outcome with early stroke treatment: pooled analysis of ATLANTIS, ECASS, and NINDS rt-PA stroke trials. Lancet 2004;363:768–74.
37. Gropen TI, Gagliano PJ, Blake CA, et al. NYSDOH Stroke Center Designation Project Workgroup. Quality improvement in acute stroke: the New York State Stroke Center Designation Project. Neurology 2006;67:88–93.
38. Lansberg MG, Schrooten M, Bluhmki E, et al. Treatment time-specific number needed to treat estimates for tissue plasminogen activator therapy in acute stroke based on shifts over the entire range of the Modified Rankin Scale. Stroke 2009; 40:2079–84.
39. Demchuk AM, Tanne D, Hill MD, et al. Predictors of good outcome after intravenous tPA for acute ischemic stroke. Neurology 2001;57:474–80.
40. Khatri P, Abruzzo T, Yeatts SD, et al. Good clinical outcome after ischemic stroke with successful revascularization is time-dependent. Neurology 2009;73: 1066–72.
41. Clark WM, Albers GW, Madden KP, et al. Recombinant tissue-type plasminogen activator (alteplase) for ischemic stroke 3 to 5 hours after symptom onset: the ATLANTIS study-a randomized controlled trial. JAMA 1999;282:2019–26.
42. Ebinger M, Iwanga T, Prosser JF, et al. Clinical-diffusion mismatch and benefit from thrombolysis 3 to 6 h after acute stroke. Stroke 2009;40(7):2572–4.
43. Hacke W, Kaste M, Bluhmki E, et al. Thrombolysis with alteplase 3 to 4.5 hours after acute ischemic stroke. N Engl J Med 2008;359:1317–29.
44. del Zoppo GJ, Saver JL, jauch EC, et al. Expansion of the time window for treatment of acute ischemic stroke with intravenous tissue plasminogen activator. A science advisory from the American Heart Association/American Stroke Association. Stroke 2009;40:2945–8.
45. Broderick J. Combined intravenous and intra-arterial r-TPA versus intra-arterial recanalization for acute ischemic stroke: the interventional management of stroke study. Stroke 2004;35:904–11.
46. Bhatia R, Hill MD, Shobha N, et al. Low rates of acute recanalization with intravenous recombinant tissue plasminogen activator in ischemic stroke. Stroke 2010; 41:2254–8.
47. Sharma VK, Teoh HL, Wong LY, et al. Recanalization therapies in acute ischemic stroke: pharmacological agents, devices, and combinations. Stroke Res Treat 2010;2010:1–8 pii: 672064.

48. Lewandowski CA, Frankel M, Tomsick TA, et al. Combined intravenous and intra-arterial r-TPA for acute ischemic stroke: emergency management of stroke (EMS) bridging trial. Stroke 1999;30:2598–605.
49. del Zoppo GJ, Higashida RT, Furlan AJ, et al. PROACT: a phase II randomized trial of recombinant pro-urokinase by direct arterial delivery in acute middle cerebral artery stroke. Stroke 1998;29:4–11.
50. Furlan A, Higashida R, Wechsler L, et al. Intra-arterial prourokinase for acute ischemic stroke. The PROACT II study: a randomized controlled trial. JAMA 1999;282:2003–11.
51. Hacke W, Zeumer H, Ferbert A, et al. Intra-arterial thrombolytic therapy improves outcome in patients with acute vertebrobasilar occlusive disease. Stroke 1988; 19:1216–22.
52. Bonatti G, Ferro F, Haglmuller T, et al. Basilar artery thrombosis: imaging and endovascular therapy. Radiol Med 2010;115:1219–33.
53. Khan S, Rich P, Clifton A, et al. Noninvasive detection of vertebral artery stenosis. A comparison of contrast-enhanced MR angiography, CT angiography, and ultrasound. Stroke 2009;40:3499–503.
54. Montavont A, Nighaoghossian N, Derex L, et al. Intravenous r-TPA in vertebrobasilar acute infarcts. Neurology 2004;62:1854–6.
55. Lindsberg PJ, Mattle HP. Therapy of basilar artery occlusion. A systemic analysis comparing intra-arterial and intravenous thrombolysis. Stroke 2006;37:922–8.
56. Schonewill WJ, Wijman CA, Rueckert MP, et al. Treatment and outcomes of acute basilar artery occlusion in the Basilar Artery International Cooperation Study (BASICS): a prospective registry study. Lancet Neurol 2009;8:724–30.
57. Smith WS, Sung G, Saver J, et al. Mechanical thrombectomy for acute ischemic stroke. Final results of the Multi MERCI trial. Stroke 2008;39:1205–12.
58. Nogueira RG, Liebeskind DS, Sung G, et al. Predictors of good clinical outcomes, mortality, and successful revascularization in patients with acute ischemic stroke undergoing thrombectomy. Pooled analysis of the Mechanical Embolus Removal in Cerebral Ischemia (MERCI) and Multi MERCI trials. Stroke 2009;40:3777–83.
59. Zhong-Song S, Loh Y, Walker G, et al. Clinical outcomes in middle cerebral artery trunk occlusions versus secondary division occlusions after mechanical thrombectomy. Pooled analysis of the Mechanical Embolus Removal in Cerebral Ischemia (MERCI) and Multi MERCI trials. Stroke 2010;41:953–60.
60. Bose A, Henkes H, Alfke K, et al. The penumbra system: a mechanical device for the treatment of acute stroke due to thromboembolism. AJNR Am J Neuroradiol 2008;29:1409–13.
61. Kulcsar Z, Bonvin C, Pereira VM, et al. Penumbra system: a novel mechanical thrombectomy device for large-vessel occlusions in acute stroke. AJNR Am J Neuroradiol 2010;31:628–33.
62. Noser EA, Shaltoni M, Hall CE, et al. Aggressive mechanical clot disruption: a safe adjunct to thrombolytic therapy in acute stroke? Stroke 2005;36:292–6.
63. Quereshi AI, Siddiqui AM, Suri MF, et al. Aggressive mechanical clot disruption and low- dose intra-arterial third-generation thrombolytic agent for ischemic stroke: a prospective study. Neurosurgery 2002;51:1319–29.
64. Becker KJ, Brott TG. Approval of the MERCI clot retriever. A critical review. Stroke 2005;36:400–3.
65. International Stroke Trial Collaborative Group. The International Stroke Trial (IST): a randomized trial of aspirin, subcutaneous heparin, both, or neither among 19,345 patients with acute ischemic stroke. Lancet 1997;349:1569–81.

66. CAST (Chinese Acute Stroke Trial) Collaborative Group. CAST: randomized placebo- controlled trial of early aspirin use in 20,000 patients with acute ischemic stroke. Lancet 1997;349:1641–9.
67. Chen ZM, Sandercock P, Pan HC, et al. Indications for early aspirin use in acute ischemic stroke: a combined analysis of 40,000 randomized patients form the Chinese Acute Stroke Trial and the International Stroke Trial. Stroke 2000;31:1240–9.
68. Mangiacapra F, Muller O, Ntaliania A, et al. Comparison of 600 versus 300-mg clopidogrel loading dose in patients with ST-segment elevation myocardial infarction undergoing primary coronary angioplasty. Am J Cardiol 2010;106:1208–11.
69. CURRENT-OASIS 7 Investigators. Dose comparisons of clopidogrel and aspirin in acute coronary syndromes. N Engl J Med 2010;363:930–42.
70. The Publications Committee for the Trial of ORG 10172 in Acute Stroke Treatment (TOAST) Investigators. Low molecular weight heparinoid, ORG 10172 (danaparoid), and outcome after acute ischemic stroke. JAMA 1998;279:1265–72.
71. Bath PM, Iddenden R, Bath FJ. Low-molecular-weight heparins and heparinoids in acute ischemic stroke. A meta-analysis of randomized controlled trials. Stroke 2000;31:1770–8.
72. Berge E, Abdelnoor M, Nakstad PH, et al. Low molecular-weight heparin versus aspirin in patients with acute ischaemic stroke and atrial fibrillation: a double-blind randomized study. Lancet 2000;355:1205–10.
73. The Amadeus Investigators. Comparison of idraparinux with vitamin K antagonists for prevention of thromboembolism in patients with atrial fibrillation: a randomized, open-label, non-inferiority trial. Lancet 2008;371:315–21.
74. The Stroke Risk in Atrial Fibrillation Working Group. Independent predictors of stroke in patients with atrial fibrillation. Neurology 2007;69:546–54.
75. Camerlingo M, Salvi P, Belloni G, et al. Intravenous heparin started within 3 hours after onset of symptoms as a treatment for acute nonlacunar hemispheric cerebral infarctions. Stroke 2005;36:2415–20.
76. Moonis M, Fisher M. Considering the role of heparin and low-molecular-weight heparins in acute ischemic stroke. Stroke 2002;33:1927–33.
77. Hallevi H, Albright KC, Martin-Schild S, et al. Anticoagulation after cardioembolic stroke. To bridge or not to bridge? Arch Neurol 2008;65:1169–73.
78. Georgiadis D, Arnold M, von Buedingen HC, et al. Aspirin vs anticoagulation in carotid artery dissection. Neurology 2009;72:1810–5.
79. Stam J. Thrombosis of cerebral veins and sinuses. N Engl J Med 2005;352: 1791–8.
80. Levine JS, Branch DW, Rauch J. The antiphospholipid antibody syndrome. N Engl J Med 2002;346:752–63.
81. Bousser MG. Cerebral venous thrombosis: diagnosis and management. J Neurol 2000;247(4):252–8.
82. Francis CW, Blinc A, Lee S, et al. Ultrasound accelerates transport of recombinant tissue plasminogen activator into clots. Ultrasound Med Biol 1995;21: 419–24.
83. Alexandrov AV, Molina CA, Grotta JC, et al. Ultrasound- enhanced systemic thrombolysis for acute ischemic stroke. N Engl J Med 2004;351:2170–8.
84. Eggers J, Koch B, Meyer K, et al. Effect of ultrasound on thrombolysis of middle cerebral artery occlusion. Ann Neurol 2003;53:797–800.
85. Dinia L, Rubiera M, Ribo M, et al. Reperfusion after stroke sonothrombolysis with microbubbles may predict intracranial bleeding. Neurology 2009;73:775–80.
86. Ali LK, Saver JL. The ischemic stroke patient who worsens: new assessment and management approaches. Rev Neurol Dis 2007;4:85–91.

87. Hacke W, Schwab S, Horn M, et al. "Malignant" middle cerebral artery territory infarction: clinical course and prognostic signs. Arch Neurol 1996;53:309–15.
88. Bereczki D, Mihalka L, Szatmari S, et al. Mannitol in acute stroke. Case fatality at 30 days and 1 year. Stroke 2003;34:1730–5.
89. Schwarz S, Georgiadis D, Aschoff A, et al. Effects of hypertonic (10%) saline in patients with raised intracranial pressure after stroke. Stroke 2002;33:136–40.
90. Barutzky J, Schwab S. Antiedema therapy in ischemic stroke. Stroke 2007;38: 3084–94.
91. Schwab S, Georgiadis D, Berrouschot J, et al. Feasibility and safety of moderate hypothermia after massive hemispheric infarction. Stroke 2001;32:2033–5.
92. Vahedi K, Hofmeijer J, Juettler E, et al. Early decompressive surgery in malignant infarction of the middle cerebral artery: a pooled analysis of three randomized controlled trials. Lancet Neurol 2007;6:215–22.
93. Pfefferkorn T, Eppinger U, Linn J, et al. Long-term outcome after suboccipital decompressive craniectomy for malignant cerebellar infarction. Stroke 2009;40: 3045–50.

Intracranial Hemorrhage: Diagnosis and Management

William David Freeman, MD[a,b,*], Maria I. Aguilar, MD[c]

KEYWORDS

- Intracranial hemorrhage • Intracerebral hemorrhage
- Intraparenchymal hemorrhage • Subarachnoid hemorrhage
- Subdural hemorrhage • Epidural hematoma

Intracranial hemorrhage (ICH) is defined as bleeding within the intracranial vault. ICH subtypes are further defined by the anatomic site of the bleeding (**Fig. 1**). Intraparenchymal hemorrhage (IPH) is defined as bleeding within the brain parenchyma, which can be spontaneous or posttraumatic. Subarachnoid hemorrhage (SAH) signifies blood within the subarachnoid space and is commonly from a ruptured intracranial aneurysm (aneurysmal SAH) or trauma. Subdural hematoma (SDH) indicates bleeding underneath the dural membrane, whereas epidural hematoma (EDH) indicates bleeding exterior to the dura. Intraventricular hemorrhage (IVH) indicates blood within the ventricular system, which normally contains cerebrospinal fluid. This article reviews the approach to the diagnosis and general management of ICH, followed by a focused discussion of specialized ICH subtype management for IPH, SAH, SDH, EDH, and IVH.

DIAGNOSIS OF ICH

ICH is diagnosed through a combination of history, physical examination, and, most commonly, noncontrast CT examination of the brain,[1–3] which discloses the anatomic bleeding location. The approach to ICH diagnosis should begin with a detailed history

Disclosures: The authors report no conflict of interest or funding for this manuscript.

[a] Department of Neurology, Mayo Clinic Florida, 4500 San Pablo Road, Cannaday 2 East Neurology, Jacksonville, FL 32224, USA
[b] Department of Critical Care, Mayo Clinic Florida, 4500 San Pablo Road, Cannaday 2 East Neurology, Jacksonville, FL 32224, USA
[c] Department of Neurology, Mayo Clinic Arizona, 5777 East Mayo Boulevard, Phoenix, AZ 85054, USA
* Corresponding author. Department of Neurology, Mayo Clinic Florida, 4500 San Pablo Road, Cannaday 2 East Neurology, Jacksonville, FL 32224.
E-mail address: freeman.william1@mayo.edu

Neurol Clin 30 (2012) 211–240
doi:10.1016/j.ncl.2011.09.002 **neurologic.theclinics.com**
0733-8619/12/$ – see front matter

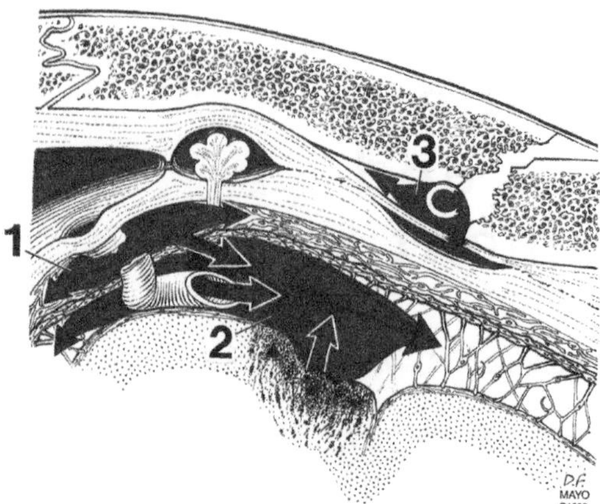

Fig. 1. Different ICH anatomic locations. (1) Bleeding within the subdural location, which is typically from torn bridging veins, that drain spinal fluid into the draining dural venous sinuses. (2) Bleeding within the subarachnoid space from either the brain cortex (cortical IPH or cortical contusion if traumatic) or a ruptured artery, such as ruptured aneurysm or pial vessel. (3) Skull-fracture ruptures the middle meningeal artery in the epidural space near fractured skull causing epidural hematoma, which can cause downward displacement of brain with hematoma expansion but may stop at skull suture lines (*far upper left*).

if available. If the patient cannot provide the history because of unconsciousness or altered mental state, a witness or other historian should be interviewed. Important historical clues include time and activity of onset if sudden deficits appeared, or loss of consciousness, fall, or presence or absence of seizure at onset. If the patient was "found down," and unresponsive by a witness, a description of the scene is often useful. Other historical information that should be collected includes medications, such as antithrombotic agents or anticoagulants; medical and surgical history; allergies; family history; and social history such as drug or alcohol use.

Laboratory values that should be checked in patients with ICH include a complete blood cell count, electrolytes, blood urea nitrogen, and creatinine (**Box 1**).[1–3] Serum glucose is reasonable to screen for hypoglycemia. A 12-lead electrocardiogram is useful to screen for arrhythmias, heart block, or myocardial ischemic changes. Coagulation parameters, including prothrombin time, activated partial thromboplastin time, and international normalized ratio (INR) are particularly useful in patients taking warfarin or heparin anticoagulation. Patients suspected of having sepsis and disseminated intravascular coagulation may have abnormal coagulation function tests, thrombocytopenia, leukocytosis/leucopenia, and additional fibrinogen and fibrin split products, and D-dimer levels should be checked. A pregnancy test is reasonable to perform in women of childbearing age before radiographs or CT scans are considered.[1–3] A drug screen may be useful in patients with hypertensive IPH from amphetamines or cocaine, or in those found unresponsive from barbiturate or opiate overdose with secondary traumatic ICH.

A stat noncontrast head CT can provide clues regarding the primary cause of ICH if the history is unclear. **Table 1** provides differential diagnoses for patients with ICH based on the initial history and CT findings. Traumatic ICH may have a telltale or characteristic "coup–countercoup" (eg, left occipital head injury creates right frontal contusion) ICH pattern that is caused by acceleration-deceleration forces of the brain tissue

Box 1
Recommended tests in patients with acute ICH

Radiology
- Stat noncontrast head CT

Electrocardiogram

Laboratory
- Complete blood cell count with platelet count
- Prothrombin time with INR
- Activated partial thromboplastin time
- Serum glucose
- Electrolytes
- Blood urea nitrogen and creatinine
- Pregnancy test in women of childbearing age
- Drugs of abuse screen (eg, opiates, barbiturates, benzodiazepines, cocaine, amphetamine)
- Troponin (or creatine kinase isoenzymes [CK-MB] if renal impairment)

Data from Refs.[1–3]

against a hard skull interior or surface edges, such as the dura matter. In severe traumatic brain injury, diffuse hemorrhage from shearing of the brain across several bony intracranial landmarks, tearing of bridging veins, cortical hemorrhage or contusions, and possibly skull fractures may occur (**Fig. 2**A–F).

Traumatic ICH

Patients with significant head and neck trauma or who are suspected of having this trauma should have the cervical spine immobilized until cleared by a neurosurgeon. Patients with trauma or evidence of bruising around the eyes ("raccoon eyes") should be examined carefully for a cerebrospinal fluid leak from the nose. Similarly, patients with bruising around the posterior ear or mastoid ("battle sign") should have careful inspection for a cerebrospinal fluid leak around the external auditory canal. If the cranial CT bone windows show a skull fracture (eg, **Fig. 2**B) or base of skull fracture, consultation with a neurosurgeon or otolaryngologist may be necessary. Patients with unstable facial fractures or base of skull fractures should have caution applied with any instrumentation to the nose (eg, nasogastric tubes) unless approved or placed by a specialist. Patients with cervical spine trauma should have the neck immobilized until cleared by the neurosurgeon, and doll's eyes (oculocephalic) responses deferred because of risk of cervical manipulation until then. If oculovestibular responses need to be tested in these patients, cold water calorics can be used instead. Patients with cervical spine trauma should still be tested within these limitations for spinal cord injury.

Neurosurgical consultation is advised when a mass effect, ongoing herniation, or obstructive hydrocephalus is present. Each ICH subtype is discussed further in the following sections. Patients with ICH are typically admitted to the intensive care unit (ICU) for frequent hemodynamic and neurologic monitoring.

Table 1
Differential diagnosis of ICH through history, initial noncontrast CT, and additional diagnostic imaging

Cause	Clues to Diagnosis	Initial CT Findings	Additional/Useful Imaging
Hypertensive IPH	History of hypertension, cardiomegaly on electrocardiogram, left ventricular hypertrophy	Basal ganglia/deep IPH	MRI with gradient echo with deep hemosiderin changes
Traumatic ICH	Facial or other bodily trauma signs or history	Cortical, coup, or contrecoup pattern of ICH, traumatic SAH pattern	MRI showing diffuse gradient echo changes consistent with diffuse axonal injury, or diffusion tensor imaging
Cerebral amyloid angiopathy	History of cognitive decline or prior IPH	Lobar IPH/SAH, may occur with anticoagulation[4]	MRI with gradient echo changes in the cortical-subcortical locations Present in up to 15% of patients older than 70 years
AVM	Headache, seizure, focal deficit	IPH ± IVH, or SAH, calcification on CT	CT angiogram or DSA
Cavernous angioma	Headache, seizure, focal deficit	IPH ± IVH, or SAH, calcification on CT if chronic	MRI with "bloom artifact" on gradient echo consistent with areas of older microhemorrhage (hemosiderin)
Aneurysm	Thunderclap headache, stupor/coma, meningismus, focal deficit	Characteristic SAH pattern	CTA and/or DSA showing intracranial aneurysm
CVT/SST	Thrombotic history	Cortical infarct or hemorrhage, sometimes bilateral; delta sign or cord sign	CTV, MRV, or DSA showing cortical vein thrombus, sagittal sinus thrombosis, other dural sinus thrombosis

Hemorrhagic tumor	Metastatic tumor history or newly diagnosed; weight loss	Vasogenic edema surrounding hemorrhage seen on CT	MRI with contrast shows ring-enhancing tumor and hemorrhage; body imaging may reveal other metastatic lesions
SDH	Fall or trauma typical, or minor trauma in the setting of anticoagulation	CT shows convexity hematoma, beyond suture lines	MRI may reveal chronic subdural hematomas or hygromas that are small or contralateral
EDH	Trauma to the temporal head region	Lens-shaped hematoma respecting suture lines	Repeat CT may be useful if abrupt neurologic deterioration occurs for surgery
Pituitary (hemorrhagic) apoplexy	Headache, obtundation, cranial nerve (III, IV, VI), shock	Initial CT may appear negative unless attention paid to sella, sometimes faint SAH around the sella	MRI with contrast, with emphasis on sella turcica/pituitary gland Pituitary apoplexy can also be infarction, which can later hemorrhage
Hemorrhagic Infarct	Clinical history of sudden stroke deficit, sometimes with major improvement; seizure from recanalization of occluded vessel	Cortical arterial territory with hemorrhagic infarct pattern (hemorrhage is around rim of vascular margins or gyri and sulci)	MRI with gradient echo showing hemosiderin around cortical infarct margins, MRA sometimes shows recanalized arterial segment (hemorrhage is from reperfusion injury)

Abbreviations: AVM, arteriovenous malformation; BPH, epidural hematoma; CAA, cerebral amyloid angiopathy; CTA, CT angiogram; CTV, CT venogram; CVT, cerebral vein thrombosis; DSA, digital subtraction angiogram; MRA, magnetic resonance angiogram; MRV, magnetic resonance venogram; SST, sagittal sinus thrombosis.

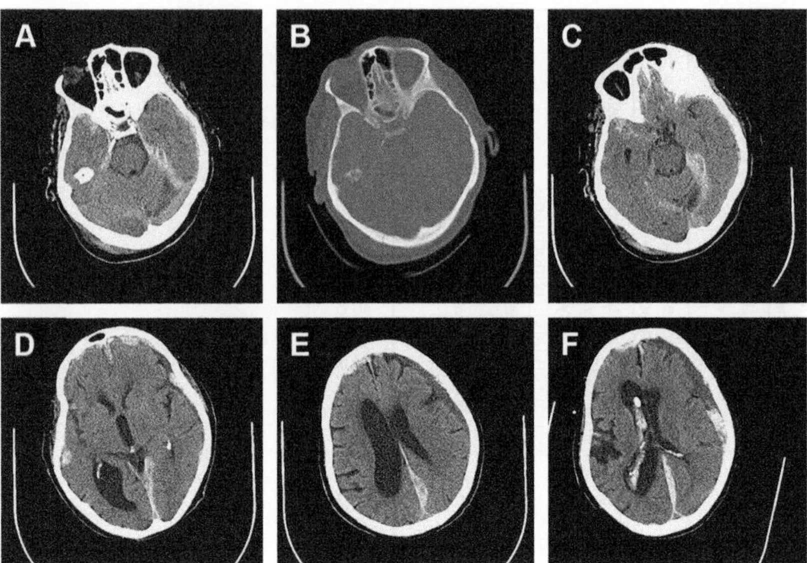

Fig. 2. Traumatic ICH in an 80-year-old woman with a witnessed fall at home. The family member stated that she fell straight backward and head hit her head on the floor, which made a sound like "a watermelon hit the ground." The patient arrived in the emergency department with a GCS of E1M2V1 (intubated) with intact pupillary, corneal, and cough brainstem reflexes. (*A*) Bitemporal hemorrhagic parenchymal contusions with SAH, right occipital cephalohematoma, with underlying right occipital lobe hypodense cerebral edema, left temporal lobe convexity SDH, and left tentorial SDH (*upper left*). (*B*) Nondisplaced right occipital bone fracture relative to **Fig. 1**A (*upper middle*). (*C*) Bifrontal (medial frontal, olfactory region) hemorrhagic parenchymal contusions with subarachnoid blood, right middle cerebral artery region SAH, which is small in comparison to most true aneurysmal SAH and in fact traumatic in origin (*upper right*). Left greater than right tentorial subdural hemorrhage is seen, consistent with acceleration-deceleration injury to the right occipital head region, and left convexity subdural hemorrhage. (*D*) Bifrontal hemorrhagic contusions (cortical parenchymal) and SAH (right sylvian fissure), and subdural hemorrhage (bihemispheric convexities and bifalcine) (*bottom left*). (*E*) Bifrontal hemorrhagic contusions, right greater than left, subdural hemorrhage left hemispheric convexity, and posterior falx cerebri (*bottom middle*). (*F*) CT scan 6 hours after images shown in **Fig. 1**A–D (*bottom right*), status postplacement of right external ventricular drain with IVH and enlarging left hemispheric convexity-acute SDH.

GENERAL MANAGEMENT OF ICH

After ICH is diagnosed, patients should be triaged according to level of consciousness, using tools such as the Glasgow Coma Scale (GCS) or other similar scale, and screened for airway protection and impending respiratory failure (**Table 2**). Patients with ICH in a coma (GCS <8) are at risk for aspirating upper-airway or gastrointestinal contents into the lungs, leading to aspiration pneumonia or acute respiratory distress syndrome. If a patient with ICH is not protecting their airway (eg, GCS <8, no gag response, or in respiratory failure from another cause, such as pulmonary contusion or chronic obstructive pulmonary disease), rapid sequence intubation (RSI) protocol is suggested.[5,6] RSI protocol is essentially preoxygenation, Sellick maneuver

Table 2
Simplified initial management ('ABC's Mnemonic) of patients with ICH

Letter	Management	Level of Evidence (AHA)
A	Airway: GCS <8: consider intubation with RSI protocol	Class I
B	Blood pressure control (see **Box 2**)	Class II
C	CPP (control ICP if elevated): HOB elevation 30°–45°	Class II
D	DVT prevention with pneumatic compression devices until bleeding stops, then consider subcutaneous UFH or LMWH	Class II
E	Early mobilization	Class I
F	Fever (core temperature >38.0°C–38.3°C)	Class I
G	Glucose target >140–185 mg/dL, use insulin Avoid hypoglycemia	Class I

Abbreviations: AHA, American Heart Association; CPP, cerebral perfusion pressure; DVT, deep vein thrombosis; GCS, Glasgow Coma Scale; HOB, head of bed; ICP, intracranial pressure; LMWH, low-molecular-weight heparin; RSI, rapid sequence intubation; UFH, unfractionated heparin.

Data from Refs.[1–3,5,6]

(pressure applied to the larynx to compress the esophagus to prevent reflux of gastrointestinal contents into the lungs during intubation), and premedication with drugs that blunt the sympathetic response to laryngoscopy and intubation that could cause an unsafe rise in intracranial pressure.[6] These RSI drugs include intravenous lidocaine and muscle relaxants. If cervical trauma is known or suspected, these patients may need fiberoptic intubation because of immobilization of the cervical spine in a cervical collar by a skilled airway provider. Patients who are alert or drowsy (eg, GCS 12–14) but have intact airway protective reflexes (gag, cough) with no signs of impending respiratory failure should be monitored for neurologic deterioration and subsequent airway compromise and admitted to an ICU. If a patient with ICH deteriorates to a comatose state (GCS$\leq$8), similar airway management should be implemented. Stuporous (eg, GCS 9–11) patients with ICH should be monitored closely for airway and respiratory compromise, and discretion used regarding intubation depending on the complete clinical scenario.

Blood pressure assessment and management should occur during the initial evaluation of patients with ICH (see **Table 2**), and whether the patient has raised intracranial pressure and will need neurosurgical intervention such as placement of an intracranial pressure monitor should be determined. Raising the patient's head of bed to 30° to 45° and ensuring the patient's neck is straight in midline and without constricting tape around the neck if intubated can help optimize intracranial pressure through optimizing jugular venous outflow. Elevating the head of bed also reduces the risk of aspiration pneumonia.

The initial approach to acute blood pressure management is shown in **Table 3**. Blood pressure should be tailored to each patient's blood pressure history and their particular ICH subtype (see **Table 3**). For most patients with ICH without intracranial pressure concerns, maintaining a mean arterial pressure of 60 to 65 mm Hg is the minimum.[2,3,5] If an intracranial pressure monitor is placed for raised intracranial pressure, then cerebral perfusion pressure should be maintained around a minimum of approximately 65 mm Hg.[2,3,5] Patients with chronic hypertension have rightward shifted cerebral autoregulation and may be accustomed to a higher baseline mean arterial pressure than normotensive patients. Oral antihypertensive medications are

Table 3
Initial blood pressure management for patients with ICH

ICH	Initial Blood Pressure Management	Additional Notes
IPH	Reduce SBP if >180 mm Hg or MAP >130 mm Hg using short-acting agents If raised ICP suspected, ask for neurosurgical placement of ICP monitor or EVD, maintain CPP >60 mm Hg Monitor neurologic examination q15 min until stable and gradually de-escalate monitoring per local ICU protocol	Correct any underlying coagulopathy stat If IVH (especially high-grade) present, increased odds of hydrocephalus and possible need of ventriculostomy, ICP monitoring
aSAH	Reduce SBP if >160 mm Hg or MAP >130 mm Hg using short-acting agents If raised ICP suspected, ask for neurosurgical placement of ICP monitor or EVD, maintain CPP >60 mm Hg Monitor neurologic examination q15min until stable and gradually de-escalate monitoring per local ICU protocol	Secure aneurysm to prevent rebleeding if possible Monitor for vasospasm and allow permissive hypertension (eg, up to 160 mm Hg SBP) if safe (aneurysm secure), especially during vasospasm peak window Maintain normal volume status (euvolemia) until vasospasm occurs then initiate HHH for secured aSAH
t-ICH	If raised ICP suspected, ask for neurosurgical placement of ICP monitor or EVD, maintain MAP/CPP >60–65 mm Hg Monitor neurologic examination q15min until stable and gradually de-escalate monitoring per local ICU protocol	Neurosurgical evaluation if surgical operable lesion or condition is identified

Abbreviations: aSAH, aneurysmal SAH; CPP, cerebral perfusion pressure (CPP = MAP - ICP); EVD, external ventricular drain; HHH, hypervolemic, hypertensive, hemodilution; ICP, intracranial pressure; MAP, mean arterial pressure; SBP, systolic blood pressure; t-ICH, traumatic ICH (eg, traumatic SAH, SDH, or EDH).

Data from Refs.[1–3,5,6]

typically held during the first 24 hours, and short-acting agents such as labetolol, hydralazine, enalprilat, nicardipine, or esmolol drips are used as needed to control mean arterial pressure/cerebral perfusion pressure within specified targets (see **Table 3**). However, caution is advised regarding holding β-blockers and clonidine in patients with known coronary disease, because of the risk for β-blocker withdrawal and rebound hypertension, respectively. In these patients, sometimes holding or halving the dose with ICU-level blood pressure monitoring is required for making informed decision about these medications. IPH and SAH blood pressures are discussed later.

Other management issues for patients with ICH include central nervous system (CNS) complications and non-CNS organ complications (**Boxes 2** and **3**). ICH growth is a significant concern and present in up to one-third of patients with IPH within 24 hours,[7] and is associated with neurologic deterioration. Patients with traumatic ICH may also have hemorrhagic expansion because of ongoing bleeding sources, such as torn bridging veins in SDH or cortical contusions (see **Fig. 2**F). EDH and aneurysmal SAH are particularly concerning because they represent arterial bleeding sources at a higher pressure than venous bleeding sources and can have rapid and dramatic deterioration. Patients with ICH on anticoagulants such as warfarin or antiplatelet

Box 2
CNS and non-CNS organ complications of ICH

CNS complications

- ICH growth and herniation
- IVH extension and hydrocephalus
- Raised intracranial pressure
- Cerebral edema
- Autonomic dysfunction: Cushing reflex from raised intracranial pressure, paroxysmal autonomic instability activity (with or without dystonia)
- Seizures: convulsive or nonconvulsive seizures or status epilepticus
- Neurologic deficits: hemiparesis, ataxia, coma, sensory loss, cognitive deficits, brainstem deficits

Non-CNS organ complications of ICH

- Cardiac: troponin leak, acute myocardial infarction from underlying coronary disease, electrocardiogram changes (QTc prolongation, ST- or T-wave changes, U waves, arrhythmias)
- Pulmonary: aspiration pneumonia, CNS breathing patterns (eg, ataxic [Biot], cluster, Cheyne-Stokes, hyperventilation, pneumotaxic), respiratory failure, acute respiratory distress syndrome, neurogenic pulmonary edema
- Gastrointestinal: Cushing ulcer and gastrointestinal hemorrhage, ileus, gastroparesis
- Neuroendocrine: hyponatremia, syndrome of inappropriate antidiuretic hormone release, cerebral salt wasting, relative adrenal insufficiency from central hypothalamic dysautoregulation
- Hematologic: deep vein thrombosis and pulmonary embolism
- Skin: decubitus

Modified from Freeman WD, Dawson SB, Flemming KD. The ABC's of stroke complications. Semin Neurol 2010;30(5):501–10; with permission.

agents such as aspirin or clopidogrel are also at risk for significant ICH expansion,[8] especially if the hemostatic deficit is not reversed. Reversal of anticoagulants in the setting of ICH is recommended.[9] Patients with mechanical heart valves and those at high risk for embolism pose a short-term embolic risk, which must be weighed against the risk of ICH expansion, herniation, and death. Restarting anticoagulants

Box 3
Antiepileptic drug prophylaxis for patients with ICH

- Patients with severe traumatic brain injury (GCS $\leq$8): 7 days (not after unless seizure occurs)
- Witnessed seizure or status epilepticus during hospitalization (or nonconvulsive seizure on electroencephalogram): duration varies according to clinical situation
- Lobar IPH: optional

Data from Refs.[1–3,5]

after the acute phase of ICH is outside the scope of this article. Antithrombotic reversal, however, is discussed later.

Treatment of Raised Intracranial Pressure (Intracranial Hypertension)

Methods to control raised intracranial pressure include head of bed elevation (30°–45°), mannitol (0.25–1 g/kg intravenously as needed), intravenous furosemide, transient hyperventilation, and sedation and paralysis. Ventriculostomy placement is suggested to drain cerebrospinal fluid from symptomatic obstructive hydrocephalus in patients with IPH with IVH extension, or patients with hydrocephalus from aneurysmal SAH.[3] Use of hypertonic saline (HTS) either as a 3% or 23.4% infusion in 15- to 30-mL boluses is increasing as a treatment option for reducing intracranial pressure. Recent studies show HTS may be as effective as mannitol for reducing intracranial pressure and with similar safety in brain-injured patients.[10–12] Hypertonic (3%) saline/acetate was studied in 27 patients with cerebral edema and raised intracranial pressure, 8 of whom had spontaneous IPH.[13] HTS infusion raised serum sodium concentrations to 145 to 155 mmol/L and reduced intracranial pressure in patients with traumatic brain injury and postoperative brain edema but not in patients with IPH or cerebral infarction. Suarez and colleagues[14] also retrospectively studied 20 patients (1 with basal ganglia IPH) with intracranial hypertension refractory to standard intracranial pressure management, including mannitol (1 g/kg), who were treated with 30 mL intravenous boluses of 23.4% saline (8008 mOsm/L). Approximately 80% of these patients experienced a decrease in intracranial pressure by at least 50% of the pretreatment value in 20 to 30 minutes. In a dog model of IPH, HTS (3% and 23.4%) was equally as effective as 1 g/kg of mannitol in reducing intracranial pressure.[11] A longer duration of effect was also noted with HTS compared with mannitol.

Overall, considerable debate remains regarding whether one agent (HTS or mannitol) is superior to the other. Theoretical considerations exist about mannitol extravasating across a leaky blood-brain barrier and worsening brain edema and intracranial pressure because mannitol's reflection coefficient (ie, ability to dissolve into injured brain tissue and back) is 0.9 compared with 1.0 for HTS. These theoretical considerations have not been seen in clinical practice per se, although mannitol should be used with caution in patients with end-stage renal disease who are dialysis-dependent, unless dialysis is planned after treatment, because it is renally excreted and works via an osmotic diuretic mechanism. Another important consideration is the ability to give mannitol via a peripheral intravenous line rather than as a 3% or 23.4% infusion, which should be given via a central venous catheter or equivalent given the high tonicity and risk of peripheral venous thrombophlebitis. Mannitol also may crystallize in the bag, which can be offset by the use of a crystalline filter on the intravenous tubing system.

If hypertonic/hyperosmolar agents such as mannitol or HTS are used to control intracranial pressure, frequent measurement of plasma osmolality and/or serum sodium is suggested (eg, serum sodium every 4–6 hours). If sodium exceeds 150 to 155 mmol/L, holding these agents is advised until these values trend back toward a more normal range (eg, 145 mmol/L). Management of fluid balance and type of total fluids in these patients is extremely important. Avoidance of intravenous free water (D5W) or hypotonic fluids (eg, 1/2 normal saline) is advised because a leaky blood-brain barrier typically exists in some form in patients with ICH, and can pass into injured brain and worsen cerebral edema and intracranial pressure. If patients become severely hypernatremic (eg, serum sodium>160 mmol/L), careful and slow correction is advised to avoid rebound intracranial hypertension and cerebral edema. Enteral free water is absorbed more slowly and can be administered via a nasogastric tube while monitoring serum sodium.

If intracranial pressure remains refractory to hyperosmolar/hypertonic agents (osmotherapy), other options include sedation, neuromuscular blockade, barbiturate-induced coma, and transient hyperventilation (partial pressure of carbon dioxide, 30–35 mm Hg) until discussion with the neurosurgeon regarding whether a role exists for structural management, such as craniotomy or decompressive craniectomy. Hypothermia is also effective for cerebral edema irrespective of cause[15] when used in a mild to moderate range (ie, 32°C–24°C). However, questions data regarding outcomes and safety remain.

Treatment of Seizures

For patients with severe traumatic brain injury with ICH with a GCS score of 8 or less, the Brain Trauma Organization recommends antiepileptic drug (AED) prophylaxis against seizures for 7 days, such as with phenytoin.[5] This recommendation is because these patients have a higher incidence of seizures in the first week, but therapy beyond 7 days has not been proven to be efficacious. AEDs should be given in patients who have experienced a witnessed seizure for a duration, as deemed appropriate by the treating physician.[2,3,5] Otherwise, AED prophylaxis is not routinely advised unless a seizure occurs. If a seizure occurs, most physicians treat patients acutely with intravenous lorazepam and follow with a loading dose infusion of fos-phenytoin or phenytoin (15–20 mg/kg) along with daily maintenance dosing to prevent seizure recurrence. If no further seizures occur after 1 month, AED therapy can be discontinued.[1–3] Prolonged AED therapy is considered on a case-by case basis. Nonconvulsive seizure and nonconvulsive status epilepticus occur in 10% to 20% of patients with ICH in the neurological ICU,[16] and are difficult to detect clinically unless motor manifestations are seen. Some neurological ICUs use continuous electroencephalography monitoring to improve detection of nonconvulsive seizure and nonconvulsive status epilepticus.

Gastrointestinal Stress Ulcer Prophylaxis and Nutrition

Patients with ICH are at risk for Cushing (stress) ulcers and gastrointestinal hemorrhage. Stress ulcer prophylaxis is recommended with either enteral or intravenous H_2-blocking agents, such as famotidine or ranitidine. Proton pump inhibitors such as omeprazole may be used if H_2-blocking agents are not available during hospitalization. Nutrition should be started if the patient is cleared from an aspiration risk standpoint. However, if the patient is unable to take in food by mouth safely and is at risk for aspiration, nutrition is typically started within the first week of hospitalization via an enteral feeding tube, unless a contraindication exists, such as bowel obstruction or perforated viscus, with intravenous fluid support provided temporarily. Enteral feeding is preferable over intravenous total parenteral nutrition.

Temperature, Fever, and Shivering

Normothermia is defined as 98.6°F (37°C). Fever (temperature, ≥38°C) in brain-injured patients worsens clinical outcomes compared with those without fever.[17–20] Fever increases the body's basal metabolic rate[21] and raises the cerebral metabolic rate of oxygen ($CMRO_2$), which creates a relative catabolic state. A febrile (temperature, ≥38°C –38.3°C) patient with ICH should be examined for a source of infection and, when clinically appropriate, undergo laboratory and microbiological testing of invasive lines, central lines, and urinary Foley tubes. If an external ventricular drain (EVD) is present, cerebrospinal fluid analysis and culture should be considered. A chest radiograph may be helpful to confirm pulmonary infection, especially in patients on mechanical ventilation. Other occult sources of infection include sinusitis, acalculous cholecystitis, and some medications. Fever of neurologic origin is considered a diagnosis of exclusion but is common after stroke, especially hemorrhagic stroke (eg, subarachnoid or intraventricular blood). Fever may also be from the systemic inflammatory response syndrome associated with critical illness.

Febrile patients with ICH should receive acetaminophen assuming no contraindication is present, such as hepatic impairment. For patients with ICH and fever that is refractory to acetaminophen and has no infectious cause, thermoregulatory interventions may be necessary, such as use of a cooling blanket or cooling devices to obtain normothermia (ie, 37°C).[17,19,22,23] In one study, patients treated with a cooling pad device had a 75% reduction in fever and more time normothermic compared with those treated with a conventional cooling blanket,[22] but the pad caused more shivering than the blanket. Other interventions include infusion of cool fluids or, in mechanically ventilated patients, increasing sedative-analgesic medication (eg, propofol, fentanyl). Reported side effects from cooling include vasoconstriction (particularly extremities), adrenergic hyperactivation,[23] and postoperative myocardial events.

Shivering is an autonomic reflex response to cooling[23] to cause thermogenesis and raise body temperature, which also raises the basal metabolic rate and $CMRO_2$ similar to fever.[21] Shivering can be difficult to control in patients not under general anesthesia, and may require multimodal treatment.[22,23] Drugs such as thiopental and fentanyl reduce $CMRO_2$ and may also reduce shivering. Meperidine is a good antishiver medication, and can be combined with a dexmedetomidine infusion or buspirone enterally for additive or synergistic effects in lowering the shiver threshold.[23] Meperidine, however, can cause sedation and CNS toxicity (eg, seizures) and should be used with caution. In intubated, mechanically ventilated patients with ICH, refractory fever, shiver, and raised intracranial pressure, treatment may require a combination of acetaminophen, a cooling device, adequate sedation, and neuromuscular blocking agents as a last resort.

Management of ICH on Antithrombotics

The most common coagulopathic ICH encountered is associated with warfarin or coumarins, given their widespread use. Warfarin-related spontaneous ICH (WICH) occurs in only 7 to 10,000 patients annually[24] or approximately every one in five cases of spontaneous ICH. WICH are thought to be larger[8] and continue to grow after 24 hours compared with spontaneous ICH in patients not taking anticoagulants. One-month mortality is approximately 50% in patients with WICH[25] compared with approximately 40% in patients not undergoing anticoagulation therapy.[26,27] The intensity of anticoagulation (eg, INR) also contributes to hematoma expansion and worse outcomes.[8] Therefore patients with symptomatic WICH with an INR greater than 1.3 should undergo emergent anticoagulation reversal,[1,2] which was reviewed in recent guidelines and summarized in **Table 4**. Other antithrombotic agents may be associated with ICH, and reversal of these agents is also addressed in **Table 4**. A more detailed discussion on management of coagulopathic ICH is outside the scope of this article, but has been provided elsewhere.[28]

IPH

Spontaneous IPH is twice as common as SAH but is equally as deadly,[1] with a 1-month mortality of 40%.[26,27] The incidence of spontaneous IPH is between 37,000 and 50,000 patients per year in the United States.[1,2] IPH is a medical emergency

Table 4
Treatment for antithrombotic-associated intracranial bleeding

Antithrombotic Agent	Treatment
Warfarin	Discontinue warfarin Give 10 mg of intravenous vitamin K[a] slowly over 30 minutes[29–32] Give PCC or rFVIIa over FFP if available[2] If PCC and rFVIIa are unavailable, give approximately 15 mL/kg of FFP[2,33–35] Check coagulation parameters frequently after treatment (eg, PT/PTT Q6 h × 24 h) then daily until anticoagulation is reversed
Tissue plasminogen activator (t-PA)	Intravenous platelet transfusion ("sixpack," or one single-donor unit) Cryoprecipitate that contains factor VIII to rapidly correct the systemic fibrinolytic state created by t-PA
Antiplatelet (aspirin, clopidogrel)	Unknown DDAVP or platelet transfusion
Dabigatran	Unknown antidote[36–39] Discontinue dabigatran Hydrate (renally excreted)
Heparin	Protamine, 1 mg per 100 U heparin[1,2]

Abbreviations: DDAVP, 1-deamino-8-D-arginine vasopressin; FFP, fresh frozen plasma; PCC, prothrombin complex concentrate; rFVIIa, recombinant factor VIIa.

[a] Intravenous vitamin K carries an approximate 3/10,000 risk of anaphylaxis and uncertain risk (possibly rare) of anaphylactoid reaction.[30,31]

Data from Refs.[1,2,29–35]

that requires emergent evaluation and management for optimal patient survival. Risk factors for IPH include increasing age, especially older than 85 years; hypertension; INR intensity greater than 3.5; cerebral amyloid angiopathy; renal failure; and prior stroke (hemorrhagic or ischemic). Neuroimaging factors predictive of IPH include leukoaraiosis, evidence of recent or prior stroke (ischemic or hemorrhagic), and the presence of cerebral microbleeds.[40–43]

IPH location and pattern of bleeding are important clues to the underlying disease (see **Table 1**). Anatomically speaking, IPH generally occurs in either a deep or a lobar location. Deep IPH (**Fig. 3**) include the caudate, thalamus, putamen, globus pallidus (basal ganglia or ganglionic ICH), internal capsule, and other deep white matter loci. In contrast, lobar IPH (**Fig. 4**) is defined as bleeding within the cortical-subcortical cerebral hemisphere. Lobar IPH is attributed to cerebral amyloid angiopathy in approximately one-third of patients.[44] Advancing age is an important risk factor for IPH occurring at all locations. Other causes of nontraumatic IPH include bleeding from arteriovenous malformations, aneurysms, cavernous angiomas, moyamoya disease, venous sinus thrombosis, venous angiomas, neoplasm, abscess, drug use (eg, cocaine), and, rarely, vasculitis (see **Table 1**).[18]

Chronic hypertension causes pathologic changes within cerebral blood vessels called *lipohyalinosis*, a process affecting small penetrating arteries or arterioles 50 to 200 μm in diameter, especially at branch points, and contributing to the formation of microaneurysms that can hemorrhage, as originally described by Charcot and Bouchard and subsequent investigators.[45–47] Hypertension has a 0.5 attributable risk for

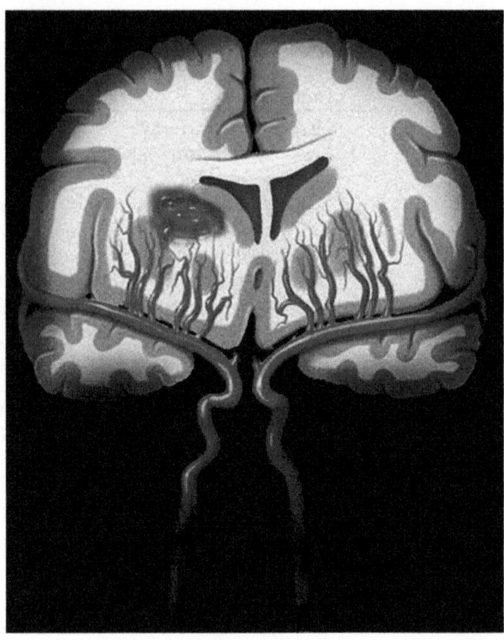

Fig. 3. Deep IPH (deep or ganglionic IPH) within the right basal ganglia below the right caudate nucleus from a ruptured penetrating blood vessel caused by chronic uncontrolled hypertension (eg, Charcot-Bouchard microaneurysm).

deep IPH, suggesting that hypertension causes approximately half of the cases of deep (nonlobar) IPHs,[44] which means the other half are from other causes. Recent MRI with gradient echo sequencing has shown microhemorrhages (**Fig. 5**) in similar locations to these vessels.[41–43]

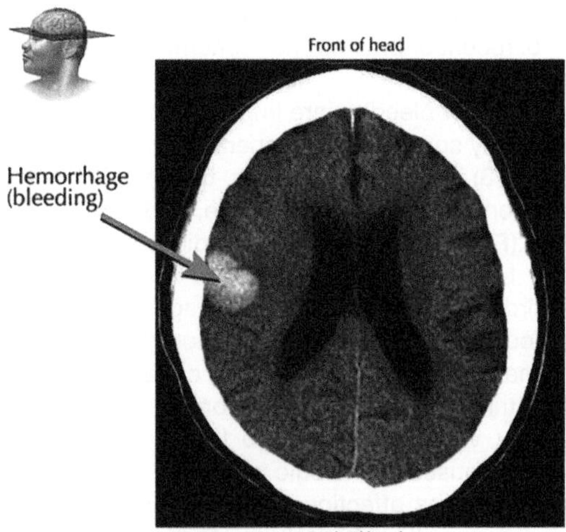

Fig. 4. Lobar IPH. Noncontrast cranial CT scan showing a right cortical-subcortical (lobar) hematoma and orientation in sagittal plane (*upper left*).

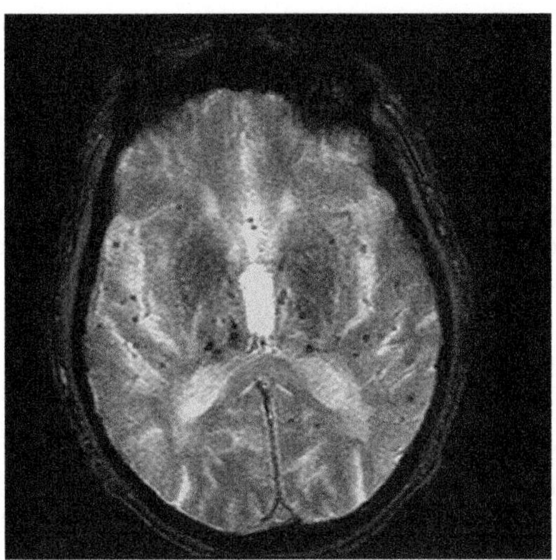

Fig. 5. Gradient echo MRI showing numerous punctate microhemorrhages (*black dots*), as often seen in cerebral amyloid angiopathy when in lobar locations. Deep microhemorrhage deposits can also be seen in chronic hypertension and patients with chronic small vessel disease.

Cerebral amyloid angiopathy (CAA) is increasingly recognized as a disorder leading to spontaneous IPH. CAA is caused by amyloid protein deposition within the walls of blood vessels in cortical-subcortical locations. Amyloid-laden blood vessels are fragile and prone to bleed. CAA affects leptomeningeal blood vessels covering the surface of the brain (ie, pial blood vessels), which can cause spontaneous cortical SAH[48] and superficial siderosis. Patients with CAA may also experience recurrent transient ischemic attack (TIA)–like spells from microhemorrhage deposits or superficial siderosis. These microhemorrhages are seen on MRI with gradient echo in up to 15% of patients older than 70 years.[49] These asymptomatic microhemorrhages also may predict future larger IPH (macrohemorrhage)[43] events.

Clinical Presentation and Medical Management of Patients with IPH

Patients with IPH present with sudden onset of alteration of consciousness, vomiting, headache, or focal neurologic deficits. The extent of neurologic deficits depends on the area of brain or brainstem affected. A patient may become unconsciousness or rapidly comatose because of massive IPH, elevated intracranial pressure, hydrocephalus, brainstem compression, nonconvulsive seizure, or postictal state. Because of the acuity and severity of presentation, most patients with IPH are brought to the emergency department for evaluation.

IPH is diagnosed using the same approach as described earlier for patients with ICH. Some centers use the National Institutes of Health (NIH) stroke scale in their initial, rapid neurologic examination, whereas others obtain a GCS score to gauge level of responsiveness and to measure possible neurologic deterioration. MRI has at least similar sensitivity for detecting ICH as CT. However, CT remains the preferred diagnostic test for detecting ICH and IPH at most hospitals because of its rapid acquisition time, widespread availability, and high sensitivity. Standard laboratory tests in the acute setting for patients with IPH are shown in **Box 1**. Cranial CT imaging in acute IPH typically shows a spherical or ellipsoid hyperdense (ie, bright or white) accumulation of intraparenchymal blood (**Fig. 6**A). Extension of the hematoma into the ventricles is common (see **Fig. 6**B, C) and can cause dilated ventricles (hydrocephalus).

Patients with IPH should be admitted to an ICU for monitoring and management of airway, respiratory function, and blood pressure; avoidance of fever; and careful glucose and electrolyte regulation. Preventing certain medical complications during hospitalization is also crucial, including pneumonia, deep venous thrombosis, pulmonary embolism, and sacral and pressure ulcers (ie, decubitus). Specific management issues are subsequently discussed.

Treatment of hypertension in IPH

Current guidelines for acute IPH target an arterial systolic blood pressure (SBP) of greater than 180 mm Hg or mean arterial pressure greater than 130 to 150 mm Hg (see **Table 3**).[1,2] When raised intracranial pressure is suspected, placement of an intracranial pressure monitor is suggested and an SBP greater than 180 should be treated with either intermittent or continuous antihypertensive medications, while maintaining a cerebral perfusion pressure of at least 60 mm Hg. For patients without raised intracranial pressure, SBP greater than 180 mm Hg should be treated to lower it to approximately 160 mm Hg, or to a mean arterial pressure of approximately 110 mm Hg. Considerable debate remains whether high or low arterial blood pressures contribute to intracerebral bleeding and hematoma expansion, and whether lower

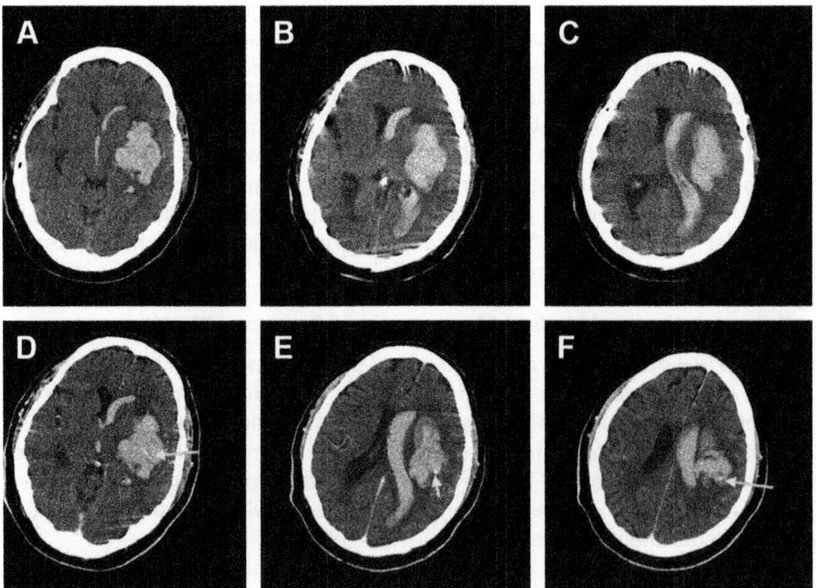

Fig. 6. Hypertensive deep IPH with IVH extension and contrast extravasation. (*A*) Left basal ganglia IPH with mass effect and midline shift from left to right, and IVH with the left frontal horn and third ventricle. (*B*) Higher slice cut with IPH, third-ventricle IVH, and left lateral ventricular IVH. (*C*) "Casted" left lateral ventricle from IPH extending into the ipsilateral ventricle. (*D–F*) The 'spot sign' (*red arrows*) described with contrast extravasation within the IPH. Whether this site of contrast leak represents the original arteriolar vessel bleeding source of the IPH, damaged blood-brain barrier with contrast leak, or secondary torn vessels injured during an expanding IPH remains unknown.

blood pressure may cause perihematomal ischemia. This controversy has led to a "chicken or the egg" analogy about whether the ICH is the cause of the acute hypertension response or is the effect as a physiologic response similar to Cushing reflex to maintain brain perfusion.

Recent data suggest the acute hypertensive response in patients with IPH typically declines approximately 2 mm Hg of mean arterial pressure per hour within 6 hours of acute IPH before reaching a plateau by 24 hours.[50,51] Because blood pressure declines naturally after acute IPH, overaggressive treatment may be unwise, and short-acting intravenous medications such as labetalol, esmolol, and enalaprilat are typically administered.[1,2] The particular antihypertensive agent chosen should be individualized based on hemodynamic parameters of the patient and other comorbidities (eg, tachycardia and hypertension may be treated with labetolol or esmolol, whereas isolated severe hypertension should be treated with hydralazine or nicardipine). Debate remains regarding whether rapid reduction in blood pressure after IPH would be injurious to perihematomal brain similar to large-vessel ischemic stroke models.

The completed phase II multicenter trials, Antihypertensive Treatment in Acute Cerebral Hemorrhage (ATACH) and the Intensive Blood Pressure Reduction in Acute Cerebral Hemorrhage Trial (INTERACT)[51,52] suggest there may be a lower blood pressure threshold (eg, 140 mm Hg systolic) for antihypertensive treatment than current guidelines recommend. Currently, two large phase III trials are underway, ATACH II and INTERACT II, targeting lower systolic ranges of 120 to 140 mm Hg or less for SBP in IPH based on these trials' previous data showing preliminary safety.

Hematoma volume and growth

IPH volume (cm^3) is a powerful predictor of 30-day mortality[27] and can be easily calculated using the formula ABC/2,[53] where A and B are the largest perpendicular diameters of the hematoma in centimeters (cm), and C is the number of vertical CT slices multiplied by the slice thickness (cm) (**Fig. 7**). IPH growth (volume increase of at least

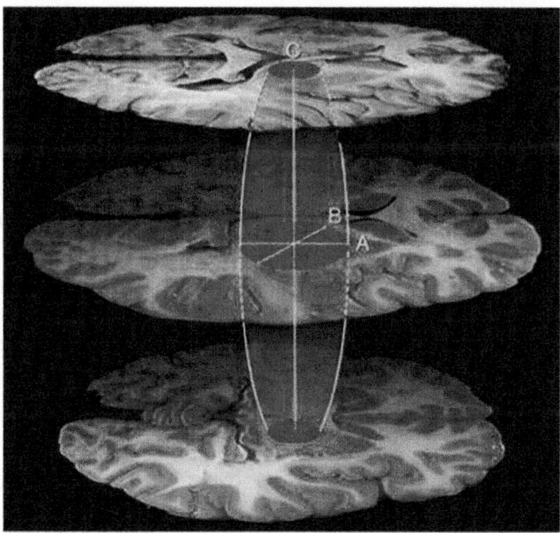

Fig. 7. ABC/2 IPH hematoma calculation of hematoma volume. The visually largest CT slice with IPH hematoma is identified, then A and B are diameters of the IPH measured in centimeters. The number of vertical slices of IPH seen is defined as C. C is multiplied by slice thickness. For example, if A and B are both 3 cm, and C is three slices vertically with 5 mm per CT slice cut, then ABC/2 = (3 cm × 3 cm × (3 slices × 0.5 cm))/2 = 13.5/2 = 6.75 cm^3

33%) occurs in approximately 38% of patients, with 26% of hematoma growth occurring between the baseline and 1-hour CT scan, and the remaining 12% of patients with IPH growth between the 1- and 20-hour CT scans.[7] IPH growth is associated with clinical neurologic deterioration.[7] Factors associated with hematoma growth include presentation within 6 hours of ictus, contrast extravasation (see **Fig. 6**D, E), antiplatelet or anticoagulant therapy, platelet count less than 100,000/μL, and liver disease.[54–56] Patients taking antiplatelet agents (eg, aspirin, clopidogrel, ticlopidine) or warfarin must stop the medication. If the platelet count is less than 50,000/μL in the setting of acute IPH, platelet transfusion may be considered, although evidence-based data supporting this are lacking. Recent data by Naidech and colleagues[57] show that patients with IPH who have impaired platelet function have a higher rate of subsequent IPH growth. This finding raises the question whether 1-deamino-8-D-arginine vasopressin (DDAVP) or platelet transfusion would help reduce IPH hematoma growth.

Treatment to reduce IPH growth: blood pressure control and recombinant factor VIIa
Because IPH volume correlates strongly with mortality, reducing hematoma growth and volume are logical targets for therapeutic intervention. It seems intuitive that hypertension could contribute to IPH growth, but limited data support a cause-and-effect relationship. Kazui and colleagues[55] found that SBP greater than 200 mm Hg at admission correlated with hematoma expansion, but this relationship was not observed in two other studies.[7,54] Additional studies have shown reduced hematoma enlargement in acute IPH when SBP was treated to 150 mm Hg or less.[51,52,56] Two of these trials, ATACH[51] and INTERACT,[52] focused on safety and CT evidence of hematoma growth. The hope is that these phase III trials will answer specifically whether aggressive blood pressure control (eg, SBP between 120 and 140 mm Hg) reduces hematoma growth and improves clinical outcomes. Based on these ongoing trials, current guidelines (eg, from the American Heart Association [AHA])[2] suggest treatment only if SBP is greater than 180 mm Hg, and assuming no increased intracranial pressure is suspected.

Mayer and colleagues[58] studied the effect of hemostatic drug recombinant factor VIIa on slowing early hematoma growth. Recombinant factor VIIa (rFVIIa or Novoseven) is a cloned product of endogenous activated coagulation factor VII and only has a U.S. Food and Drug Administration (FDA) label indication for bleeding episodes in hemophiliac patients associated with factor inhibitors.[59] In the phase II multicenter study by Mayer and colleagues,[58] 399 patients with acute IPH were randomized to receive placebo or 40 μg/kg, 80 μg/kg, or 160 μg/kg of rFVIIa within 1 hour after IPH was diagnosed on baseline CT scan. The primary outcome of the study was to assess IPH growth at 24 hours. The study found a dose-dependent effect on reducing hematoma growth, with a mean increase of 29%, 16%, 14%, and 11% in the placebo, 40 μg/kg, 80 μg/kg, and 160 μg/kg dose arms, respectively (P = .01). Clinical outcomes were secondary measurements by the modified Rankin Scale (mRS). The mRS outcome measure was assessed at 90 days and showed that 69% of placebo-treated patients were either dead or severely disabled (modified Rankin Scale score 4–6), compared with 49% to 55% for the rFVIIa-treated patients (P = .004). Mortality at 90 days was 29% for placebo-treated patients compared with 18% in rFVIIa-treated patients. Thromboembolic events of myocardial infarction or ischemic stroke occurred in 7% of rFVIIa-treated patients compared with 2% of placebo-treated patients (P = .12). In more than 170,000 doses of rFVIIa administered to hemophiliac patients for whom the drug was originally manufactured, only 17 serious thromboembolic complications were reported[54] as comparison. Hemophiliac patients are typically younger with fewer vascular risk factors than patients with IPH in the rFVIIa study. Another important issue is the cost of rFVIIa, which is approximately $1020 to $1369 per 1.2-mg vial.[60]

In 2008, a subsequent phase III multicenter trial was reported[61] for acute IPH using rFVIIa among 841 randomized patients. In this study, 268 patients received placebo, whereas the other 297 patients received either 20 μg/kg intravenously of rFVIIa (276 patients) or 80 μg/kg intravenously of rFVIIa within 4 hours after symptomatic stroke onset. The primary end point was poor outcome, defined as severe disability or death according to the modified Rankin scale 90 days after stroke onset. The mean increase in IPH volume at 24 hours was 26% in the placebo group, 18% in the 20-μg/kg rFVIIa group ($P = .09$), and 11% in the 80-μg/kg group ($P<.001$). IPH volume growth was reduced by 2.6 mL (95% CI, −0.3–5.5; $P = .08$) in the group receiving 20 μg/kg of rFVIIa, and 3.8 mL (95% CI, 0.9–6.7; $P = .009$) in the group receiving 80 μg/kg, compared with the placebo group. No significant difference was seen in the proportion of patients with poor clinical outcome (24% in the placebo group, 26% in the 20-μg/kg rFVIIa group, and 29% in 80-μg/kg group). The frequency of thromboembolic events was similar in the three groups, but the arterial events were more frequent in patients receiving 80 μg/kg of rFVIIa compared with the placebo group (9% vs 4%; $P = .04$). Therefore, rFVIIa seems to reduce IPH hematoma growth but did not improve survival or functional outcome. Based on this information, the FDA did not approve rFVIIa for a label indication for IPH. Based on these data, the authors do not recommend rFVIIa outside of a clinical trial.

Perihematoma edema

Three phases of perihematomal edema occur after IPH.[62] The first phase occurs within hours and involves separation of clot and plasma (clot retraction). The second phase occurs over the next 2 days and involves plasma protein extravasation, activation of the coagulation cascade and complement, and an inflammatory process triggered by fibrin and thrombin. The third phase (after the third day) involves erythrocyte lysis and hemoglobin-mediated neuronal toxicity. Perihematoma edema volume increases up to 75% of the hematoma size in patients with hyperacute IPH, and strongly predicts functional outcome.[63,64]

Surgical Management

A meta-analysis of seven surgical trials for supratentorial IPH showed no benefit with surgery.[65] The most recent and largest study, the Surgical Trial in Intracerebral Hemorrhage (STICH) trial was an international, prospective, randomized trial comparing early surgery (n = 503) and initial conservative management (n = 530) in 1033 patients with spontaneous supratentorial IPH for whom best treatment was deemed uncertain.[66] The study end point was favorable clinical outcome, which was defined as good recovery or moderate disability on the Glasgow Outcome Scale. No significant difference was seen between groups, with favorable outcome achieved in 26% of patients randomized to early surgery compared with 24% of patients randomized to conservative treatment ($P = .414$). The authors concluded that early surgical evacuation of IPH showed no overall benefit compared with conservative medical therapy.

STICH had some limitations that should be noted. First, 73% of patients who underwent very early surgery (n = 339) did not undergo surgery until 12 hours from randomization, and only 16% (n = 74) underwent surgery within 12 hours of ictus. Most patients (>75%) underwent frank craniotomy with hematoma evacuation, but other less-invasive techniques were used, including minimally invasive methods such as endoscopic methods of hematoma evacuation.

Established indications for potential neurosurgical intervention are shown in **Box 4**, which include comatose patients with transtentorial herniation, those with significant IVH and hydrocephalus, and those with symptomatic cerebellar ICH (AHA).

Newer surgical therapies

Although the STICH trial suggested no benefit of surgical treatment in supratentorial IPH, several newer surgical methods are being reported. Nishihara and colleagues[67] report use of novel transparent endoscopic tools for hematoma evacuation treated within 24 hours of IPH onset via a burr-hole approach in 82 patients. Vespa and colleagues[68] report a pilot study of IPH evacuation using a frameless stereotactic aspiration and thrombolysis method using recombinant tissue plasminogen activator (rt-PA) in 28 patients with ICH, and found a 77% reduction in ICH volume after surgery. IPH volume was reduced, but no significant difference was seen in mortality between surgical (56%) and nonsurgical patients (59%) at 180 days. Murthy and colleagues[69] performed decompressive craniectomy and IPH clot evacuation for large hemispheric IPH (volume>48 cm^3) in 12 patients. Eleven (91.6%) patients survived to discharge, and 6 had good functional outcome (modified Rankin Scale score, 0–3). An NIH-sponsored safety study Minimally Invasive Surgery plus tPA for Intracerebral Hemorrhaghe Evacuation (MISTIE) is investigating minimally invasive surgery in combination with rt-PA for IPH removal.[70]

Prognosis After IPH

Poor-prognostic variables in IPH include IPH volume greater than 30 cm^3, age older than 80 years, infratentorial location, low presenting GCS score, and the presence of intraventricular blood.[71] These variables were combined in a composite scale called the *ICH score* by Hemphill and colleagues[71] to estimate 30-day mortality, and were derived from a multivariate regression analysis study of patients with IPH, Mortality increases with increasing ICH total score (ICH score of 0–6 ranges from 0%–100% mortality).

SAH: DIAGNOSIS AND MANAGEMENT

Aneurysmal SAH is typically characterized by an explosive or "thunderclap headache," which is instantaneously maximal at onset. The headache of aneurysmal SAH is fairly distinct in patients who are able to provide history, but it is typically the "worst headache of one's life" even among those with migraines and other headache disorders. Aneurysmal SAH headache should be considered in the evaluation of patients with a "worst or first" headache, but most headaches are instantaneously

Box 4
Indications for neurosurgical consultation or intervention in patients with IPH-IVH

- GCS score of 8 or less with transtentorial herniation
- Significant IVH or hydrocephalus
- 3 cm or more of posterior fossa or symptomatic cerebellar ICH evacuation (ventricular cerebrospinal fluid drainage alone not recommended)

Data from Morgenstern LB, Hemphill JC, Anderson C, et al. Association/American Stroke Association Guideline for Healthcare Professionals From the American Heart Guidelines for the Management of Spontaneous Intracerebral Hemorrhage. Stroke 2010;41:2108–29. doi: 10.1161/STR.0b013e3181ec611b.

maximal in pain at onset. Patients with aneurysmal SAH may also have transient loss of consciousness from an acute spike in intracranial pressure and a drop in cerebral perfusion pressure (transient intracranial circulation arrest), or from acute diffuse vasoconstriction of the cerebral arteries. The longer duration of intracranial bleeding and lack of intracranial circulatory flow can lead to global cerebral edema, which can lead to refractory intracranial hypertension and death. Patients who have lesser forms of intracranial SAH bleeding and who survive to seek medical attention often present to an emergency department. A noncontrast head CT is warranted immediately.[3] The CT scan in aneurysmal SAH typically shows a star-shaped pattern of intracranial bleeding around the basal cisterns, around the Circle of Willis vessels, and in front of the brainstem (**Fig. 8**A, B); sometimes IPH with SAH blood (see **Fig. 8**C); and, less commonly, subdural or epidural blood. Associated extension of SAH blood into ventricles may be present, leading to obstructive (noncommunicating) hydrocephalus or communicating hydrocephalus from occlusion of the arachnoid granulations. Both forms of hydrocephalus can lead to increased hydrostatic pressure within the brain and increased intracranial pressure, leading to depressed cerebral perfusion pressure and, if unchecked, eventual cessation of intracranial flow and brain death.

Patients should undergo a CT angiogram or diagnostic cerebral angiogram to identify the aneurysm as soon as possible. Once the location of the aneurysm is identified, the configuration and the aneurysm's dome-to-neck ratio and other factors dictate treatment with either endovascular coiling (**Fig. 9**) with platinum coils or craniotomy with base clipping of the aneurysm.

Patients with aneurysmal SAH and symptomatic hydrocephalus should have an EVD placed to measure intracranial pressure and calculate cerebral perfusion pressure. The zero point of the EVD and the arterial line should be at the same level, which is at the foramen of Monro (approximately the level of the tragus at the ear) for accurate cerebral perfusion pressure calculation.[72,73] Once the aneurysm is secure,

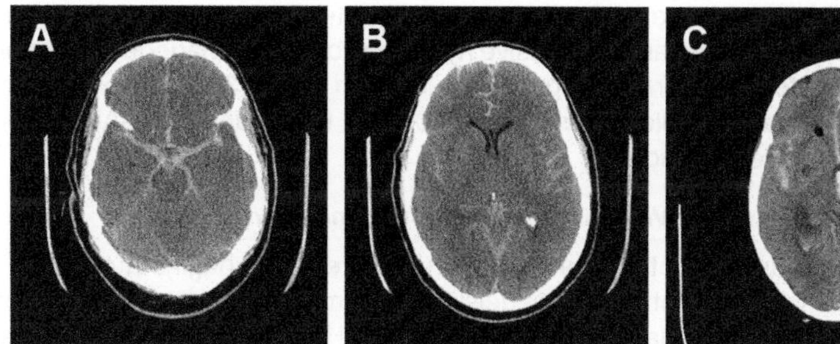

Fig. 8. Aneurysmal SAH from a ruptured anterior cerebral artery aneurysm in a 43-year-old man who presented as a GCS 6-E1M4V1 and was intubated at another hospital and sent to the authors' hospital, where he was noted to be GCS 4-E1M2V1T with extensor posturing. (*A*) SAH blood in the typical star-shaped pattern commonly seen in aneurysmal SAHs, which are spaces normally filled with cerebrospinal fluid and represent a path of least resistance for blood to travel after aneurysm rupture. (*B*) The same patient's CT at a higher level with blood over the convexities. (*C*) SAH blood from a 60-year-old patient with a ruptured anterior communicating artery aneurysm, which ruptured anteriorly and caused a focal left frontal lobe hematoma from the pressure jet of blood and the direction of the SAH blood coming out of the aneurysm. Third-ventricular IVH extension is also seen, and a small amount of right intraventricular air from surgery. The key finding is the presence of diffuse SAH blood along with the left frontal lobe hematoma, which should raise the suspicion of aneurysmal origin.

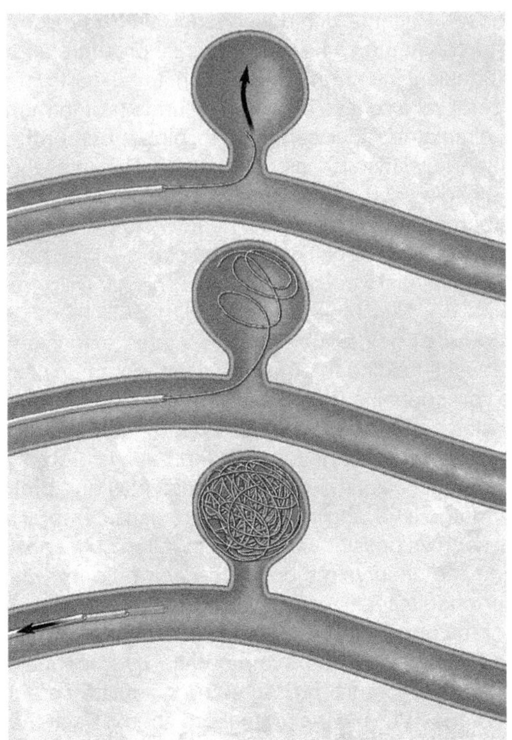

Fig. 9. Artistic representation of an intracranial aneurysm coiled with detachable platinum coils.

post–aneurysmal SAH management is typically predicated on maintaining euvolemia (or normal fluid balance state) and permissive hypertension to allow adequate cerebral perfusion. Immediate blood pressure goals are listed in **Table 3**. However, extreme hypertension (cerebral perfusion pressure, >120–130) in aneurysmal SAH beyond autoregulation is typically avoided.

Vasospasm (Delayed Arterial Vessel Narrowing After Aneurysmal SAH)

Aneurysmal SAH is unique in that the aneurysm rupture event begins a cascade of events intracranially that potentially cause delayed ischemic neurologic deficits. These deficits span an average 21 days post–aneurysmal SAH but peaks between days 7 and 14, with vasospasm risk being proportional to the amount of SAH blood seen on the initial CT scan (ie, Fisher Grade).[74,75] Nimodipine enterally, 60 mg every 4 hours for 21 days, is the standard prophylactic medication for vasospasm prevention, and for making sure patients with aneurysmal SAH do not become dehydrated or volume-depleted. Detailed review of vasospasm management and hypervolemic hypertensive hemodilution therapy is outside the scope of this article, but is addressed elsewhere.[76,77]

Patients with aneurysmal SAH can develop a host of CNS and non-CNS organ complications (see **Box 2**). Hyponatremia is common after aneurysmal SAH and may be from so-called cerebral salt wasting, which is a poorly understood natriuresis that occurs after aneurysmal SAH and other intracranial CNS disorders. Syndrome of inappropriate antidiuretic hormone hypersecretion may also occur. Other unique complications seen in aneurysmal SAH include takotsubo stress cardiomyopathy, which can be seen with troponin leak and cause left apical ballooning on echocardiogram. It represents a potentially reversible cardiomyopathy in terms of ejection fraction compared with coronary disease–based infarction of the myocardium. Takotsubo cardiomyopathy may complicate hypervolemic hypertensive hemodilution management because of heart failure and pulmonary edema.

SDH AND EDH

SDH or EDH are associated with a significant 30-day mortality of at least 40% to 60% (**Fig. 10**).[77–80] SDH is typically caused by tearing of bridging veins between the brain and skull, either from trauma or sometimes spontaneously in elderly patients or those on anticoagulation. EDH, however, typically occurs from tearing of the middle meningeal artery from a blow to the temporal bone just above the zygomatic process, which represents a relative weak or thin spot on the human skull. A fracture or trauma to this area injures the middle meningeal artery and can cause arterial bleeding. The initial blow may cause transient loss of consciousness followed by a lucid interval, followed by a rapid neurologic deterioration from massive arterial bleeding and expansion of the EDH, herniation, and death. For both SDH and EDH, delay of operative intervention worsens outcomes.[77–80] Indications for EDH surgery described by Bullock and colleagues[79] and the Surgical Management of Traumatic Brain Injury Author Group state that an EDH greater than 30 cm^3 should be surgically evacuated regardless of the patient's GCS score, and that comatose patients with acute EDH (GCS<9) with anisocoria should undergo surgical evacuation as soon as possible. Patients with nonoperable, medically managed EDH are those with a GCS score greater than 8 without focal deficit, EDH volume less than 30 cm^3, maximal EDH thickness less than 15 mm, and less than a 5-mm midline shift. These nonoperable patients require serial CT scanning and close neurologic observation in a neurosurgical center.

Other important complications to consider, particularly in patients with SDH, are seizures, especially those in nonconvulsive form, which may occur in up to 20% of patients with acute SDH.[81] Cerebral or cortical edema also can occur with either, but cortical edema from SDH can cause TIA-like phenomena that are negative on MRI, and electroencephalogram should be considered. The authors have observed that sometimes patients with acute SDH experience a transient response to dexamethasone (eg, 4 mg intravenously every 6 hours) presumably from a forme fruste of cortical vasogenic edema, although little to no literature supports this.[82]

PRIMARY AND SECONDARY IVH AND HYDROCEPHALUS

IVH results from either primary bleeding within the ventricle (primary IVH) or secondarily from ICH that expands into the ventricle (secondary IVH). The estimated incidence of IVH is 22,000 patients per year.[83] Approximately one-third of IVHs are secondary, meaning bleeding from the parenchyma or another location leaked into the ventricle. Primary IVH is not as common as secondary IVH and is defined by blood only within the ventricles. The differential diagnosis of primary IVH includes aneurysm, arteriovenous malformation, trauma, coagulopathy, choroid plexus tumor, and ependymal lesion. Secondary IVH is caused by spontaneous IPH with IVH extension approximately half the time (see **Fig. 6**A–C)[83] and aneurysm 10% to 30% of the time (**Fig. 8**C). Traumatic IVH should be considered when the history or findings support trauma (see **Fig. 2**F).

The pathophysiology of IVH is in causing obstruction of the cerebrospinal fluid flow by blockage of the ventricular pathways (obstructive or noncommunicating

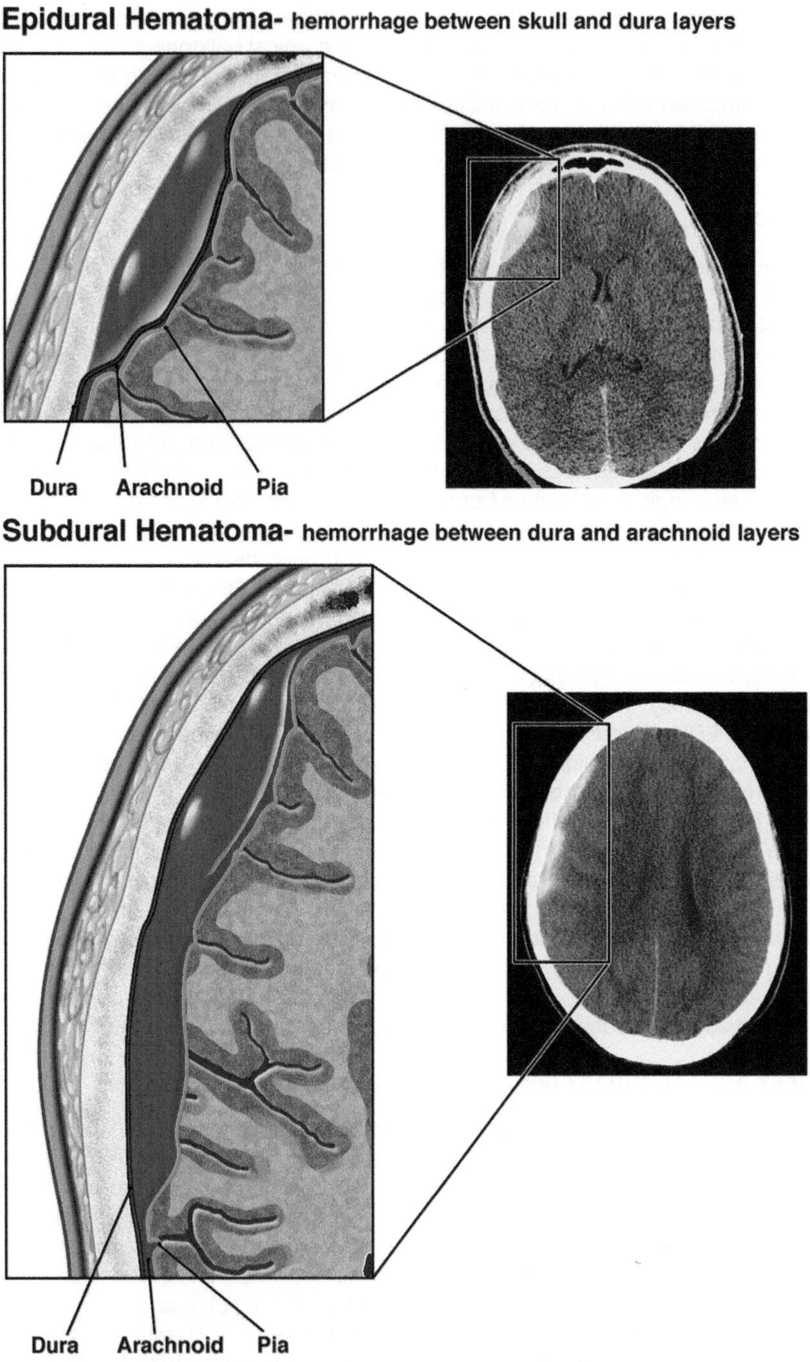

Epidural Hematoma- hemorrhage between skull and dura layers
Dura
Arachnoid
Pia
Subdural Hematoma- hemorrhage between dura and arachnoid layers
Dura
Arachnoid
Pia

Fig. 10. SDH and EDH shown in artistic diagrams and on CT. SDHs look crescentic, like a crescent moon, and do not respect cranial suture lines because SDH are below the dura mater (subdural). EDHs, however, are lens-shaped and typically respect cranial suture lines because they are above the dura.

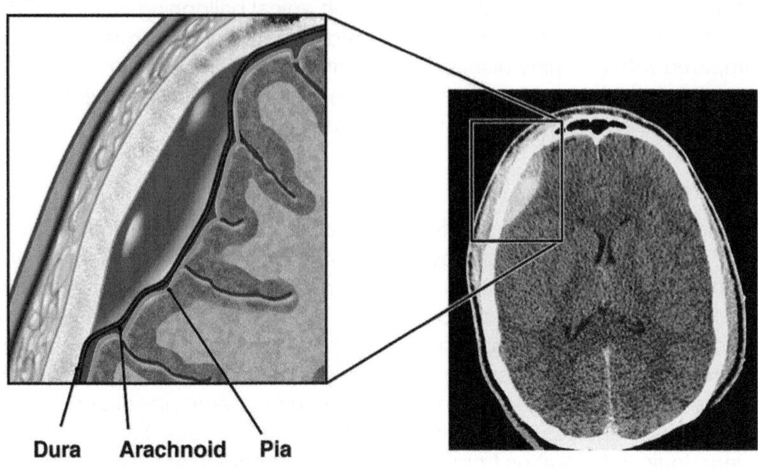

hydrocephalus) or of the tiny arachnoid granulations that normally drain cerebrospinal fluid into the draining veins from the head into the jugular venous sinuses (ie, communicating or nonobstructive hydrocephalus). IVH also causes localized inflammation, which can cause neurologic dysfunction and localized irritation of the surrounding brain tissue. Both types of hydrocephalus lead to an increase in hydrostatic pressure and increased intracranial pressure, which lowers cerebral perfusion pressure defined by the difference between the mean arterial pressure and the intracranial pressure (eg, cerebral perfusion pressure = mean arterial pressure − intracranial pressure). Hydrocephalus can be acute or delayed and lead to cognitive deficits, spasticity, incontinence, and gait dysfunction.

Standard treatment for IVH with acute obstructive hydrocephalus includes placement of a cerebrospinal fluid drain via external ventriculostomy.[83] The volume of IVH is an independent predictor of mortality[6] similar to IPH volume,[84,85] and is up to 40% to 80% by 1 month. A study of urokinase placed in the ventricles of patients with IVH via ventriculostomy expedited clot resolution within the ventricles,[84] and may improve 30-day mortality.[84–88] However, rebleeding into the ventricles with urokinase treatment occurred in approximately 6% of patients. Some institutions are using rt-PA off-label[83] in efforts to expedite IVH clot resolution. A large, multicenter, prospective phase III trial (clot lysis: evaluating accelerated resolution [CLEAR] IVH) is investigating the optimal dose of intraventricular rt-PA to expedite removal of IVH.[70] The results of this pivotal trial will help determine whether this becomes an FDA-approved (label indication) drug for patients with IVH. Medical management of patients with IVH includes raising the head of bed, optimizing cerebral perfusion pressure (via an intracranial pressure monitor), and osmotherapy as needed.

SUMMARY

ICH is a neurologic emergency because of its high 1-month mortality, and may require neurosurgical intervention. Patients with ICH should be triaged rapidly and efficiently based on airway and respiratory function and level of consciousness. Patient history and noncontrast CT often yield clues to assist in diagnosing the underlying cause of the ICH. Specialized management of each ICH subtype depends on correct diagnosis. Indications for surgical intervention include a GCS score of 8 or less in potentially salvagable patients with either traumatic ICH or IPH with herniation (although deep IPH surgery has not been proven superior to optimal medical management), comatose patients with SDH or EDH with anisocoria, those with an EDH volume greater than 30 cm^3, and those with symptomatic cerebellar IPH with mass effect or hydrocephalus. Medical and critical care management of patients with ICH, including optimizing cerebral perfusion pressure, oxygenation, and metabolic status (avoidance of fever and optimal nutrition), and preventing infections, deep vein thrombosis, and decubitus and gastrointestinal stress ulcers, will improve the chances of survival in patients with ICH.

REFERENCES

1. Broderick JP, Connelly S, Feldman E, et al. Guidelines for the management of spontaneous intracerebral hemorrhage in adults: 2007 Update: A Guideline From the American Heart Association/American Stroke Association Stroke Council, High Blood Pressure Research Council, and the Quality of Care and Outcomes in Research Interdisciplinary Working Group: The American Academy of Neurology affirms the value of this guideline as an educational tool for neurologists. Stroke 2007;38:2001.

2. Morgenstern LB, Hemphill JC, Anderson C, et al. Association/American Stroke Association Guideline for Healthcare Professionals From the American Heart Guidelines for the Management of Spontaneous Intracerebral Hemorrhage. Stroke 2010;41:2108–29. DOI: 10.1161/STR.0b013e3181ec611b.
3. Bederson JB, Connolly ES Jr, Batjer HH, et al. American Heart Association Guidelines for the management of aneurysmal subarachnoid hemorrhage: a statement for healthcare professionals from a special writing group of the Stroke Council, American Heart Association. Stroke 2009;40(3):994–1025.
4. Lee SH, Ryu WS, Roh JK. Cerebral microbleeds are a risk factor for warfarin-related intracerebral hemorrhage. Neurology 2009;72(2):171–6.
5. Brain Trauma Organization Guidelines for TBI and ICH. Guidelines for the Management of Severe Traumatic Brain Injury. 3rd edition. Available at: https://www.braintrauma.org/coma-guidelines/. Accessed September 29, 2011.
6. Reynolds SF, Heffner J. Airway management of the critically ill patient: rapid-sequence intubation. Chest 2005;127(4):1397–412.
7. Brott T, Broderick JP, Kothari R, et al. Early hemorrhage growth in patients with intracerebral hemorrhage. Stroke 1997;28:1–5.
8. Rosand J, Eckman MH, Knudsen KA, et al. The effect of warfarin and intensity of anticoagulation on outcome of intracerebral hemorrhage. Arch Intern Med 2004; 164:880–4.
9. Aguilar MI, Hart RG, Kase CS, et al. Treatment of warfarin-associated intracerebral hemorrhage: literature review and expert opinion. Mayo Clin Proc 2007; 82(1):82–92.
10. Larive LL, Rhoney DH, Parker D Jr, et al. Introducing hypertonic saline for cerebral edema: an academic center experience. Neurocrit Care 2004;1(4):435–40.
11. Qureshi AI, Wilson DA, Traystman RJ. Treatment of elevated intracranial pressure in experimental intracerebral hemorrhage: comparison between mannitol and hypertonic saline. Neurosurgery 1999;44(5):1055–63.
12. Ogden AT, Mayer SA, Connolly ES Jr. Hyperosmolar agents in neurosurgical practice: the evolving role of hypertonic saline. Neurosurgery 2005; 57(2):207–15.
13. Qureshi AI, Suarez JI, Bhardwaj A, et al. Use of hypertonic (3%) saline/acetate infusion in the treatment of cerebral edema: effect on intracranial pressure and lateral displacement of the brain. Crit Care Med 1998;26:440–6.
14. Suarez JI, Qureshi AI, Bhardwaj A, et al. Treatment of refractory intracranial hypertension with 23.4% saline. Crit Care Med 1998;26:1118–22.
15. Polderman K. Induced hypothermia and fever control for prevention and treatment of neurological injuries. Lancet 2008;371:1955–69.
16. Rossetti AO, Oddo M. The neuro-ICU patient and electroencephalography paroxysms: if and when to treat. Curr Opin Crit Care 2010. [Epub ahead of print].
17. Carhuapoma JR, Gupta K, Coplin WM, et al. Treatment of refractory fever in the neurosciences critical care unit using a novel, water-circulating cooling device. A single-center pilot experience. J Neurosurg Anesthesiol 2003;15(4):313–8.
18. Diringer MN, Neurocritical Care Fever Reduction Trial Group. Treatment of fever in the neurologic intensive care unit with a catheter-based heat exchange system. Crit Care Med 2004;32(2):559–64.
19. Leira R, Davalos A, Silva Y, et al, Stroke Project, Cerebrovascular Diseases Group of the Spanish Neurological Society. Early neurologic deterioration in intracerebral hemorrhage: predictors and associated factors. Neurology 2004;63(3):461–7.
20. Marion DW. Controlled normothermia in neurologic intensive care. Crit Care Med 2004;32(Suppl 2):S43–5.

21. Ritter AM, Robertson CS. Cerebral metabolism. Neurosurg Clin N Am 1994;5(4):633–45.
22. Mayer SA, Kowalski RG, Presciutti M, et al. Clinical trial of a novel surface cooling system for fever control in neurocritical care patients. Crit Care Med 2004;32(12):2508–15.
23. Doufas AG, Sessler DI. Physiology and clinical relevance of induced hypothermia. Neurocrit Care 2004;1(4):489–98.
24. Hart RG, Tonarelli SB, Pearce LA. Avoiding central nervous system bleeding during antithrombotic therapy: recent data and ideas. Stroke 2005;36(7):1588–93.
25. Sjoblom L, Hardemark HG, Lindgren A, et al. Management and prognostic features of intracerebral hemorrhage during anticoagulant therapy: a Swedish multicenter study. Stroke 2001;32:2567–74.
26. Broderick JP, Brott TG, Tomsick T, et al. Intracerebral hemorrhage more than twice as common as subarachnoid hemorrhage. J Neurosurg 1993;78:188–91.
27. Aguilar MI, Freeman WD. Treatment of coagulopathy in intracranial hemorrhage. Curr Treat Options Neurol 2010;12(2):113–28.
28. Broderick JP, Brott TG, Duldner JE, et al. Volume of intracerebral hemorrhage: a powerful and easy-to-use predictor of 30-day mortality. Stroke 1993;24:987–93.
29. AquaMEPHYTON. Physician's Desk Reference, PDR.net; 2001.
30. Riegert-Johnson DL, Volcheck GW. The incidence of anaphylaxis following intravenous phytonadione (vitamin K1): a 5-year retrospective review. Ann Allergy Asthma Immunol 2002;89(4):400–6.
31. Fiore LD, Scola MA, Cantillon CE, et al. Anaphylactoid reactions to vitamin K. J Thromb Thrombolysis 2001;11(2):175–83.
32. Freeman WD, Aguilar MI. Management of warfarin-related intracerebral hemorrhage. Expert Rev Neurother 2008;8(2):271–90.
33. Ansell J, Hirsh J, Hylek E, et al. Pharmacology and management of the vitamin K antagonists: American College of Chest Physicians Evidence-Based Clinical Practice Guidelines (8th edition). Chest 2008;133:160S–98S.
34. Olson JD. Mechanisms of hemostasis. Effect on intracerebral hemorrhage. Stroke 1993;24(Suppl 12):I109–14.
35. Schulman S. Clinical practice. Care of patients receiving long-term anticoagulant therapy. N Engl J Med 2003;349:675–83.
36. Dabigatran [package insert]. Rhein (Germany): Boehringer Ingelheim.
37. Connolly SJ, Ezekowitz MD, Yusuf S, et al, RELY Trial Investigators. Dabigatran versus warfarin in patients with atrial fibrillation. N Engl J Med 2009;361:1139–51.
38. Drug information unit request. Boehringer Ingelheim Pharmaceuticals, Inc.
39. van Ryn J, Stangier J, Haertter S, et al. Dabigatran etexilate—a novel, reversible, oral direct thrombin inhibitor: interpretation of coagulation assays and reversal of anticoagulant activity. Thromb Haemost 2010;103:1116–27.
40. Smith EE, Rosand J, Knudsen KA, et al. Leukoaraiosis is associated with warfarin-related hemorrhage following ischemic stroke. Neurology 2002;59:193–7.
41. Jeerakathil T, Wolf PA, Beiser A, et al. Cerebral microbleeds: prevalence and associations with cardiovascular risk factors in the Framingham Study. Stroke 2004;35:1831–5.
42. Nighoghossian N, Hermier M, Adeleine P, et al. Old microbleeds are a potential risk factor for cerebral bleeding after ischemic stroke: a gradient-echo T2*-weighted brain MRI study. Stroke 2002;33:735–42.

43. Lee SH, Bae HJ, Kwon SJ, et al. Cerebral Microbleeds are regionally associated with intracerebral hemorrhage. Neurology 2004;62:72–6.
44. Woo D, Sauerbeck LR, Kissela BM, et al. Genetic and environmental risk factors for intracerebral hemorrhage. Stroke 2002;33:1190–6.
45. Qureshi AI, Tuhrim S, Broderick JP, et al. Spontaneous intracerebral hemorrhage. N Engl J Med 2001;344(19):1450–60.
46. Fisher CM. Pathological observations in hypertensive cerebral hemorrhage. J Neuropathol Exp Neurol 1971;30:536–50.
47. Garcia JH, Ho KL. Pathology of hypertensive cerebral arteriopathy. Neurosurg Clin N Am 1992;3:497–507.
48. Greenberg SM, Eng JA, Ning M, et al. Hemorrhage burden predicts recurrent intracerebral after lobar hemorrhage. Stroke 2004;35:1415–20.
49. Walker DA, Rubino F. Routine use of gradient-echo MRI to screen for cerebral amyloid angiopathy in elderly patients. Am J Roentgenol 2004;182(6):1547–50.
50. Qureshi AI, Bliwise DL, Bliwise NG, et al. Rate of 24-hour blood pressure decline and mortality after spontaneous intracerebral hemorrhage: a retrospective analysis with a random effects regression model. Crit Care Med 1999;27(3):480–5.
51. Antihypertensive Treatment of Acute Cerebral Hemorrhage (ATACH) investigators. Antihypertensive treatment of acute cerebral hemorrhage. Crit Care Med 2010;38(2):637–48.
52. Anderson CS, Huang Y, Wang JG, et al. INTERACT Investigators. Intensive Blood Pressure Reduction in Acute Cerebral Haemorrhage trial (INTERACT): a randomised pilot trial. Lancet Neurol 2008;7(5):391–9.
53. Kothari RU, Brott T, Broderick JP, et al. The ABCs of measuring intracerebral hemorrhage volumes. Stroke 1996;27:1304–5.
54. Toyoda K, Okada Y, Minematsu K, et al. Antiplatelet therapy contributes to acute deterioration of intracerebral hemorrhage. Neurology 2005;65:1000–4.
55. Kazui S, Minematsu K, Yamamoto H, et al. Predisposing factors to enlargement of spontaneous intracerebral hemorrhage. Stroke 1997;28:2370–5.
56. Ohwaki K, Yano E, Nagashima H, et al. Blood pressure management in acute intracerebral hemorrhage: relationship between elevated blood pressure and hematoma enlargement. Stroke 2004;35:1364–7.
57. Naidech AM, Bendok BR, Garg RK, et al. Reduced platelet activity is associated with more intraventricular hemorrhage. Neurosurgery 2009;65(4):684–8.
58. Mayer SA, Brun NC, Begtrup K, et al, Recombinant Activated Factor VII Intracerebral Hemorrhage Trial Investigators. Recombinant activated factor VII for acute intracerebral hemorrhage. N Engl J Med 2005;352(8):777–85.
59. NovoSeven. [Package Insert].
60. Fewel ME, Park P. The emerging role of recombinant-activated factor VII in neurocritical care. Neurocrit Care 2004;1:19–30.
61. Mayer SA, Brun NC, Begtrup K, et al. Efficacy and safety of recombinant activated factor VII for acute intracerebral hemorrhage. N Engl J Med 2008;358(20):2127–37.
62. Xi G, Keep RF, Hoff JT. Pathophysiology of brain edema formation. Neurosurg Clin N Am 2002;13(3):371–83.
63. Gebel JM, Jauch EC, Brott TG, et al. Relative edema volume is a predictor of outcome in patients with hyperacute spontaneous intracerebral hemorrhage. Stroke 2002;33:2636–41.
64. Gebel JM, Jauch EC, Brott TG, et al. Natural history of perihematomal edema in patients with hyperacute spontaneous intracerebral hemorrhage. Stroke 2002;33:2631–5.

65. Fernandes HM, Gregson B, Siddique S, et al. Surgery in intracerebral hemorrhage. The uncertainty continues. Stroke 2000;31(10):2511–6.
66. Mendelow AD, Gregson BA, Fernandes HM, et al, STICH investigators. Early surgery versus initial conservative treatment in patients with spontaneous supratentorial intracerebral haematomas in the International Surgical Trial in Intracerebral Haemorrhage (STICH): a randomised trial. Lancet 2005;365(9457):387–97.
67. Nishihara T, Nagata K, Tanaka S, et al. Newly developed endoscopic instruments for the removal of intracerebral hematoma. Neurocrit Care 2005;2:67–74.
68. Vespa P, McArthur D, Miller C, et al. Frameless stereotactic aspiration and thrombolysis of deep intracerebral hemorrhage is associated with reduction of hemorrhage volume and neurologic improvement. Neurocrit Care 2005;2:274–81.
69. Murthy JM, Chowdary GV, Murthy TV, et al. Decompressive craniectomy with clot evacuation in large hemispheric hypertensive intracerebral hemorrhage. Neurocrit Care 2005;2:258–62.
70. Hanley DF, Hacke W. Ongoing studies: from critical care and emergency medicine neurology in stroke. Stroke 2005;36:205.
71. Hemphill JC, Bonovich DC, Besmertis L, et al. The ICH score: a simple, reliable grading scale for intracerebral hemorrhage. Stroke 2001;32:891–7.
72. Nates JL, Niggemeyer LE, Anderson MB, et al. Cerebral perfusion pressure monitoring alert! [letter]. Crit Care Med 1997;25:895–6.
73. Rose JC, Mayer SA. Optimizing blood pressure in neurological emergencies. Neurocrit Care 2004;1(3):287–99.
74. Kistler JP, Crowell RM, Davis KR, et al. The relation of cerebral vasospasm to the extent and location of subarachnoid blood visualized by CT scan: a prospective study. Neurology 1983;33(4):424–36.
75. Macdonald RL, Pluta RM, Zhang JH. Cerebral vasospasm after subarachnoid hemorrhage: the emerging revolution. Nat Clin Pract Neurol 2007;3(5):256–63.
76. Ullman JS, Bederson JB. Hypertensive, hypervolemic, hemodilutional therapy for aneurysmal subarachnoid hemorrhage. Is it efficacious? Yes. Crit Care Clin 1996;12(3):697–707.
77. Bullock MR, Chesnut R, Ghajar J, et al. Surgical management of acute subdural hematomas. Neurosurgery 2006;58:S16–24 [discussion: Si-iv].
78. Bullock MR, Chesnut R, Ghajar J, et al, Surgical Management of Traumatic Brain Injury Author Group. Surgical management of acute epidural hematomas. Neurosurgery 2006;58(Suppl 3):S7–15 [discussion: Si-iv].
79. Koc RK, Akdemir H, Oktem IS, et al. Acute subdural hematoma: outcome and outcome prediction. Neurosurg Rev 1997;20(4):239–44.
80. Wilberger JE Jr, Harris M, Diamond DL. Acute subdural hematoma: morbidity, mortality, and operative timing. J Neurosurg 1991;74(2):212–8.
81. Rabinstein AA, Chung SY, Rudzinski LA, et al. Seizures after evacuation of subdural hematomas: incidence, risk factors, and functional impact. J Neurosurg 2010;112(2):455–60.
82. Bender MB, Christoff N. Nonsurgical treatment of subdural hematomas. Arch Neurol 1974;31(2):73–9.
83. Engelhard HH, Andrews CO, Slavin KV, et al. Current management of intraventricular hemorrhage. Surg Neurol 2003;60:15–22.
84. Naff NJ, Carhuapoma JR, Williams MA, et al. Treatment of intraventricular hemorrhage with urokinase: effects on 30-Day survival. Stroke 2000;31(4):841–7.

85. Akdemir H, Selcuklu A, Pasaoglu A, et al. Treatment of severe intraventricular hemorrhage by intraventricular infusion of urokinase. Neurosurg Rev 1995; 18(2):95–100.
86. Coplin WM, Vinas FC, Agris JM, et al. A cohort study of the safety and feasibility of intraventricular urokinase for nonaneurysmal spontaneous intraventricular hemorrhage. Stroke 1998;29(8):1573–9.
87. Tung MY, Ong PL, Seow WT, et al. A study on the efficacy of intraventricular urokinase in the treatment of intraventricular haemorrhage. Br J Neurosurg 1998;12(3): 234–9.
88. Naff NJ, Hanley DF, Keyl PM, et al. Intraventricular thrombolysis speeds blood clot resolution: results of a pilot, prospective, randomized double-blind, controlled trial. Neurosurgery 2004;54(3):577–83.

Head and Spinal Cord Injury: Diagnosis and Management

Prashant Chittiboina, MD, MPH[a], Hugo Cuellar-Saenz, MD[b], Christina Notarianni, MD[a], Raul Cardenas, MD[c], Bharat Guthikonda, MD[a,*]

KEYWORDS

- Traumatic brain injury • Intracranial pressure • Management
- Cerebrovascular injury • Pediatric • Spinal cord injury
- Vertebral injury

INTRACRANIAL PRESSURE MANAGEMENT

In modern neurotraumatology, intracranial pressure (ICP) management is a central tenet. The incidence of raised ICP or intracranial hypertension (ICHTN) is very high in modern neurotrauma units. In patients with demonstrable mass lesions, up to 63% may have ICHTN. By contrast, up to 13% of patients with a normal initial computed tomogram of head (CT Head) may have ICHTN.[1] Elevated ICP, in turn, is an independent predictor of worse outcomes in patients with severe traumatic brain injury (TBI).[2–4] Increased ICP is also directly related to increased mortality in such patients.[2] In patients with sustained ICHTN, control of ICP within thresholds leads to improved outcomes.[5] In addition, inability to control ICP is a predictor of poor outcomes.[1] Since the 1970s, significant reductions in morbidity and mortality have been achieved in patients with severe TBI with intensive management protocols. ICP control is an integral part of management protocols.[6]

Pathophysiology

In TBI, ICHTN can be caused by various factors. Cerebrospinal fluid (CSF) parameters may be responsible for up to one-third of ICP elevation; predominantly due to a decrease in CSF absorption and an increased resistance to outflow. Vascular factors

[a] Department of Neurosurgery, Louisiana State University Health Sciences Center in Shreveport, 1501 King's Highway, Shreveport, LA 71130, USA
[b] Division of Neuro-Interventional Surgery, Louisiana State University Health Sciences Center in Shreveport, 1501 King's Highway, Shreveport, LA 71130, USA
[c] Department of Neurosurgery, University of Texas Health Sciences Center in Houston, 6431 Fannin, Suite 7.146, Houston, TX 77030, USA
* Corresponding author.
E-mail address: bguthi@lsuhsc.edu

Neurol Clin 30 (2012) 241–276
doi:10.1016/j.ncl.2011.09.001 neurologic.theclinics.com
0733-8619/12/$ – see front matter

may be responsible for the remaining two-thirds. Vascular factors include an increase in cerebral blood volume (CBV) via hyperemia, vasogenic edema due to damaged blood-brain barrier (BBB), cytotoxic edema, and ischemic edema.[7] Hyperemia and edema may lead to changes in compliance of brain, leading to an abnormal volume-pressure response in the intracranial cavity.[8] Brain compliance is represented by the pressure-volume index (PVI). In practical terms PVI can be understood as the amount of volume that must be added or removed to change the ICP tenfold (**Fig. 1**).[9] The normal PVI is 26 $\pm$ 4 mL, that is, 26 mL of volume raises ICP from 1 to 10 mm Hg. The same volume will also raise the ICP from 10 to 100 mm Hg.[10] Changes in PVI can occur in TBI independent of edema.[11] Changes in CSF outflow resistance may play an important role in altered PVI in addition to hyperemia and edema.

Indications for ICP Monitoring

With ubiquitous availability of imaging methods, most patients with severe TBI undergo imaging with CT Head at the time of presentation. Despite the advances in imaging technology, the presence of ICHTN cannot be reliably predicted by imaging studies alone.[12] The current recommendations regarding indications for ICP monitoring include all salvageable patients with a severe TBI (defined as Glasgow Coma Scale [GCS] score of 3–8 after resuscitation) and an abnormal computed tomography (CT) scan (defined as presence of hematomas, contusions, swelling, herniation, or compressed basal cisterns). Monitoring is also indicated in patients with severe TBI with a normal CT scan if 2 or more of the following are present: age over 40 years, unilateral or bilateral motor posturing, or systolic blood pressure less than 90 mm Hg.[6] The effect of untreated ICHTN on outcomes is unknown. However, implementation of protocol-based ICP management leads to improvements in outcomes.[13] In addition, an increased frequency of monitoring has also been associated with improved outcomes.[14] Prophylactic treatments without an ICP monitor, such as hyperventilation, mannitol, barbiturates, and paralysis, may result in poor outcomes. ICP monitoring is thus recommended in severe TBI because it leads to improved outcomes.[6]

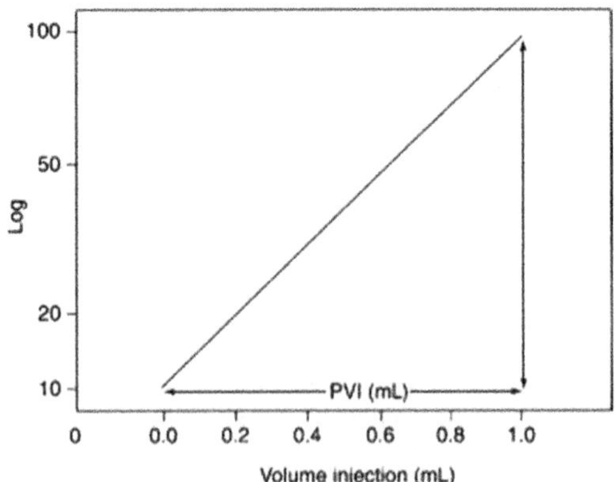

Fig. 1. The pressure-volume index (PVI) is plotted as a straight line on a semilogarithmic scale. This graph shows the relationship between pressure and volume in the cerebrospinal fluid space. (*From* Marmarou A, Beaumont A. Physiology of the Cerebrospinal Fluid and Intracranial Pressure. In: Winn HR, editor. Youman's Neurological Surgery. 4th edition. Elsevier Health Sciences; 2004. p.75–194; with permission.)

Goals of ICP Management

The debate regarding the numerical threshold for initiating therapy in monitored patients is ongoing. Based on available data, the current recommendation places the ICP threshold at 20 mm Hg.[15] Both lower and higher thresholds have been proposed.[2,16] In a large prospective study, logistic regression techniques were used to analyze the effect on ICP outcomes of increments of 5 mm Hg. A threshold at 20 mm Hg had the highest predictive value for outcomes.[2] Although there is no consensus on a definite threshold for treatment, groups reviewing the literature to suggest guidelines have settled on 20 to 25 mm Hg as a threshold for treatment. In the United States, recommendations by the Brain Trauma Foundation (BTF) suggest a treatment threshold of 20 mm Hg.[15] The European Brain Injury Consortium suggests that "...generally ICP elevations above 20–25 mm Hg should be treated."[17] For the pediatric population, although lower thresholds have been suggested, the current recommendations continue to support a threshold of 20 mm Hg.[18]

Approach to ICP Management

Current recommendations

Many well-designed clinical and experimental studies have approached the issue of ICP management in TBI. Consensus groups including a large body of practicing neurosurgeons, traumatologists, and intensivists have attempted to suggest guidelines based on current available evidence. The BTF published the third edition of evidence-based guidelines in 2007.[19] Based on the strength of available evidence, levels of recommendations are classified as Level I, II, and III. Level I recommendations are based on the strongest evidence for effectiveness, and represent principles of patient management that reflect a high degree of clinical certainty. Level II recommendations reflect a moderate degree of clinical certainty. For Level III recommendations, the degree of clinical certainty is not established.[20] Guidelines for the management of pediatric TBI were published in 2003 as consensus statements by a varied group of surgical and pediatric societies. The recommendations are classed as Standards, Guidelines, and Options, based on degrees of certainty. Standards are accepted principles of patient management that reflect a high degree of clinical certainty; Guidelines are a particular strategy or range of management strategies that reflect a moderate clinical certainty. Options are the remaining strategies for patient management for which there is unclear clinical certainty.[21–23] **Table 1** presents an overview of the current recommendations for management of ICP in TBI.

General measures for patients with TBI in neurotrauma units

The general methods include airway control, breathing, circulation (ABC protocol), normovolemia, sedation, analgesia, posture, temperature, and seizure prophylaxis (**Table 2**). These measures ensure adequate control of ICP in addition to ensuring adequate cerebral perfusion pressure (CPP). Adequate ventilation must be maintained to keep the Sao_2 above 90%, and mean arterial pressure should be maintained above 90 mm Hg.[47] Normal saline or hypertonic saline (3%–7.5% NaCl) may be used to maintain volume status. Sedative and analgesic medications frequently aid maintenance of ICP by blunting the effects of nursing care. Although useful in the short term in the intensive care unit (ICU) for managing patients with TBI, the effects of propofol on long-term prognosis remain unknown.[48] Posture is maintained to ensure adequate CPP while reducing ICP. The head is kept straight to prevent venous kinking[49] and the head of bed is elevated to 30°. Keeping the head of bed flat has been

Table 1
Current state of evidence-based recommendations for the management of ICP in TBI

Topic	Consensus Group	Recommendation	Level of Recommendation
Indications for ICP monitoring	BTF[6]	ICP should be monitored in all salvageable patients with a severe TBI (GCS score of 3–8 after resuscitation) and an abnormal CT scan. An abnormal CT scan of the head is one that reveals hematomas, contusions, swelling, herniation, or compressed basal cisterns	Class II
		ICP monitoring is indicated in patients with severe TBI with a normal CT scan if 2 or more of the following features are noted at admission: age over 40 y, unilateral or bilateral motor posturing, or systolic blood pressure ≤90 mm Hg	Class III
	Pediatric[24]	ICP monitoring is appropriate in infants and children with severe TBI (GCS score ≤8)	Options
	EBIC[17]	None	N/A
ICP threshold	BTF[15]	Treatment should be initiated with ICP thresholds above 20 mm Hg	Level II
	Pediatric[18]	Treatment for intracranial hypertension, defined as a pathologic elevation in ICP, should begin at an ICP of 20 mm Hg	Options
	EBIC[17]	ICP elevations above 20–25 mm Hg should be treated	N/A
ICP monitoring technology	BTF[6]	The available technologies are ranked as follows: 1. Intraventricular devices: fluid-coupled catheter with an external strain gauge 2. Intraventricular devices: micro strain gauge or fiber-optic 3. Parenchymal pressure transducer devices 4. Subdural devices 5. Subarachnoid fluid-coupled devices 6. Epidural devices	
	Pediatric[25]	In pediatric patients who require ICP monitoring, a ventricular catheter or an external strain gauge transducer or catheter tip pressure transducer device is an accurate and reliable method of monitoring ICP. A ventriculostomy catheter device also enables therapeutic CSF drainage	Options
	EBIC[17]	None	N/A

(*continued on next page*)

Table 1
(*continued*)

Topic	Consensus Group	Recommendation	Level of Recommendation
Hyperosmolar therapy	BTF[26]	Mannitol is effective for control of raised ICP at doses of 0.25 g/kg to 1 g/kg body weight. Arterial hypotension (systolic blood pressure ≤90 mm Hg) should be avoided	Level II
		Restrict mannitol use before ICP monitoring to patients with signs of transtentorial herniation or progressive neurologic deterioration not attributable to extracranial causes	Level III
	Pediatric[27]	Hypertonic saline is effective for control of increased ICP after severe head injury. Effective doses as a continuous infusion of 3% saline range between 0.1 and 1.0 mL/kg of body weight per hour, administered on a sliding scale. The minimum dose needed to maintain ICP ≤ 20 mm Hg should be used. Mannitol is effective for control of increased ICP after severe TBI. Effective bolus doses range from 0.25 g/kg body weight to 1 g/kg body weight	Options
		Euvolemia should be maintained by fluid replacement. A Foley catheter is recommended in these patients to avoid bladder rupture	
		Serum osmolarity should be maintained below 320 mOsm/L with mannitol use, whereas a level of 360 mOsm/L appears to be tolerated with hypertonic saline, even when used in combination with mannitol	
		The choice of mannitol or hypertonic saline as a first-line hyperosmolar agent should be left to the treating physician	
	EBIC[17]	Preferably mannitol given repeatedly in bolus infusions, or as indicated by monitoring	N/A
		Serum osmolarity should be maintained at ≤315 mOsm/L	
		Other agents, such as glycerol or sorbitol, are not advocated	
		If osmotherapy has an insufficient effect, furosemide can be given additionally	

(*continued on next page*)

Table 1
(*continued*)

Topic	Consensus Group	Recommendation	Level of Recommendation
Hyperventilation	BTF[28]	Prophylactic hyperventilation ($Paco_2$ of 25 mm Hg or less) is not recommended	Level II
		Hyperventilation is recommended as a temporizing measure for the reduction of elevated ICP	Level III
		Hyperventilation should be avoided during the first 24 h after injury when CBF is often critically reduced	
		If hyperventilation is used, jugular venous oxygen saturation (Sjo_2) or brain tissue oxygen tension ($Pbro_2$) measurements are recommended to monitor oxygen delivery	
	Pediatric[29]	Mild or prophylactic hyperventilation ($Paco_2 \leq 35$ mm Hg) in children should be avoided	Options
		Mild hyperventilation ($Paco_2$ 30–35 mm Hg) may be considered for longer periods for intracranial hypertension refractory to sedation and analgesia, neuromuscular blockade, cerebrospinal fluid drainage, and hyperosmolar therapy	
		Aggressive hyperventilation ($Paco_2$ ≤ 30 mm Hg) may be considered as a second tier option in the setting of refractory hypertension. CBF, jugular venous oxygen saturation, or brain tissue oxygen monitoring is suggested to help identify cerebral ischemia in this setting	
		Aggressive hyperventilation therapy titrated to clinical effect may be necessary for brief periods in cases of cerebral herniation or acute neurologic deterioration	
	EBIC[17]	If other methods of ICP control fail, more intensive hyperventilation ($Paco_2 \leq 30$ mm Hg) may be used, preferably with monitoring of cerebral oxygenation to detect cerebral ischemia	N/A

(*continued on next page*)

Table 1
(*continued*)

Topic	Consensus Group	Recommendation	Level of Recommendation
Anesthetics, analgesics, and sedatives	BTF[30]	Prophylactic administration of barbiturates to induce burst-suppression EEG is not recommended High-dose barbiturate administration is recommended to control elevated ICP refractory to maximum standard medical and surgical treatment. Hemodynamic stability is essential before and during barbiturate therapy Propofol is recommended for the control of ICP, but not for improvement in mortality or 6-mo outcome. High-dose propofol can produce significant morbidity	Level II
	Pediatric[31–46]	High-dose barbiturate therapy may be considered in hemodynamically stable patients with salvageable severe head injury and refractory intracranial hypertension If high-dose barbiturate therapy is used to treat refractory intracranial hypertension, appropriate hemodynamic monitoring and cardiovascular support are essential	Options
	EBIC	Sedation and analgesia are accepted methods of management of ICP	N/A

Abbreviations: BTF, Brain Trauma Foundation; CBF, cerebral blood flow; CT, computed tomography; EBIC, European Brain Injury Consortium; EEG, electroencephalography; GCS, Glasgow Coma Scale; ICP, intracranial pressure; N/A, not available; TBI, traumatic brain injury.

shown to increase ICP, whereas a higher elevation may lead to a reduced CPP.[50] Seizures may occur in up to 17% of patients with TBI. The risk seems to increase with the severity of injury.[51] Seizures may increase the cerebral metabolic rate acutely and lead to raised ICP. However, the effect of seizures on long-term outcomes remains unclear.[52] The current guidelines suggest the use of anticonvulsants to prevent early seizures after TBI. The use of anticonvulsants may not improve either the rate of late seizures or neurologic outcomes.[53]

Specific measures for management of raised ICP

CSF drainage Ventriculostomies are frequently inserted in patients with TBI.[54] CSF drainage for ICP management is performed typically by releasing a few milliliters of CSF into the drainage bag. Immediate reduction in ICP is seen with drainage of fluid. Although CSF drainage decreases ICP in the short term, there is no improvement in cerebral circulation or oxygenation. The effect of CSF drainage on long-term outcomes remains unclear.[50]

Table 2
General measures of managing patients with severe TBI in neurotrauma units

General Measure	Intervention	Level of Evidence
Airway	Secure early in the following patients: GCS <9, signs of respiratory distress, declining O_2 saturation (<90%), increasing O_2 requirement (Fio_2 >50%), labored breathing Rising Pco_2 (>45 mm Hg) in patients without COPD Patient unable to clear out secretions due to respiratory/oropharyngeal weakness Patients with severe agitation requiring sedation that may compromise	N/A
Breathing	Maintain Pao_2 between 80 and 120 mm Hg, $Paco_2$ 35–40 mm Hg, Sao_2 >90%	Level II
Circulation	Maintain euvolemia with goal CVP >5 mm Hg 0.9% NaCl at 1–3 mL/kg/h maintenance fluid 0.9% NaCl 0.5–1.0 L IV bolus as needed Maintain MAP >70 mm Hg and/or SBP >90 mm Hg Phenylephrine infusion at 10–1000 μg/min Norepinephrine infusion at 2–100 μg/min Dopamine infusion at 10–1000 μg/min Epinephrine infusion at 1–12 μg/min	N/A
Posture	HOB elevation, keep head at 30° (except in large ischemic stroke) Keep neck straight to prevent venous kinking	N/A
Temperature	Keep temperature below 38°C Acetaminophen 650 mg PO/PR every 4 h Cooling blanket Surface cooling Endovascular cooling	N/A
Sedation and analgesia	Propofol IV drip at 0.1–5 mg/kg/h Fentanyl IV drip at 50–200 μg/h Morphine 2–4 mg IVP every 2–4 h as needed Ativan 1–2 mg IVP every 4–6 h as needed	Level II
Seizure prophylaxis	Phenytoin (or fosphenytoin) 1 g LD IV then 100 mg every 8 h for 7 d Levetiracetam 500 mg PO twice a day for 7 d	Level II

The goals of therapy include maintenance of adequate ICP and CPP. Levels of evidence as determined by the BTF recommendations.

Abbreviations: COPD, chronic obstructive pulmonary disease; CVP, central venous pressure; HOB, head of bed; IV, intravenous; IVP, intravenous perfusion; LD, loading dose; MAP, mean arterial pressure; N/A, not available; PO, by mouth; PR, per rectum; SBP, systolic blood pressure.

Data from Bratton SL, Chestnut RM, Ghajar J, et al. Guidelines for the management of severe traumatic brain injury. XI. Anesthetics, analgesics, and sedatives. J Neurotrauma 2007;24(Suppl 1):S71–6.

Pharmacologic therapy Hyperosmolar therapy remains the cornerstone for ICP management in modern neurotrauma units. Hyperosmolar therapy including mannitol and hypertonic saline are used in 73% to 83% of units taking care of patients with severe TBI.[54] The use of corticosteroids in acute TBI to control ICP is not recommended,[55] and this practice is falling out of favor.[54] Opioids, midazolam, and barbiturates have been used to control ICP. Bolus opioid infusions may actually result in raised ICP by raising cerebral blood flow (CBF). Although they are routinely used to maintain analgesia (fentanyl and remifentanyl), their use to control spikes in ICP is not recommended. Both midazolam and barbiturates have no effect on ICP. In addition, midazolam may decrease mean arterial pressure and CPP.[56]

Mannitol Mannitol is an isomer of sorbitol. Although it is commonly thought that mannitol acts by drawing excess fluid from the cranial cavity, the precise mechanism of action is unknown.[56] The immediate reduction in ICP probably results from a reduction of blood viscosity and plasma expansion. The effect lasts for 3 to 4 hours. It is typically administered in doses ranging from 0.25 to 1 mg/kg,[26,57] though there might be some support for using higher doses.[56] Monitoring of serum osmolarity is recommended when administering mannitol. The effectiveness of mannitol in reducing ICP is related to the osmolarity. In addition, serum osmolarity greater than 320 mOsm may predispose to renal failure.[58]

Hypertonic saline Hypertonic saline (3%–7.5% NaCl solution) is being increasingly used in neurotrauma units for the management if ICP. In addition to a reduction in ICP, hypertonic saline also expands the intravascular volume, increases cardiac output, improves CPP, and improves absorption of CSF.[59] The mechanism of action for hypertonic saline is likely attributable to a hyperosmolar effect. Hypertonic saline may have advantages over mannitol when used in severe TBI. Unlike mannitol, repeated administration does not diminish the ICP-lowering effect, and does not cause a rebound increase in ICP. It may also be used during intractable ICHTN unresponsive to mannitol and barbiturates.[60] There is strong evidence that hypertonic saline is superior to mannitol in its ability to lower ICP.[56] Hypertonic saline may be used as a continuous infusion of 3% solution or in bolus doses of 7.5% to 23.5% solution. Continuous infusions are typically given at a rate of 0.1 to 1.0 mL/kg/h.

Barbiturates Barbiturates induce a suppression of cerebral metabolic rate. In patients with an intact flow-metabolism coupling, a reduction in the metabolic rate leads to a reduction in blood flow and consequently reduced ICP.[59] In addition, barbiturates offer protection during episodes of cerebral hypoxia.[61] Barbiturates are used less frequently for ICP control than other modalities,[54] partly because of the conflicting evidence regarding the effect of barbiturates in improving outcomes in TBI.[56] Systemic hypotension is a constant companion to barbiturate use, and these agents may also cause cardiac depression, sepsis, electrolyte abnormalities, and renal dysfunction.[59] At present, barbiturate therapy for management of ICP is recommended for refractory ICHTN only. Attention must be given to prevent hemodynamic instability.[30,56,62] When used in clinical situations, pentobarbital is given as an infusion at the rate of 1 to 8 mg/kg/h with loading doses of 1 to 5 mg every 15 minutes to achieve acute control of ICP. Alternatively, thiopental may be used at the rate of 1 to 6 mg/kg/h with bolus doses of 300 to 400 mg every 30 minutes (total 4 g over 1–5 hours).[59] There is no difference between these agents when used to control ICP.[56]

Chemical paralysis In ICHTN due to agitation, posturing, or coughing, nondepolarizing muscle paralytics may reduce ICP acutely. Paralytics are used along with sedatives and analgesics in ventilated patients.[63] With the use of paralytics neurologic status cannot be easily assessed, and necessitates withholding paralytics daily for assessment. Routine paralytic use in all patients with TBI is not recommended, due to increased incidence of extracranial adverse effects such as pneumonia and sepsis. The use of paralytics has also been associated with an increased length of stay in the ICU and an increased incidence of critical illness myopathy.[64,65]

Hyperventilation Hyperventilation induces hypocapnia, leading to cerebral vasoconstriction. The subsequent reduction in CBV causes a reduction in ICP. An increased oxygen extraction compensates for a reduction in flow, thereby preserving normal metabolic processes to continue.[50] Aggressive hyperventilation to reduce $Paco_2$ to less than 25 mm Hg had been the cornerstone of ICP management for more than 2 decades. However, recent studies have questioned the use of chronic hyperventilation. Evidence for inadequate increase in oxygen extraction[66] may mean that hyperventilation may predispose to cerebral ischemia.[28,67] This finding has been confirmed in metabolic imaging of patients undergoing hyperventilation. Despite improvements in ICP and CPP, larger volumes of severely hypoperfused regions have been observed with hyperventilation.[68] Chronic hyperventilation leads to significantly worse outcomes, although some of this effect may be attenuated with the use of tromethamine (THAM) intravenously (dose: THAM [ml] = body weight [kg] × base deficit).[69] At present, hyperventilation is only recommended as a temporizing measure for the reduction of ICP with measurements of jugular venous oxygen saturation (Sjo_2) or brain tissue oxygen tension ($Pbro_2$) measurements to monitor oxygen delivery. In addition, hyperventilation is avoided during the first 24 hours after injury when CBF is often critically reduced.[28]

Hypothermia Induced hypothermia reduces ICP by a reduction in the cerebral metabolic rate. In addition to a reduction of CBF, hypothermia may reduce inflammatory responses as well as glutamate and free radicals. Prolonged hypothermia may be associated with adverse effects including arrhythmias, coagulopathies, sepsis, and pneumonia.[50,59] Methods of hypothermic intervention include systemic hypothermia or selective hypothermia. Systemic hypothermia is achieved by surface cooling,[70] by endovascular catheters,[71] and occasionally by gastric lavage.[72] Alternatively, selective hypothermia is achieved by using a cooling cap or band.[73] The target temperatures may range from mild (34°–36°C) to moderate (32°–34°C) hypothermia. It is suggested that hypothermia may have higher chances of reducing mortality when cooling is maintained for more than 48 hours.[74] Hypothermia is maintained for 24 to 72 hours or longer depending on ICP response. Slow, controlled rewarming over 24 hours is critical, because of the development of rebound cerebral edema, hypotension, and electrolyte abnormalities. The current recommendations recognize that prophylactic hypothermia is not significantly associated with decreased mortality. It is noted that preliminary findings suggest a greater decrease in mortality risk is observed when target temperatures are maintained for more than 48 hours. Prophylactic hypothermia has also been associated with significantly higher Glasgow Outcome Scale scores when compared with scores for normothermic controls.[74]

Surgical therapies In cases of intractable ICHTN, removal of a section of skull is a drastic measure undertaken to control ICP.[75] Decompressive craniectomy involves removing a large portion of skull in the absence of a large mass-occupying lesion such as subdural hematoma, epidural hematoma, or cerebral contusion. Decompression results in an immediate drop in ICP, but is only performed after all other measures have been exhausted.[50] Recently there has been an increased interest in assessing the outcomes following decompressive craniectomy for intractable ICHTN. When compared with early, prophylactic surgery, improved outcomes were observed when decompression was performed in response to intractable ICHTN.[76] The timing for performing decompression is critical. The emphasis is on performing the decompression before irreversible ischemic damage occurs.[77] Although the immediate goal of reducing ICP is met in most patients (85%),[75] the effect on outcomes remains to be clarified.[50] Due to the surgical, drastic nature of the procedure, there is a paucity of randomized controlled trial (RCT) data regarding efficacy and safety. The two published randomized studies report on the importance of timing (early) and size (larger) of decompressive craniectomy in patients with severe TBI.[78,79] At present, there is strong evidence that decompressive craniectomy reduces elevated ICP immediately after surgery but does not improve long-term outcomes in children. There is also moderate evidence, based on one RCT, that a larger bone flap results in greater reduction of ICP, with limited evidence that patients with a GCS less than 6 show no improvement. There was conflicting evidence as to whether a decompressive craniectomy affects long-term outcomes.[50,78,79]

CEREBROVASCULAR TRAUMA

Traumatic injury to the intracranial or extracranial vasculature is rare and can be life threatening. Vascular trauma can be caused by either blunt or penetrating injuries. The incidence of cerebrovascular trauma has been reported as between 0.1% and 1.55%.[75–79] The cervical carotid artery is more frequently involved then the vertebral artery.[77,79,80] Blunt trauma is more common than penetrating injuries, and motor vehicle accidents remain the most common cause of blunt trauma, accounting for 40% to 70% of cases.[75] Mortality for blunt carotid trauma has been reported as between 20% and 40%.[81] Cerebrovascular injury can range from a simple intimal tear to a complete transaction of the vessel. Both arterial and venous sides of the vasculature can be affected. On the arterial side, dissections, traumatic aneurysms, or arteriovenous fistulae may develop. On the venous side, one may encounter a dural sinus tear or venous thrombosis.[82]

Traumatic Dissection

An arterial dissection begins with a small intimal tear, allowing blood to enter the wall of the artery, splitting its layers, and resulting in a stenosis, irregularity of the wall or, occasionally, an aneurysmal dilatation.[82,83] Dissections occur in approximately 1% of all patients with blunt force trauma.[84] Intracranial dissections are rare; if present, they involve the supraclinoid segment of the internal carotid artery (ICA).[82] Extracranial dissections are the most common, and carotid involvement is twice as likely to occur than vertebral artery involvement.[79] Carotid injury is usually associated with TBI and/or basal skull fractures, whereas vertebral dissections are associated with cervical spine fractures.[85] There are several other risk factors and accompanying physical findings that may be present in traumatic dissections.[86] Screening protocols have been developed to identify patients at risk (**Box 1**).[75,80] The use of screening protocols combined with imaging studies has led to an increase in the identification of these lesions. Contrast-enhanced CT and magnetic resonance (MR) imaging might demonstrate an intramural thrombus, narrowing of the arterial lumen, and/or an intimal flap, pointing to the presence of a true and false lumen; there may also be parenchymal cerebral or cerebellar changes.[78,87] Angiographically, dissections present with an irregular lumen with stenosis or occlusion, intimal flaps, tapering of the lumen of the ICA or slow flow from the ICA to the middle cerebral artery.[88,89] The degree of luminal compromise can range from a mild irregularity to a complete occlusion. At the carotid level, dissections usually spare the bulb, differentiating this from atherosclerotic disease (**Fig. 2**).[88] Carotid dissections usually occur at the cervical and petrous segments whereas vertebral dissections occur at the V3 segment, where the vertebral artery enters the foramen magnum and is not protected by bony foramina.[90,91]

Box 1
Screening protocols for blunt cerebrovascular trauma

Denver Criteria

Cervical spine fracture

Unexplained neurologic deficit

Skull base fracture into carotid canal

LeFort II or III fracture

Expanding cervical hematoma

Cervical bruit

Ischemic stroke on secondary CT scan

Head trauma with GCS <6

Near hanging with anoxic injury

Memphis Criteria

Cervical spine fracture

Unexplained neurologic deficit

Skull base fracture into carotid canal

LeFort II or III fracture

Horner syndrome

Neck soft-tissue injury

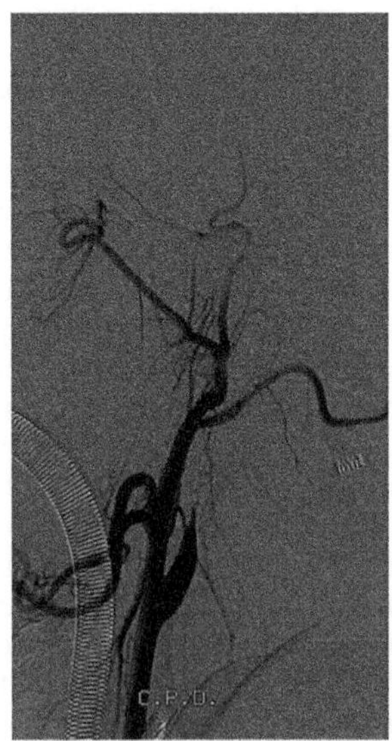

Fig. 2. Cervical carotid dissection. Digital subtraction angiography showing tapering of the proximal third of the right internal carotid artery with complete occlusion above the carotid bulb.

Management is primarily aimed at preventing thromboembolic complications and maintaining patency of the involved artery.[92,93] Whereas 85% of spontaneous dissections improve or resolve on follow-up studies, only 55% of trauma-related dissections improve and 25% will progress to complete occlusion.[94] The data on the management for blunt cerebrovascular trauma are limited. Most investigators agree that some form of antithrombotic treatment is appropriate. Intravenous heparin is the most widely reported regimen, with complication rates ranging from 8% to 16%[77,80,95–97] and 30% to 36% in patients who harbor some kind of contraindication for anticoagulant therapy.[98,99] Recent recommendations describe a target partial thromboplastin time of 40 to 50 seconds.[80,100]

Antiplatelet therapy (single or dual with clopidogrel) is an alternative that may avoid the risks associated with systemic heparinization.[96,99,101,102] Several studies have reported similar or better neurologic outcomes in comparison with heparin.[98,99,101] At present, endovascular or surgical interventions are reserved for patients who have resilient or recurrent symptoms despite medical management. Endovascular interventions are the nonmedical treatment of choice, and options include stenting, with balloon or self-expandable stents, and/or intra-arterial thrombolysis for acute strokes.

Traumatic Aneurysms

Traumatic aneurysms are rare lesions caused by dissection or rupture of the arterial wall as a result of blunt or penetrating trauma. Wall damage forms a contained hematoma or “pseudoaneurysm.” These lesions account for fewer than 1% of all intracranial aneurysms in adults, but their proportion increases in children to about 20%.[103,104] Intracranial traumatic aneurysms can be located at the skull base (petrous, cavernous, supraclinoid segments), subcortical (close to falx or tentorium), or be distally associated with skull fractures or hematomas.[82,97] The most common site involved is the cavernous segment of the ICA, which is associated with base-of-the-skull fractures. Extracranial traumatic aneurysms also occur secondary to blunt, penetrating, or iatrogenic trauma.[105] Blunt trauma is commonly caused by rotatory hyperextension, strangulation, or fracture of the mandible. Penetrating trauma–related aneurysms are more common, and result from stabbing or gunshot wounds.[106]

Traumatic intracranial aneurysms may present symptoms acutely or in a delayed fashion, even weeks after the event.[107,108] These lesions often present with intracranial hemorrhage (intraparenchymal, subdural, intraventricular, or subarachnoid), with some cases causing life-threatening epistaxis due to bleeding of the ICA into the sphenoid sinus.[107,109–111]

Diagnosis of traumatic aneurysms relies on a high level of clinical suspicion. A trauma patient who presents with delayed or unexplained neurologic deterioration, unusual location of cerebral hemorrhage, and/or large epistaxis warrants further investigation. Although CT angiography is a valid imaging study, further angiographic investigation is still necessary.[112,113] The presence of a skull-base fracture involving the carotid canal also should raise suspicion for a traumatic pseudoaneurysm.[114] Time between trauma and the rupture of the aneurysm can range from days to months; half of the cases present with rupture within 3 weeks.[115–117] Certain angiographic features can point to the traumatic origin of an aneurysm, delayed filling and emptying of the aneurysm, location (peripheral and away from branching points), irregular contour, absence of a neck, and/or the history of the patient (**Fig. 3**).[82,118]

Treatment is recommended in all traumatic intracranial aneurysms because mortality rates range between 34% and 54%.[86,115–117,119–122] Treatment strategy should consider that this “aneurysm” is an extravascular pouch and that the walls are made by thrombus and not arterial wall layers, making it more fragile.[82,123–125]

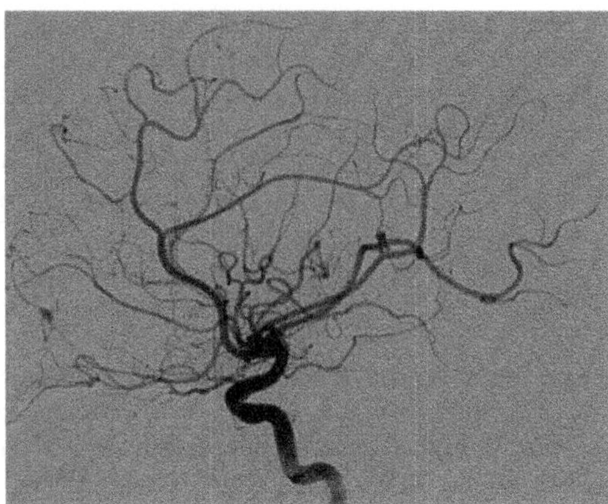

Fig. 3. Traumatic pseudoaneurysm. Lateral digital subtraction angiography showing a distal frontal pseudoaneurysm of the anterior cerebral artery. The aneurysm is distally located, irregular in shape, and away from branching points in a patient with history of head trauma.

The goal of treatment should be immediate proximal occlusion of the parent artery by embolization (coils, balloons, glue) or surgical vessel occlusion.[82,86,126] Endovascular occlusion of the parent vessel, selective embolization of the aneurysm, and stent placement have shown favorable results in the treatment of traumatic aneurysms.[104,105,123,127–129]

Traumatic Arteriovenous Fistulae

An arteriovenous fistula (AVF) is an abnormal communication between an artery and a vein, and tends to occur where these two structures are in close proximity. Direct carotid cavernous fistulae (CCF) are the most common traumatic AVF, and are usually secondary to a skull-base fracture; however, iatrogenic AVF after transsphenoid surgery might also be encountered.[77,82,86] The fistula develops when the ICA and/or its meningeal branches tear within the cavernous sinus, producing a direct communication with the cavernous sinus.[130]

Clinical findings include objective vascular bruit, pulsating exophthalmos, chemosis, and ophthalmoplegia.[131] Loss of vision may occur, secondary to increased intraocular pressure related to venous congestion.[132]

Imaging should include a high-resolution CT scan to assess for fractures. Approximately 75% of all patients have a skull-base fracture associated with CCF, and the incidence of a CCF in a patient with a sphenoid bone fracture is around 3% to 5%.[133–136] CT angiography or MR angiography usually can confirm the diagnosis; findings include enlargement and early enhancement of the cavernous sinus and superior ophthalmic vein. Angiography is necessary to accurately define the location of the defect and to look for high-risk features such as retrograde cortical venous drainage, which entails a high risk for hemorrhage and warrants early treatment.[82,104,137] Endovascular management is the treatment of choice; intervention can be performed using coils and/or liquid embolic material, covered stent repair, or ICA occlusion (**Fig. 4**).[104,105,124,138–141]

Traumatic Venous Lesions

Traumatic venous lesions are often overlooked, and might be more frequent than is reported.[8] Venous thrombosis may develop following penetrating or blunt trauma

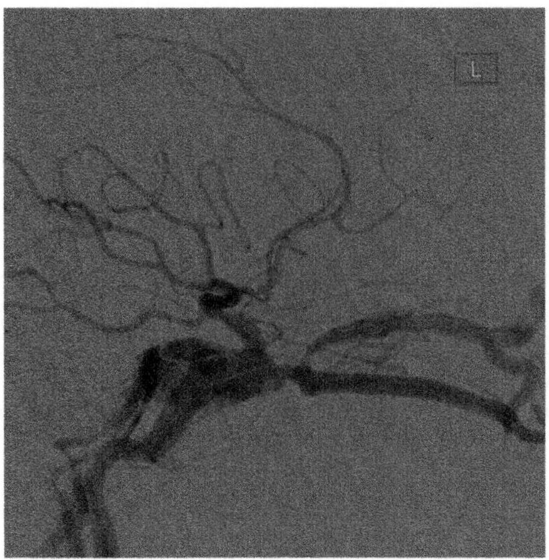

Fig. 4. Direct carotid cavernous fistula. Lateral digital subtraction angiography of the left internal carotid artery showing a direct communication with the cavernous sinus with venous drainage to the superior and inferior ophthalmic veins and inferior petrosal sinus. The patient had a history of base skull fracture after a motor vehicle accident.

due to tear or laceration of dural sinuses, fractures, extrinsic compression, or increased pressure.[139,142–144] An acute blood clot or thrombus might extend, leading to venous hypertension and increased ICP.[145] The clinical presentation is variable but often includes headaches, seizures, visual disturbances, and/or papilledema, among others.[145] Clinical presentation is closely related to location and extent of the cerebral venous thrombosis (CVT). If CVT is suspected clinically, imaging is needed for confirmation.[146] Acute thrombosis within the dural sinuses can be identified as a high-attenuation lesion on nonenhanced CT. If thrombosis of the superior sagittal sinus occurs, a triangular filling defect (empty delta sign) can be seen on postcontrast images. MR imaging is the modality of choice for CVT; it may be difficult to recognize an acute thrombus on conventional sequences, and early changes, such as edema and gyral swelling, are subtle.[146] Stroke lesions that do not correspond to an arterial territory suggest CVT; hemorrhage often is an accompanying factor.[82,146,147] On angiography there may be a delayed transit time, filling of collateral veins, or nonvisualization of the affected structure.[82,137]

Treatment is aimed at avoiding the progression of the thrombosis. Intravenous heparin is considered standard therapy.[148,149] Patients who present with rapidly progressive thrombosis should be considered for endovascular management. Direct thrombolytic infusion by a percutaneous or retrograde venous approach is feasible, with the potential benefit of avoiding systemic hemorrhagic effects caused by intravenous heparinization.[150–154]

NEUROSURGICAL TRAUMA IN CHILDREN

Trauma is the leading cause of death in children 18 years and younger. The major determinant of morbidity and mortality in pediatric trauma is TBI. TBI is broadly defined as an alteration of brain function caused by an external force. It can range from mild or concussive to severe or comatose. There are approximately half a million emergency department visits for TBI in children of age 0 to 14 years each year (**Table 3**).

Table 3
Estimated average annual numbers of TBI-related emergency department visits, hospitalizations, and deaths by age group, United States, 2002 to 2006

Age Group	Emergency Department Visits	Hospitalizations	Deaths	Total
Children (0–14 years)	473,947	35,136	2174	511,527
Older adults (≥65 years)	141,998	81,499	14,347	237,844

The estimated average annual number of TBIs that occur among children aged 0 to 14 years is 511,257. By contrast, the number of TBIs in adults aged 65 years and older is 237,844. TBI-related emergency department visits accounted for a larger proportion in children (92.7%) than in older adults (59.7%).

Data from Eisenberg HM, Frankowski RF, Contant CF, et al. High-dose barbiturate control of elevated intracranial pressure in patients with severe head injury. J Neurosurg 1988;69(1):15–23.

Falls are the major external force causing TBI in children, especially those aged 0 to 4 years, followed by events in which a child is struck by or against an object, including collision with a moving or stationary object (**Fig. 5**). TBI is often referred to as a "silent epidemic" because complications, such as memory and learning difficulties, that result from TBI are not always immediately apparent.[155] This section discusses the diagnosis and management of the most common neurosurgical injuries that can occur as a result of the primary impact in TBI.

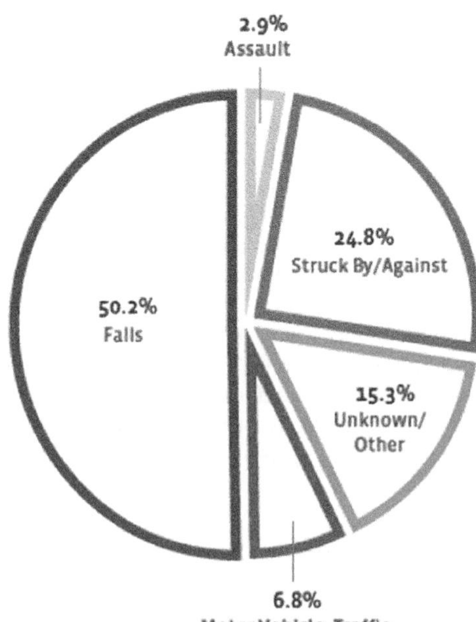

Fig. 5. Estimated average percentage of annual traumatic brain injury-combined emergency department visits, hospitalizations, and deaths among children 0 to 14 years, by external cause, United States, 2002 to 2006.

Skull Fractures

Skull fractures (**Fig. 6**) can occur in up to 20% of children with head injuries, yet the majority will not require any intervention. However, the presence of a fracture on imaging studies should raise concern of an underlying brain injury; therefore a CT scan is the best tool for initial diagnosis and management. Plain skull radiographs, while very good for diagnosing fractures, are unable to show underlying brain injury or hemorrhage that may need immediate attention. Most fractures in children are closed, simple, linear fractures involving the parietal bone that will heal without intervention. Approximately 25% of skull fractures will be depressed because of a focal impact on the skull.[156,157] These fractures most commonly involve the parietal bone and will be greenstick fractures, whereby the bone is connected but fixed in a new depressed position. Examination will reveal subgaleal swelling and tenderness. In infants and young children a fracture line may be palpable, and in depressed fractures a small dent may be felt. Treatment of depressed greenstick skull fractures in infants remains somewhat controversial. Without intervention, many of these fractures will elevate over time, due to rapid intracranial and skull growth. However, if the depression is large or if it does not improve with observation, surgical elevation of the fracture should be performed. In older children and adolescents, depressed fractures should be elevated surgically if the fragment is depressed 1 cm or more from the skull.[158,159]

Growing Skull Fractures (Leptomeningeal Cyst)

With complex, comminuted skull fractures, laceration of the dura with or without underlying injury to the cortex can occur. When dural lacerations occur with these complex fractures, a child can be at risk for the development of a growing skull fracture (**Fig. 7**). The pathogenesis of the growing fracture is from CSF pulsations through the lacerated dura causing herniation of the cerebral cortex into the epidural space.[160] This process causes the fracture sites to push apart, often with resorption of the fractured bone. Such a situation most frequently occurs in children younger than 2 years, in whom brain growth is extremely rapid. Children will present with pulsatile masses or fluid collections at the site of the fracture, and CT scan will demonstrate herniation of cerebral tissue with increased separation of the fractured bone. All will require surgical repair of the lacerated dura with plating of the fracture site.

Intracranial Hemorrhage

Intracranial hemorrhage can be classified as extra-axial or intra-axial. Extra-axial hemorrhages are located beneath the skull but outside of the cerebral cortex, whereas

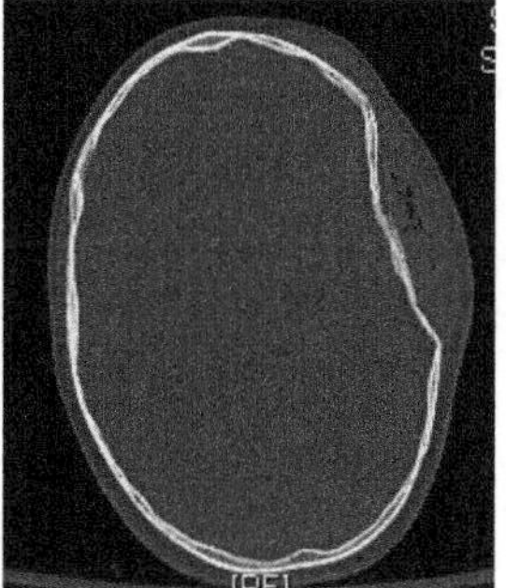

Fig. 6. Noncontrast computed tomography (CT) scan of bone window, showing left frontotemporal depressed skull fracture.

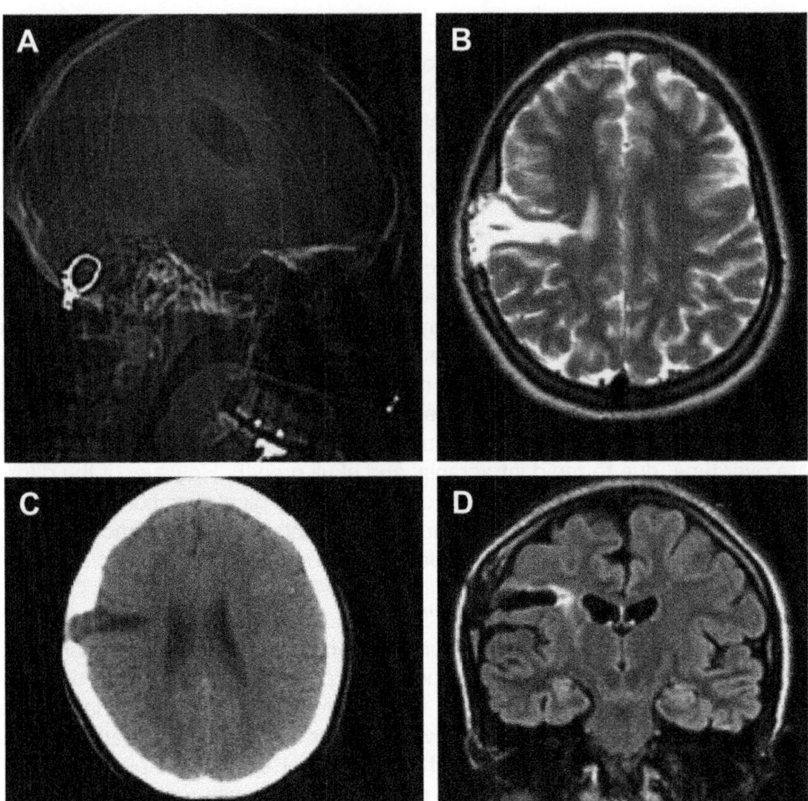

Fig. 7. CT of the brain revealed a skull defect on the localizing sagittal image (*A*), with axial views demonstrating underlying gliosis and demarcated volume loss within the lateral right sensorimotor cortex (*B*). The cerebral volume loss and bony defect are striking on the subsequent axial T2-weighted (*C*) and coronal fluid-attenuated inversion recovery (*D*) magnetic resonance imaging sequences.

intra-axial hemorrhages are within the cerebral cortex. All present with similar signs and symptoms such as headache, nausea, vomiting, hemiplegia or hemiparesis, and altered mental status, indicating raised ICP. CT scan is the best and quickest imaging study to assess for these injuries in the acute trauma setting.

Epidural Hematoma

Epidural hematomas are hemorrhages located between the skull and the dura (**Fig. 8**). These hematomas are most frequently located in the supratentorial region, usually in the temporal area. Most often these hemorrhages occur from rupture and bleeding of the middle meningeal artery, which runs just under the temporal bone in the area of the pterion. Frequently the patient will have a lucid interval after the initial injury, followed by a quick decline in his or her neurologic examination. Almost all patients will require emergent surgical evacuation because these hematomas can rapidly expand, causing mass effect and possible cerebral herniation.

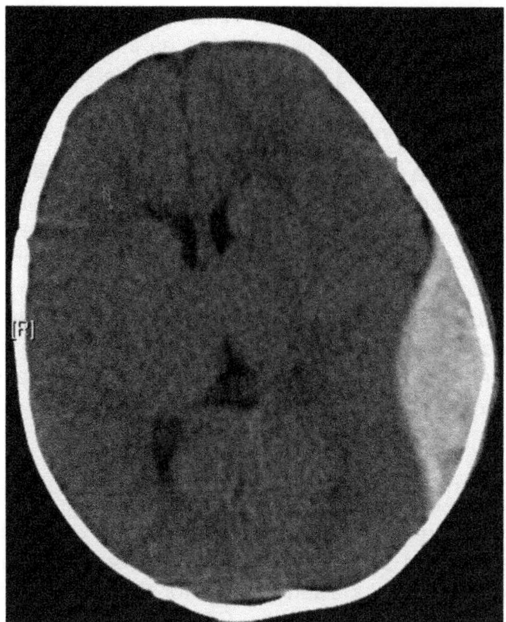

Fig. 8. Non contrast CT scan showing left-sided epidural hematoma.

Subdural Hematoma

A subdural hematoma is a hemorrhage that occurs between the dura and the pial surface of the brain (**Fig. 9**). It is often a result of tearing of bridging veins on the surface of the cortex that drain to a venous sinus. Often these patients have more severe brain

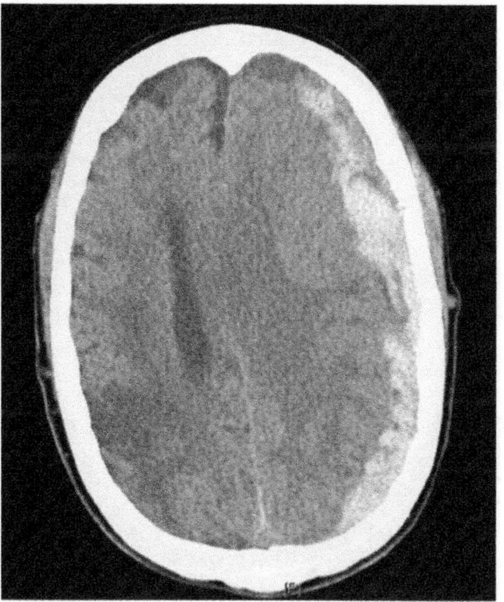

Fig. 9. Noncontrast CT scan showing large left-sided subdural hematoma with mass effect and midline shift.

injury and are comatose shortly after the initial injury. Surgical management with urgent evacuation of the clot is usually required, as these hemorrhages can cause significant mass effect and midline shift, with possible cerebral herniation.

Intracerebral Hemorrhage (Cerebral Contusions)

These contusions are areas of bleeding within the cortex itself (**Fig. 10**). Such hemorrhages are relatively uncommon in infants after trauma. Older children develop cerebral contusions most often from acceleration/deceleration injuries, most commonly in the frontal and temporal lobes. Cerebral contusions can be observed and conservatively managed if they remain small; this requires serial imaging and neurologic examination to monitor the patient. Some contusions will blossom over the first 24 to 48 hours after the initial injury. If a cerebral contusion becomes large and/or exhibits significant mass effect on the surrounding brain and is easily accessible, surgical evacuation of the intracerebral hemorrhage may be necessary.

Diffuse Axonal Injury

Diffuse axonal injury (DAI) is a shearing injury to the axons located in the deep white matter, arising from severe deceleration injuries. Children with DAI are unconscious on arrival at the hospital, and CT does not show any evidence of significant intracranial pathology. Other symptoms include abnormal motor signs, even decorticate or decerebrate posturing, and papillary dysfunction. CT scans do not readily show DAI, and MR imaging is much more sensitive. MR imaging will reveal multifocal hyperintense foci at the gray-white interfaces, corpus callosum, and brainstem on T2-weighted images.[161] Treatment involves ICP monitoring and clinical examination, although most DAI patients will have normal ICP. Recovery from DAI is variable among patients, and can take weeks to months. Factors associated with a poor outcome in DAI are bilateral unreactive pupils, multiple corpus callosum or brainstem lesions, and older age.[162]

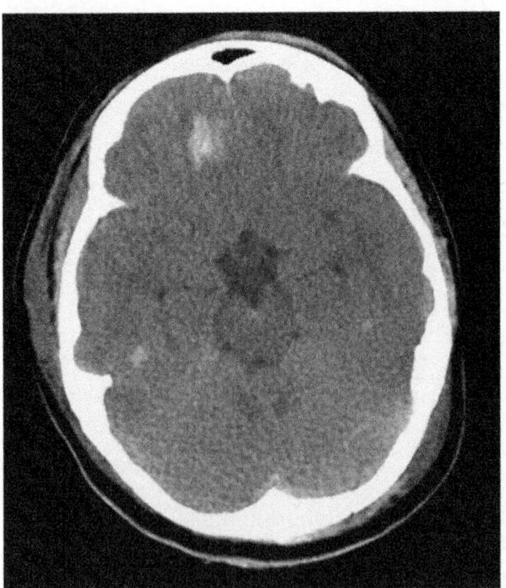

Fig. 10. Noncontrast CT scan showing right frontal intracerebral hemorrhage and punctate bilateral temporal lobe hemorrhages.

Spinal Cord Injury Without Radiographic Abnormality

Spinal cord injury without radiographic abnormality (SCIWORA) is a common and difficult problem attributable to lack of radiographic abnormalities. It has a wide range of incidence, 5% to 70%, most likely due to a varied clinical awareness of the syndrome.[163] Patients with true SCIWORA have spinal cord injury and have a detailed radiologic evaluation, including plain radiographs, flexion/extension views, CT and MR studies, which do not show any structural cause for the spinal cord injury. SCIWORA accounts for up to two-thirds of severe cervical injuries in children younger than 8 years, and is most common in the upper cervical and thoracic regions of the spinal cord.[164] The elasticity of the pediatric spine allows for a transient subluxation at the time of injury and elastic recoil to a normal alignment at presentation. Children with this injury may have a fracture through the cartilaginous endplates, which cannot be visualized on plain films or an unrecognized interspinous ligamentous injury. Flexion/extension views in an awake patient may demonstrate these underlying injuries. Most patients will present acutely with a complete cord injury, but some patients may present in a delayed fashion up to 4 days after the initial injury.[164] Treatment of SCIWORA includes spinal immobilization, usually a cervical collar, for 3 months.[165] Before immobilization is discontinued, dynamic films, namely flexion/extension radiographs, should be obtained to confirm spinal stability. Neurologic outcome is based on the presence and degree of spinal cord signal changes at the time of injury.[156,157,164,166] Those patients with no evidence of cord signal changes have an excellent chance for full neurologic recovery. Patients with signal changes consistent with edema or microhemorrhages are associated with significant improvement of function with time. Cord disruption or frank hematomyelia is most often associated with severe neurologic injury and poor chance of recovery of function.[156,157]

SPINAL CORD INJURY

Acute traumatic spinal cord injury (SCI) remains one of the most devastating events that can occur in an individual. Not only is SCI associated with the obvious harsh physical setbacks of the injury itself, but also permanently affects the individual's social, economic, and psychological realms. According to the National Spinal Cord Injury Statistical Center in Birmingham, Alabama, it is estimated that the annual incidence of SCI, not including those who die at the scene of the accident, is approximately 40 cases per million population in the United Sates (or approximately 12,000 new cases each year). Since 2005, motor vehicle crashes have accounted for approximately 42% of reported SCI cases (**Fig. 11**).

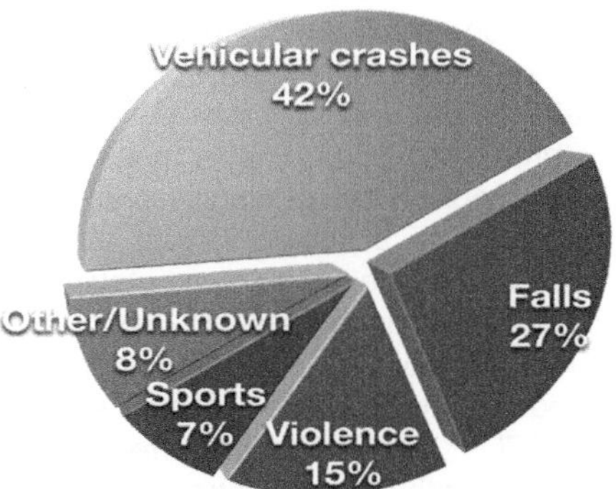

Fig. 11. Causes of spinal cord injury in the United States.

The average age at the time of injury is 39.5 years, and about 77.8% of these injuries occur in males. Incomplete tetraplegia is the most common type of SCI, followed in frequency by complete paraplegia, complete tetraplegia, and incomplete paraplegia. In economic terms the lifetime costs incurred by an individual with SCI range from $500,000 to $3 million, depending on the extent of the injury and the age of the injured patient (not including the loss of wages and so forth). In total, about $4 billion is spent annually on the acute treatment and chronic care of SCI-injured individuals.[167]

Diagnosis of SCI

The diagnosis of SCI is usually not established until the patient is transferred to the emergency department and is evaluated by a physician. Secondary to this, all patients who are victims of a significant trauma, trauma patients with loss of consciousness, and minor trauma victims with complaints referable to the spine or spinal cord should be treated as having an SCI by the field team until proved otherwise. Other clues that might point toward SCI are the presence of abdominal breathing, inability to move any one limb, numbness or tingling in any dermatomal distribution, or the occurrence of priapism. Management on the field should include, in addition to the mandatory ABCs, immobilization before extrication to prevent any active or passive movements of the spine, maintenance of blood pressure, maintenance of oxygenation, and caution with intubation with uncleared cervical spines.[168]

Once in the emergency department, the initial evaluation and stabilization should take place by the trauma team in the original restraints from the field. When the patient is deemed stable, transfer to the CT scanner for further imaging should take place, still in the original restraints from the field.

The patient should then be examined and the images should be evaluated. The American Spinal Cord Injury Association has defined a grading system for SCI based on neurologic function. The injury, regardless of its etiology, is always classified in terms that describe the retained neurologic function of the injured patient. The classification's nomenclature spans the letters A through E (**Fig. 12**).

Pathophysiology of SCI

There are two known phases of SCI pathophysiology: primary and secondary. The initial traumatic event that physically disrupts the anatomic structures involved in the injury accounts for the primary phase of the insult. The most common form of acute SCI is a compressive-contusive type injury, whereby the displaced elements of the supporting vertebral structures exert force on the neural elements causing the immediate injury, and often sustained compression. The subsequent events that rapidly follow this mechanical disruption include phenomena such as cellular edema, vascular dysfunction, ischemia, excitotoxicity, inflammation, and cell death, and encompass the secondary phase (**Table 4**). As data on these mechanisms continue to amass, our understanding of the processes influencing secondary injury increases, and this has led to the adoption of neuroprotective strategies in an attempt to attenuate these noxious effects. For example, the acknowledgment that ongoing ischemia may worsen secondary damage has led to the implementation of clinical guidelines to promote spinal cord perfusion and aggressively avoid hypotension through an elevated mean arterial pressure. However, few of these research efforts have been able to drive a pharmacologic agent from the preclinical stages into clinically relevant remedies for patients with SCI.[169] All of the drugs currently in use have failed to show substantive benefit, with only methylprednisolone showing modest success in the 1990 landmark study.[170] Nevertheless, the risk for complications related to its use

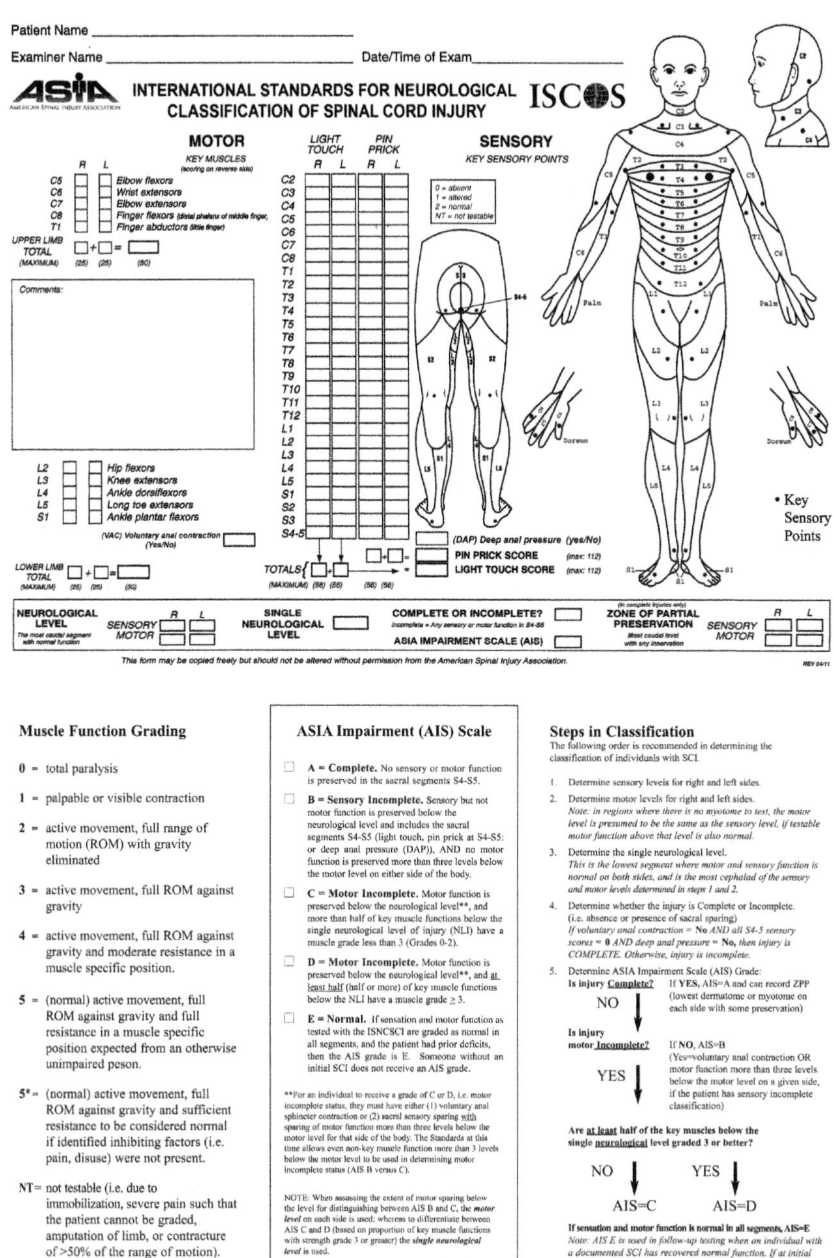

Patient Name ______________________

Examiner Name ______________________ Date/Time of Exam ______________________

ASIA — AMERICAN SPINAL INJURY ASSOCIATION

INTERNATIONAL STANDARDS FOR NEUROLOGICAL CLASSIFICATION OF SPINAL CORD INJURY

ISCOS

MOTOR

KEY MUSCLES (scoring on reverse side)

	R	L	
C5			Elbow flexors
C6			Wrist extensors
C7			Elbow extensors
C8			Finger flexors (distal phalanx of middle finger)
T1			Finger abductors (little finger)

UPPER LIMB TOTAL (MAXIMUM) ☐+☐=☐ (25) (25) (50)

Comments:

	R	L	
L2			Hip flexors
L3			Knee extensors
L4			Ankle dorsiflexors
L5			Long toe extensors
S1			Ankle plantar flexors

(VAC) Voluntary anal contraction (Yes/No) ☐

LOWER LIMB TOTAL (MAXIMUM) ☐+☐=☐ (25) (25) (50)

SENSORY

KEY SENSORY POINTS

LIGHT TOUCH R L — PIN PRICK R L

C2, C3, C4, C5, C6, C7, C8, T1, T2, T3, T4, T5, T6, T7, T8, T9, T10, T11, T12, L1, L2, L3, L4, L5, S1, S2, S3, S4-5

0 = absent
1 = altered
2 = normal
NT = not testable

TOTALS{☐+☐ ☐+☐ (MAXIMUM) (56) (56) (56) (56)

(DAP) Deep anal pressure (Yes/No) ☐

PIN PRICK SCORE (max: 112) ☐

LIGHT TOUCH SCORE (max: 112) ☐

NEUROLOGICAL LEVEL (The most caudal segment with normal function) — SENSORY R ☐ L ☐; MOTOR R ☐ L ☐

SINGLE NEUROLOGICAL LEVEL ☐

COMPLETE OR INCOMPLETE? ☐ (Incomplete = Any sensory or motor function in S4-S5)

ASIA IMPAIRMENT SCALE (AIS) ☐

ZONE OF PARTIAL PRESERVATION (In complete injuries only) (Most caudal level with any innervation) — SENSORY R ☐ L ☐; MOTOR R ☐ L ☐

This form may be copied freely but should not be altered without permission from the American Spinal Injury Association.

REV 04/11

Muscle Function Grading

0 = total paralysis

1 = palpable or visible contraction

2 = active movement, full range of motion (ROM) with gravity eliminated

3 = active movement, full ROM against gravity

4 = active movement, full ROM against gravity and moderate resistance in a muscle specific position.

5 = (normal) active movement, full ROM against gravity and full resistance in a muscle specific position expected from an otherwise unimpaired peson.

5* = (normal) active movement, full ROM against gravity and sufficient resistance to be considered normal if identified inhibiting factors (i.e. pain, disuse) were not present.

NT= not testable (i.e. due to immobilization, severe pain such that the patient cannot be graded, amputation of limb, or contracture of >50% of the range of motion).

ASIA Impairment (AIS) Scale

☐ **A = Complete.** No sensory or motor function is preserved in the sacral segments S4-S5.

☐ **B = Sensory Incomplete.** Sensory but not motor function is preserved below the neurological level and includes the sacral segments S4-S5 (light touch, pin prick at S4-S5: or deep anal pressure (DAP)), AND no motor function is preserved more than three levels below the motor level on either side of the body.

☐ **C = Motor Incomplete.** Motor function is preserved below the neurological level**, and more than half of key muscle functions below the single neurological level of injury (NLI) have a muscle grade less than 3 (Grades 0-2).

☐ **D = Motor Incomplete.** Motor function is preserved below the neurological level**, and at least half (half or more) of key muscle functions below the NLI have a muscle grade ≥ 3.

☐ **E = Normal.** If sensation and motor function as tested with the ISNCSCI are graded as normal in all segments, and the patient had prior deficits, then the AIS grade is E. Someone without an initial SCI does not receive an AIS grade.

**For an individual to receive a grade of C or D, i.e. motor incomplete status, they must have either (1) voluntary anal sphincter contraction or (2) sacral sensory sparing with sparing of motor function more than three levels below the motor level for that side of the body. The Standards at this time allows even non-key muscle function more than 3 levels below the motor level to be used in determining motor incomplete status (AIS B versus C).

NOTE: When assessing the extent of motor sparing below the level for distinguishing between AIS B and C, the ***motor level*** on each side is used; whereas to differentiate between AIS C and D (based on proportion of key muscle functions with strength grade 3 or greater) the ***single neurological level*** is used.

Steps in Classification

The following order is recommended in determining the classification of individuals with SCI.

1. Determine sensory levels for right and left sides.
2. Determine motor levels for right and left sides.
   Note: in regions where there is no myotome to test, the motor level is presumed to be the same as the sensory level, if testable motor function above that level is also normal.
3. Determine the single neurological level.
   This is the lowest segment where motor and sensory function is normal on both sides, and is the most cephalad of the sensory and motor levels determined in steps 1 and 2.
4. Determine whether the injury is Complete or Incomplete.
   (i.e. absence or presence of sacral sparing)
   If voluntary anal contraction = **No** *AND all S4-5 sensory scores =* **0** *AND deep anal pressure =* **No,** *then injury is COMPLETE. Otherwise, injury is incomplete.*
5. Determine ASIA Impairment Scale (AIS) Grade:
   Is injury Complete? If **YES,** AIS=A and can record ZPP (lowest dermatome or myotome on each side with some preservation)
   NO ↓
   Is injury motor Incomplete? If **NO,** AIS=B (Yes=voluntary anal contraction OR motor function more than three levels below the motor level on a given side, if the patient has sensory incomplete classification)
   YES ↓
   Are at least half of the key muscles below the single neurological level graded 3 or better?
   NO ↓ AIS=C   YES ↓ AIS=D

If sensation and motor function is normal in all segments, AIS=E
Note: AIS E is used in follow-up testing when an individual with a documented SCI has recovered normal function. If at initial testing no deficits are found, the individual is neurologically intact; the ASIA Impairment Scale does not apply.

Fig. 12. American Spinal Cord Injury Association (ASIA) scoring sheet for the patient with spinal cord injury. (*Courtesy of* American Spinal Injury Association, Atlanta, GA; with permission.)

Table 4
Secondary SCI timetable

Time After SCI	Injury Phase	Phases and Key Events	
		Key Processes and Events	**Therapeutic Aims**
≤2 h	Primary Immediate	Mechanical Injury Traumatic axonal severing Gray matter hemorrhage Hemorrhagic necrosis Microglial activation Release of factors (IL-1β, TNF-α, IL-6 and others)	Neuroprotection
≤48 h	Early Acute	Vasogenic edema Cytotoxic edema Lipid peroxidation Glutamate mediated excitotoxicity Continued hemorrhage Continued necrosis Neutrophil invasion Peak BBB permeability Early demyelination Neuronal death Axonal swelling Systemic shock Spinal shock Hypotension Hypoxia	Neuroprotection Immune modulation Cell-based remyelination Glial scar degradation
≤2 wk	Secondary subacute	Macrophage infiltration Reactive astrocytosis BBB repair Resolution of edema	
≤6 mo	Intermediate	Continued formation of glial scar Cyst formation Lesion stabilization	Glial scar degradation
≥6 mo	Chronic/late	Prolonged Wallerian degeneration Persistence of spared, demyelinated axons Potential structural and functional plasticity of spared spinal cord tissue	Rehabilitation Neuroprosthesis

Abbreviations: BBB, blood-brain barrier; IL, interleukin; TNF, tumor necrosis factor.

has found its detractors, and its widespread use as the standard of care has been questioned.[171,172]

Timing of Intervention

There has long been a debate regarding the optimal time to intervene in patients with acute SCI. Preclinical data dating back from the 1970s demonstrated in animal studies that injury to the spinal cord could be worsened by sustained compression. The damage caused by such an insult can be attenuated by decompressive surgery, thereby relieving the pressure being applied to the spinal cord.[173–180] There is, however, no clear consensus regarding the optimal timing of decompressive surgery after SCI, but it is evident that there is no increased morbidity in early decompression.[181,182] In addition, an article by Furlan and colleagues[183] published the opinion of a panel of 10 experts who recommended that "surgical decompression of the injured spinal cord is performed within 24hrs when medically feasible." This opinion seems to echo the current standard used in their practice by a large proportion of the international spine community.[184] Thus, although not definitely proved with class I data, the preclinical evidence as well as lower-quality clinical studies seem to favor early decompression. It is imperative to reiterate that the benefit of early decompression in the setting of SCI is contingent on the presence of ongoing spinal cord compression.

Radiologic Evaluation

Having access to imaging modalities such as radiography, CT, and MR imaging to quantify the amount of compression is imperative to be able to both diagnose SCI and determine the patients' potential for benefit from early surgical intervention. Measurements such as anteroposterior (AP) canal diameter, transverse canal diameter, canal area, and the ratio between AP diameter and transverse diameter have been used in the past, and are described in the literature as useful tools in determining spinal canal compromise.[185–189] However, the most reliable means to quantify spinal cord compression was set forth in a study by Fehlings and colleagues.[190] This method calculates maximal spinal cord compression by comparing the AP cord diameter at the level of maximum injury with the AP cord diameter at nearest normal levels above and below.

Surgical Decision Making

Important considerations when assessing whether a patient with spinal trauma requires surgery include the presence of spinal cord compression and a neurologic deficit. However, additional concepts to be taken into account that will help decide on how to steer the therapeutic decision making must include the mechanism of injury, the presence or absence of biomechanical instability, osteoligamentous integrity and fracture configuration. Several investigators have attempted to incorporate some or all of these elements to create a comprehensive spinal trauma classification system for use in the clinical realm. However, no single system has gained widespread use. Two novel classification systems for spinal trauma have been recently developed by members of the Spine Trauma Study Group (STSG). The first, known as the Subaxial Cervical Spine Injury Classification (SLIC), addresses injuries to the subaxial cervical spine. The second, contributed by the STSG and known as the Thoracolumbar Injury Classification and Severity Score (TLICS), addresses spinal injuries at the thoracolumbar junction based on an algorithm virtually identical to SLIC. The investigators have recommended that patients with an SLIC or a TLICS score of less than 4 should be treated nonoperatively, those with an SLIC or a TLICS score of greater than 4 should be treated operatively, and those with an SLIC or a TLICS score of exactly 4 can be managed with or without surgery at the discretion of the clinical management team (**Table 5**).[191,192] The combination of radiographic and clinical information gathered on the individual patient will determine the necessity of operative intervention; however, the surgeon involved will still need to make a decision as to the type of operation to be performed. This decision is largely based on the location of the primary pathology. However, there seems to be a degree of discretion on the surgeon's behalf to interpret the evidence, his or her personal experience, and his or her proficiency at

Table 5
Subaxial and thoracolumbar classification systems

Injury Variable	Weighed Severity Points for SLIC	Weighed Severity Points for TLICS
Morphology		
No abnormality	0	0
Compression	1	1
Distraction	3	3
Rotation/Translation	4	4
Discoligamentous Complex Integrity		
Intact	0	0
Indeterminate	1	2
Disrupted	2	3
Neurologic Status		
Intact	0	0
Root injury	1	2
Complete/conus cord injury	2	3
Incomplete cord injury	3	2
Cord compression with neural deficit/cauda equina	+1	3

Abbreviations: SLIC, Subaxial Cervical Spine Injury Classification; TLICS, Thoracolumbar Injury Classification and Severity Score.

executing a certain approach over another, to formulate what would be the best modality of treatment for a particular patient.

REFERENCES

1. Narayan RK, Kishore PR, Becker DP, et al. Intracranial pressure: to monitor or not to monitor? A review of our experience with severe head injury. J Neurosurg 1982;56(5):650–9.
2. Schreiber MA, Aoki N, Scott BG, et al. Determinants of mortality in patients with severe blunt head injury. Arch Surg 2002;137(3):285–90.
3. Marmarou A, Anderson RL, Ward JD, et al. Impact of ICP instability and hypotension on outcome in patients with severe head trauma. J Neurosurg (Special Supplements) 1991;75(1s):S59–66.
4. Becker DP, Miller JD, Ward JD, et al. The outcome from severe head injury with early diagnosis and intensive management. J Neurosurg 1977;47(4):491–502.
5. Eisenberg HM, Frankowski RF, Contant CF, et al. High-dose barbiturate control of elevated intracranial pressure in patients with severe head injury. J Neurosurg 1988;69(1):15–23.
6. Bratton SL, Chestnut RM, Ghajar J, et al. Guidelines for the management of severe traumatic brain injury. VI. Indications for intracranial pressure monitoring. J Neurotrauma 2007;24(Suppl 1):S37–44.
7. Marmarou A, Maset AL, Ward JD, et al. Contribution of CSF and vascular factors to elevation of ICP in severely head-injured patients. J Neurosurg 1987;66(6):883–90.
8. Ursino M, Lodi CA, Rossi S, et al. Intracranial pressure dynamics in patients with acute brain damage. J Appl Physiol 1997;82(4):1270–82.
9. Marmarou A, Shulman K, Rosende RM. A nonlinear analysis of the cerebrospinal fluid system and intracranial pressure dynamics. J Neurosurg 1978;48(3):332–44.

10. Shapiro K, Marmarou A, Shulman K. Characterization of clinical CSF dynamics and neural axis compliance using the pressure-volume index: I. The normal pressure-volume index. Ann Neurol 1980;7(6):508–14.
11. Schuhmann MU, Thomas S, Hans VH, et al. CSF dynamics in a rodent model of closed head injury. Acta Neurochir Suppl 1998;71:300–2.
12. Miller MT, Pasquale M, Kurek S, et al. Initial head computed tomographic scan characteristics have a linear relationship with initial intracranial pressure after trauma. J Trauma 2004;56(5):967–72 [discussion: 972–3].
13. Palmer S, Bader MK, Qureshi A, et al. The impact on outcomes in a community hospital setting of using the AANS traumatic brain injury guidelines. Americans Associations for Neurologic Surgeons. J Trauma 2001;50(4): 657–64.
14. Bulger EM, Nathens AB, Rivara FP, et al. Management of severe head injury: institutional variations in care and effect on outcome. Crit Care Med 2002; 30(8):1870–6.
15. Bratton SL, Chestnut RM, Ghajar J, et al. Guidelines for the management of severe traumatic brain injury. VIII. Intracranial pressure thresholds. J Neurotrauma 2007;24(Suppl 1):S55–8.
16. Ratanalert S, Phuenpathom N, Saeheng S, et al. ICP threshold in CPP management of severe head injury patients. Surg Neurol 2004;61(5):429–34 [discussion: 434–5].
17. Maas AI, Dearden M, Teasdale GM, et al. EBIC-guidelines for management of severe head injury in adults. European Brain Injury Consortium. Acta Neurochir (Wien) 1997;139(4):286–94.
18. Adelson PD, Bratton SL, Carney NA, et al. Guidelines for the acute medical management of severe traumatic brain injury in infants, children, and adolescents. Chapter 6. Threshold for treatment of intracranial hypertension. Pediatr Crit Care Med 2003;4(Suppl 3):S25–7.
19. Carney NA, Ghajar J. Guidelines for the management of severe traumatic brain injury. Introduction. J Neurotrauma 2007;24(Suppl 1):S1–2.
20. Carney NA. Guidelines for the management of severe traumatic brain injury. Methods. J Neurotrauma 2007;24(Suppl 1):S3–6.
21. Adelson PD, Bratton SL, Carney NA, et al. Guidelines for the acute medical management of severe traumatic brain injury in infants, children, and adolescents. Chapter 1. Introduction. Pediatr Crit Care Med 2003;4(Suppl 3): S2–4.
22. Bratton SL, Chestnut RM, Ghajar J, et al. Guidelines for the management of severe traumatic brain injury. I. Blood pressure and oxygenation. J Neurotrauma 2007;24(Suppl 1):S7–13.
23. Kelly DF, Goodale DB, Williams J, et al. Propofol in the treatment of moderate and severe head injury: a randomized, prospective double-blinded pilot trial. J Neurosurg 1999;90(6):1042–52.
24. Adelson PD, Bratton SL, Carney NA, et al. Guidelines for the acute medical management of severe traumatic brain injury in infants, children, and adolescents. Chapter 5. Indications for intracranial pressure monitoring in pediatric patients with severe traumatic brain injury. Pediatr Crit Care Med 2003; 4(Suppl 3):S19–24.
25. Adelson PD, Bratton SL, Carney NA, et al. Guidelines for the acute medical management of severe traumatic brain injury in infants, children, and adolescents. Chapter 7. Intracranial pressure monitoring technology. Pediatr Crit Care Med 2003;4(Suppl 3):S28–30.

26. Hung OR, Hare GM, Brien S. Head elevation reduces head-rotation associated increased ICP in patients with intracranial tumours. Can J Anaesth 2000;47(5): 415–20.
27. Adelson PD, Bratton SL, Carney NA, et al. Guidelines for the acute medical management of severe traumatic brain injury in infants, children, and adolescents. Chapter 11. Use of hyperosmolar therapy in the management of severe pediatric traumatic brain injury. Pediatr Crit Care Med 2003;4(Suppl 3):S40–4.
28. Annegers JF, Hauser WA, Coan SP, et al. A population-based study of seizures after traumatic brain injuries. N Engl J Med 1998;338(1):20–4.
29. Adelson PD, Bratton SL, Carney NA, et al. Guidelines for the acute medical management of severe traumatic brain injury in infants, children, and adolescents. Chapter 12. Use of hyperventilation in the acute management of severe pediatric traumatic brain injury. Pediatr Crit Care Med 2003;4(Suppl 3):S45–8.
30. Bratton SL, Chestnut RM, Ghajar J, et al. Guidelines for the management of severe traumatic brain injury. XIII. Antiseizure prophylaxis. J Neurotrauma 2007;24(Suppl 1):S83–6.
31. Adelson PD, Bratton SL, Carney NA, et al. Guidelines for the acute medical management of severe traumatic brain injury in infants, children, and adolescents. Chapter 13. The use of barbiturates in the control of intracranial hypertension in severe pediatric traumatic brain injury. Pediatr Crit Care Med 2003; 4(Suppl 3):S49–52.
32. Rhoney DH, Parker D. Considerations in fluids and electrolytes after traumatic brain injury. Nutr Clin Pract 2006;21(5):462–78.
33. Clifton GL, Miller ER, Choi SC, et al. Fluid thresholds and outcome from severe brain injury. Crit Care Med 2002;30(4):739–45.
34. Piek J, Chesnut RM, Marshall LF, et al. Extracranial complications of severe head injury. J Neurosurg 1992;77(6):901–7.
35. Ramming S, Shackford SR, Zhuang J, et al. The relationship of fluid balance and sodium administration to cerebral edema formation and intracranial pressure in a porcine model of brain injury. J Trauma 1994;37(5):705–13.
36. Fletcher JJ, Bergman K, Blostein PA, et al. Fluid balance, complications, and brain tissue oxygen tension monitoring following severe traumatic brain injury. Neurocrit Care 2010;13(1):47–56.
37. Schmoker JD, Shackford SR, Wald SL, et al. An analysis of the relationship between fluid and sodium administration and intracranial pressure after head injury. J Trauma 1992;33(3):476–81.
38. York J, Arrillaga A, Graham R, et al. Fluid resuscitation of patients with multiple injuries and severe closed head injury: experience with an aggressive fluid resuscitation strategy. J Trauma 2000;48(3):376–9 [discussion: 379–80].
39. Zornow MH, Prough DS. Fluid management in patients with traumatic brain injury. New Horiz 1995;3(3):488–98.
40. Cole CD, Gottfried ON, Liu JK, et al. Hyponatremia in the neurosurgical patient: diagnosis and management. Neurosurg Focus 2004;16(4):E9.
41. Rivkees SA. Differentiating appropriate antidiuretic hormone secretion, inappropriate antidiuretic hormone secretion and cerebral salt wasting: the common, uncommon, and misnamed. Curr Opin Pediatr 2008;20(4):448–52.
42. Zafonte RD, Mann NR. Cerebral salt wasting syndrome in brain injury patients: a potential cause of hyponatremia. Arch Phys Med Rehabil 1997; 78(5):540–2.
43. Zygun DA. Sodium and brain injury: do we know what we are doing? Crit Care 2009;13(5):184.

44. Aiyagari V, Deibert E, Diringer MN. Hypernatremia in the neurologic intensive care unit: how high is too high? J Crit Care 2006;21(2):163–72.
45. Maggiore U, Picetti E, Antonucci E, et al. The relation between the incidence of hypernatremia and mortality in patients with severe traumatic brain injury. Crit Care 2009;13(4):R110.
46. Wong MF, Chin NM, Lew TW. Diabetes insipidus in neurosurgical patients. Ann Acad Med Singap 1998;27(3):340–3.
47. Bratton SL, Chestnut RM, Ghajar J, et al. Guidelines for the management of severe traumatic brain injury. XV. Steroids. J Neurotrauma 2007;24(Suppl 1):S91–5.
48. Meyer MJ, Megyesi J, Meythaler J, et al. Acute management of acquired brain injury part II: an evidence-based review of pharmacological interventions. Brain Inj 2010;24(5):706–21.
49. Bratton SL, Chestnut RM, Ghajar J, et al. Guidelines for the management of severe traumatic brain injury. II. Hyperosmolar therapy. J Neurotrauma 2007;24(Suppl 1):S14–20.
50. Diringer MN, Zazulia AR. Osmotic therapy: fact and fiction. Neurocrit Care 2004;1(2):219–33.
51. Latorre JG, Greer DM. Management of acute intracranial hypertension: a review. Neurologist 2009;15(4):193–207.
52. Horn P, Münch E, Vajkoczy P, et al. Hypertonic saline solution for control of elevated intracranial pressure in patients with exhausted response to mannitol and barbiturates. Neurol Res 1999;21(8):758–64.
53. Smith AL. Barbiturate protection in cerebral hypoxia. Anesthesiology 1977;47(3):285–93.
54. Schramm WM, Jesenko R, Bartunek A, et al. Effects of cisatracurium on cerebral and cardiovascular hemodynamics in patients with severe brain injury. Acta Anaesthesiol Scand 1997;41(10):1319–23.
55. Hsiang JK, Chesnut RM, Crisp CB, et al. Early, routine paralysis for intracranial pressure control in severe head injury: is it necessary? Crit Care Med 1994;22(9):1471–6.
56. Nates JL, Cooper DJ, Day B, et al. Acute weakness syndromes in critically ill patients–a reappraisal. Anaesth Intensive Care 1997;25(5):502–13.
57. Meyer MJ, Megyesi J, Meythaler J, et al. Acute management of acquired brain injury part I: an evidence-based review of non-pharmacological interventions. Brain Inj 2010;24(5):694–705.
58. Oertel M, Kelly DF, Lee JH, et al. Efficacy of hyperventilation, blood pressure elevation, and metabolic suppression therapy in controlling intracranial pressure after head injury. J Neurosurg 2002;97(5):1045–53.
59. Bratton SL, Chestnut RM, Ghajar J, et al. Guidelines for the management of severe traumatic brain injury. XI. Anesthetics, analgesics, and sedatives. J Neurotrauma 2007;24(Suppl 1):S71–6.
60. Bratton SL, Chestnut RM, Ghajar J, et al. Guidelines for the management of severe traumatic brain injury. XIV. Hyperventilation. J Neurotrauma 2007;24(Suppl 1):S87–90.
61. Coles JP, Minhas PS, Fryer TD, et al. Effect of hyperventilation on cerebral blood flow in traumatic head injury: clinical relevance and monitoring correlates. Crit Care Med 2002;30(9):1950–9.
62. Ghajar J, Hariri RJ, Narayan RK, et al. Survey of critical care management of comatose, head-injured patients in the United States. Crit Care Med 1995;23(3):560–7.

63. Muizelaar JP, Marmarou A, Ward JD, et al. Adverse effects of prolonged hyperventilation in patients with severe head injury: a randomized clinical trial. J Neurosurg 1991;75(5):731–9.
64. Kammersgaard LP, Rasmussen BH, Jørgensen HS, et al. Feasibility and safety of inducing modest hypothermia in awake patients with acute stroke through surface cooling: a case-control study: the Copenhagen Stroke Study. Stroke 2000;31(9):2251–6.
65. Tokutomi T, Morimoto K, Miyagi T, et al. Optimal temperature for the management of severe traumatic brain injury: effect of hypothermia on intracranial pressure, systemic and intracranial hemodynamics, and metabolism. Neurosurgery 2007;61(Suppl 1):256–65 [discussion: 265–6].
66. Marion DW, Obrist WD, Carlier PM, et al. The use of moderate therapeutic hypothermia for patients with severe head injuries: a preliminary report. J Neurosurg 1993;79(3):354–62.
67. Lee ST, Lui TN, Wong CW, et al. Early seizures after severe closed head injury. Can J Neurol Sci 1997;24(1):40–3.
68. Liu WG, Qiu WS, Zhang Y, et al. Effects of selective brain cooling in patients with severe traumatic brain injury: a preliminary study. J Int Med Res 2006;34(1): 58–64.
69. Bratton SL, Chestnut RM, Ghajar J, et al. Guidelines for the management of severe traumatic brain injury. III. Prophylactic hypothermia. J Neurotrauma 2007;24(Suppl 1):S21–5.
70. Aarabi B, Hesdorffer DC, Ahn ES, et al. Outcome following decompressive craniectomy for malignant swelling due to severe head injury. J Neurosurg 2006; 104(4):469–79.
71. Albanèse J, Leone M, Alliez J-R, et al. Decompressive craniectomy for severe traumatic brain injury: evaluation of the effects at one year. Crit Care Med 2003;31(10):2535–8.
72. Guerra WK, Gaab MR, Dietz H, et al. Surgical decompression for traumatic brain swelling: indications and results. J Neurosurg 1999;90(2):187–96.
73. Taylor A, Butt W, Rosenfeld J, et al. A randomized trial of very early decompressive craniectomy in children with traumatic brain injury and sustained intracranial hypertension. Childs Nerv Syst 2001;17(3):154–62.
74. Jiang JY, Xu W, Li WP, et al. Efficacy of standard trauma craniectomy for refractory intracranial hypertension with severe traumatic brain injury: a multicenter, prospective, randomized controlled study. J Neurotrauma 2005;22(6): 623–8.
75. Biffl WL, Moore EE, Ryu RK, et al. The unrecognized epidemic of blunt carotid arterial injuries: early diagnosis improves neurologic outcome. Ann Surg 1998; 228(4):462–70.
76. Cothren CC, Moore EE, Ray CE, et al. Screening for blunt cerebrovascular injuries is cost-effective. Am J Surg 2005;190(6):845–9.
77. Miller PR, Fabian TC, Bee TK, et al. Blunt cerebrovascular injuries: diagnosis and treatment. J Trauma 2001;51(2):279–85 [discussion: 285–6].
78. Nedeltchev K, Baumgartner RW. Traumatic cervical artery dissection. Front Neurol Neurosci 2005;20:54–63.
79. Risgaard O, Sugrue M, D'Amours S, et al. Blunt cerebrovascular injury: an evaluation from a major trauma centre. ANZ J Surg 2007;77(8):686–9.
80. Miller PR, Fabian TC, Croce MA, et al. Prospective screening for blunt cerebrovascular injuries: analysis of diagnostic modalities and outcomes. Ann Surg 2002;236(3):386–93 [discussion: 393–5].

81. Gomez CR, May AK, Terry JB, et al. Endovascular therapy of traumatic injuries of the extracranial cerebral arteries. Crit Care Clin 1999;15(4):789–809.
82. Krings T, Geibprasert S, Lasjaunias PL. Cerebrovascular trauma. Eur Radiol 2008;18(8):1531–45.
83. Zhao WY, Krings T, Alvarez H, et al. Management of spontaneous haemorrhagic intracranial vertebrobasilar dissection: review of 21 consecutive cases. Acta Neurochir (Wien) 2007;149(6):585–96 [discussion: 596].
84. Hughes KM, Collier B, Greene KA, et al. Traumatic carotid artery dissection: a significant incidental finding. Am Surg 2000;66(11):1023–7.
85. Wei CW, Montanera W, Selchen D, et al. Blunt cerebrovascular injuries: diagnosis and management outcomes. Can J Neurol Sci 2010;37(5):574–9.
86. Fusco MR, Harrigan MR. Cerebrovascular dissections: a review part II. Blunt cerebrovascular injury. Neurosurgery. Available at: http://www.ncbi.nlm.nih.gov/entrez/query.fcgi?cmd=Retrieve&db=PubMed&dopt=Citation&list_uids=21135751. Accessed June 15, 2011.
87. Nunez DB, Berkmen T. Imaging of blunt cerebrovascular injuries. Eur J Radiol 2006;59(3):317–26.
88. Hart RG, Easton JD. Dissections of cervical and cerebral arteries. Neurol Clin 1983;1(1):155–82.
89. Mokri B, Piepgras DG, Houser OW. Traumatic dissections of the extracranial internal carotid artery. J Neurosurg 1988;68(2):189–97.
90. Golueke P, Sclafani S, Phillips T, et al. Vertebral artery injury—diagnosis and management. J Trauma 1987;27(8):856–65.
91. Friedman D, Flanders A, Thomas C, et al. Vertebral artery injury after acute cervical spine trauma: rate of occurrence as detected by MR angiography and assessment of clinical consequences. AJR Am J Roentgenol 1995;164(2):443–7 [discussion: 448–9].
92. Benninger DH, Gandjour J, Georgiadis D, et al. Benign long-term outcome of conservatively treated cervical aneurysms due to carotid dissection. Neurology 2007;69(5):486–7.
93. Cothren CC, Moore EE, Biffl WL, et al. Anticoagulation is the gold standard therapy for blunt carotid injuries to reduce stroke rate. Arch Surg 2004;139(5):540–5 [discussion: 545–6].
94. Sturzenegger M. Spontaneous internal carotid artery dissection: early diagnosis and management in 44 patients. J Neurol 1995;242(4):231–8.
95. Biffl WL, Ray CE, Moore EE, et al. Treatment-related outcomes from blunt cerebrovascular injuries: importance of routine follow-up arteriography. Ann Surg 2002;235(5):699–706 [discussion: 706–7].
96. Eachempati SR, Vaslef SN, Sebastian MW, et al. Blunt vascular injuries of the head and neck: is heparinization necessary? J Trauma 1998;45(6):997–1004.
97. Fabian TC, Patton JH, Croce MA, et al. Blunt carotid injury. Importance of early diagnosis and anticoagulant therapy. Ann Surg 1996;223(5):513–22 [discussion: 522–5].
98. Stein DM, Boswell S, Sliker CW, et al. Blunt cerebrovascular injuries: does treatment always matter? J Trauma 2009;66(1):132–43 [discussion: 143–4].
99. Wahl WL, Brandt MM, Thompson BG, et al. Antiplatelet therapy: an alternative to heparin for blunt carotid injury. J Trauma 2002;52(5):896–901.
100. Cothren CC, Moore EE. Blunt cerebrovascular injuries. Clinics (Sao Paulo) 2005;60(6):489–96.

101. Cothren CC, Biffl WL, Moore EE, et al. Treatment for blunt cerebrovascular injuries: equivalence of anticoagulation and antiplatelet agents. Arch Surg 2009;144(7):685–90.
102. Edwards NM, Fabian TC, Claridge JA, et al. Antithrombotic therapy and endovascular stents are effective treatment for blunt carotid injuries: results from longterm followup. J Am Coll Surg 2007;204(5):1007–13 [discussion: 1014–5].
103. Lasjaunias P, Wuppalapati S, Alvarez H, et al. Intracranial aneurysms in children aged under 15 years: review of 59 consecutive children with 75 aneurysms. Childs Nerv Syst 2005;21(6):437–50.
104. McGuinness BJ, Moriarty M, Hope JK. Interventional radiology in the treatment of intracranial vascular injuries and fistulae. Injury 2008;39(11):1242–8.
105. Diaz-Daza O, Arraiza FJ, Barkley JM, et al. Endovascular therapy of traumatic vascular lesions of the head and neck. Cardiovasc Intervent Radiol 2003; 26(3):213–21.
106. Jones RF, Terrell JC, Salyer KE. Penetrating wounds of the neck: an analysis of 274 cases. J Trauma 1967;7(2):228–37.
107. Hemphill JC, Gress DR, Halbach VV. Endovascular therapy of traumatic injuries of the intracranial cerebral arteries. Crit Care Clin 1999;15(4):811–29.
108. Yang TC, Lo YL, Huang YC, et al. Traumatic anterior cerebral artery aneurysm following blunt craniofacial trauma. Eur Neurol 2007;58(4):239–45.
109. Chambers EF, Rosenbaum AE, Norman D, et al. Traumatic aneurysms of cavernous internal carotid artery with secondary epistaxis. AJNR Am J Neuroradiol 1981;2(5):405–9.
110. Chen D, Concus AP, Halbach VV, et al. Epistaxis originating from traumatic pseudoaneurysm of the internal carotid artery: diagnosis and endovascular therapy. Laryngoscope 1998;108(3):326–31.
111. Han MH, Sung MW, Chang KH, et al. Traumatic pseudoaneurysm of the intracavernous ICA presenting with massive epistaxis: imaging diagnosis and endovascular treatment. Laryngoscope 1994;104(3 Pt 1):370–7.
112. Cohen JE, Gomori JM, Segal R, et al. Results of endovascular treatment of traumatic intracranial aneurysms. Neurosurgery 2008;63(3):476–85 [discussion: 485–6].
113. Dubey A, Sung WS, Chen YY, et al. Traumatic intracranial aneurysm: a brief review. J Clin Neurosci 2008;15(6):609–12.
114. Resnick DK, Subach BR, Marion DW. The significance of carotid canal involvement in basilar cranial fracture. Neurosurgery 1997;40(6):1177–81.
115. Asari S, Nakamura S, Yamada O, et al. Traumatic aneurysm of peripheral cerebral arteries. Report of two cases. J Neurosurg 1977;46(6):795–803.
116. Buckingham MJ, Crone KR, Ball WS, et al. Traumatic intracranial aneurysms in childhood: two cases and a review of the literature. Neurosurgery 1988;22(2): 398–408.
117. Fleischer AS, Patton JM, Tindall GT. Cerebral aneurysms of traumatic origin. Surg Neurol 1975;4(2):233–9.
118. Schuster JM, Santiago P, Elliott JP, et al. Acute traumatic posteroinferior cerebellar artery aneurysms: report of three cases. Neurosurgery 1999;45(6): 1465–7 [discussion: 1467–8].
119. Holmes B, Harbaugh RE. Traumatic intracranial aneurysms: a contemporary review. J Trauma 1993;35(6):855–60.
120. Parkinson D, West M. Traumatic intracranial aneurysms. J Neurosurg 1980; 52(1):11–20.

121. Uzan M, Cantasdemir M, Seckin MS, et al. Traumatic intracranial carotid tree aneurysms. Neurosurgery 1998;43(6):1314–20 [discussion: 1320–2].
122. Ventureyra EC, Higgins MJ. Traumatic intracranial aneurysms in childhood and adolescence. Case reports and review of the literature. Childs Nerv Syst 1994; 10(6):361–79.
123. Cohen JE, Rajz G, Itshayek E, et al. Endovascular management of traumatic and iatrogenic aneurysms of the pericallosal artery. Report of two cases. J Neurosurg 2005;102(3):555–7.
124. Joo JY, Ahn JY, Chung YS, et al. Therapeutic endovascular treatments for traumatic carotid artery injuries. J Trauma 2005;58(6):1159–66.
125. Levy ML, Rezai A, Masri LS, et al. The significance of subarachnoid hemorrhage after penetrating craniocerebral injury: correlations with angiography and outcome in a civilian population. Neurosurgery 1993;32(4):532–40.
126. Haddad FS, Haddad GF, Taha J. Traumatic intracranial aneurysms caused by missiles: their presentation and management. Neurosurgery 1991;28(1):1–7.
127. Cox MW, Whittaker DR, Martinez C, et al. Traumatic pseudoaneurysms of the head and neck: early endovascular intervention. J Vasc Surg 2007;46(6): 1227–33.
128. Eckard DA, O'Boynick PL, McPherson CM, et al. Coil occlusion of the parent artery for treatment of symptomatic peripheral intracranial aneurysms. AJNR Am J Neuroradiol 2000;21(1):137–42.
129. Maras D, Lioupis C, Magoufis G, et al. Covered stent-graft treatment of traumatic internal carotid artery pseudoaneurysms: a review. Cardiovasc Intervent Radiol 2006;29(6):958–68.
130. Love L, Marsan RE. Carotid cavernous fistula. Angiology 1974;25(4):231–6.
131. Desal H, Leaute F, Auffray-Calvier E, et al. Direct carotid-cavernous fistula. Clinical, radiologic and therapeutic studies. Apropos of 49 cases. J Neuroradiol 1997;24(2):141–54 [in French].
132. de Keizer R. Carotid-cavernous and orbital arteriovenous fistulas: ocular features, diagnostic and hemodynamic considerations in relation to visual impairment and morbidity. Orbit 2003;22(2):121–42.
133. Fabian TS, Woody JD, Ciraulo DL, et al. Posttraumatic carotid cavernous fistula: frequency analysis of signs, symptoms, and disability outcomes after angiographic embolization. J Trauma 1999;47(2):275–81.
134. Liang W, Xiaofeng Y, Weiguo L, et al. Traumatic carotid cavernous fistula accompanying basilar skull fracture: a study on the incidence of traumatic carotid cavernous fistula in the patients with basilar skull fracture and the prognostic analysis about traumatic carotid cavernous fistula. J Trauma 2007;63(5): 1014–20 [discussion: 1020].
135. Unger JM, Gentry LR, Grossman JE. Sphenoid fractures: prevalence, sites, and significance. Radiology 1990;175(1):175–80.
136. West OC, Mirvis SE, Shanmuganathan K. Transsphenoid basilar skull fracture: CT patterns. Radiology 1993;188(2):329–38.
137. Gaskill-Shipley MF, Tomsick TA. Angiography in the evaluation of head and neck trauma. Neuroimaging Clin N Am 1996;6(3):607–24.
138. Kocer N, Kizilkilic O, Albayram S, et al. Treatment of iatrogenic internal carotid artery laceration and carotid cavernous fistula with endovascular stent-graft placement. AJNR Am J Neuroradiol 2002;23(3):442–6.
139. Archondakis E, Pero G, Valvassori L, et al. Angiographic follow-up of traumatic carotid cavernous fistulas treated with endovascular stent graft placement. AJNR Am J Neuroradiol 2007;28(2):342–7.

140. Luo CB, Teng MM, Chang FC, et al. Traumatic indirect carotid cavernous fistulas: angioarchitectures and results of transarterial embolization by liquid adhesives in 11 patients. Surg Neurol 2009;71(2):216–22.
141. van Rooij WJ, Sluzewski M, Slob MJ, et al. Predictive value of angiographic testing for tolerance to therapeutic occlusion of the carotid artery. AJNR Am J Neuroradiol 2005;26(1):175–8.
142. Hasso AN, Lasjaunias P, Thompson JR, et al. Venous occlusions of the cavernous area—a complication of crushing fractures of the sphenoid bone. Radiology 1979;132(2):375–9.
143. Meier U, Gartner F, Knopf W, et al. The traumatic dural sinus injury—a clinical study. Acta Neurochir (Wien) 1992;119(1–4):91–3.
144. Taha JM, Crone KR, Berger TS, et al. Sigmoid sinus thrombosis after closed head injury in children. Neurosurgery 1993;32(4):541–5 [discussion: 545–6].
145. Kinal ME. Traumatic thrombosis of dural venous sinuses in closed head injury. J Neurosurg 1967;27(142):145.
146. Lee SK, terBrugge KG. Cerebral venous thrombosis in adults: the role of imaging evaluation and management. Neuroimaging Clin N Am 2003;13(1):139–52.
147. Ducreux D, Oppenheim C, Vandamme X, et al. Diffusion-weighted imaging patterns of brain damage associated with cerebral venous thrombosis. AJNR Am J Neuroradiol 2001;22(2):261–8.
148. Ameri A, Bousser MG. Cerebral venous thrombosis. Neurol Clin 1992;10(1):87–111.
149. Bousser MG. Cerebral venous thrombosis: nothing, heparin, or local thrombolysis? Stroke 1999;30(3):481–3.
150. Barnwell SL, Higashida RT, Halbach VV, et al. Direct endovascular thrombolytic therapy for dural sinus thrombosis. Neurosurgery 1991;28(1):135–42.
151. Higashida RT, Helmer E, Halbach VV, et al. Direct thrombolytic therapy for superior sagittal sinus thrombosis. AJNR Am J Neuroradiol 1989;10(Suppl 5):S4–6.
152. Horowitz M, Purdy P, Unwin H, et al. Treatment of dural sinus thrombosis using selective catheterization and urokinase. Ann Neurol 1995;38(1):58–67.
153. Scott JA, Pascuzzi RM, Hall PV, et al. Treatment of dural sinus thrombosis with local urokinase infusion. Case report. J Neurosurg 1988;68(2):284–7.
154. Tsai FY, Higashida RT, Matovich V, et al. Acute thrombosis of the intracranial dural sinus: direct thrombolytic treatment. AJNR Am J Neuroradiol 1992;13(4):1137–41.
155. Faul M, Xu L, Wald M, et al. Traumatic brain injury in the United States: emergency department visits, hospitalizations, and deaths, 2002-2006. Centers for Disease Control; 2010. p. 74. Available at: http://www.cdc.gov/TraumaticBrainInjury/. Accessed June 11, 2011.
156. Choux M. Incidence, diagnosis and management of skull fractures. In: Raimondi AJ, Choux M, Rocco CD, editors. Head injuries in the newborn and infant. Düsseldorf (Germany): Springer-Verlag; 1986. p. 163–92.
157. Harwood-Nash DC, Hendrick EB, Hudson AR. The significance of skull fractures in children. A study of 1,187 patients. Radiology 1971;101(1):151–6.
158. Davis PC, Reisner A, Hudgins PA, et al. Spinal injuries in children: role of MR. AJNR Am J Neuroradiol 1993;14(3):607–17.
159. Steinbok P, Flodmark O, Martens D, et al. Management of simple depressed skull fractures in children. J Neurosurg 1987;66(4):506–10.
160. Muhonen MG, Piper JG, Menezes AH. Pathogenesis and treatment of growing skull fractures. Surg Neurol 1995;43(4):367–72 [discussion: 372–3].

161. Patterson A. Craniocerebral trauma. In: Osborn AG, editor. Diagnostic neuroradiology. St. Louis (MO): Mosby; 1994. p. 200–35.
162. Rosa CM, Luigi B, Antonio D, et al. Early prognosis after severe traumatic brain injury with minor or absent computed tomography scan lesions. J Trauma 2011; 70(2):447–51.
163. Adelson PD, Resnick DK. Spinal cord injury in children. In: Albright AL, Pollack IF, Adelson PD, editors. Principles and practice of pediatric neurosurgery. New York (NY): Thieme; 1999. p. 965–73.
164. Pang D, Wilberger JE Jr. Spinal cord injury without radiographic abnormalities in children. J Neurosurg 1982;57(1):114–29.
165. Pang D, Pollack IF. Spinal cord injury without radiographic abnormality in children—the SCIWORA syndrome. J Trauma 1989;29(5):654–64.
166. Ramón S, Domínguez R, Ramírez L, et al. Clinical and magnetic resonance imaging correlation in acute spinal cord injury. Spinal Cord 1997;35(10): 664–73.
167. Baptiste DC, Fehlings MG. Emerging drugs for spinal cord injury. Expert Opin Emerg Drugs 2008;13(1):63–80.
168. Anon. Spinal cord injury facts and figures at a glance. J Spinal Cord Med 2010; 33(4):439–40.
169. Anon. The Consortium for Spinal Cord Medicine. Early acute management in adults with spinal cord injury: a clinical practice guideline for health care providers. Washington, DC: Paralyzed Veterans of America; 2009.
170. Bracken MB, Shepard MJ, Collins WF, et al. A randomized, controlled trial of methylprednisolone or naloxone in the treatment of acute spinal-cord injury. Results of the Second National Acute Spinal Cord Injury Study. N Engl J Med 1990;322(20):1405–11.
171. Bracken MB, Shepard MJ, Holford TR, et al. Administration of methylprednisolone for 24 or 48 hours or tirilazad mesylate for 48 hours in the treatment of acute spinal cord injury. Results of the Third National Acute Spinal Cord Injury Randomized Controlled Trial. National Acute Spinal Cord Injury Study. JAMA 1997;277(20):1597–604.
172. Hurlbert RJ. Methylprednisolone for acute spinal cord injury: an inappropriate standard of care. J Neurosurg 2000;93(Suppl 1):1–7.
173. Delamarter RB, Sherman JE, Carr JB. 1991 Volvo Award in experimental studies. Cauda equina syndrome: neurologic recovery following immediate, early, or late decompression. Spine 1991;16(9):1022–9.
174. Carlson GD, Minato Y, Okada A, et al. Early time-dependent decompression for spinal cord injury: vascular mechanisms of recovery. J Neurotrauma 1997; 14(12):951–62.
175. Delamarter RB, Sherman J, Carr JB. Pathophysiology of spinal cord injury. Recovery after immediate and delayed decompression. J Bone Joint Surg Am 1995;77(7):1042–9.
176. Brodkey JS, Richards DE, Blasingame JP, et al. Reversible spinal cord trauma in cats. Additive effects of direct pressure and ischemia. J Neurosurg 1972;37(5): 591–3.
177. Carlson GD, Gorden CD, Oliff HS, et al. Sustained spinal cord compression: part I: time-dependent effect on long-term pathophysiology. J Bone Joint Surg Am 2003;85(1):86–94.
178. Dimar JR, Glassman SD, Raque GH, et al. The influence of spinal canal narrowing and timing of decompression on neurologic recovery after spinal cord contusion in a rat model. Spine 1999;24(16):1623–33.

179. Cadotte DW, Singh A, Fehlings MG. The timing of surgical decompression for spinal cord injury. F1000 Med Rep 2010;2:67.
180. Dolan EJ, Tator CH, Endrenyi L. The value of decompression for acute experimental spinal cord compression injury. J Neurosurg 1980;53(6):749–55.
181. Levi L, Wolf A, Rigamonti D, et al. Anterior decompression in cervical spine trauma: does the timing of surgery affect the outcome? Neurosurgery 1991; 29(2):216–22.
182. Campagnolo DI, Esquieres RE, Kopacz KJ. Effect of timing of stabilization on length of stay and medical complications following spinal cord injury. J Spinal Cord Med 1997;20(3):331–4.
183. Furlan JC, Noonan V, Cadotte DW, et al. Timing of decompressive surgery of spinal cord after traumatic spinal cord injury: an evidence-based examination of pre-clinical and clinical studies. J Neurotrauma 2010. Available at: http://www.ncbi.nlm.nih.gov/pubmed/20001726. Accessed March 11, 2011.
184. Fehlings MG, Rabin D, Sears W, et al. Current practice in the timing of surgical intervention in spinal cord injury. Spine 2010;35(Suppl 21):S166–73.
185. Denno JJ, Meadows GR. Early diagnosis of cervical spondylotic myelopathy. A useful clinical sign. Spine 1991;16(12):1353–5.
186. Edwards WC, LaRocca H. The developmental segmental sagittal diameter of the cervical spinal canal in patients with cervical spondylosis. Spine 1983; 8(1):20–7.
187. Eismont FJ, Clifford S, Goldberg M, et al. Cervical sagittal spinal canal size in spine injury. Spine 1984;9(7):663–6.
188. Matsuura P, Waters RL, Adkins RH, et al. Comparison of computerized tomography parameters of the cervical spine in normal control subjects and spinal cord-injured patients. J Bone Joint Surg Am 1989;71(2):183–8.
189. Stanley JH, Schabel SI, Frey GD, et al. Quantitative analysis of the cervical spinal canal by computed tomography. Neuroradiology 1986;28(2):139–43.
190. Fehlings MG, Rao SC, Tator CH, et al. The optimal radiologic method for assessing spinal canal compromise and cord compression in patients with cervical spinal cord injury. Part II: results of a multicenter study. Spine 1999;24(6): 605–13.
191. Vaccaro AR, Hulbert RJ, Patel AA, et al. The subaxial cervical spine injury classification system: a novel approach to recognize the importance of morphology, neurology, and integrity of the disco-ligamentous complex. Spine 2007;32(21): 2365–74.
192. Vaccaro AR, Lehman RA, Hurlbert RJ, et al. A new classification of thoracolumbar injuries: the importance of injury morphology, the integrity of the posterior ligamentous complex, and neurologic status. Spine 2005;30(20):2325–33.

Acute Neurologic Effects of Alcohol and Drugs

Harold W. Goforth, MD[a,b,*], Francisco Fernandez, MD[c]

KEYWORDS

• Alcohol • Drugs • Neurologic • Stimulant • Toxicology
• Opioids

Neurologic effects of acute drug intoxication are varied, and this article discusses the acute neurologic effects of certain drugs as well as associated treatments and guidelines to management.

STIMULANTS

Acute intoxication and neurologic complication from stimulants are strikingly similar. Stimulants include various substances such as cocaine; crack; amphetamine; 3,4-methylenedioxymethamphetamine (MDMA; best known as ecstasy); ephedrine; phenylpropanolamine; and methylphenidate.[1] Acute intoxication is characterized by a "high" feeling with euphoria that mimics a manic episode. It is typically associated with autonomic hyperactivity. Route of administration includes snorting, smoking, and intravenous injection. Although all inhibit the reuptake of dopamine, norepinephrine, and serotonin, the prevailing thought on cocaine's effects are through dopaminergic effects.[2] Stimulant intoxication includes[3]

1. Recent use of a stimulant
2. A clinically significant maladaptive behavioral or psychological change that develops shortly after the use of the stimulant
3. Two or more of the following physical symptoms
   a. Tachycardia
   b. Pupillary dilatation
   c. Altered blood pressure
   d. Chills or perspiration
   e. Nausea and/or vomiting

[a] Durham Veterans Affairs Medical Center, 508 Fulton Street, Mailstop #116A, Durham, NC 27705, USA
[b] Duke University Medical Center, DUMC 3309, Durham, NC 27710, USA
[c] University of South Florida, 3515 East Fletcher Avenue, Tampa, FL 33613, USA
* Corresponding author. Duke University Medical Center, DUMC 3309, Durham, NC 27710.
E-mail address: harold.goforth@duke.edu

Neurol Clin 30 (2012) 277–284
doi:10.1016/j.ncl.2011.09.015
0733-8619/12/$ – see front matter Published by Elsevier Inc.

f. Evidence of weight loss
g. Psychomotor agitation
h. Chest pain, cardiac arrhythmias
i. Confusion, seizures, dyskinesias, dystonias, or coma.

The symptoms observed are not caused by a general medical condition or better accounted by another mental disorder.

Severe intoxication is most commonly associated with seizures, cardiac arrhythmias, hyperpyrexia, and vasoconstriction leading to increased risk for myocardial infarction, stroke, and even death.[4,5]

METHAMPHETAMINE

Acute intoxication due to methamphetamine is similar to that caused by stimulants; however, there are fewer issues with seizures and cerebrovascular disease than with cocaine.[1,6] The euphoric high, hyperpyrexia, autonomic hyperactivity, and cardiopulmonary effects are similar. Unlike cocaine and other stimulants, acute coronary syndromes are more common than acute cerebrovascular complications.[7] Nonetheless, damage to the small blood vessels of the brain, resulting in stroke and paralysis, can also occur.[8] Many users of methamphetamine suffer from cognitive impairment, which can be of sufficient severity to cause a dementing illness[9] and chronic psychosis.[10]

MARIHUANA

Marihuana use produces a short period of intoxication or high characterized by variably psychosensory experiences (eg, hallucinations, paranoia, inhibition, and impaired cognition).[11] The cognitive impairment may last for hours after using marihuana. Other than the psychosensory and cognitive changes, no acute neurologic complications are seen with marihuana use.

INHALANTS

Inhalants encompass a wide range of pharmacologically diverse substances inclusive of volatile solvents, nitrous oxide, and volatile alkyl nitrites.[12] Signs and symptoms of inhalant intoxication include dizziness, nystagmus, euphoria, dysarthria, gait disturbance, tremor, depressed reflexes, generalized weakness, stupor, and/or coma.[3] In the differential diagnostic process, the recent use of inhalant products, inhalant odor and residue, and periorbital rash are diagnostic.[13,14] Inhalant-induced delirium is common and should be treated accordingly whether or not severe behavioral disturbances are present.[15] Care should be taken to avoid routine use of sedatives, such as the benzodiazepines, in conjunction with a neuroleptic, which may result in further depression of central nervous system (CNS) function.

KETAMINE AND PHENCYCLIDINE

Both phencyclidine and ketamine are arylcyclohexylamine-dissociative anesthetics that are similar to hallucinogens in their effects.[16] Ketamine is a short-acting derivative of phencyclidine. Both these anesthetics produce profound changes in consciousness and perceptual distortions that are popular among teenagers and young adults to enhance sensory experiences at clubs and rave parties.[17] Although both produce a dissociative psychotic state, phencyclidine is more likely to lead to a dangerous and violent behavior.[18] Acute phencyclidine intoxication can be distinguished from phencyclidine intoxication delirium by the presence of vertical and/or horizontal nystagmus, ataxia, and slurred speech.[3] Convulsions and dystonias may occur and may herald progression to coma and death.[1]

SEROTONERGIC HALLUCINOGENS

This group of agents is best known as psychedelic drugs producing psychotomimetic experiences that are presumed by some to be "enlightening." Lysergic acid diethylamide (LSD) is one such agent that alters perception, mood, and thought.[16] LSD has limited sympathomimetic effects, and there are some case reports of it causing large vessel occlusions.[1] Coagulopathies may occur but only in massive doses.[19] The most common adverse clinical effects of LSD are bad trips, flashbacks, and persistent psychosis.[16] Similar complications can occur with psilocybin (also known as magic mushrooms); however, these are much less frequent because the physiologic effects of this hallucinogen are less pronounced. Mescaline (commonly referred to as peyote) is another phenethylamine hallucinogen, which like psilocybin has limited, if any, neurologic complications.

MDMA is the most consequential of this group of drugs.[1] MDMA is structurally related to both amphetamines and mescaline. Thus, sympathomimetic symptoms abound. Also, a propensity for serotonin syndrome is common. Major neurologic complications probably secondary to its sympathomimetic effects include delirium, headache, irritability, nystagmus, intracranial hemorrhage, venous sinus thrombosis, and herniation.[20]

SEDATIVE HYPNOTICS

Although all these CNS depressants share a common mechanism of action through the brain's inhibitory neurotransmitter γ-aminobutyric acid (GABA), they are really 3 distinct groups: benzodiazepines, barbiturates, and nonbenzodiazepine hypnotics.[21] These hypnotics are clinically useful for anxiety, insomnia, muscle relaxants, seizures, and detoxification from alcohol. Acute neurologic effects are similar to alcohol.[22] Although benzodiazepines have a wide therapeutic index, barbiturates do not. With large ingestions, CNS depression and consequent cardiorespiratory depression, anoxia, and anoxic encephalopathy are the only acute neurologic complications from sedative hypnotics.

ALCOHOL

Alcohol (ethanol) produces multiple acute neurologic effects, including incoordination, anxiolysis, cognitive changes, and modulation of locomotor activity. The GABAergic system plays a central role in modulating alcohol's effects, especially on the anxiolytic, motor, amnestic, and hypnotic features produced with acute intoxication. Acute intoxication can also produce amnestic periods during which the ability of a person to perform high-level tasks is preserved. However, flumazenil does not seem to counteract ethanol's actions. Other potential neurologic systems involved in producing ethanol's acute CNS effects include the serotonergic system, glutamatergic changes with chronic use, and the dopaminergic system in reinforcing the pleasurable effects of alcohol.[23]

Alcohol withdrawal is characterized by delirium in severe forms, but tremulousness and autonomic instability are consistent features. Untreated alcohol withdrawal delirium has been noted to have a mortality of up to 25%, so appropriate recognition and treatment are imperative. Alcohol withdrawal seizures in 1 to 3 days after cessation of alcohol use are not infrequent but in most cases do not require specific antiseizure therapy other than standard measures for treating alcohol withdrawal. Treatment of alcohol withdrawal involves administration and tapering of GABAergic substances such as benzodiazepines or barbiturates. The most commonly used agents include chlordiazepoxide, diazepam, or lorazepam, with large doses at times being required to adequately control withdrawal.[24]

Wernicke-Korsakoff syndrome has been clearly linked with nutritional deficiency of thiamine as occurs in alcoholism due to dietary neglect. Wernicke syndrome is characterized by confusion, ataxia, and ophthalmoplegia. It is important to recognize this condition because it may be partially reversible with thiamine repletion. Alternatively, this condition may evolve to become Korsakoff psychosis involving permanent retrograde and anterograde amnesias with confabulation and psychosis. Wernicke syndrome seems to have a low prevalence (0.4%–2.8% of reported autopsies), but the disorder is highly underreported and underdiagnosed. Treatment of Wernicke syndrome involves the administration of high-dose parenteral thiamine. Recent guidelines support doses of thiamine, 500 mg intravenously every 8 hours for a minimum of 3 days or until there is a plateau with regard to clinical improvement. Administration of high doses takes advantage of both a passive diffusion gradient of thiamine across the blood-brain barrier (BBB) as well as the active transport of thiamine across the BBB.[25]

Central pontine myelinolysis (CPM) can occur in a variety of contexts, but particular risk factors include dialysis, liver failure, advanced cancer, cachexia, sepsis, dehydration, acute pancreatitis, chronic alcoholism, vitamin B6 deficiency, and electrolyte disturbances. Chronic alcohol use is a particular risk factor for this condition, and long-term alcoholics have been noted to be perhaps less symptomatic after rapid correction of hyponatremia than others, demanding a high clinical index of suspicion to adequately diagnose. The mechanisms of CPM are poorly understood but probably relate to the osmotic injury to the vascular endothelium producing vasogenic edema and brain dehydration. During correction of electrolyte abnormalities, it is important to only gently correct hyponatremia at a rate not to exceed 10 mmol sodium per liter in a 24-hour period and less than 18 mmol sodium per liter in the initial 48-hour period.[26]

Alcoholic polyneuropathy most typically occurs after long-term alcohol use, but its sequelae can present acutely, such as falls or worsening autonomic dysfunction. There is a direct toxic effect of alcohol on autonomic and peripheral nerves but can also be secondary to nutrient deficiencies, which are common in alcoholics because of decreased dietary intake and diminished gastrointestinal absorption. Common nutritional deficiencies in alcoholics include thiamine, riboflavin, pyridoxine, folate, and cyanocobalamin deficiencies. The clinical manifestation of alcoholic neuropathy mimics those seen with thiamine, pyridoxine, and cyanocobalamin deficiencies and affects the muscular, cardiovascular, gastrointestinal, and nervous systems. Initial presentations of alcoholic polyneuropathy are typically observed in the lower extremities and affects both sensory and/or motor systems but can extend into the upper extremities and involve the autonomic system as well. Axonal degeneration and reductions in myelination are commonly observed. Treatment involves cessation of alcohol use and multivitamin supplementation.[27]

Alcoholic myopathy can present acutely and involve severe rhabdomyolysis, threatening renal failure. In addition, such myopathy has been linked in part to the electrolyte disturbances common among alcoholics, including hypophosphatemia, hypokalemia, and hypomagnesemia. Treatment is primarily supportive with careful attention toward prevention of secondary organ dysfunction due to rhabdomyolysis or electrolyte complications.[28]

With chronic alcohol use, the liver deteriorates and develops fibrosis, that is, cirrhosis. At some point, the liver is unable to clear naturally occurring toxins such as ammonia and native GABAergic molecules, which can severely affect cognitive and neurologic functions known as hepatic encephalopathy. Altered mental status, asterixis, and coma can all occur, and, although elevated levels of ammonia are supportive, they are not required for diagnosis. Hepatic coma sequelae include coarse tremor, choreoathetotic movements, dysarthria, ataxia, and hepatocerebral degeneration. The mainstay of treatment of hepatic encephalopathy is supportive and involves administration of lactulose, titrated to produce 3 to 5 soft bowel movements daily. Alternatively, oral neomycin or rifaximin can be used as well to reduce bowel flora, but care must be taken with neomycin because it can cause sensorineural hearing loss, despite not being well absorbed orally.[29]

OPIATES

Heroin remains popular as a primary drug in substance abuse treatment admissions in the northeastern United States, but opioid abuse has also largely grown with easier access to prescribed opioids. Recent abuse indicators for other opiates are increasing

Table 1
Neurologic symptoms and syndromes associated with substance use

Compartment	Symptoms/Syndrome	Cause
Peripheral nerves	Femoral/median neuropathy	Direct trauma from needle
	Mononeuropathies: single and multiple	Compressive neuropathies arising from prolonged coma, especially lateral popliteal and ulnar nerve but also sciatic
	Botulism	Skin popping due to deep intradermal injecting drug use
	Guillain-Barré syndrome	Use of n-hexane as well as possible comorbid HIV-AIDS
	Plexopathy	Either due to ischemia or compression damage
Spinal cord	Compression	Extradural abscess, discitis, osteomyelitis
	Anterior cord syndrome	Cord infarction from infective endocarditis, vasculitis, and vasospasm
	Intrinsic cord lesion	Acute hemorrhage, abscess
Brain	Encephalopathy	Meningoencephalitis (urgent lumbar puncture), direct drug effect, postanoxic, vasculitis, metabolic, head injury
	Intracerebral hemorrhage	Hypertensive surge, with underlying arteriovenous malformation, septic arteritis, mycotic aneurysm, vasculitis
	Meningitis	Infective endocarditis, atypical organisms, HIV
	Seizures	Direct drug effect, hypertensive crisis, abscess or empyema, stroke, meningoencephalitis, metabolic
	Stroke and infarcts	Vasospasm, embolism, dissection, vasculitis
	Subacute focal deficit	Abscesses, subdural empyema, progressive multifocal leukoencephalopathy, HIV/AIDS
	Subarachnoid hemorrhage	Hypertensive surges, coexisting arteriovenous malformation or aneurysm, mycotic aneurysm, vasculitis

Data from Enevoldson TP. Recreational drugs and their neurologic consequences. J Neurol Neurosurg Psychiatry 2004;75(Suppl 3):9–15.

because of diversion and theft of pharmaceutical supplies. Recent abuse indicators for oxycodone, hydrocodone, methadone, and fentanyl suggest increased rates of drug diversion and abuse of prescription opiates, especially oxycodone and hydrocodone, whereas the prevalence of heroin use has appeared to remain relatively stable.[30] Clinical states of opioid intoxication and withdrawal are common. Both human immunodeficiency virus (HIV) and hepatitis C virus are efficiently transmitted via the intravenous route with the sharing of needles. Other infectious complications of intravenous drug abuse include endocarditis, septicemia, and joint infections. See **Table 1** for additional details.

Opiate receptors are found predominantly in the CNS, the gastrointestinal tract, and peripheral tissues. There are 3 classes of opiate receptors, including μ, δ, and κ, and the μ receptors are generally thought to be responsible for supraspinal analgesia. Opiates more commonly cause dysphoria than euphoria, and iatrogenic addiction in individuals without a preexisting addiction history is rare. Physiologic effects of opiate intoxication include dysphoria; somnolence; diminished respiratory rate; and, in overdose, death.[31] Treatment involves administration of an opioid antagonist (naloxone) and supportive therapy until the patient's body has sufficiently eliminated the substance for safe discontinuation of the opioid antagonist.[32]

Conversely, opioid withdrawal is associated with irritability, anxiety, rhinorrhea, diaphoresis, diarrhea, piloerection, and nausea/vomiting. Treatment is supportive as opioid withdrawal is not considered life threatening in the absence of extenuating circumstances but can be quite miserable for the patient. Use of clonidine and antispasmodic agents are common, and patients can be referred to opioid substitution centers for methadone or buprenorphine.[33]

SUMMARY

As with other neurologic emergencies, physicians and other clinicians have important roles to play in the acute phases of intoxication and withdrawal from drugs and alcohol. Routine screening, particularly for adolescents and young adults, are important. Early and aggressive treatment of overdose, misuse, or abuse are key in preventing long-term neurobehavioral complications from cerebrovascular and cardiovascular events as well as psychiatric comorbidities, violent crime, and spread of HIV-AIDS and hepatitis C. Advances in the neurosciences hold promise for new treatments, and the next decade promises to be most important in translating these findings into promising treatments and prevention.

REFERENCES

1. Enevoldson TP. Recreational drugs and their neurological consequences. J Neurol Neurosurg Psychiatry 2004;75(Suppl 3):9–15.
2. Nestler EJ. The neurobiology of cocaine addiction. Sci Pract Perspect 2005;3:4–10.
3. American Psychiatric Association. Diagnostic and statistical manual of mental disorders, 4th edition, text revision (DSM-IV TR). Washington, DC: American Psychiatric Association Press; 2000.
4. Benzaquen BS, Cohen V, Eisenberg MJ. Effects of cocaine on the coronary arteries. Am Heart J 2001;142:402–10.
5. Johnson BA, Devous MS, Ruiz P, et al. Treatment advances for cocaine induced ischemic stroke: focus on dihydropyridine class calcium channel antagonists. Am J Psychiatry 2001;158:1191–8.

6. Rawson R, Gonzalez R, Ling W. Methamphetamine abuse and dependence: an update. Dir Psychiatry 2006;26(10):131–44.
7. Mooney L, Glasner-Edwards S, Rawson RA, et al. Medical effects of methamphetamine use. In: Roll JM, Rawson RA, Ling W, et al, editors. Methamphetamine addiction: from basic science to treatment. New York: Guilford Press; 2009. p. 117–42.
8. Wang G, Volkow N, Chang L, et al. Partial recovery of human brain metabolism in methamphetamine abusers after protracted abstinence. Am J Psychiatry 2004; 161:242–8.
9. Simon SL, Domier C, Carnell J, et al. Cognitive impairment in individuals currently using methamphetamine. Am J Addict 2000;9(3):222–31.
10. Meredith CW, Jaffe C, Ang-Lee K, et al. Implications of chronic methamphetamine use: a literature review. Harv Rev Psychiatry 2005;13(3):141–54.
11. Johns A. Psychiatric effects of cannabis. Br J Psychiatry 2001;178:116–22.
12. Williams JF, Storck M. Inhalant abuse. Pediatrics 2007;119:1009–17.
13. Sakai JT, Hall SK, Mikulich-Gilbertson SK, et al. Inhalant use, abuse, and dependence among adolescent patients: commonly comorbid problems. J Am Acad Child Adolesc Psychiatry 2004;43:1080–8.
14. Flanagan RJ, Ives RJ. Volatile substance abuse. Bull Narc 1994;46:49–78.
15. Hernandez-Avila CA, Ortega-Soto HA, Jasso A, et al. Treatment of inhalant-induced psychotic disorder with carbamazepine versus haloperidol. Psychiatr Serv 1998;49:812–5.
16. Abraham HD, Aldridge AM, Gogia P. The psychopharmacology of hallucinogens. Neuropsychopharmacology 1996;14:285–98.
17. Weaver MF, Scholl SH. Hallucinogens and club drugs. In: Galanter M, Kleber HD, editors. Textbook of substance abuse treatment. 4th edition. Washington, DC: American Psychiatric Publishing; 2008. p. 191–200. Chapter 14.
18. Mars-Simon PA, Weiler M, Santangelo MA, et al. Analysis of sexual disparity of violent behavior in PCP intoxication. Vet Hum Toxicol 1988;30:53–5.
19. Klock J, Boerner U, Becker C. Coma, hyperthermia, and bleeding associated with massive LSD overdose. West J Med 1973;20:183–8.
20. Gahlinger P. Club drugs: MDMA, gamma-hydroxybutyrate, rohypnol, and ketamine. Am Fam Physician 2004;69(11):2619–26.
21. Roy Byrne P, Cowley D. Benzodiazepines in clinical practice: risks and benefits. Clinical practice series: 17. Washington, DC: American Psychiatric Press; 1991.
22. Schukit MA, Greenblatt D, Irwin M, et al. Reactions to ethanol and diazepam in health young men. J Stud Alcohol 1991;52:180–7.
23. Tabakoff BH. Alcohol: neurobiology. In: Lowinson JH, Ruiz P, Millman RB, et al, editors. Substance abuse: a comprehensive textbook. Baltimore (MD): Williams & Wilkins; 1992.
24. Hughes JR. Alcohol withdrawal seizures. Epilepsy Behav 2009;15(2):92–7.
25. Sechi GP, Serra A. Wernicke's encephalopathy: new clinical settings and recent advances in diagnosis and management. Lancet Neurol 2007;6:442–55.
26. Yoon B, Shim Y, Chung S. Central pontine and extrapontine myelinolysis after alcohol withdrawal. Alcohol Alcohol 2008;43(6):647–9.
27. Peters TJ, Kotowicz J, Nyka W, et al. Treatment of alcoholic polyneuropathy with vitamin B complex: a randomized controlled trial. Alcohol Alcohol 2006;41(6): 636–42.
28. Pall HS, Williams AC, Heath DA, et al. Hypomagnesaemia causing myopathy and hypocalcaemia in an alcoholic. Postgrad Med J 1987;63(742):665–7.

29. Lizardi-Cervera J, Almeda P, Guevara L, et al. Hepatic encephalopathy: a review. Ann Hepatol 2003;2(3):122–30.
30. NIDA. NIDA epidemiologic trends in drug abuse, proceedings of the community epidemiology work group: highlights and executive summary. U.S.D.o.H.a.H. Service. National Institutes of Health; 2008.
31. Lipman AJ. Opioid pharmacotherapy. In: Warfield CB, Bajwa ZH, editors. Principles and practice of pain medicine. New York: McGraw Hill Publishers; 2004. p. 583–600.
32. Goldfrank LR, Weisman RS. Opioids. In: Goldfrank LR, Flomenbaum NE, Lewin NA, et al, editors. Goldfrank's toxicologic emergencies. 5th edition. Norwalk (CT): Appleton & Lange; 1994. p. 769–83.
33. Kosten TR, O'Connor PG. Management of drug and alcohol withdrawal. N Engl J Med 2003;348:1786–95.

Acute Demyelinating Disorders: Emergencies and Management

Reem F. Bunyan, MD, MS[a], Junger Tang, MD[b], Brian Weinshenker, MD, FRCP(C)[c,*]

KEYWORDS

- CNS inflammatory demyelinating disease • Multiple sclerosis
- Acute disseminated encephalomyelitis • Neuromyelitis optica
- Acute demyelination • Apheresis

Central nervous system (CNS) demyelinating diseases are typically chronic disorders. Episodic relapses, a hallmark of the early phase of the disease, are usually mild and remit spontaneously or following a brief course of corticosteroids. Attacks of CNS demyelinating disease occasionally present with serious and emergent neurologic complications, either directly because of inflammation and destruction of brain or spinal cord tissue or because of secondary complications; these complications may result from brain edema that leads to mass effect and occasional brain herniation syndromes, or from systemic disturbances attributable to the function of the specific structures affected by the lesions, including pulmonary edema and respiratory failure. These complications may occur in the context of prototypic MS but are even more likely in the setting of alternative demyelinating disease contexts (eg, acute disseminated encephalomyelitis [ADEM], or neuromyelitis optica [NMO], tumefactive forms of MS, including Baló concentric sclerosis, and Marburg variant).

This article reviews the spectrum of acute emergent presentations of demyelinating disease and the importance of identification of the demyelinating disease context in which they occur to evaluate prognosis and institute effective long-term management. With emergency presentations, which are unusual in CNS demyelinating disease, consideration of other conditions that may mimic demyelinating disease is

---

Financial disclosure/conflict of interest: The authors have nothing to disclose.
[a] Department of Neurology, Neurosciences Center, King Fahad Specialist Hospital Dammam, Dammam, Saudi Arabia
[b] MS Treatment and Research Center at the Minneapolis Clinic of Neurology, Golden Valley, MN, USA
[c] Department of Neurology, Mayo Clinic, 200 First Street Southwest, Rochester, MN 55905, USA
* Corresponding author.
E-mail address: wein@mayo.edu

Neurol Clin 30 (2012) 285–307
doi:10.1016/j.ncl.2011.09.013
neurologic.theclinics.com

critical. Clinicians should be aware of the myriad of mimics and the "red flags" that suggest a diagnosis other than demyelinating disease that may require specific treatment. Investigation should be individualized based on the index of suspicion for specific diagnoses suggested by these "red flags." Guided by the index of suspicion, investigations, including cerebrospinal fluid (CSF) analysis, magnetic resonance imaging (MRI), magnetic resonance spectroscopy (MRS), and, occasionally, brain/spinal cord biopsy, are helpful in excluding neoplasms (gliomatosis, lymphoma), vasculitis, sarcoidosis, and infections, such as progressive multifocal leukoencephalopathy, among other disease entities.

Treatment options for acute demyelinating disease (corticosteroids, plasmapheresis, intravenous immunoglobulin [IVIG], and immunosuppression) are reviewed, largely in the context of acute management. Potential neurologic and medical complications that may occasionally occur in the context of demyelinating disease, including brain herniation, posterior reversible encephalopathy syndrome (PRES), respiratory failure, neurogenic pulmonary edema, and acute heart failure are summarized, along with their management.

OVERVIEW OF INFLAMMATORY DEMYELINATING DISEASE

The spectrum of CNS inflammatory demyelinating diseases (CNS IDDs) is broad. The commonest variant is prototypic multiple sclerosis (MS), but other variants are relatively more likely to present with severe clinical deficits and emergency complications, including ADEM, NMO, and less common variants such as Baló concentric sclerosis, the Marburg variant of MS, and tumefactive MS.[1] The boundaries between some of these entities are becoming better defined, in particular those that distinguish NMO from MS; however, some of these entities are much less well distinguished and intermediate phenotypes may defy accurate classification. Clinicopathological differences among these various conditions lead to different emergent presentations; however, the treatment of these emergency conditions is often the same regardless of phenotype, although the prognosis and long-term management may vary.

Dissemination in space coupled with dissemination in time is a time-honored concept in the field of MS; however, at initial presentation, these criteria may not be satisfied. It is often necessary to establish a working diagnosis of demyelinating disease at the first presentation, especially when it presents with severe disability or some other emergency complication. The inflammatory demyelinating lesions are pathologically heterogeneous. Although biopsy is not a commonly applied investigation when making a diagnosis, biopsy may be indicated for patients who present atypically (eg, with a large lesion with mass effect, or with atypical multifocal disease simulating vasculitis, gliomatosis cerebri, or other CNS pathologies). ADEM and NMO are usually pathologically distinguishable from prototypic MS and from one another.[2,3] Prototypic MS has been classified immunopathologically into 4 separate patterns of demyelination.[4] Patterns I and II suggest an immune-mediated attack, either cellular (pattern I) or antibody-mediated (pattern II), whereas patterns III and IV suggest a primary oligodendrogliopathy. The specific pattern may dictate responsiveness to certain immunotherapies. For example, patients with pattern II pathology, characterized by immunoglobulin deposition and terminal membrane attack complement activation, respond favorably to therapeutic plasma exchange.[5]

Acute Disseminated Encephalomyelitis

ADEM has classically been described as a monophasic illness most common in children who have had an antecedent viral illness or immunization.[6–9] Recurrent or relapsing forms have been described, although how these are distinguished from MS remains controversial.[10,11] Patients with ADEM commonly report a preceding nonspecific upper respiratory infection.[1] Specific infections that have been associated with ADEM include herpes virus infections (Epstein-Barr virus, cytomegalovirus, herpes simplex virus, and varicella zoster virus), influenza A and B, rubella, mumps, and HIV. Immunizations for varicella, influenza, diphtheria-tetanus, polio, and rabies occasionally precede ADEM.[12] Perivenous distribution of inflammation and demyelination are usually present in ADEM, whereas confluent demyelination occurs in acute MS, including tumefactive forms. Hemorrhagic variants (acute hemorrhagic leukoencephalitis, Hurst disease) are thought to be severe variants of ADEM.[13] **Fig. 1** shows an example of MRI findings in ADEM. Oligoclonal bands are less likely to be present in the CSF of patients with ADEM than in patients with MS.[8]

The proposed consensus definitions by the International Pediatric MS Study Group for monophasic ADEM require encephalopathy as part of a polysymptomatic presentation, in large part because its presence discriminates between MS and ADEM; however, encephalopathy may be seen in acute variants of MS and should not be considered as diagnostic of ADEM.[11] Encephalopathy may present as behavioral changes, including confusion, irritability, and restlessness. Alternatively, ADEM may result in altered consciousness producing lethargy and drowsiness, or in more severe cases, obtundation, stupor, and coma that may require airway protection and can be fatal directly owing to cerebral herniation or to a supervening medical complication in some instances. The development of fever, headaches, seizures, and meningeal signs may reflect a meningoencephalitis and is more common in pediatric cases. Manifestations of ADEM may include optic neuritis or transverse myelitis.

High-dose intravenous corticosteroids are widely used as initial treatment for ADEM. The typical dose is intravenous methylprednisolone 30 mg/kg per day (maximum of 1000 mg/d) in children and 1000 mg per day in adult patients.[9] Infusions are typically given for 3 to 5 consecutive days followed by an optional oral steroid taper over 2 to 3 weeks. Management in corticosteroid-refractory cases is not well established; based on its proven efficacy in a randomized clinical trial of acute, severe demyelinating disease (class I evidence), we recommend plasma exchange 1.0 to 1.5 plasma volumes per exchange, 7 treatments over 2-weeks.[14,15] The use of plasma exchange has recently been systematically reviewed by the American Academy of Neurology and the American Society for Apheresis and found to be appropriate for the treatment of acute fulminant demyelinating CNS disease.[16,17] IVIG, 1 to 2 g/kg given in 1 dose or divided over 3 to 5 days has also been reported as an effective treatment.[18]

Neuromyelitis Optica

NMO (or Devic disease) was historically diagnosed in patients who experienced severe bilateral optic neuritis and transverse myelitis that developed concurrently or occurred sequentially within weeks of one another. In Asia, optic-spinal MS (OSMS) was recognized as a relapsing variant with special predilection for optic nerves and spinal cord, distinct from classical MS. A potential relationship of OSMS to NMO was recognized, but that relationship remained unclear. In the early twenty-first century, a pathogenic antibody (NMO–immunoglobulin G [NMO-IgG]) specifically reactive to aquaporin-4, a water channel protein on astrocyte foot processes, was found to distinguish NMO and many cases of OSMS from prototypic MS.[19] The revised diagnostic criteria by Wingerchuk and colleagues[20] in 2006 incorporate serum NMO-IgG antibody seropositivity as 1 of 3 supportive criteria in addition to requiring optic neuritis and myelitis to have occurred. NMO spectrum disorders (NMOSDs),

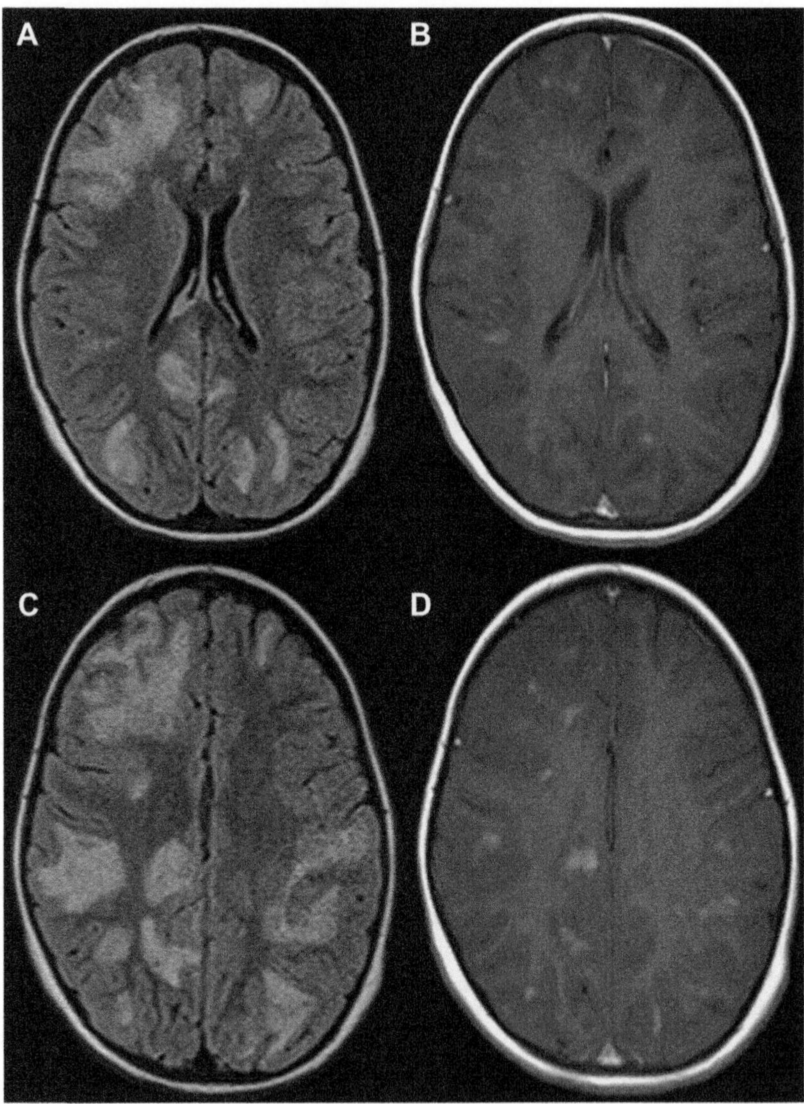

Fig. 1. Acute disseminated encephalomyelitis. (*A*) Axial fluid-attenuated inversion recovery (FLAIR) image showing multiple large indistinct homogeneous T2 signal abnormalities. (*B*) Axial T1 postcontrast image showing multiple enhancing lesions. (*C–D*) Same as (*A*) and (*B*) but at a more rostral level. (*Courtesy of* Dr Moses Rodriguez, Mayo Clinic, Rochester, MN.)

such as recurrent optic neuritis or recurrent longitudinally extensive transverse myelitis (LETM) in patients seropositive for NMO-IgG who do not satisfy the full NMO criteria, are increasingly being recognized and studied, as are patients with NMOSD with characteristic brain lesions for NMO, such as hypothalmic lesions associated with a symptomatic form of narcolepsy.

The vast majority of patients with NMO diagnosed by contemporary diagnostic criteria have a relapsing course.[21] Relapses are often, although not invariably, more severe and are associated with more severe visual and sensorimotor deficits than

MS relapses; typically, myelitis is accompanied by a longitudinally extensive lesion on MRI of the spinal cord that spans 3 or more vertebral segments; patients often have a complete transverse myelitis with severe, and sometimes symmetric motor and sensory findings below the highest involved spinal level. However, the NMO spectrum includes a variety of brain and brainstem lesions, the most common and characteristic of which is intractable nausea with vomiting or hiccups associated with lesions in the area postrema in the floor of the fourth ventricle.[22] Emergencies occurring in the setting of NMO exacerbations include neurogenic respiratory failure owing to upper cervical cord and brainstem involvement, as discussed later in this article. Hypothalamic involvement that has been documented in NMO may cause hypothermia and a symptomatic form of narcolepsy associated with profound somnolence.[23] PRES has been identified in a series of patients with NMOSD that may be caused by vasogenic edema secondary to impairment of water flux as a result of aquaporin-4 autoimmunity and may present a self-limiting, reversible coma or cortical blindness.[24]

Acute NMO exacerbations are routinely treated with high-dose intravenous corticosteroids.[25] A typical course of treatment is methylprednisolone 1000 mg intravenously daily for 5 days with an optional oral prednisone taper. Patients failing to respond to corticosteroids benefit from plasma exchange, as reviewed in several articles including the recently released management guidelines by the European Federation of Neurologic Societies.[25–27]

Traditional MS treatments, such as β-interferon drugs, have generally been ineffective and, according to some publications, actually deleterious in patients with NMO and are not usually recommended.[28,29] In 2 Japanese studies that involved interferon β-1b subcutaneous injections given every other day, one showed no significant reduction in relapse rates whereas the other found an increase in severe attacks of optic neuritis and transverse myelitis.[30,31] Long-term treatment options include azathioprine (2–3 mg/kg/d) in conjunction with prednisone (1 mg/kg/d for 6 months and then tapered),[26] mycophenolate mofetil (2000 mg daily) combined with prednisone for 6 months,[32] and rituximab (1000 mg intravenously administered twice 2 weeks apart, repeated every 6 months).[33]

Acute Multiple Sclerosis (Marburg Variant)

A fulminant case of MS was described by Otto Marburg in 1906 that is now considered to be an example of a variant form of MS.[34] Marburg described a 30-year-old woman who died 26 days after presenting with headaches, vomiting, confusion, left hemiparesis, gait unsteadiness, and a left extensor plantar response. This eponymously named variant is a monophasic illness with rapid progression that may lead to death from rapidly destructive brain pathology within a few weeks of onset.

The Marburg variant of MS is distinguished from ADEM, despite its overlapping clinical presentation, by the greater asymmetry of lesions, greater tendency to produce focal neurologic findings (eg, hemiparesis, aphasia), and lesser tendency to cause encephalopathy; it is most definitively distinguished pathologically, however. Lesions associated with the Marburg variant lack perivenous demyelination characteristic of ADEM.[35] The large demyelinating lesions are also more destructive than those seen with ADEM or classical MS in terms of myelin loss and axonal injury.

Brainstem involvement with attendant quadriparesis, ophthalmoplegia, ataxia, dysarthria, and dysphagia may prove fatal.[36] Aspiration pneumonia with potentially life-threatening consequences may result from impaired control of secretions; however, much of the morbidity in survivors reflects the severe destructive nature of the supratentorial lesions that predominate in this condition. Hemiparesis and seizures may result from cerebral hemispheric lesions. A decompressive hemicraniectomy was recently performed in a patient with the Marburg variant who developed subfalcine and uncal herniation in the setting of increased intracranial pressure secondary to the presence of large, active supratentorial lesions.[37]

Treatments recommended for this rare condition are high-dose intravenous corticosteroids and immunosuppressants, such as cyclophosphamide.[36] We recommend plasma exchange based on its favorable results in other fulminant cases of MS.

Baló Concentric Sclerosis

Baló concentric sclerosis is a tumefactive type of demyelinating disease characterized pathologically or radiologically based on a whorled pattern of demyelination of varying degrees; typically, it results in a solitary tumorlike lesion, and cerebral and brainstem locations have been reported. Similar to the Marburg variant of MS, Baló concentric sclerosis is usually characterized by a monophasic rapidly progressive course that can result in death within months.[38] **Fig. 2** shows a characteristic Baló lesion with concentric rings. Causes of mortality include cerebral herniation and pneumonia often secondary to aspiration in the setting of bulbar dysfunction. Brainstem lesions may cause diplopia, dysarthria, dysphagia, opththalmoplegia, and ataxia. A patient with cerebral hemispheric lesions may present with hemiparesis and hypoesthesia reminiscent of cerebral infarction.[39]

Young adults are most commonly affected, with the upper age range of published cases approaching the sixth decade of life. The distinctive onion bulblike concentric rings of demyelination and myelination that are best seen by MRI have also been found in patients with prototypic MS and ADEM, and the boundaries between MS and Baló disease are not entirely clear.[40]

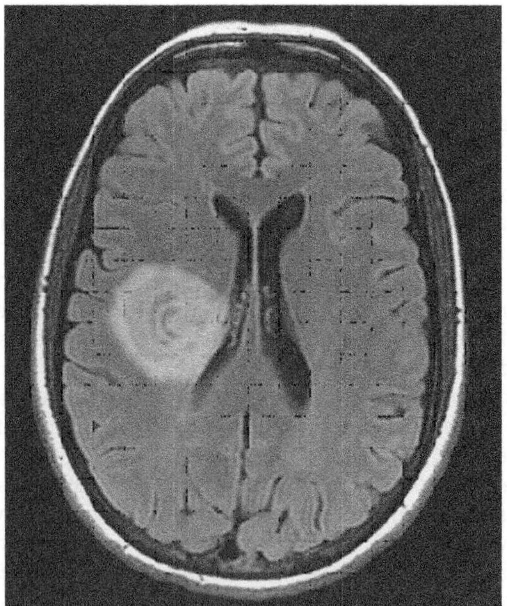

Fig. 2. Baló concentric sclerosis. Axial FLAIR image showing a lesion with a concentric ring pattern in the right centrum semiovale. (*Courtesy of* Dr John Corboy, University of Colorado, Denver, CO.)

Intravenous methylprednisolone in one antemortem case was followed by clinical improvement.[41] In another case, a 16-year-old boy with a biopsy suggestive of Baló concentric sclerosis was treated with adrenocorticotropic hormone and intravenous cyclophosphamide. Improvement was observed after 2 weeks, although the investigators questioned whether the patient may have had ADEM.[42] The patient was later treated with azathioprine. Although optimal management is unclear, treatments used for acute attacks of MS seem to be most appropriate.

Tumefactive Multiple Sclerosis

MS lesions with atypical radiological features bearing a tumorlike appearance are labeled as having tumefactive MS. These radiological features include diameter greater than 2.0 cm, vasogenic edema, mass effect, and partially open ring enhancement (**Fig. 3**).[43] Other diagnoses should be carefully considered before making a diagnosis of tumefactive MS, including high-grade glioma, metastasis, or primary CNS lymphoma. Magnetic resonance spectroscopy or a stereotactic brain biopsy may be helpful (see Demyelinating Disease Mimics and Investigations section). An open-ring sign (incomplete ring of gadolinium enhancement with the nonenhancing section of the ring typically abutting the deep gray matter or cortical ribbon), when present, may distinguish demyelinating disease from a neoplasm; the sensitivity and specificity of this sign are imperfect.[44] An accurate histopathological determination of the MRI abnormality in question can be challenging, but is critical. A highly cellular lesion with atypical astrocytes, some with nuclear debris mimicking mitotic figures (Creutzfeldt cells), as seen in acute demyelinating disease, may lead to misdiagnosis in inexperienced hands as glioblastoma; inappropriate irradiation of an MS lesion may exacerbate demyelinating disease.[45,46]

Tumefactive cerebral hemispheric lesions may produce mass effect, resulting in midline shift and transtentorial herniation.[47] Cerebral herniation may lead to a decreased level of consciousness with eventual progression to stupor, coma, and then death. Such lesions may result in apraxia, aphasia, and cortical blindness.[43] Seizures and

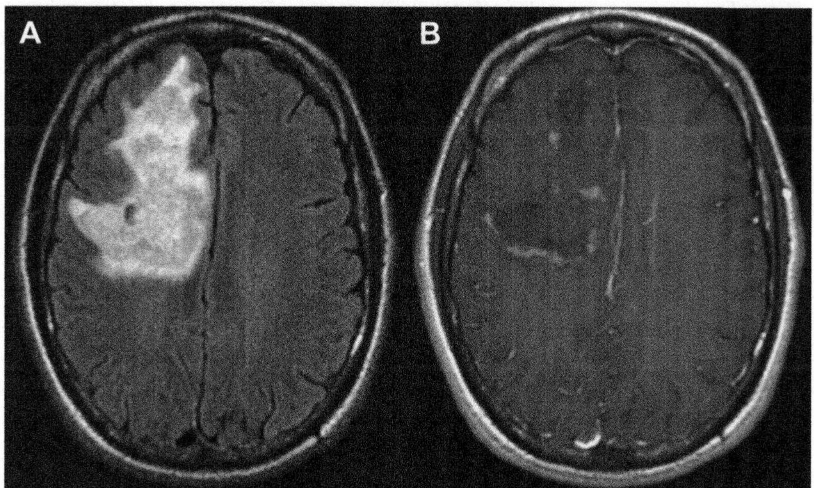

Fig. 3. Tumefactive MS. (*A*) Axial FLAIR image showing a large right frontal lesion with T2 signal abnormality including a small resolving focus of hemorrhage at a biopsy site. (*B*) Axial T1 postcontrast image showing incomplete ring enhancement. (*Courtesy of* Dr Istvan Pirko, Mayo Clinic, Rochester, MN.)

encephalopathy less commonly occur. Brainstem lesions can cause quadriparesis, ophthalmoplegia, and bulbar dysfunction in the form of dysarthria or dysphagia.

A large retrospective study of biopsy-confirmed CNS IDD included 168 patients.[43] **Table 1** summarizes symptoms at disease onset; most had polysymptomatic presentation. All but 13 (7.7%) of the patients had a prebiopsy MRI lesion greater than 2.0 cm in diameter. The median age at onset was 37 years, and the median time to the second attack was nearly 5 years. Half of patients ultimately had recurrent attacks leading to a diagnosis of relapsing-remitting MS, whereas a quarter remained monophasic. Compared with a population-based MS cohort matched for disease duration, the average Expanded Disability Status Scale score in those longer than 10 years from onset in the tumefactive MS group (1.5) was better than the population-based MS group (3.5), justifying aggressive rescue therapy even in critically ill patients.

High-dose intravenous corticosteroids are normally used for the initial treatment of tumefactive MS. In refractory cases, plasmapheresis may be effective.[48,49]

DEMYELINATING DISEASE MIMICS AND INVESTIGATIONS

The differential diagnosis of suspect demyelinating disease is usually of "acute leukoencephalopathies" that are acute or subacute diseases that affect the white matter of the CNS that preferentially, but not exclusively, target the brain.[1] Acute demyelinating disease may also present primarily as acute myelopathy, the differential diagnosis of which will be discussed separately later in this article. Leukoencephalopathy and myelopathy may occur simultaneously, and when this occurs, a diagnosis of demyelinating disease is more likely, although it does not exclude other diseases. Typically, clinicians consider a diagnosis of demyelinating disease when there is prominent involvement of long-fiber tracts and/or optic nerves; however, patients with acute leukoencephalopathies can present primarily or exclusively with symptoms often associated with diseases affecting gray matter, such as coma, cognitive impairment, or seizures. MRI has revolutionized the recognition of acute leukoencephalopathies that present with atypical symptoms by revealing pathology that is confined to or principally affects white matter. Radiologically, brain involvement in demyelinating disease can be unifocal, multifocal, or diffuse. In this section, situations where white matter disease is both the predominant and the causative lesion for the clinical state is considered and not situations wherein extensive

Table 1
Neurologic symptoms at presentation of tumefactive MS

Symptom	%
Motor	50%
Cognitive	43%
Sensory	36%
Cerebellar	31%
Brainstem	24%
Visual field defect	10%
Seizure	6%
Optic neuritis	~5%[a]
Bowel/bladder/sexual dysfunction	~5%[a]

[a] Estimated from bar graph.

Data from Lucchinetti CF, Gavrilova RH, Metz I, et al. Clinical and radiographic spectrum of pathologically confirmed tumefactive multiple sclerosis. Brain 2008;131;1759–75.

ischemic, degenerative white matter changes are detected on MRI scan and thought to be incidental to the clinical presentation. Furthermore, situations where white matter changes are a result of extensive vasogenic cerebral edema reflecting an underlying focal cerebral lesion (eg, cerebral edema in a patient with a meningioma) are not considered.

The differential diagnosis of an acute leukoencephalopathy often focuses on acute inflammatory demyelinating diseases of the CNS; however, a large variety of other conditions in a variety of categories may mimic idiopathic inflammatory disease of the CNS, which may also be unifocal, and some multifocal or diffuse. **Box 1** shows the major conditions to be considered in the differential diagnosis are ischemic vascular conditions, including vasculitis and other noninflammatory vasculopathies, tumors (lymphoma and glioma), infectious disorders, toxic exposures, and other inflammatory disorders including paraneoplastic disorders and autoimmune encephalopathies.

Although a detailed discussion of all of the entities summarized in **Box 1** is beyond the scope of this article, we focus on the general approach, concentrating on recognizing "red flags" that suggest a diagnosis other than inflammatory demyelinating disease. These red flags are broadly classified into 4 groups:

1. Demographic and other risk factors: for example, cardiovascular risk factors (consider embolic strokes); preexisting cancer (consider metastases, coagulopathy or paraneoplastic disorder); known systemic autoimmune disease (consider vasculitis or other direct complication of autoimmune disease; note, however, that NMO frequently coexists with other autoimmune disease; coexisting systemic lupus erythematosus or Sjogren syndrome does not "rule out" NMO); phenotypic features of mitochondrial disorder (short stature, hearing loss, retinitis pigmentosa, migrainelike headaches, seizures)
2. Specific neurologic symptoms, especially ones atypical for demyelinating disease: for example, hearing loss (suggests Susac syndrome, the MRI of which is characteristic but frequently leads to misdiagnosis as ADEM because of the presentation with encephalopathy and multifocal nature of lesions with predilection for the corpus callosum); coexisting migraine (suggests cerebral autosomal dominant arteriopathy with subcortical ischemic leukoencephalopathy [CADASIL], antiphospholipid antibody syndrome or mitochondrial encephalomyopathy)
3. Specific non-CNS syndrome: for example, mucocutaneous ulcers (suggests Behcet syndrome); livedo reticularis (suggests antiphospholipid antibody syndrome); peripheral neuropathy (suggests B12 deficiency, sarcoidosis, or systemic vasculitis)
4. Imaging features. Acute demyelinating lesions are usually not single lesions, they exert relatively little mass effect, and they often manifest an "open ring" pattern of enhancement (discontinuity of a ring of gadolinium enhancement along the "trailing edge" of a tumefactive lesion, which, when present, is helpful in suggesting that demyelinating disease is the pathology). Red flags include prominent mass effect (suggests tumor, infection); homogeneous pattern of enhancement in some/most lesions (suggests neurosarcoidosis or lymphoma); lack of enhancement in an acute lesion (suggests progressive multifocal leukoencephalopathy, ischemia, paraneoplastic disorder, although can be seen occasionally in ADEM and does not rule out demyelinating disease).

A general approach to the differential diagnosis is shown in **Fig. 4**. As illustrated, the index of suspicion for an alternative diagnosis and the entity suspected based on the 4 categories of "red flags" outlined previously is a critical first step. Often, it is necessary

Box 1
Differential diagnosis of acute leukoencephalopathy

1. Inflammatory
    a. Idiopathic inflammatory demyelinating disease
    b. Drug-induced inflammatory demyelinating disease (- 5FU/levamisole[a]; TNFα scavengers)
    c. Behcet syndrome
    d. Hashimoto (autoimmune) encephalopathy[a]
    e. Other (eg, SLE, Sjogren syndrome)
    f. Neurosarcoidosis
2. Ischemic/Vascular
    a. Thromboembolic (cardiac, arterial, paradoxic)
    b. Vasculopathy
        i. Moyamoya
        ii. Retinocochlear vasculopathy of Susac
        iii. CADASIL
    c. Vasculitis
        i. Systemic
        ii. Primary CNS
        iii. Drug-induced
        iv. Infection-associated
    d. Venous infarction owing to venous sinus thrombosis
    e. Other
        i. Degos disease[a]
3. Metabolic/Nutritional
    a. Mitochondrial encephalomyopathy
    b. Vitamin B12 deficiency
    c. Central pontine myelinolysis
4. Infectious
    a. Cerebritis/abscess
    b. Viral encephalitis
    c. Progressive multifocal leukoencephalopathy
    d. Whipple disease[a]
    e. HIV
        i. Primary infection
        ii. Opportunistic infection
    f. SSPE and other slow viral illnesses[a]
    g. Neurosyphilis
5. Postinfectious
6. Radiation induced

7. Toxic
   a. Chemotherapy
      i. Methotrexate
      ii. Nitrous oxide (produces acute B12 deficiency)
   b. Solvents
   c. Carbon monoxide
   d. Clioquinol[a]
   e. Lead
8. Genetic
   a. Mitochondrial encephalopathy
   b. CADASIL[a]
9. Oncologic
   a. Neoplastic
      i. CNS glioma
      ii. Gliomatosis cerebri
      iii. Primary CNS lymphoma
      iv. Intravascular lymphoma (neoplastic angioendotheliomatosis)
   b. Paraneoplastic-limbic encephalitis
      i. Progressive spasticity and dementia associated with anti-amphiphysin antibodies[a]
      ii. Brainstem encephalitis
10. Miscellaneous
   a. Posterior reversible leukoencephalopathy
   b. CLIPPERS (Chronic lymphocytic inflammation with pontine perivascular enhancement responsive to steroids)[a]

Abbreviations: 5FU, 5 fluorouracil; CADASIL, cerebral autosomal dominant arteriopathy with subcortical ischemic leukoencephalopathy; CNS, central nervous system; HIV, human immunodeficiency virus; SLE, systemic lupus erythematosus; SSPE, subacute sclerosis panencephalitis; TNF, tumor necrosis factor.

[a] Entities currently thought to be rare, although some are recently recognized and accurate estimates of their occurrence are unavailable.

Data from Weinshenker BG, Lucchinetti CF. Acute leukoencephalopathies: Differential diagnosis and investigation. Neurologist 1998;4:148–66.

to begin treatment before alternative diagnoses can be excluded with certainty. There are relatively few contraindications to brief courses of high-dose corticosteroids, which may also benefit neoplasms, systemic autoimmune disorders, and other potential mimics, although they could potentially exacerbate some entities, such as progressive multifocal leukoencephalopathy. Conversely, response to corticosteroids should be interpreted conservatively and not considered as diagnostic of inflammatory demyelinating disease. Many disease entities, including lymphoma, cerebral edema of any cause, and even cord compression, may benefit from corticosteroids. Rapid and dramatic benefit with remission is suggestive of demyelinating disease in a clinically suspicious context, however. Identification of red flags and targeted investigation

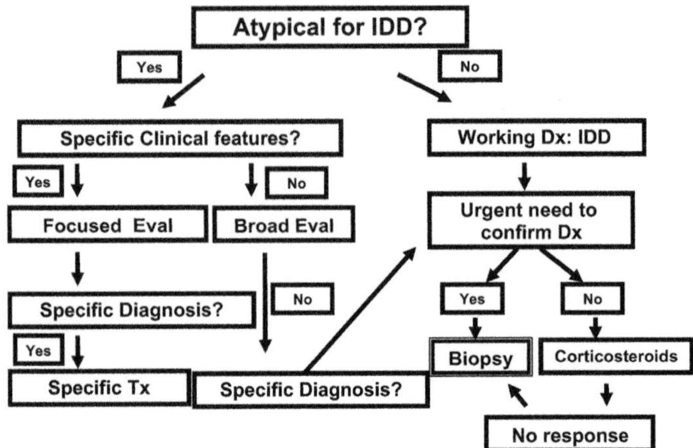

Fig. 4. Diagnostic algorithm. DX, diagnosis; Eval, evaluation; Tx, treatment.

with relatively noninvasive tests based on high index of suspicion of a given diagnosis is preferred; however, when a patient is rapidly deteriorating or when corticosteroids fail and a patient has severe neurologic disability, a brain biopsy is often the most definitive way to establish a diagnosis of demyelinating disease when an adequate biopsy can be safely obtained (difficult or impossible for some brainstem and spinal cord lesions or deep cerebral lesions) of an acute, typically gadolinium-enhancing lesion. When the situation is less acute, a variety of ancillary investigations shown in **Table 2** may be informative, although when the index of suspicion is low, these investigations often do not yield a diagnosis when ordered as a broad panel to rule out a variety of potential mimics.

Neuroimaging has acquired recent interest as a tool to distinguish neoplasms from tumefactive demyelinating disease.[50–53] Indeed, in some pediatric metabolic disorders and mitochondrial disorders, the findings on MRS may be diagnostic.[52] The findings in demyelinating disease evolve over the course of the lesion[54] and are nonspecific.[55] In general, there is an increase in choline, lipids, and myoinositol, reflecting myelin breakdown, an increase in lactate reflecting inflammation, and a decrease in *N*-acetylaspartate reflecting neuronal injury.[52] The findings overlap with those seen in ischemic and neoplastic disorders, however. A persistent reduction in *N*-acetylaspartate accompanied by sustained reduction in magnetization transfer ratio, reflecting myelin loss, is suggestive of demyelination, but acute decreases in *N*-acetylaspartate may be transient and recovery may occur as a result of resolution of edema.[54] Recently, increased levels of glutamate and glutamine have also been reported in demyelinating lesions.[50,51] Another recently observed imaging characteristic of demyelinating disease, although perhaps not entirely specific, has been peripheral lesion restriction on diffusion-weighted imaging.[51] These techniques should be used in the context of a multimodal approach of MR that includes conventional MRI (including analysis of gadolinium enhancement and diffusion-weighted imaging) and advanced MR techniques, including magnetization transfer, diffusion tensor imaging, and spectroscopy.

Brain biopsy may be diagnostic of acute demyelinating disease, but may be misinterpreted. Acute demyelinating lesions are typically hypercellular, and therefore may be misdiagnosed as brain tumors. The key features are the typical presence of large numbers of foamy macrophages with myelin debris, perivascular inflammatory cells,

Table 2
Non-MRI diagnostic evaluation of leukoencephalopathy of unknown cause

Source	Test	Reason
CSF	IgG index	Inflammatory demyelinating (MS)
	Oligoclonal bands	SSPE
		HIV
		Other Infection
	Measles antibody titer	SSPE
	PCR	Whipple disease
	Tropheryma whippelii	PML
	JC virus	Viral encephalitis
	Other (HSV, CMV, VZV)	
	Lactate/Pyruvate	Mitochondrial encephalopathy
Echocardiogram		Endocarditis
		Cardioembolic source
		Potential for paradoxic embolism
Ophthalmologic examination, including fluorescein angiography	Evidence of retinal vasculitis?	Susac syndrome
		Other vasculitis (eg, Eale disease)
	Evidence of uveitis/pars planitis?	MS
		Sarcoidosis
		Lymphoma
Cerebral angiography		Vasculitis
		Vasculopathy (eg, moyamoya disease)
		Atheroembolic disease
		Venous sinus thrombosis
Other biopsies	Conjunctiva	Sarcoidosis
	Small bowel	Whipple disease
	Skin	Systemic lupus erythematosus
		Vasculitis
		CADASIL

Abbreviations: CADASIL, cerebral autosomal dominant arteriopathy with subcortical ischemic leukoencephalopathy; CMV, cytomegalovirus; HIV, human immunodeficiency virus; HSV, herpes simplex virus; IgG, immunoglobulin G; JC, initials of patients in whom causative virus for PML first discovered; MRI, magnetic resonance imaging; MS, multiple sclerosis; PCR, polymerase chain reaction; PML, progressive multifocal leukoencephalopathy; SSPE, subacute sclerosing panencephalitis; VZV, varicella zoster virus.

and an intimate admixture of histiocytes with reactive astrocytes, occasionally with Creutzfeldt cells, which are prominent astrocytes with nuclear debris that may be mistaken for mitotic figures (see previous discussion of tumefactive demyelinating disease). Neuromyelitis optica lesions have some overlapping characteristics but are notable for the prominence of neutrophils and eosinophils in these lesions, prominent gray matter involvement, prominent perivascular complement and immunoglobulin,[3] and selective loss of immunoreactive aquaporin-4 in acute lesions.[56] As long-term treatment of NMO differs from MS, it is important to differentiate NMO from MS. ADEM lesions typically lack confluent demyelination but have prominent perivascular mononuclear inflammation; demyelination is typically mild and surrounds the zones of perivascular inflammation.[2] Although acute disseminated encephalomyelitis may be associated with severe encephalopathy or coma, it typically causes less necrosis and the long-term outcome in survivors is favorable. Approximately 30% of cases are misdiagnosed, however, based on current clinical criteria, as ADEM is ultimately diagnosed with a fulminant form of MS, and it is precisely in such cases that an early diagnosis and aggressive early immunosuppression may be most needed. Brain biopsy may show specific abnormalities leading to alternative diagnoses, either with standard staining techniques (eg, granulomas, vasculitis, neoplasms) or with special immunopathological stains, such as staining for light chain immunoglobulin fragments to detect lymphoma, or with other special pathologic techniques, such as in situ hybridization for JC virus for progressive multifocal leukoencephalopathy.

Inflammatory demyelinating disease may present with an acute myelitis leading to paraplegia or quadriplegia, urinary retention, and occasionally respiratory failure. The most important item in the evaluation is to rule out structural causes of myelopathy with MRI.[57] The presence of a symptomatic intrinsic spinal cord lesion still has a broad differential diagnosis, which includes infectious myelitis as may occur with certain herpes viruses, such as varicella zoster; other inflammatory disorders, such as sarcoidosis; vascular disorders (vasculitis, embolic infarction, including cholesterol embolism, hypoperfusion syndromes, hemorrhage, and venous hypertension in association with arteriovenous fistula); neoplasms (glioma and ependymoma are the most frequent); paraneoplastic disorders often presenting as progressive “tractopathy”; structural disorders, such as syringomyelia; and occasionally metabolic disorders, such as B12 or copper deficiency. Differential diagnosis, as is true for leukoencephalopathies, depends on index of suspicion. Often corticosteroid treatment is urgently necessary for presumptive inflammatory demyelinating transverse myelitis before a final diagnosis. In addition to MRI, helpful investigations include CSF analysis (IgG index, oligoclonal bands, cell count, polymerase chain reaction [PCR] when viral infection suspected); serology (NMO-IgG for NMO spectrum disorder; SSA/Ro and SSB/La, which are also associated with NMO-associated myelopathy and increase risk of recurrent myelitis; antinuclear antibody; antiphospholipid antibody); B12 and methylmalonic acid and copper in patients with posterior column sensory syndrome suggestive of subacute combined degeneration of the cord; chest CT scan is indicated when neurosarcoidosis is suspected.

MANAGEMENT OF CNS INFLAMMATORY DEMYELINATING DISEASE EMERGENCIES

Management of patients' CNS IDD emergencies can be divided into 3 categories: supportive care, acute remission-inducing therapy, and therapy of associated complication.

Supportive Care

Patients with severe attacks of CNS IDD may deteriorate rapidly, requiring airway support or mechanical ventilation. Although a detailed discussion of respiratory and other supportive care is beyond the scope of this article, it is appropriate to emphasize that aggressive *supportive care* is recommended because of the high frequency of reversibility of acute neurologic deficits experienced by patients with IDD. Critically ill patients are at risk of pressure ulcers, deep venous thrombosis, or respiratory or urinary tract infections; management requires a multidisciplinary team.

Acute Remission-Inducing Treatment

Therapy for the severe attack of CNS IDD generally consists of corticosteroids and plasma exchange. Intravenous corticosteroids are indicated for patients with a suspected severe or catastrophic demyelinating event even before defining the specific type of underlying CNS IDD, such as distinguishing between ADEM from acute severe MS or a severe attack of MS or between MS or NMO. High-dose methylprednisolone, typically 1 g daily intravenously for 3 to 5 days, is recommended for acute MS attacks.[58] There are no controlled studies that specifically aimed at studying the efficacy of corticosteroids in catastrophic CNS IDD. It is widely thought that patients with acute severe MS (Marburg variant) usually die of their illness based on the literature, but this is likely the result of reporting biases of fatal cases. This impression has led to therapeutic nihilism; however, we have treated patients who have survived and experience prolonged quiescent periods if they survive their acute or subacute illness. Corticosteroids have rapid onset of action. They reduce inflammatory edema by reducing capillary permeability as early as 8 hours after administration.[59] The radiological accompaniment is a reduction in gadolinium enhancement on MRI. Corticosteroids induce monocytopenia, and reduce the number of CD4 lymphocytes and B cells. In addition, they reduce proinflammatory cytokines.[59] Animal models show that glucocorticoids may prevent axonal injury when administered early in the disease.[60]

Plasma exchange (PLEX) is now widely accepted to be an effective treatment of severe attacks of CNS IDD, and perhaps the treatment of choice. Its efficacy in this context is supported by one randomized controlled trial (class I evidence) for effectiveness of PLEX in severe acute demyelinating attacks of MS, ADEM, transverse myelitis, and NMO. Plasma exchange is achieved by separation of plasma from the cellular blood elements, discarding plasma, and replacing it with colloid fluid. In the United States, the process is accomplished typically with a centrifuge device, although a variety of filtration devices, occasionally followed by a second selective form of filtration or immunoadsorption, are used outside of the United States to accomplish similar or more complete Ig removal; PLEX may require placement of a double-lumen central venous catheter, although it can be accomplished via large-bore peripheral venous catheters if venous access is satisfactory. Evidence for efficacy of PLEX in severe CNS IDD was robustly demonstrated by Weinshenker and colleagues[14] in a randomized controlled crossover study of 22 patients with severe attacks of CNS IDD who failed to respond to intravenous corticosteroids, including those with transverse myelitis, ADEM, NMO, and MS. Patients were randomized to 7 sessions of true versus sham exchanges over 14 days. Nine patients experienced moderate to marked improvement, 8 of whom received true PLEX and 1 sham therapy. After crossover, 3 of 8 who had received sham exchange in the first treatment period and had not improved, experienced moderate to marked improvement after receiving active treatment in the second treatment period, whereas none of the 6 patients who failed active plasma exchange improved after crossing over to sham treatment. Several subsequent uncontrolled prospective or retrospective studies that followed this one confirmed this finding in patients with severe attacks of CNS IDD, including transverse myelitis, MS, and NMO. Keegan and colleagues[5] retrospectively studied patients treated with PLEX and found 59 patients with severe episodes of CNS IDD, including 22 patients with MS, 10 with NMO, and 10 with ADEM. The investigators found that 44.1% of patients showed moderate or marked response and that early therapy (within 20 days of symptom onset), male sex, and preservation of tendon reflexes predicted a positive response. Llufriu and colleagues[61] conducted a retrospective study of 41 patients with CNS IDD episodes treated with PLEX. Thirty-nine percent of patients showed improvement at hospital discharge and 63% at 6-month follow-up. The mechanism of action of PLEX is suspected to be the result of removal of humoral circulating factors, although alterations in T-cell behavior following PLEX have also been documented. In NMO, antibodies to the dominant CNS water channel AQP-4 (NMO IgG) have been shown to be pathogenic in the disease. Therefore, removal of this antibody and complement might explain its therapeutic efficacy in NMO. In addition, other humoral factors, including proinflammatory cytokines and chemokines, likely have an important role. On the other hand, MS is associated with cellular and humoral mechanisms and the exact mechanism of PLEX efficacy in acute MS attacks is uncertain, although the presence of antibody and complement in biopsies from patients undergoing plasma exchange showed strong concordance with favorable response.[5] Complications of PLEX in general relate to the venous access (risk of sepsis or accidental arterial puncture), hypotension, or citrate toxicity; angiotensin-converting inhibitor medications may cause systemic reactions, such as flushing, hypotension, and dyspnea owing to impaired bradykinin metabolism in patients treated with immunoadsorption. There are no PLEX-related complications that are unique to patients with CNS IDD.

The role of cyclophosphamide in treatment of severe attacks of CNS IDD has not been studied systematically. A retrospective study of patients with transverse myelitis showed improvement in outcome.[62] The study, however, was limited by the retrospective nature, variability in baseline patient characteristics, and nonstratification of patients based on specific underlying cause of transverse myelitis (MS, NMO, isolated transverse myelitis). Cyclophosphamide may have a role in chronic therapy once patients recover the severe attack in patients at risk of relapse.

Pradhan and colleagues[63] reported a series of 4 children (ages 1, 4, 12, and 14 years) with ADEM who did not respond to intravenous corticosteroids and subsequently following treatment with IVIG improved markedly. All 4 patients were in critical care units with encephalopathy and quadripersis and showed response to therapy within 2 to 3 days of IVIG therapy and were able to ambulate over 10 to 14 days.

The need for and choice of a chronic immunotherapy of CNS IDD is determined by the underlying demyelinating disease context; for example, immunomodulatory therapies effective for MS are not effective for NMO. A detailed discussion of chronic maintenance immunotherapy is beyond the scope of this article.

Emergency Complications

The potential medical complications of CNS IDD are diverse, as shown in **Box 2**. They may result from unique functions related to the site of the lesion (eg, neurogenic pulmonary edema with certain brainstem lesions), may result from particularly severe inflammation (eg, mass effect and cerebral herniation), or may reflect a unique pathophysiology of a specific inflammatory demyelinating disease (eg, posterior reversible encephalopathy in the context of NMO owing to disruption of brain water channel function). Management of these complications is generally the same as for that of the same complications in other settings, but also involves management of the underlying inflammatory demyelination, as described in the previous section on management of demyelinating emergencies.

Box 2
Emergency complications of CNS IDD

Raised intracranial pressure and cerebral herniation

Neurogenic pulmonary edema

Myocardial dysfunction

Hypothermia

Posterior reversible encephalopathy syndrome

Aspiration pneumonia

Large CNS inflammatory demyelinating lesions may result in cerebral edema and consequently raised intracranial pressure (ICP) in the setting of tumefactive multiple sclerosis or acute severe multiple sclerosis (Marburg variant), or in diffuse CNS IDD (ADEM). This complication should be treated aggressively with measures to reduce ICP, including elevation of head of the bed, fluid restriction, blood pressure control, hyperventilation (to a target pCO_2 28–32 mm Hg), intravenous mannitol (1.0–1.5 g/kg of 20% solution rapid infusion), and, when necessary, with phenobarbital coma and/or hypothermia.

Table 3 summarizes several reported cases with resistant focal cerebral edema treated with hemicraniectomy that include focal tumefactive lesions that occurred in the context of different types of CNS IDD.[37,47,64,65] The development of raised ICP occurred at different tempos and the management of raised ICP and of the primary CNS IDD differed in these cases. Mass effect is uncommon in CNS IDD, but may occur with tumefactive demyelinating lesions, acute severe MS, or ADEM. The reasons why certain patients with CNS IDD experience mass effect is unknown. The clinical outcome relates to the degree of injury and is a combined effect of the cerebral edema and raised ICP and primary pathologic process of the demyelinating disease. Hemicraniectomy should be considered in patients with tumefactive lesions with refractory raised ICP as a life-saving measure.

Respiratory failure may occur in patients with inflammatory demyelinating disease. Patients with NMO or MS with lesions involving the brainstem and cervical cord may develop neurogenic respiratory failure. Respiratory failure in the context of an acute attack is less common in patients with multiple sclerosis, who typically develop respiratory failure in the setting of severe chronic preexisting disability.[66,67] Mechanical ventilation is indicated in these patients with catastrophic brainstem attacks, while aggressive treatment for underlying inflammatory demyelinating disease is administered. Respiratory failure in patients with MS is often caused by aspiration pneumonia in patients with chronic progressive disease; mechanical ventilation and tracheostomy in these patients is associated with overall improved survival.

Neurogenic pulmonary edema may occur in patients with head and/or neck injury, subarachnoid hemorrhage, seizures, brain tumors, and Reye syndrome. The most well recognized lesion in the setting of IDD associated with neurogenic pulmonary edema is a lesion of the nucleus tractus solitarius located in the medulla oblongata accompanied by neurologic signs of medullary involvement, such as rotary nystagmus, dysphonia, unilateral paralysis of the soft palate, mental status changes, diplopia, or hemifacial numbness.[68,69] It may, however, occur as a solitary manifestation of a lesion in this location.[70] A single patient with MS is reported to have developed unilateral neurogenic pulmonary edema responsive to intravenous steroid therapy.[71] Animal models show that lesions of the nucleus of the tractus solitarius cause increased pulmonary arterial pressure and pulmonary lymph flow resulting in pulmonary edema.[72] The pathophysiology underlying this rare complication is likely multifactorial and includes altered vascular permeability and abnormal myocardial function owing to alteration in central sympathetic output. Other possible causes include proinflammatory cytokines and chemokines (tumor necrosis factor α, interleukin-1β, and interleukin-6) that may be induced by acute neurologic disorders. Focal structural lesions have been implicated in neurogenic pulmonary edema, such as lesions of the preoptic chiasm that are believed to cause pulmonary edema as a release phenomenon as a result of loss of the inhibitory effect of the preoptic chiasm.[73]

Acute heart failure is another rare complication of MS[74,75] that may result in pulmonary edema or cardiogenic shock. It is attributed to variation in sympathetic tone as has been invoked as a potential explanation of pulmonary edema. One reported patient

Table 3
Hemicraniectomy experience for cerebral herniation in central nervous system demyelinating disease

Author/Year	Age, y/ Gender	Interval (Onset-Craniectomy)	Symptom Onset	MRI Findings	Therapy Before Hemicraniectomy	Therapy Following Hemicraniectomy	Outcome/Interval from Hemicraniectomy
Ahmed et al,[65] 2010	38 F	2 d	Ataxia, hemiparesis, coma	Monofocal	Mannitol, dexamethasone	Intravenous methylprednisolone pulse therapy	Minimal deficit (Interval NS)
Von Stuckrad-Barre et al,[64] 2003	34 F	6 d	Hemiplegia	Monofocal	Intravenous methylprednisolone, midazolam, mannitol	Intravenous immunoglobulin	Minimal deficit (3 mo)
Nilsson et al,[47] 2009	50 F	2 wk	Seizures, dysphasia, hemiparesis	Multifocal	Betamethasone	High-dose intravenous corticosteroids pulse therapy	Minimal deficit (6 wk)
González Sánchez et al,[37] 2010	31 F	NS	Coma	Monofocal	PLEX, IVIG, barbiturate coma	No further treatment	Minimal deficit (3 mo)

Abbreviations: IVIG, intravenous immunoglobulin; NS, not specified; PLEX, Plasma exchange.

had myocardial impairment in addition to unilateral pulmonary edema associated with severe left ventricular dysfunction on transthoracic echocardiography.[71] She was treated with aggressive diuresis in addition to intravenous steroid therapy and improved within 24 hours. Another study reported acute heart failure in a 19-year-old woman with a 3-week history of progressive bulbar symptoms and MRI evidence of multiple T2 hyperintensities.[74] She developed acute cardiac failure and cardiogenic shock with signs of multiorgan failure. The patient was treated with implantation of a left ventricular assist device. Myocardial function recovered spontaneously after 2.5 months and the device was successfully explanted. There was no histopathological evidence of myocarditis. Eight weeks later, the patient had a clinical relapse of MS. Whether this is complication is similar in pathogenesis to stress cardiomyopathy (Takotsubo cardiomyopathy) is unclear.

Hypothermia is an uncommon and easily unrecognized complication that typically occurs in patients with advanced MS and manifests as episodic encephalopathy (**Box 3**).[76,77] Typically, hypothermia occurs in patients with advanced disability in the setting of chronic demyelinating disease and not in the setting of an acute inflammatory attack. Body temperature may decline to as low as 29°C and thus a thermometer capable of reliably recording hypothermia is essential to make the diagnosis. Lower temperatures are often associated with other systemic symptoms, such as thrombocytopenia, coagulopathy, or neurologic symptoms, such as delusions, dysarthria, bradycardia, and/or miosis.[76] Patients with hypothermia demonstrated MRI abnormalities in the hypothalamic region.[76,78] Severe episodes may lead to death. Subacute onset of neurologic decline is typical. Patients respond to rewarming within 48 hours.[78] Recurrent episodes were reported to respond to steroid therapy, perhaps suggesting an underlying inflammatory etiology.

PRES is a clinical-radiographic condition of multiple symptoms, including seizures, encephalopathy, headache, and visual symptoms, such as cortical blindness, associated with reversible areas of subcortical brain edema on MRI. Lesions occur preferentially in the posterior areas of the brain. It occurs in hypertensive emergencies and is associated with eclampsia. It was reported in a recent series of 5 patients with NMO, which likely reflects excess occurrence in this subtype of IDD. The postulated pathophysiology in this context is thought to relate to depletion of aquaporin-4 (AQP4) water channels, which is known to occur when cells are exposed to NMO-IgG in the absence of complement.[79] Autopsy samples show extensive loss of AQP4 regardless of lesion stage in the spinal cord lesions of patients with NMO.[56] AQP4 knock out mice are prone to vasogenic edema. PRES is treated with supportive care and corticosteroids to reduce inflammatory activity of NMO; most lesions resolve within 7 days.[24]

Box 3
Vignette: hypothermia presenting as encephalopathy in a patient with secondary progressive MS

A 60-year-old man with MS for more than 20 years with a secondary progressive course presented with slowness of thinking and speech that progressed to coma. He had a persistent core body temperature of 32°C. After improving upon rewarming, he experienced recurrence of symptoms with subsequent drops in core body temperature. His optimal body temperature was 35°C and once the temperature dropped below 33°C, he developed slowness of speech and thinking. Neurologic examination revealed mild cognitive impairment. He had bilateral internuclear ophthalmoplegia, mild cerebellar dysarthria, cerebellar incoordination in the upper extremities, and paraplegia. Head MRI showed chronic MS lesions with no evidence of contrast enhancement.

REFERENCES

1. Weinshenker BG, Lucchinetti CF. Acute leukoencephalopathies: differential diagnosis and investigation. Neurologist 1998;4(3):148–66.
2. Young NP, Weinshenker BG, Parisi JE, et al. Perivenous demyelination: association with clinically defined acute disseminated encephalomyelitis and comparison with pathologically confirmed multiple sclerosis. Brain 2010;133:333–48.
3. Lucchinetti CF, Mandler RN, McGavern D, et al. A role for humoral mechanisms in the pathogenesis of Devic's neuromyelitis optica. Brain 2002;125:1450–61.
4. Lucchinetti CF, Bruck W, Lassmann H. Evidence for pathogenic heterogeneity in multiple sclerosis. Ann Neurol 2004;56:308.
5. Keegan M, König F, McClelland R, et al. Relation between humoral pathological changes in multiple sclerosis and response to therapeutic plasma exchange. Lancet 2005;366:579–82.
6. Tenembaum S, Chitnis T, Ness J, et al. Acute disseminated encephalomyelitis. Neurology 2007;68:S23–36.
7. Menge T, Hemmer B, Nessler S, et al. Acute disseminated encephalomyelitis: an update. Arch Neurol 2005;62:1673–80.
8. de Seze J. Multiple sclerosis: clinical aspects, acute disseminated encephalomyelitis, neuromyellitis optica and other inflammatory variants. Rev Neurol 2007;163: 647–50.
9. Young NP, Weinshenker BG, Lucchinetti CF. Acute disseminated encephalomyelitis: current understanding and controversies. Semin Neurol 2008;28:84–94.
10. Poser CM, Brinar VV. Disseminated encephalomyelitis and multiple sclerosis: two different diseases—a critical review. Acta Neurol Scand 2007;116:201–6.
11. Krupp LB, Banwell B, Tenembaum S. Consensus definitions proposed for pediatric multiple sclerosis and related disorders. Neurology 2007;68:S7–12.
12. Sonneville R, Klein I, de Broucker T, et al. Post-infectious encephalitis in adults: diagnosis and management. J Infect 2009;58:321–8.
13. Hart MN, Earle KM. Haemorrhagic and perivenous encephalitis: a clinical-pathological review of 38 cases. J Neurol Neurosurg Psychiatry 1975;38:585–91.
14. Weinshenker BG, O'Brien PC, Petterson TM, et al. A randomized trial of plasma exchange in acute central nervous system inflammatory demyelinating disease. Ann Neurol 1999;46:878–86.
15. Dodick DW, Silber MH, Noseworthy JH, et al. Acute disseminated encephalomyelitis after accidental injection of a hog vaccine: successful treatment with plasmapheresis. Mayo Clin Proc 1998;73:1193–5.
16. Cortese I, Chaudhry V, So YT, et al. Evidence-based guideline update: plasmapheresis in neurologic disorders: report of the Therapeutics and Technology Assessment Subcommittee of the American Academy of Neurology. Neurology 2011;76:294–300.
17. Weinstein R. Therapeutic apheresis in neurological disorders: a survey of the evidence in support of current category I and II indications for therapeutic plasma exchange. J Clin Apher 2008;23:196–201.
18. Marchioni E, Marinou-Aktipi K, Uggetti C, et al. Effectiveness of intravenous immunoglobulin treatment in adult patients with steroid-resistant monophasic or recurrent acute disseminated encephalomyelitis. J Neurol 2002;249:100–4.
19. Lennon VA, Kryzer TJ, Pittock SJ, et al. IgG marker of optic-spinal multiple sclerosis binds to the aquaporin-4 water channel. J Exp Med 2005;202:473–7.
20. Wingerchuk DM, Lennon VA, Pittock SJ, et al. Revised diagnostic criteria for neuromyelitis optica. Neurology 2006;66(10):1485–9.

21. Wingerchuk DM, Hogancamp WF, O'Brien PC, et al. The clinical course of neuromyelitis optica (Devic's syndrome). Neurology 1999;53:1107–14.
22. Popescu BF, Lennon VA, Parisi JE, et al. Neuromyelitis optica unique area postrema lesions: nausea, vomiting, and pathogenic implications. Neurology 2011; 76:1229–37.
23. Poppe AY, Lapierre Y, Melancon D, et al. Neuromyelitis optica with hypothalamic involvement. Mult Scler 2005;11:617–21.
24. Magaña SM, Matiello M, Pittock SJ, et al. Posterior reversible encephalopathy syndrome in neuromyelitis optica spectrum disorders. Neurology 2009;72:712–7.
25. Wingerchuk DM, Weinshenker BG. Neuromyelitis optica. Curr Treat Options Neurol 2008;10:55–66.
26. Wingerchuk DM. Diagnosis and treatment of neuromyelitis optica. Neurologist 2007;13:2–11.
27. Sellner J, Boggild M, Clanet M, et al. EFNS guidelines on diagnosis and management of neuromyelitis optica. Eur J Neurol 2010;17:1019–32.
28. Shimizu J, Hatanaka Y, Hasegawa M, et al. IFNbeta-1b may severely exacerbate Japanese optic-spinal MS in neuromyelitis optica spectrum. Neurology 2010;75: 1423–7.
29. Weinshenker BG, Wingerchuk DM. Japanese optic-spinal MS: is it MS or neuromyelitis optica and does the answer dictate treatment? Neurology 2010;75:1404–5.
30. Tanaka M, Tanaka K, Komori M. Interferon-beta(1b) treatment in neuromyelitis optica. Eur Neurol 2009;62:167–70.
31. Warabi Y, Matsumoto Y, Hayashi H. Interferon beta-1b exacerbates multiple sclerosis with severe optic nerve and spinal cord demyelination. J Neurol Sci 2007; 252:57–61.
32. Jacob A, Matiello M, Weinshenker BG, et al. Treatment of neuromyelitis optica with mycophenolate mofetil: retrospective analysis of 24 patients. Arch Neurol 2009;66:1128–33.
33. Jacob A, Weinshenker BG, Violich I, et al. Treatment of neuromyelitis optica with rituximab: retrospective analysis of 25 patients. Arch Neurol 2008;65:1443–8.
34. Marburg O. Die sogenannte "acute Multiple Sklerose". Jahrb Neurol Psychiatr 1906;27:211–312.
35. Mendez MF, Pogacar S. Malignant monophasic multiple sclerosis or "Marburg's disease". Neurology 1988;38:1153–5.
36. Johnson MD, Lavin P, Whetsell WO Jr. Fulminant monophasic multiple sclerosis, Marburg's type. J Neurol Neurosurg Psychiatry 1990;53:918–21.
37. González Sánchez JJ, Nora JE, de Notaris M, et al. A case of malignant monophasic multiple sclerosis (Marburg's disease type) successfully treated with decompressive hemicraniectomy. J Neurol Neurosurg Psychiatr 2010;81(9): 1056–7.
38. Capello E, Mancardi GL. Marburg type and Balo's concentric sclerosis: rare and acute variants of multiple sclerosis. Neurol Sci 2004;25(Suppl 4):S361–3.
39. Mowry EM, Woo JH, Ances BM. Balo's concentric sclerosis presenting as a stroke-like syndrome. Nat Clin Pract Neurol 2007;3:349–54.
40. Canellas AR, Gols AR, Izquierdo JR, et al. Idiopathic inflammatory-demyelinating diseases of the central nervous system. Neuroradiology 2007;49:393–409.
41. Spiegel M, Kruger H, Hofmann E, et al. MRI study of Balo's concentric sclerosis before and after immunosuppressive therapy. J Neurol 1989;236:487–8.
42. Louboutin JP, Elie B. Treatment of Balo's concentric sclerosis with immunosuppressive drugs followed by multimodality evoked potentials and MRI. Muscle Nerve 1995;18:1478–80.

43. Lucchinetti CF, Gavrilova RH, Metz I, et al. Clinical and radiographic spectrum of pathologically confirmed tumefactive multiple sclerosis. Brain 2008;131: 1759–75.
44. Masdeu JC, Quinto C, Olivera C, et al. Open-ring imaging sign: highly specific for atypical brain demyelination. Neurology 2000;54:1427–33.
45. Creutzfeldt HG. Zur Frage der sogenannten akuten multiplen Sklerose (Encephalomeyelitis disseminata non purulenta scleroticans acuta). Zugleich Mitteilung einer besonderen Entstehungsart von Riesenzellen. Arch Psych 1923;68: 485–517.
46. Miller RC, Lachance DH, Lucchinetti CF, et al. Multiple sclerosis, brain radiotherapy, and risk of neurotoxicity: the Mayo Clinic experience. Int J Radiat Oncol Biol Phys 2006;66:1178–86.
47. Nilsson P, Larsson EM, Kahlon B, et al. Tumefactive demyelinating disease treated with decompressive craniectomy. Eur J Neurol 2009;16(5):639–42.
48. Mao-Draayer Y, Braff S, Pendlebury W, et al. Treatment of steroid-unresponsive tumefactive demyelinating disease with plasma exchange. Neurology 2002;59: 1074–7.
49. Paus S, Promse A, Schmidt S, et al. Treatment of steroid-unresponsive tumefactive demyelinating disease with plasma exchange. Neurology 2003;61:1022 [author reply: 1022].
50. Masu K, Beppu T, Fujiwara S, et al. Proton magnetic resonance spectroscopy and diffusion-weighted imaging of tumefactive demyelinating plaque. Neurol Med Chir (Tokyo) 2009;49:430–3.
51. Malhotra HS, Jain KK, Agarwal A, et al. Characterization of tumefactive demyelinating lesions using MR imaging and in-vivo proton MR spectroscopy. Mult Scler 2009;15:193–203.
52. Cecil KM, Kos RS. Magnetic resonance spectroscopy and metabolic imaging in white matter diseases and pediatric disorders. Top Magn Reson Imaging 2006; 17:275–93.
53. Hesselink JR. Differential diagnostic approach to MR imaging of white matter diseases. Top Magn Reson Imaging 2006;17:243–63.
54. Enzinger C, Strasser-Fuchs S, Ropele S, et al. Tumefactive demyelinating lesions: conventional and advanced magnetic resonance imaging. Mult Scler 2005;11: 135–9.
55. Law M, Meltzer DE, Cha S. Spectroscopic magnetic resonance imaging of a tumefactive demyelinating lesion. Neuroradiology 2002;44:986–9.
56. Roemer SF, Parisi JE, Lennon VA, et al. Pattern-specific loss of aquaporin-4 immunoreactivity distinguishes neuromyelitis optica from multiple sclerosis. Brain 2007;130:1194–205.
57. Schmalstieg WF, Weinshenker BG. Approach to acute or subacute myelopathy. Neurology 2010;75:S2–8.
58. Fox R, Kinkel R. High dose methylprednisolone in the treatment of multiple sclerosis. In: Cohen JA, Rudick RA, editors. Multiple sclerosis therapeutics. London (UK): Informa; 2007. p. 515–34.
59. Andersson PB, Goodkin DE. Glucocorticosteroid therapy for multiple sclerosis: a critical review. J Neurol Sci 1998;160:16–25.
60. Smith KJ, Kapoor R, Hall SM, et al. Electrically active axons degenerate when exposed to nitric oxide. Ann Neurol 2001;49:470–6.
61. Llufriu S, Castillo J, Blanco Y, et al. Plasma exchange for acute attacks of CNS demyelination: predictors of improvement at 6 months. Neurology 2009;73: 949–53.

62. Greenberg BM, Thomas KP, Krishnan C, et al. Idiopathic transverse myelitis: corticosteroids, plasma exchange, or cyclophosphamide. Neurology 2007;68: 1614–7.
63. Pradhan S, Gupta RP, Shashank S, et al. Intravenous immunoglobulin therapy in acute disseminated encephalomyelitis. J Neurol Sci 1999;165:56–61.
64. von Stuckrad-Barre S, Klippel E, Foerch C, et al. Hemicraniectomy as a successful treatment of mass effect in acute disseminated encephalomyelitis. Neurology 2003;61:420–1.
65. Ahmed AI, Eynon CA, Kinton L, et al. Decompressive craniectomy for acute disseminated encephalomyelitis. Neurocrit Care 2010;13:393–5.
66. Pittock SJ, Weinshenker BG, Wijdicks EF. Mechanical ventilation and tracheostomy in multiple sclerosis. J Neurol Neurosurg Psychiatr 2004;75:1331–3.
67. Berlin L, Kurtzke JF, Guthrie TC. Acute respiratory failure in multiple sclerosis and its management. AMA Arch Neurol Psychiatry 1953;69:394–5.
68. Simon RP, Gean-Marton AD, Sander JE. Medullary lesion inducing pulmonary edema: a magnetic resonance imaging study. Ann Neurol 1991;30:727–30.
69. Gentiloni N, Schiavino D, Della Corte F, et al. Neurogenic pulmonary edema: a presenting symptom in multiple sclerosis. Ital J Neurol Sci 1992;13:435–8.
70. Crawley F, Saddeh I, Barker S, et al. Acute pulmonary oedema: presenting symptom of multiple sclerosis. Mult Scler 2001;7:71–2.
71. Makaryus JN, Kapphahn S, Makaryus AN. Unilateral neurogenic pulmonary oedema and severe left ventricular dysfunction secondary to acute multiple sclerosis exacerbation. Heart Lung Circ 2009;18:155–8.
72. Darragh TM, Simon RP. Nucleus tractus solitarius lesions elevate pulmonary arterial pressure and lymph flow. Ann Neurol 1985;17:565–9.
73. Maire FW, Patton HD. Neural structures involved in the genesis of preoptic pulmonary edema, gastric erosions and behavior changes. Am J Physiol 1956;184: 345–50.
74. Kjellman UW, Hallgren P, Bergh CH, et al. Weaning from mechanical support in a patient with acute heart failure and multiple sclerosis. Ann Thorac Surg 2000; 69:628–30.
75. Melin J, Usenius JP, Fogelholm R. Left ventricular failure and pulmonary edema in acute multiple sclerosis. Acta Neurol Scand 1996;93:315–7.
76. Weiss N, Hasboun D, Demeret S, et al. Paroxysmal hypothermia as a clinical feature of multiple sclerosis. Neurology 2009;72:193–5.
77. Linker RA, Mohr A, Cepek L, et al. Core hypothermia in multiple sclerosis: case report with magnetic resonance imaging localization of a thalamic lesion. Mult Scler 2006;12:112–5.
78. White KD, Scoones DJ, Newman PK. Hypothermia in multiple sclerosis. J Neurol Neurosurg Psychiatr 1996;61:369–75.
79. Hinson SR, Pittock SJ, Lucchinetti CF, et al. Pathogenic potential of IgG binding to water channel extracellular domain in neuromyelitis optica. Neurology 2007;69: 2221–31.

Drug-Induced Movement Disorders: Emergencies and Management

Bradley J. Robottom, MD[a], Lisa M. Shulman, MD[b], William J. Weiner, MD[b,*]

KEYWORDS

• Movement disorders • Emergency • Dystonia
• Parkinsonism • Drug-induced • Tremor

Movement disorders often have an insidious onset and slow progression, and are not often associated with emergency situations. However, neurologists may be called on to diagnose and treat evolving movement disorders or acute complications of existing diseases in the emergency room or intensive care unit. Such situations meet the working definition of an "emergency," a rapidly evolving disorder (hours to days) in which the failure to diagnose and treat may lead to significant morbidity or mortality.[1] Because the key to diagnosis in movement disorders is recognition, key features that help to distinguish each movement disorder are presented in **Table 1**. This article discusses rapidly evolving situations that may require emergency intervention. Several of the disorders discussed are rare, so treatment guidelines are often not based on randomized, double-blind, placebo-controlled trials.

NEUROLEPTIC MALIGNANT SYNDROME

Neuroleptic malignant syndrome (NMS), first described in 1960,[2] is an iatrogenic disorder resulting from exposure to drugs that block dopamine receptors. Although most cases are caused by neuroleptics (both typical and atypical, even clozapine),[3–6] other medications such as prochlorperazine, metoclopramide, amoxapine, tetrabenazine, droperidal, lithium, and promethazine are also implicated.[7–11] Diagnostic criteria

---

The authors do not have any financial conflicts of interest in regards to the content of this article.

[a] Durham Office, 4111 Ben Franklin Boulevard, Durham, NC 27704, USA
[b] Department of Neurology, University of Maryland School of Medicine, 110 South Paca Street, Third Floor, Baltimore, MD 21201, USA
* Corresponding author.
E-mail address: Wweiner@som.umaryland.edu

Neurol Clin 30 (2012) 309–320
doi:10.1016/j.ncl.2011.09.007 **neurologic.theclinics.com**

Table 1
Clinical definitions of movement disorders

Myoclonus	• Sudden, brief, shocklike movements • May be due to muscle contraction (positive myoclonus) or loss of muscle tone (negative myoclonus or asterixis)
Dystonia	• Involuntary sustained muscle contractions that produce twisting or squeezing movements • Often accompanied by abnormal posture
Parkinsonism	• Cardinal features include bradykinesia, rigidity, tremor, and postural instability • All features need not be present • Drug-induced parkinsonism is often symmetric and may lack tremor
Tremor	• Rhythmic, oscillatory movement produced by alternating or synchronous contractions of antagonist muscles
Tics	• Brief, paroxysmal movements or vocalizations sometimes accompanied by premonitory urge • May be stereotyped • Unlike other hyperkinetic movements, may be voluntarily suppressed for a short period of time
Chorea	• Involuntary, irregular, purposeless movements that "flow" into one another in a random fashion • Rapid, large-amplitude proximal movements that are sometimes described as "flinging," are referred to as ballism, and represent an extreme end of the spectrum of chorea

integrating clinical and laboratory features (**Table 2**) have been developed.[12] Newer consensus guidelines that include expert opinion from psychiatrists, neurologists, anesthesiologists, and emergency medicine specialists are in development.[13] Because the incidence of NMS is low (0.2%),[14] a high index of suspicion is necessary to make the appropriate diagnosis. NMS is important to consider in any patient with acute-onset parkinsonism and fever because it is life threatening (mortality rate 5%–20%). Young and middle-aged men appear to be at higher risk.[15] Postpartum women may also have an elevated risk.[16] Case reports of identical twins with NMS suggest that there may be genetic susceptibility as well.[17]

NMS is a clinical syndrome comprising fever, rigidity, mental status change, autonomic dysfunction, and other movement disorders (tremor, dystonia, and myoclonus). Key laboratory abnormalities include leukocytosis and elevated creatine phosphokinase. In addition, acute-phase reactants including albumin and serum iron are decreased.[18] Symptoms often begin after initiation or an increase in neuroleptic dose.[3] NMS increases in severity over 48 to 72 hours and lasts 2 to 14 days.[19] Medical

Table 2
Diagnostic criteria for NMS

Criteria	Feature
Major	Fever, rigidity, elevated creatine phosphokinase level
Minor	Tachycardia, abnormal blood pressure, tachypnea, altered consciousness, diaphoresis, leukocytosis

The presence of all 3 major, or 2 major and 4 minor criteria, indicates a high likelihood of NMS in the appropriate clinical context.

complications can be chronic and irreversible and include renal failure from rhabdomyolysis, respiratory failure from decreased chest wall compliance, aspiration pneumonia, and other complications of immobility such as deep venous thrombosis and pressure ulcers. Pulmonary embolism, pneumonia, or renal failure may result in death.

No prospective, randomized trials exist for NMS. Key steps in treatment include withdrawal of the causative agent and treatment with dopaminergic agents. Bromocriptine has been used most often and is considered the drug of choice[20]; however, other dopaminergic agents including carbidopa/levodopa, ropinirole, and pramipexole are likely effective. Dantrolene, a nonspecific muscle relaxant, reduces muscular rigidity and minimizes rhabdomyolysis if the dopaminergic agent does not reverse the symptoms.[21] Combination therapy has been found to be safe and effective,[20] and treatment should continue for 7 to 10 days depending on the half-life of the causative agent. One-third of patients may relapse if neuroleptics are restarted too early, so waiting at least 2 weeks after NMS has cleared is good practice.[22] In patients who require acute treatment of psychosis, electroconvulsive therapy has been successful.[23]

PARKINSONISM-HYPERPYREXIA SYNDROME

Parkinsonism-hyperpyrexia syndrome (PHS) may be indistinguishable from NMS except that it occurs in patients with preexisting parkinsonism. PHS occurs in patients with Parkinson disease (PD) who abruptly withdraw or reduce dopaminergic medications. It was first reported in the context of abrupt discontinuation of antiparkinsonian medications during "levodopa holidays" in the 1980s.[24–26] Although levodopa holidays are no longer recommended, patient noncompliance or abrupt changes in medication replicate that scenario. Aggressive medication adjustments are not uncommon, particularly after deep brain stimulation surgery (DBS) in PD. Clinicians must realize that PHS is a potential complication and that DBS does not protect the patient from PHS.[27] Although abrupt withdrawal of first-line antiparkinsonian medication (carbidopa/levodopa and dopamine agonists) is the typical scenario for PHS, discontinuation of amantadine or tolcapone has also been reported as causative.[28,29] Rapidly switching between dopamine agonists may also lead to PHS.[30] Dehydration and metabolic disturbances may also precipitate it.[31] Treatment involves supportive measures and reinstituting dopaminergic therapy. Bromocriptine and dantrolene may be added as additional therapy. High-dose intravenous methylprednisolone has been proposed as adjunctive therapy, and appears to be effective based on one small, randomized trial.[32] Despite treatment, permanent worsening of PD and fatalities have been reported.[33]

SEROTONIN SYNDROME

Any drug that enhances serotonergic transmission can precipitate serotonin syndrome (SS), which has the core clinical features of fever, myoclonus, and altered mental status.[34] SS was first described in 1960 in patients receiving monoamine oxidase inhibitor (MAO-I) monotherapy,[35] but is now encountered in patients taking 2 or more drugs with serotonergic actions (tricyclic antidepressants or selective serotonin reuptake inhibitors [SSRI] in combination with nonselective MAO-I) (**Box 1**).[36] Although selective MAO-B inhibitors (rasagiline, selegiline) do carry a warning regarding their use in combination with SSRIs, the agents are routinely used together in PD patients with only rare reports of SS occurring.[37] An underrecognized causative agent of SS is fentanyl, a widely used anesthetic that is a direct serotonin agonist. When used in patients taking SSRIs, it has the potential to cause SS.[38,39] Many of

Box 1
Drugs reported to cause serotonin syndrome

Monoamine oxidase inhibitors

Selective serotonin reuptake inhibitors

Serotonin and norepinephrine reuptake inhibitors

Tricyclic antidepressants

L-Tryptophan

Buspirone

Opiates (except morphine)

Lithium

Triptans

3,4-Methylenedioxymethamphetamine (ecstasy)

Lysergic acid diethylamide (LSD)

Amphetamines

Cocaine

the clinical features overlap with NMS; however, SS may have additional clinical features such as myoclonus, hyperreflexia, seizures, and mood alteration (restlessness, elevated mood).[40] This overlap may relate to the impact that elevated serotonin levels have on lowering dopamine levels. Treatment consists of discontinuation of the causative agent, supportive therapy, and cyproheptadine for severe cases. Cyproheptadine, an antihistamine and serotonin antagonist, is given in divided doses up to a maximum dose of 32 mg/d.[41] SS may resolve quickly[42] or can be fatal. Two case reports have been published detailing the use of electroconvulsive therapy for the treatment of refractory SS.[43] As with NMS and PHS, the rarity and seriousness of SS precludes large, randomized trials.

ACUTE DYSTONIC REACTION

Acute dystonic reaction is most commonly seen after exposure to dopamine receptor blockers, both neuroleptics and antiemetics. Dystonia begins within 24 hours of exposure, and 90% of reactions occur within 5 days.[44] Acute dystonic reactions are less common than tardive dyskinesia or drug-induced parkinsonism, affecting approximately 6% of patients exposed to "typical" neuroleptics and 1% to 2% of those exposed to "atypical" neuroleptics.[45] Clinical manifestations are diverse, usually affecting the head and neck. Laryngeal dystonia, blepharospasm, cervical dystonia, oculogyric crisis, and focal limb dystonia have all been reported. Acute dystonic reactions are more common in young men,[46] whereas tardive dyskinesia and drug-induced parkinsonism are more common in the elderly.[45] Concomitant alcohol abuse may increase the risk of developing acute dystonic reactions and akathisia.[47,48] Treatment with an intravenous anticholinergic agent such as benztropine (1–2 mg) or with diphenhydramine (25–50 mg) is very effective (**Table 3**). Because of the possibility of a reoccurrence, a short oral course of an anticholinergic (4–7 days) may be necessary.[45] After an acute dystonic reaction, patients are at higher risk for future dystonic reactions when exposed to other dopamine receptor blockers.[49]

Table 3
Treatment of hyperkinetic movement disorders

Movement Disorder	Medication Class	Medication	Initial Daily Dose (mg)	Recommended Maximum Daily Dose (mg)
Chorea	Neuroleptic	Haloperidol	0.5	8
		Risperidone	0.5	6
	Dopamine-depleting agent[a]	Tetrabenazine	12.5	75
	Benzodiazepine	Clonazepam	0.5	6
Myoclonus	Anticonvulsant	Valproic acid	750	Titrate to serum level
		Levetiracetam	500	3000
		Primidone[a]	12.5	750
	Benzodiazepine	Clonazepam	0.5	6
Tics	Neuroleptic	Haloperidol	0.5	8
		Risperidone	0.5	6
	Dopamine-depleting agent[a]	Tetrabenazine	12.5	75
	Antihypertensive[a]	Clonidine	0.1	0.6
		Guanfacine	1	3
Acute dystonic reaction	Anticholinergic	Benztropine	1	6
		Diphenhydramine	25	400

[a] These agents are generally not helpful in acute treatment but can be given with a neuroleptic that could eventually be discontinued.

COCAINE AND AMPHETAMINES

Cocaine and amphetamines both enhance neurotransmission of monoamines (dopamine, norepinephrine, and serotonin). Cocaine blocks neurotransmitter reuptake at the synaptic nerve endings[50] while amphetamines increase release of neurotransmitters from synaptic nerve endings.[51] Chronic use of these psychostimulants can lead to stereotypic motor behaviors, tics, dystonia, chorea, and myoclonus.[52–54] Amphetamine use is highly associated with punding behaviors (complex prolonged, purposeless, and stereotyped behavior),[55] while chorea is well described in cocaine users ("crack dancing").[56] While abnormal movements usually appear during intoxication, they may persist for days or weeks, and have been described during withdrawal.[57–60] In patients with tic disorders, psychostimulants have the potential to lead to an acute worsening[61–63]; this has not been proved in a randomized treatment trial of methylphenidate in children with attention-deficit/hyperactivity disorder and tic disorders.[64] No specific treatment is available for neurologic complications of psychostimulant toxicity.

3,4-METHYLENEDIOXYMETHAMPHETAMINE

3,4-Methylenedioxymethamphetamine, or ecstasy, is a "designer drug" that has effects similar to those of psychostimulants and hallucinogens.[51] Side effects can include a variety of neurologic symptoms including anxiety, tremor, ataxia, rigidity, myoclonus, and nystagmus.[65,66] Of importance, ecstasy may also cause seizures and malignant hyperthermia.[67] It should be considered in the differential diagnosis of both NMS and SS. The mechanism of hyperthermia in ecstasy overdose may be attributable to massive serotonin release, and there are many similarities to the symptoms seen in classic SS as well as NMS.[68] Treatment is generally supportive, though aggressive measures should be taken to prevent extreme hyperthermia. In case reports, dantrolene has been effective in the treatment of ecstasy overdose complicated by hyperthermia (>40°C).[69]

OPIOIDS

Opioids are prescribed commonly for the treatment of pain, but are also frequently abused. When used at typical doses, opioids may cause myoclonus and reduce the seizure threshold.[70] One prescription opioid, meperidine, has a much higher likelihood of adverse neurologic effects and is of particular interest. Meperidine may cause a variety of neuropsychiatric adverse effects including agitation, delirium, hallucinations, seizure, tremor, and myoclonus.[71,72] In addition, meperidine may contribute to the development of SS in patients taking tricyclic antidepressants, SSRIs, or serotonin and norepinephrine reuptake inhibitors.[73–75]

MOTOR FLUCTUATIONS AND DYSKINESIA IN PARKINSON DISEASE

Motor fluctuations are common in advanced PD, seen in 40% of patients by 4 to 6 years with an increasing frequency of 10% per year.[76] Generally not dangerous, motor fluctuations are one of the more common disease-specific reasons for which patients seek emergency treatment. During "off" periods, prominent rigidity, bradykinesia, and postural instability may develop, making it impossible for the patients to care for themselves or to walk. Psychiatric features may become pronounced, including depressed mood, anxiety, and, panic. Dysautonomia including tachycardia, diaphoresis, and variations in blood pressure may occur.[77] While "off" periods do not usually result in a visit to the emergency department, some situations lead to emergency evaluation. Patients with suddenly worsening "off" periods associated with new symptoms (eg, freezing, unpredictable, or prolonged "off" periods) are more likely to seek urgent evaluation.[77] In these situations investigation should search for a potential cause of the abrupt change. A careful compilation of medication history is necessary to ensure that no changes have been made to the antiparkinsonian regimen. Patients should also be questioned about the addition of medications to their regimen, particularly dopamine receptor blockers (antipsychotics and antiemetics), as exposure to dopamine receptor antagonists may lead to abrupt deterioration in PD. Concurrent infection (urinary tract infection, pneumonia) or metabolic derangement should be considered. In a patient with falls and abruptly worsening PD, subdural hematoma should be considered.[78]

Levodopa-induced dyskinesia (LID) is usually not dangerous and is most often managed in the outpatient setting. However, severe LID may lead to rhabdomyolysis and dehydration.[77] Generalized LID may be complicated by involvement of respiratory muscles, with patients reporting symptoms of dyspnea, tachypnea, chest wall discomfort, and involuntary grunting.[79] Failure to recognize respiratory dyskinesia may lead to unnecessary testing. Greater emphasis on medical and medication history may improve the diagnosis of respiratory dyskinesia in the emergency setting. Treatment of dyskinesia should include lowering (or holding) levodopa dosage. Benzodiazepines may be useful to treat concomitant anxiety. Neuroleptics should not be used. Long-term management for chronic dyskinesia may involve the addition of amantadine or DBS.[80]

PSYCHOSIS IN PARKINSON DISEASE

Psychosis in PD is a common reason for inpatient admission and is a strong predictor of nursing home placement.[81] It is more commonly encountered in PD with dementia

(PDD), occurring in 45% to 64% of patients.[82,83] Visual hallucinations are more common than auditory hallucinations, and usually consist of complex, formed visual images, often of unknown but nonthreatening people.[84] Paranoid delusions may accompany hallucinations, and constitute a greater problem. Hallucinations and mild delusions may be treated at home, but paranoia may become extreme and require hospitalization. PD psychosis may be precipitated by metabolic derangements, infections (urinary tract infection, pneumonia), and changes in drug therapy, including addition of any dopaminergics or anticholinergics.

Emergency treatment of psychosis requires a multifaceted approach. The patient's living conditions need to be assessed to determine whether hospitalization is required. A thorough workup for metabolic or infectious disorders is indicated. Nonessential psychoactive medications should be discontinued. Dopaminergic drugs that are least potent with respect to motor function should be reduced (anticholinergics, amantadine, dopamine agonists, MAO-B inhibitors, catechol-*O*-methyltransferase inhibitors).[85] The daily levodopa dose may also need to be lowered. An antipsychotic medication can be started, and is often necessary to resolve psychosis. Useful antipsychotics include clozapine and quetiapine. Clozapine has the most robust evidence base.[86] Despite the lack of compelling evidence for quetiapine,[86] it is often prescribed because of clozapine's risk of agranulocytosis and the need for monitoring the complete blood count on a frequent basis. Other antipsychotics, "typical" and "atypical," may cause unacceptable worsening of motor function and should not be used for treatment of psychosis in PD.[85,86]

ACUTE PARKINSONISM

Acute or subacute onset of parkinsonism has a broad differential diagnosis. Parkinsonism as part of a primary neurodegenerative disease is insidious in onset and slowly progressive. However, when parkinsonism develops over a period of days to weeks, a secondary cause should be considered. In this situation a review of the medication list, investigation for a structural lesion, and examination for pathognomonic findings are most important. In the absence of a structural abnormality, particular attention should be given to potential medication or toxic exposures (**Table 4**).[87]

While neuroleptics (typical and atypical) and dopamine-blocking antiemetics (especially metoclopramide) are widely recognized in causing parkinsonism, other medication classes and occupational toxins have also been implicated.

Table 4
Iatrogenic and toxic causes of acute parkinsonism

Drug-induced	Neuroleptics Antiepileptics Antidepressants Chemotherapeutic agents Amiodarone Antiemetics
Toxic	1-methyl-1-4-phenyl-4-proprionoxypiperidine (MPTP) Carbon monoxide Carbon disulfide Manganese Cyanide Methanol

SUMMARY

Although movement disorders are often not regarded as emergencies, there will be situations when the neurologist will be called upon to consult emergently. A common etiology in movement disorders emergencies is that of a toxic exposure, to either prescription or illicit drugs. The workup should always include a careful record of medication and drug history. Because these cases are rare, consulting a neurologist is advisable. This article has reviewed the diagnosis and management of acute-onset movement disorders occurring secondary to drug use, drug withdrawal syndromes, and drug-induced emergencies occurring in patients with movement disorders. These disorders are uncommon and few in any randomized controlled trials that have been conducted. When possible, treatment recommendations are made based on randomized trial data; however, due to the uncommon nature of the disorders, clinical experience and literature reports form the basis for many treatment recommendations.

REFERENCES

1. Frucht SJ, Fahn S, editors. Movement disorder emergencies: diagnosis and treatment. Totowa (NJ): Humana Press; 2005. p. 1.
2. Delay J, Pichot P, Lemperiere T. Un neuroleptique majeur non phenothiazine et non reserpinique l'haloperidal dans le traitement des psychoses. Ann Med Pscyhol 1960;118:145–52 [in French].
3. Shalev A, Munitz H. The neuroleptic malignant syndrome: agent and host interaction. Acta Psychiatr Scand 1986;50:18–25.
4. Caroff SN, Mann SC. Neuroleptic malignant syndrome. Psychopharmacol Bull 1988;24:25–9.
5. Shalev A, Hermesh H, Munitz H. Mortality from neuroleptic malignant syndrome. J Clin Psychiatry 1989;50:18–25.
6. Hasan S, Buckley P. Novel antipsychotics and the neuroleptic malignant syndrome: a review and critique. Am J Psychiatry 1998;115:1113–6.
7. Caroff SN, Mann SC, Campbell EC. Neuroleptic malignant syndrome. Adverse Drug React Bull 2001;209:799–802.
8. Khan FY, Qusad MJ. Neuroleptic malignant syndrome. Neuroscience 2006;11(2):104–6.
9. Petzinger GM, Bressman SB. A case of tetrabenazine-induced neuroleptic malignant syndrome after prolonged treatment. Mov Disord 1997;12(2):246–8.
10. Washington C, Haines KA, Tam CW. Amoxipine-induced neuroleptic malignant syndrome. DICP 1989;23(9):713.
11. Gill J, Singh H, Nugent K. Acute lithium intoxication and neuroleptic malignant syndrome. Pharmacotherapy 2003;23(6):811–5.
12. Levenson JL. Neuroleptic malignant syndrome. Am J Psychiatry 1985;142(10):1137–45.
13. Gurrera R, Caroff S, Cohen A. Neuroleptic malignant syndrome diagnosis: an international consensus study using the Delphi technique. Eur Psychiatry 2010;25(Suppl 1):949.
14. Caroff SN, Mann SC. Neuroleptic malignant syndrome. Med Clin North Am 1993;77:202.
15. Kipps CM, Fung VSC, Grattan-Smith P, et al. Movement disorder emergencies. Mov Disord 2005;20(3):322–34.
16. Alexander PJ, Thomas RM, Das A. Is risk of neuroleptic malignant syndrome increased in the postpartum period? J Clin Psychiatry 1998;59(5):254–5.

17. Otani K, Horiuchi M, Kondo T, et al. Is the predisposition to neuroleptic malignant syndrome genetically transmitted. Br J Psychiatry 1991;158(1):850–3.
18. Rosebush P, Anglin R, Richards C, et al. Neuroleptic malignant syndrome and acute phase response. J Clin Psychopharmacol 2008;28:459–61.
19. Berman BD. Neuroleptic malignant syndrome: a review for neurohospitalists. The Neurohospitalist 2011;1(1):41–7.
20. Rosenberg MR, Green M. Neuroleptic malignant syndrome: review of response to therapy. Arch Intern Med 1989;149:1927–31.
21. Adnet P, Lestavel P, Krivosic-Horber R. Neuroleptic malignant syndrome. Br J Anaesth 2000;85:129–35.
22. Rosebush PI, Stewart TD, Gelenberg AJ. Twenty neuroleptic rechallenges after neuroleptic malignant syndrome in 15 patients. J Clin Psychiatry 1989;50: 295–8.
23. Caroff SN, Mann SC, Keck PE. Specific treatment of the neuroleptic malignant syndrome. Biol Psychiatry 1998;44:378–81.
24. Weiner WJ, Koller WC, Perlik S, et al. Drug holiday and management of Parkinson disease. Neurology 1980;30:1257–61.
25. Sechi G, Tanda F, Mutani R. Fatal hyperpyrexia after withdrawal from levodopa. Neurology 1984;34:249–51.
26. Friedman JH, Feinberg SS, Feldman RG. A neuroleptic malignant-like syndrome due to levodopa therapy withdrawal. JAMA 1985;15:2792–5.
27. Factor SA. Fatal parkinsonism-hyperpyrexia syndrome in a Parkinson's disease patient while actively treated with deep brain stimulation. Mov Disord 2007; 22(1):148–53.
28. Ito T, Shibata K, Watanabe A, et al. Neuroleptic malignant syndrome following withdrawal of amantadine in a patient with influenza a encephalopathy. Eur J Pediatr 2001;160(6):401.
29. Iwuagwu CU, Riley D, Bonomo RA. Neuroleptic malignant-like syndrome in an elderly patient caused by abrupt withdrawal of tolcapone, a catechol-O-methyl transferase inhibitor. Am J Med 2000;108(6):517–8.
30. Reimer J, Kuhlmann A, Muller T. Neuroleptic malignant-like syndrome after rapid switch from bromocriptine to pergolide. Parkinsonism Relat Disord 2002;9(2):115–6.
31. Kuno S, Mizuta E, Yamasaki S. Neuroleptic malignant syndrome in parkinsonian patients: risk factors. Eur Neurol 1997;38:56–9.
32. Sato Y, Asoh T, Metoki N, et al. Efficacy of methylprednisolone pulse therapy on neuroleptic malignant syndrome in Parkinson's disease. J Neurol Neurosurg Psychiatry 2003;74:574–6.
33. Factor SA, Weiner WJ. Movement disorders emergencies: adults and children. American Academy of Neurology, 61st Annual Meeting. Seattle, WA, April 25–May 2, 2009.
34. Sternbach H. The serotonin syndrome. Am J Psychiatry 1991;148:705–13.
35. Oates JA, Sjoerdsma A. Neurologic effects of tryptophan in patients receiving a monoamine oxidase inhibitor. Neurology 1960;10:1076–8.
36. Mason PJ, Morris VA, Balcezak TJ. Serotonin syndrome. Presentation of 2 cases and review of the literature. Medicine 2000;79:201–9.
37. Robottom BJ. Efficacy, safety, and patient preference of monoamine oxidase B inhibitors in the treatment of Parkinson's disease. Patient Prefer Adherence 2011;5:57–64.
38. Alkhatib AA, Peterson KA, Tuteja AK. Serotonin syndrome as a complication of fentanyl sedation during esophagogastroduodenoscopy. Dig Dis Sci 2010;55: 215–6.

39. Kirschner R, Donovan JW. Serotonin syndrome precipitated by fentanyl during procedural sedation. J Emerg Med 2010;38(4):477–80.
40. Radomski JW, Dursun SM, Reveley MA, et al. An exploratory approach to the serotonin syndrome: an update of clinical phenomenology and revised diagnostic criteria. Med Hypotheses 2000;55(3):218–24.
41. Hall M, Buckley N. Serotonin syndrome. Aust Prescr 2003;26:62–3.
42. Mills KC. Serotonin syndrome: a clinical update. Crit Care Clin 1997;13(4): 763–83.
43. Okamoto N, Sakamoto K, Nagafusa Y, et al. Electroconvulsive therapy as a potentially effective treatment for severe serotonin syndrome: two case reports. J Clin Psychopharmacol 2010;30(3):350–2.
44. Diederich NJ, Goetz CG. Drug-induced movement disorders. Neurol Clin 1998; 16(1):125–39.
45. Pierre JM. Extrapyramidal symptoms with atypical antipsychotics: incidence, prevention and management. Drug Saf 2005;28(3):191–208.
46. van Harten PN, Hock HW, Kahn RS. Acute dystonia induced by drug treatment. BMJ 1999;319:623–6.
47. Lutz EG. Neuroleptic-induced akathisia and dystonia triggered by alcohol. JAMA 1976;236:2422–3.
48. Freed E. Alcohol-triggered neuroleptic-induced tremor, rigidity, and dystonia. Med J Aust 1981;2:44–5.
49. Campbell D. The management of acute dystonic reactions. Aust Prescriber 2001; 24:19–20.
50. Lange RA, Hillis LD. Cardiovascular complications of cocaine use. N Engl J Med 2001;345:351–8.
51. Brust JCM. Substance abuse and movement disorders. Mov Disord 2010;25: 2010–20.
52. Rylander G. Psychosis and the punding and choreiform syndromes in addictions to central stimulant drugs. Psychiatry Neurol Neurchir 1972;75:203–12.
53. Derlet RW, Alberston TE. Emergency department presentation of cocaine intoxication. Ann Emerg Med 1989;18:182–6.
54. Brody SL, Slovis CM, Wrenn KD. Cocaine-related medical problems: consecutive series of 233 patients. Am J Med 1990;88:325–31.
55. Randrup A, Munkvad J. Stereotyped activities produced by amphetamine in several species and man. Psychopharmacologia 1967;11:300–10.
56. Daras M, Koppel BS, Atos-Radzion E. Cocaine-induced choreoathetoid movements (crack-dancing). Neurology 1994;44:751–2.
57. Choy-Kwong M, Lipton RB. Dystonia related to cocaine withdrawal: a case report and pathogenic hypothesis. Neurology 1989;39:996–7.
58. Kumor K. Cocaine withdrawal dystonia. Neurology 1990;40:863–4.
59. Weiner WJ, Rubinstein A, Lewin B, et al. Cocaine-induced persistent dyskinesias. Neurology 2001;56:964–5.
60. Lundh H, Tunving K. An extrapyramidal choreiform syndrome caused by amphetamine addiction. J Neurol Neurosurg Psychiatry 1981;44:728–30.
61. Pascual-Leone A, Dhuna A. Cocaine-associated multifocal tics. Neurology 1990; 40:999–1000.
62. Factor SA, Sanchez-Ramos JR, Weiner WJ, et al. Cocaine and Tourette's syndrome. Ann Neurol 1988;23:423–4.
63. Golden GS. Gilles de la Tourette's syndrome following amphetamine administration. Dev Med Child Neurol 1976;16:76–7.

64. Kurlan R. Treatment of ADHD in children with tics: a randomized controlled trial. Neurology 2001;58:527–36.
65. Brown C, Osterloh J. Multiple severe complications from recreational ingestion of MDMA (ecstasy). JAMA 1987;258:780–1.
66. Hinkelbein J, Gabel A, Volz M, et al. Suicide attempt with high dose ecstasy. Anesthetist 2003;52:51–4.
67. Regenthal R, Kruger M, Rudolf K, et al. Survival after massive "ecstasy" (MDMA) ingestion. Intensive Care Med 1999;25:640–1.
68. Ames D, Wirshing WC. Ecstasy, the serotonin syndrome, and neuroleptic malignant syndrome—a possible link? JAMA 1993;269:869–70.
69. Grunau BE, Wiens MO, Brubacher JR. Dantrolene in the treatment of MDMA-related hyperpyrexia: a systematic review. CJEM 2010;12:435–42.
70. Lauterbach EC. Hiccup and apparent myoclonus after hydrocodone: a review of the opiate-related hiccup and myoclonus literature. Clin Neuropharmacol 1999;22:87–92.
71. Hershey LA. Meperidine and central neurotoxicity. Ann Intern Med 1983;98:548–9.
72. Kaiko RF, Folwy KM, Grabinski PY, et al. Central nervous system excitatory effects of meperidine in cancer patients. Ann Neurol 1983;13:180–5.
73. Dougherty JA, Young H, Shafi T. Serotonin syndrome induced by amitriptyline, meperidine, and venlafaxine. Ann Pharmacol 2002;36:1647–8.
74. Tissot TA. Probable meperidine-induced serotonin syndrome in a patient with a history of fluoxetine use. Anesthesiology 2003;98:1511–2.
75. Latta KS, Ginsberg B, Barkin RL. Meperidine: a critical review. Am J Ther 2002;9:53–68.
76. Ahlskog JE, Muenter MD. Frequency of levodopa-related dyskinesias and motor fluctuations as estimated from the cumulative literature. Mov Disord 2001;16(3):448–58.
77. Factor SA, Molho ES. Emergency department presentations of patients with Parkinson's disease. Am J Emerg Med 2000;18(2):209–15.
78. Chou SM, Gutmann L. Deteriorating parkinsonism and subdural hematomas. Neurology 2001;57:1295.
79. Weiner WJ, Goetz CG, Nausieda PA, et al. Respiratory dyskinesias: extrapyramidal dysfunction and dyspnea. Ann Intern Med 1978;88:327–31.
80. Pahwa R, Factor SA, Lyons KE, et al. Practice parameter: treatment of Parkinson disease motor fluctuations and dyskinesia (an evidence-based review): report of the Quality Standards Subcommittee of the American Academy of Neurology. Neurology 2006;66:983–95.
81. Aarsland D, Larsen JP, Tandberg E, et al. Predictors of nursing home placement in Parkinson's disease: a population-based, prospective study. J Am Geriatr Soc 2000;48:938–42.
82. Robottom BJ, Weiner WJ. Parkinson's disease dementia. Curr Psychiatry Rev 2009;5(3):218–25.
83. Giladi N, Treves TA, Paleacu D, et al. Risk factors for dementia, depression and psychosis in long-standing Parkinson's disease. J Neural Transm 2000;107(1):59–71.
84. Mosimann UP, Rowan EN, Partington CE, et al. Characteristics of visual hallucinations in Parkinson disease dementia and dementia with Lewy bodies. Am J Geriatr Psychiatry 2006;14:153–60.
85. Friedman JH, Factor SA. Atypical antipsychotics in the treatment of drug-induced psychosis in Parkinson's disease. Mov Disord 2000;15:201–11.

86. Miyasaki JM, Shannon K, Voon V, et al. Practice parameter: evaluation and treatment of depression, psychosis, and dementia in Parkinson disease (an evidence-based review). Neurology 2006;66:996–1002.
87. Robottom BJ, Weiner WJ, Factor SA. Movement disorders emergencies part 1: hypokinetic disorders. Arch Neurol 2011;68:567–72.

Urgent and Emergent Psychiatric Disorders

Nadejda Alekseeva, MD[a], Felix Geller, MD[b], James Patterson, MD, PhD[b], Mary Fitz-Gerald, MD[b], Rita Horton, MD[b], Alireza Minagar, MD[c,*]

KEYWORDS

• Neurologic disease • Depression • Anxiety • Psychosis

In the emergency department, neurologists regularly evaluate patients exhibiting behavioral abnormalities that stem from their underlying neurologic diseases. This behavior may be the initial presence of a neurologic illness or may indicate the deterioration and progress of the disease process. In addition, many neurologic patients present with acute and potentially dangerous psychiatric symptoms that demand rapid and accurate management. Assessment, diagnosis, and treatment of patients with psychiatric manifestations in the context of neurologic illness pose a significant challenge to treating neurologists. This article discusses a general approach to assessment and treatment of some of the more common psychiatric disorders.

DEPRESSION

Depression is a frequent and prominent manifestation of neurologic disorders.[1] Common neurovegetative symptoms of depression are best remembered with the SIG: E-CAPS mnemonic: Sleep (decreased typically), Interest (decreased), Guilt (increased and/or poor self-esteem or feeling worthless), Energy (often fatigued), Concentration (decreased), Psychomotor (retardation or agitation, especially if anxiousness is present), and Suicide (depressed mood, feeling hopeless, thoughts of death or suicide). Other frequent manifestations of depression consist of decreased sexual desire or function and somatic preoccupation.[2]

Several neurologic disorders and medications are associated with depression (**Table 1**).[3–11] Ischemic stroke, particularly in patients with left frontal lobe lesions, is frequently associated with depression.[12–14] Clinical manifestations of poststroke depression range from apathy and dysthymia to major depression.[15] Clinical

[a] Department of Psychiatry, Overton Brooks VA Medical Center, Shreveport, LA, USA
[b] Department of Psychiatry, Louisiana State University Health Sciences Center, Shreveport, LA 71130, USA
[c] Department of Neurology, Louisiana State University Health Sciences Center, 1501 Kings Highway, Shreveport, LA 71130, USA
* Corresponding author.
E-mail address: aminag@lsuhsc.edu

Neurol Clin 30 (2012) 321–344
doi:10.1016/j.ncl.2011.09.003 **neurologic.theclinics.com**

Table 1
Medical conditions and medications associated with psychiatric abnormalities

Category	Disease	Depression	Anxiety	Psychosis	Mania	Aggression	Cognition
Autoimmune	Systemic lupus erythematosus	+	—	+	—	+	+
Brain	Alzheimer disease	+	+	+	—	+	+
	Calcification of basal ganglia	+	+	+	—	—	+
	Cerebral neoplasms	+	+	+	+	+	+
	Cerebrovascular accidents	+	+	+	+	+	+
	Encephalitis	+[a]	+	+	+[b]	+	+
	Epilepsy (especially temporal lobe)	+	+	+	+	+	+
	Frontotemporal lobar dementias	+	+[b]	+[b]	+[b]	+[b]	+
	Huntington disease	+	+	+	—	+	+
	Hypoxic encephalopathy	+	+	+	—	+	+
	Meningitis	—	—	+[b]	+[b]	—	+
	Mental retardation	+	+	+	+	+	+
	Migraine	+	+	—	—	—	±
	Multiple sclerosis	+	+	+	+	+	+
	Other dementias	+	+	+	—	+	+
	Parkinson disease	+	+	+[c]	+[d]	+	+
	Progressive supranuclear palsy	+	+	—	—	—	+
	Pseudobulbar palsy	+	+	—	—	—	—
	Traumatic brain injury	+	+	+	+	+	+
	Wilson disease	+	+	+	+	+	+
Cancer or Neoplasms	Pancreatic carcinoma	+	+	—	—	—	—
	Pheochromocytoma	—	+	—	—	—	—
Cardiovascular	Angina	+	+	—	—	—	—
	Arrhythmia	+	+	—	—	—	—
	Congestive heart failure	+	+	—	—	—	+
	Myocardial infarct (postmyocardial infarct)	+	+	—	—	—	+

Endocrinologic	Addison disease	+	—	+	—	—	—
	Cushing syndrome	+	+	+	+[b]	—	+
	Hypercalcemia or hyperparathyroidism	+	+	+	+[b]	—	+
	Hyperthyroidism	+	+	+	+	—	+
	Hypothyroidism	+	—	+	+[b]	+	+
Infectious	Hepatitis C virus	+[a]	—	+[a]	+[b]	—	+
	Epstein-Barr virus	+	+	+[b]	—	—	+
	HIV virus or AIDS	+	+	+	+	—	+
	Neurosyphilis	—	—	+	—	+	+
Pulmonary	Asthma	—	+	—	—	—	—
	Chronic obstructive pulmonary disease	+	+	—	—	—	+
	Pulmonary embolus	—	+	—	—	—	—
Systemic	Carcinoid syndrome	+[e]	+	—	—	—	+
	Delirium	+	+	+	—	+	+
	Hypokalemia	—	—	—	—	+	—
	Hypocalcemia	—	+	+[b]	—	—	—
	Hypoglycemia	+	+	+[b]	—	+	+
	Hyponatremia	+[f]	+[f]	+	—	—	+
	Lymphoma	+	—	—	—	—	+
	Porphyria	+	+	+	—	+	—
	Vitamin deficiency: B_{12}	+	+	+	—	—	+
	Vitamin deficiency: D	+	—	—	—	—	+
	Vitamin deficiency: folate	+	+	—	—	—	—

[a] Treatment of viral infections with interferons has been strongly linked to depression and psychosis.
[b] Many case reports.
[c] Treatment of Parkinson disease with dopaminergic agents is associated with psychosis.
[d] Treatment with deep-brain stimulation has been linked to induction of mania.
[e] Treatment (inhibition of serotonin) could cause depression, and use of SSRIs might unmask carcinoid.
[f] Treatment of anxiety or depression with SSRIs can cause hyponatremia.

manifestations of poststroke depression are significant because it increases mortality and disability[16] and interferes with functional recovery.[17] Patients with Alzheimer disease present with apathy, depression, and psychosis.[18,19] Major depression is a salient psychiatric feature of multiple sclerosis[20,21] with an approximate 50% lifetime prevalence rate. In addition, treatment of multiple sclerosis with beta-interferons is uncommonly associated with depression. Of the neurobehavioral disorders experienced by patients with Parkinson disease, depression develops in up to one-third of the patients, particularly in those with akinesia and rigidity as their prominent symptoms.[22] Depression is the most common psychiatric presentation of Huntington's disease and its presence is accompanied by an increased risk of suicide in this population.[23] Epilepsy is associated with depression and the risk of suicide is believed to be increased among epileptic patients.[24] Central nervous system (CNS) tumors are associated with depression. Depression is a well-known complication of cerebral gliomas and it has been reported in up to 93% of these patients.[25] In addition, paraneoplastic syndromes, such as limbic encephalitis,[26] may present with depression, personality changes, amnesia, anxiety, or seizures.

Patients with AIDS commonly suffer from neurologic complications (neuroAIDS), which consists of neurocognitive impairment and HIV-associated dementia.[27] AIDS patients commonly suffer from depression, which is a major differential diagnosis for HIV-associated dementia.

Certain less common neurologic diseases, such as prion diseases, also manifest with depression and anxiety. Patients with classical Creutzfeldt-Jakob disease, as well as variant CJD, present with psychiatric symptoms, such as depression and psychosis.[28] Several medications that are used to treat various medical disorders are also associated with psychiatric symptoms, including depression (see **Table 1**).

Assessment

Comprehensive assessment of neurologic patients with depression requires attention to many variables, including medical and psychiatric history, medications, neurologic examination, and laboratory values. Making a diagnosis of depression in a neurologic patient may be a difficult task because certain diagnostic criteria for depression, such as insomnia, anorexia, fatigue, and poor concentration, are also clinical features of the underlying neurologic disease.

Treatment

Treatment of depression in patients with neurologic diseases commences with identifying and treating the underlying neurologic disease and removing any offensive medications. Currently, few well-designed clinical studies have been performed on the clinical efficacy of the antidepressant agents in the context of neurologic diseases. Therefore, treating neurologists must use the general guidelines for the use of antidepressants and make an effort to use antidepressants that do not worsen existing depression or concomitant manifestations of the underlying neurologic disease.

Tricyclic antidepressants (TCAs) are older medications. Structurally, they are tertiary tricyclics, such as amitriptyline, imipramine, and doxepin, with anticholinergic, antihistaminic, and anti–$alpha_1$-adrenergic activity properties. These agents are usually effective in patients with neurologic diseases. Of various TCAs, nortriptyline is preferred due to its milder anticholinergic effects and less deleterious effect on cognition. The second group of antidepressants includes the secondary amine metabolites of amitriptyline and imipramine (nortriptyline and desipramine) with fewer side effects compared with the first group.

Newer antidepressants include the selective serotonin reuptake inhibitors (SSRIs) (eg, fluoxetine, sertraline, citalopram, and escitalopram) and selective serotonin-norepinephrine reuptake inhibitors (SNRIs) (eg, venlafaxine and duloxetine), which are used extensively due to their more acceptable side-effect profile, which includes less hypotension and anticholinergic effects. However, these medications may cause extrapyramidal side effects and sexual dysfunction. Some of the psychotropic medications, such as bupropion, may lower the seizure threshold in epileptic patients and they should be avoided in this group.[29]

It may take from 2 to 4 weeks for antidepressants to demonstrate their clinical effect. Generally, neurologic patients with depression should be treated with antidepressants for at least 1 year after remission, before the medication is tapered. Early and unplanned cessation of antidepressant can lead to relapse of depression. Another effective treatment of depression in patients with poststroke depression, epilepsy, Parkinson disease, and multiple sclerosis is electroconvulsive therapy. However, this procedure is contraindicated in patients with increased intracranial pressure. In cases of severe and treatment-resistant depression, or when the patient is suicidal, psychiatric consultation should be obtained. Neurologic patients who are suicidal must be admitted for further psychiatric treatment.

ANXIETY: CLINICAL MANIFESTATION

Anxiety is defined as a feeling of unpleasant and diffuse apprehension that may be a normal and transient response to stressful events of daily living or a persistent pathologic condition. The uneasy sense of anxiety is frequently associated with autonomic manifestations, such as headache, sweating, frequent urination, feeling of tightness in the chest, and palpitations. A significant number of patients with chronic medical disorders suffer from anxiety. Anxiety, as a symptom, presents in the context of various psychiatric disorders, such as panic disorder with agoraphobia, panic disorder due to a general medical condition, or posttraumatic stress disorder. Anxiety is a manifestation of several neurologic disorders. In epileptic patients, anxiety or fear is the most frequent ictal emotion and may be the prodromal symptom in some patients.[30] Epileptic patients develop interictal anxiety, panic attacks, and phobias, all of which adversely affect the patients' quality of life. Patients with Parkinson disease also suffer from anxiety disorders and almost half of these patients, while completing standardized questionnaires, reported significant anxiety that was not diagnosed by their treating physicians.[31] Significantly, anxiety symptoms may develop before the appearance of the motor manifestations of Parkinson disease[32] and this, in turn, may make the diagnosis more difficult. Patients with Parkinson disease may present with several different forms of anxiety disorders, including generalized anxiety disorder, social phobia, panic disorder, and obsessive-compulsive disorder. The anxiety of Parkinson disease patients often coexists with depression and is frequently associated with motor fluctuations due to on-off phenomenon with levodopa use.[33] The presence of anxiety in patients with Parkinson disease may be a psychological result of increasing disability due to the underlying neurologic disorder. Patients with ischemic strokes involving the left frontal and right temporal lobes often develop anxiety.

Assessment

The treating neurologist who assesses the neurologic patient with anxiety should consider the possibility that anxiety may be a part of the underlying neurologic disease or a side effect of the medications that the patient takes (**Table 2**).[34] Neurologic patients with anxiety need a detailed assessment.

Table 2
Medications and drugs of abuse associated with psychiatric symptoms

	Depression	Anxiety	Psychosis	Mania	Aggression
Medications					
Anticholinergics	—	+	—	—	+
Antidepressants (including SSRIs)	—	+	—	—	—
Antihypertensives (including β-blockers)	+	+	+	—	—
Baclofen	+	—	—	—	—
Barbiturates	+	+	—	—	+
Cimetidine	+	—	—	—	—
Corticosteroids	+	+	+	+	+
Decongestants	—	+	—	+	—
Digoxin	—	+	+	—	—
Estrogen	+	+	—	—	—
Insulin	—	+	—	—	—
Interferon	+	—	+	—	—
Isoniazid	—	—	+	—	—
Levodopa and other dopamine agonists	+	+	+	+	—
Neuroleptics	—	+	—	—	—
Nonsteroidal antiinflammatories	+	+	+	—	—
Opioids	+	—	—	—	—
Sympathomimetics or bronchodilators	—	+	—	+	—
Theophylline	—	+	—	—	—
Thyroid preparations	—	+	—	—	—
Drugs of Abuse					
Alcohol intoxication	+	+	+	+	+
Alcohol withdrawal	+	+	+	—	+
Amphetamine intoxication	—	+	+	—	+
Amphetamine withdrawal	+	—	—	—	—
Benzodiazepine intoxication	+	—	+	—	+
Benzodiazepine withdrawal	+	+	+	—	—
Caffeine intoxication	—	+	—	—	—
Caffeine withdrawal	—	+	—	—	—
Cocaine intoxication	—	+	+	—	+
Cocaine withdrawal	+	+	—	—	—
Marijuana intoxication	—	+	+	—	—
Opiate intoxication	+	+	—	—	—
Phencyclidine intoxication	—	+	+	+	+

Data from Frumin M, Chisholm T, Dickey CC, et al. Psychiatric and behavioral problems. Neurol Clin 1998;16(2):521–44.

Treatment

Although treatment of underlying neurologic disease often lessens anxiety, it may not eliminate it. Several agents with dissimilar mechanisms of action and side-effect profiles have been used to treat anxiety. These include antidepressants, usually with the SSRIs being first line, then moving to TCAs or monoamine oxidase inhibitors. In addition, treatment can be augmented with buspirone, SNRIs, benzodiazepines, antiepileptic agents, and atypical antipsychotics. SSRIs and TCAs may effectively reduce anxiety; however, their onset of action is slow. Buspirone, which is a non-benzodiazepine anxiolytic medication without sedative or cognitive adverse effects, is a reasonable treatment of anxiety attacks, particularly in anxious patients with cognitive decline. Benzodiazepines (particularly the short-acting, high-potency benzodiazepines) are often used for the treatment of anxiety; however, their use is restricted because they are highly addictive and may worsen interdose anxiety. Beta-blocker agents are used for treatment of peripheral autonomic manifestations, such as tachycardia and tremor. However, these medications may cause depression. Generally, pharmacologic treatment of anxiety should be initiated at low doses of the medications and continued with slow increases of the prescribed dose until therapeutic effects are observed. Neurologic patients with anxiety must avoid drinking alcohol and coffee and must not smoke because these agents may worsen anxiety. In cases of disabling anxiety, lack of a therapeutic response to the standard treatment, complicated social situations, comorbid substance use, and suicidal ideation, a psychiatric consult must be obtained. Alternative therapeutic methods, such as relaxation therapy and behavioral modification, should also be considered.

PSYCHOSIS

Psychosis is defined as an abnormal condition in which the patient loses touch with reality. Clinically, psychosis manifests with delusions, hallucinations, personality changes, and poorly organized thinking, which point toward an underlying CNS disorder. Psychotic disorders are uncommon in the primary care setting and they are observed in only up to 1% of patients and 3% of patients in the general population.[35] Medical patients most frequently develop psychosis due to organic diseases and, once they present with hallucinations, delusions, agitation, and acute alteration of sensorium, a comprehensive diagnostic work-up is warranted to identify the underlying cause.

Certain neurologic disorders may present with psychosis. These include head trauma, vascular diseases, CNS space-occupying lesions (particularly tumors), epilepsy, Wernicke-Korsakoff syndrome, B12 deficiency, CNS infections (eg, herpetic encephalitis and neurosyphilis), and neurodegenerative diseases, such as Alzheimer disease, Parkinson disease, and Pick disease. In addition, patients with acute encephalopathy or those who use illegal drugs, such as cocaine, methamphetamine, and hallucinogens, develop sudden-onset psychosis. Apart from this, several neurologic diseases characterized by dementia and parkinsonism present with psychosis and delusional beliefs.[36]

Assessment

Assessment of neurologic patients with psychosis demands a comprehensive physical and mental status evaluation. Because psychotic patients have disordered thinking processes, gathering information from family members, friends, and medical records is necessary. A review of medical records may reveal a history of psychiatric disorders, such as schizophrenia or drug abuse, which can explain the present psychotic picture.

Treatment

The initial step in treatment of the psychotic patients consists of establishing the safety of the patient and the staff. In most cases, psychotic patients must be admitted to the hospital so medical work-up and psychiatric assessment can be done. Emergent pharmacologic management of these patients includes use of intravenous or intramuscular haloperidol. Psychotic patients who are also agitated should be treated with lorazepam, which will further calm the patient. Atypical antipsychotics, such as risperidone, quetiapine, ziprasidone, and aripiprazole, are commonly used for treatment of psychotic symptoms. The treating neurologist should be familiar with the side effects of both older-generation and recent atypical antipsychotic agents. Neurologic patients with psychosis are prone to side effects, such as extrapyramidal symptoms, excessive sedation, and further confusion.

MANIA

Mania is characterized by elevated energy and mood, reduced need for sleep, pressured speech, distractibility, and impulsive behavior. Similar to other psychiatric symptoms, such as psychosis and depression, mania may stem from a psychiatric disorder, such as bipolar mood disorder, or may be secondary to an underlying neurologic disease. Manic patients can get themselves involved in high-risk behaviors, such as gambling and excessive sexual activity. A thorough list of secondary causes of mania is presented in **Box 1**.[37–44] Certain neurologic diseases, such as multiple sclerosis and epilepsy, present with either unipolar mania or bipolar mood disorder with rapid cycling. In addition, certain treatments for neurologic diseases, such as corticosteroids, may induce manic-like syndrome in some patients.

Assessment

The assessment of manic patients for underlying neurologic disease demands a detailed neurologic and mental examination with focus on any neurologic manifestations that point toward the underlying diagnosis.

Treatment

The best treatment of mania goes back to treatment of the underlying disease. However, this is usually difficult, if not impossible, because many neurologic diseases remain incurable. It is important to realize that manic patients are at high risk to commit suicide, harm other members of society, or engage in reckless behavior. Therefore, manic patients who present to the emergency room need to be admitted for further neurologic and psychiatric treatment. In nonemergency cases in which manic symptoms are mild, patients should be treated with mood-stabilizing medications, such as lithium carbonate, valproic acid, and carbamazepine.[45] Atypical antipsychotic agents may be useful in bipolar patients with manic and psychotic features. In cases in which pharmacologic treatment is ineffective or contraindicated, electroconvulsive therapy should be considered.

SUICIDE

Suicide is defined as the act in which an individual intentionally takes his or her life. Patients who attempt suicide are frequently taken to a hospital emergency department. Attempted suicide is a manifestation of many psychiatric disorders. Many neurologic patients also attempt to take their own life. Certain chronic and incurable neurologic diseases, such as Huntington disease, neuroAIDS, spinal cord injuries, and multiple sclerosis, are associated with increased suicide risk. Depression is the most frequent psychiatric disorder observed in patients with Huntington disease; the risk of suicide is elevated in this group compared with the general population. Epileptic patients are at increased risk of premature death due to suicide.[46] Certain risk factors associated with suicide are presented in **Box 2**.[47–50]

Assessment

Thorough and rapid evaluation of suicidal patients in the emergency department is necessary to ensure those at high suicide risk are admitted and treated. Suicide risk is increased in patients with a history of psychiatric disorders, those with previous suicide attempts, patients who are actively planning suicide, and patients who are found to have sustained injuries or ingested substances inconsistent with the history given by the patient.

Treatment

Establishing patient safety is the most significant step in the treatment of suicidal patients in the emergency department. If there are any concerns that the individual is at risk for taking his or her life, the patient must be admitted to the psychiatric service and be placed under suicidal observation. Sharp objects, drugs, belts, and any potentially dangerous medical equipment should be removed from the patient's room. If the patient has overdosed with a poisonous substance, the poison control center should be notified and be involved in the patient's care. If there are concerns about cardiac toxicity, the patient should be admitted in the cardiac monitoring unit. A one-to-one sitter and/or physical restraints (only if the patient is agitated) should be used to secure the patient's safety. Once the patient is medically stable and out of acute danger, treatment of the patient requires diagnosis of the underlying cause and its effective management.

NEUROLEPTIC MALIGNANT SYNDROME AND OTHER HYPERMETABOLIC SYNDROMES

Four frequently diagnosed hypermetabolic syndromes exist that manifest with hyperthermia, rigidity of muscles, and autonomic dysfunction. These include neuroleptic malignant syndrome (NMS), serotonin syndrome, lethal catatonia, and malignant hyperthermia. Various features that assist correct identification of these syndromes are presented in **Table 3**.[51]

NMS is a potentially lethal complication of neuroleptics. The incidence of NMS is less than 1% and results from decreased dopaminergic neurotransmission. NMS usually results from the initiation of a dopamine receptor blocker (ie, antipsychotic drugs) (an idiosyncratic reaction) or it may stem from discontinuation of dopamine receptor stimulator (ie, antiparkinsonian drugs). However, NMS may happen at any time during treatment of patients with neuroleptic drugs. Clinically, NMS manifests with altered sensorium (confusion, agitation, and delirium), fever, rigidity, autonomic dysfunction, tremor, and excessive sweating.[52] Factors that may increase the risk of NMS are dehydration and concurrent lithium therapy. Use of atypical antipsychotic clozapine[53] or the addition of aripiprazole to clozapine has also been associated with NMS.[54]

Serotonin syndrome is a potentially lethal condition that is associated with activation of CNS serotonin type 1A receptors due to excessive serotonin activity. It is caused by an increase in serotonin production or decrease in its metabolism that leads to a hyperserotonergic state. Coadministration of a monoamine oxidase inhibitor with an SSRI, as well as medications such as meperidine or dextromethorphan, is associated with development of serotonin syndrome. Combining an SSRI with tryptophan or lithium

Box 1
Secondary causes of mania

Neurologic

Epilepsy: temporal lobe epilepsy (most common)

Traumatic brain injury

- Right temporal or orbitalfrontal cortex lesion
- 10% of closed head injury patients meet the criteria for mania in the subsequent 12 months
- Patient commonly has comorbid seizures

Multiple sclerosis

- Risk for bipolar disorder is 2 to 13 times greater than the risk for the general population
- Steroid-induced mood lability is increased in patients with a history of depression
  - Pathologic laughing and crying occurs without mania

Dementia

- Symptoms often seem manic in nature, but mostly depression, abulia, disinhibition, aggression, and irritability

Parkinson disease

- Often idiopathic from medication

Huntington disease

- Often present before the cardinal symptoms of dementia and chorea

Fahr disease (idiopathic calcification of the basal ganglia)

Adrenoleukodystrophy or metachromatic leukodystrophy

CNS tumors

- Right-sided tumors
- Symptoms of mania are more likely to arise from basal temporal tumors

Cardiovascular

Cerebrovascular accident

- Mania occurs in less than 1% of patients
- Neurologic disease, especially cerebrovascular disease, was twice as frequent among elderly patients with late-onset mania than those with long-standing affective disorders
- Adults with late-onset mania also seem to have more frequent episodes of late-onset silent cerebral infarcts
- Symptoms are identical to those of primary mania
- Lesions in the right orbital frontal cortex and thalamus seem to be most often correlated with poststroke mania
- Examine for the possibility of seizures, especially in the temporal-parietal area

Infectious/Inflammatory

HIV and/or AIDS

Neurosyphilis

- Can display grandiose and expansive moods similar to mania

Neurocysticercosis: based on case studies

Collagen-vascular diseases
- Lupus
- Rheumatoid arthritis
- Neurosarcoidosis
  - All instances require the ruling out of delirium

Endocrine

Hypo and hyperthyroidism

Diabetes mellitus

Hypercortisolemia

Vitamin deficiencies

Carcinoid syndrome

Uremia

Hemodialysis

is also associated with serotonin syndrome. Another example is combining migraine medications, known as triptans, with SSRIs or SNRIs. Clinically, serotonin syndrome manifests as alteration of mental status, agitation, myoclonus, enhanced reflexes, diaphoresis, and tremor.[55] The presence of certain features, such as shivering and myoclonus, differentiates serotonin syndrome from NMS.

Catatonia is a syndrome that is induced by several psychiatric and medical conditions, such as schizophrenia, drug abuse or overdose, bipolar mood disorder, posttraumatic stress disorder, encephalitis, hepatic encephalopathy, and autoimmune disorders. Clinically, catatonia is recognized by the presence of cataplexy, waxy flexibility, mutism, and resistance to instructions or efforts to be moved along with off and on agitation. Catatonia can be an adverse effect of certain medications, such as neuroleptics.[56] Prominent features of lethal catatonia include significant psychomotor disturbance and fever. This form of catatonia initiates with agitation followed by rigidity, fever, mutism, and exhaustion, along with frequent delusions and hallucinations.

Malignant hyperthermia (MH), also recognized as malignant hyperpyrexia, is an uncommon, life-threatening genetic syndrome that is characterized by rigidity, hyperthermia, and metabolic acidosis. MH is triggered by exposure to certain volatile anesthetic agents and the neuromuscular blocking medication, succinylcholine. As a genetic disorder, MH is frequently inherited in an autosomal dominant pattern for which at least six genetic loci have been identified. The most significant genetic locus is the ryanodine receptor gene.

Assessment

An outline for assessment of the hypermetabolic syndromes is presented in **Table 3**.

Treatment

In most cases, patients with hypermetabolic syndromes must be admitted to the medical or intensive care services for close cardiopulmonary monitoring. Treating physicians should be on alert for certain medical complications, such as cardiac arrhythmias, hypertension, pulmonary embolus, and disseminated intravascular coagulation.

Treatment of NMS includes rapid identification and cessation of the insulting agent, hydration, and use of antipyretics to control the fever. Usually, patients with NMS require admission to the intensive care unit for close cardiorespiratory monitoring.

Box 2
Risk factors for suicide and self-injurious behavior

Patients with high risk of suicide

High-risk populations

Older age patients with self-harm behaviors

Patients with repeated self-harm behaviors resulting in significant tissue damage

Alert risk factors (*may prompt hospitalization*)

Younger age

Completion of, at least, a high school degree

Diagnosis of a psychotic disorder

Taking active precautions against discovery

Feeling hopeless, helpless, and/or worthless

Active suicidal ideation

Unremitting anxiety disorder

Recent purchase of a weapon

Impulsivity

Serial or repeated suicide attempts

Regret that one survived a suicide attempt

Beck Hopelessness Scale score greater than or equal to 9

New onset of global insomnia

Other risk factors (*may prompt close follow-up*)

Older age

Male gender

Unemployment

Mood disorders

Psychotic disorders

Substance abuse or dependence

Non-zero score on the suicide item of the Beck Depression Inventory

Previous suicide attempts

First year after an index episode of psychotic or mood disorders

Social isolation

Family history of suicide

Increasing frequency of attempts

Increasing seriousness of attempts

Disruption of important psychosocial factors (job, relationships)

History of childhood abuse (sexual, physical, mental)

Poor stress tolerance

Poor treatment compliance or ability to form a therapeutic relationship in the past

Table 3
Clinical features and treatment of NMS and other hypermetabolic syndromes

Disorder	Symptoms	Treatment
NMS	History 1. Associated with initiation or increase of antipsychotic medication; often within 1 mo of change 2. Predisposing factors a. Dehydration b. Lithium use c. Presence of a mood disorder d. Possible rapid escalation of a dose (ie, intramuscular injections) Physical examination 1. Altered mental status 2. Marked muscle rigidity, but can vary with the potency of the medication used 3. Fever 4. Autonomic instability 5. Increased white blood cell count 6. Increased C K, renal function requires monitoring 7. Delirium	Discontinuation of the offending medication Intravenous fluids Antipyretic agents Cooling blanket: must examine for paradoxic pyrexia secondary to blood vessel constriction If supportive measures are inadequate, use Dantrolene or bromocriptine Bromocriptine: 2.5 mg twice a day or three times a day orally; may increase to a total dose of 45 mg per day Dantrolene sodium 1 mg/kg/daily for a period of eight days and proceed orally for another seven days Monitor liver function for hepatotoxicity. May reduce fever from the skeletal muscle contraction Wait at least 2 wk until retrying an antipsychotic Replenish serum iron levels if needed
LC	History Maybe a variant of NMS Appears more often as a rapid onset of hyperactive, often disorganized, delirium, high fever, then progresses to exhaustion, stupor, and coma with a mortality rate up to 50% Physical examination Combination of immobility, mutism, withdrawal, negativism, posturing, grimacing, and rigidity; common for all underlying disorders Waxy flexibility, stereotypy, echolalia, echopraxia, and episodic verbigeration; more common in psychotic disorders Anorexia, electrolyte imbalance, and cyanosis Arrhythmia and cardiac arrest Low serum iron levels	Lorazepam 1–2 mg intravenously once every 4 hours Consider ECT

(*continued on next page*)

Table 3
(continued)

Disorder	Symptoms	Treatment
SS	History The addition or consumption (overdose) of a serotonergic agent or combination of multiple antidepressants Physical Exam Mental status change: confusion, anxiety, irritability, agitation, restlessness Nervous system abnormality: myoclonus, hyperreflexia, ankle clonus, tremor, incoordination, ataxia Autonomic instability Muscle rigidity Laboratory: leukocytosis, rhabdomyolysis Fluid and electrolyte abnormalities: hyponatremia, hypomagnesaemia, and hypocalcemia DIC serotonin secreting tumors are possible	Removal of the offending agent Supportive measures: IV fluids, antipyretics, antihypertensives, cardiac monitoring, benzodiazepines for myoclonic jerks If needed: cyproheptadine mirtazapine ketanserin propranolol
MH	History Administration of volatile anesthetics and neuromuscular blocking agents Family history, but variable expression Physical Examination Tachypnea Tachycardia Rigidity Acidosis Rhabdomyolysis Hyperthermia Caffeine contracture test +	Pretreat vulnerable individuals with dantrolene before administration of anesthetic agent Once condition develops: a. Termination of exposure to anesthesia b. Effective core cooling c. Dantrolene: inhibits calcium release from SR

Abbreviations: CK, createnine kinase; DIC, Disseminated intravascular coagulation; ECT, electroconvulsive therapy; IM, intramuscular; IV, intravenous; LC, lethal catatonia; MH, malignant hyperthermia; NMS, neurolpetic malignant syndrome; SR, sarcoplasmic reticulum; SS, serotonin syndrome.

Other agents, such as Sinemet (carbidopa and levodopa) and amantadine, have been used for treatment of NMS. Following recovery from NMS, there is still a chance of recurrence when psychotic patients are treated with neuroleptics. To decrease such a risk, neuroleptics should reintroduced at least 2 weeks after the complete resolution of NMS.

Treatment of serotonin syndrome also requires cessation of the precipitating drug or drugs followed by administration of serotonin antagonists, such as cyproheptadine, as well as supportive care to control agitation, autonomic instability, and hyperthermia.

In patients with lethal catatonia who are on the treatment with neuroleptics, the dose should be decreased before cessation because the psychotic patient may demonstrate worsening of the underlying psychotic syndrome. In general, neuroleptics have no place in treatment of catatonia. Lorazepam has been used for treatment of lethal catatonia.[57] Electroconvulsive therapy should be applied when the patient fails pharmacotherapy.

Dantrolene, which works on the ryanodine receptors to prevent release of calcium, is used intravenously for treatment of MH. Treatment with dantrolene should be initiated rapidly if there is any clinical suspicion before full-blown MH develops.

AGGRESSION

Aggression is a violent and hostile behavior, which may intimidate or cause pain and injury to other members of society. Assessment and management of an aggressive and agitated patient who is physically or verbally abusive and poses a threat to himself or herself, the caregivers, or other members of society, is a significant challenge to any treating neurologist. Patients with various neurologic disorders present to the emergency room with aggressive behavior. Demented patients often develop aggression. In fact, behavioral and psychological features of dementia consist of aggression, psychosis, apathy, depression, and psychomotor agitation.[58] Patients with organic brain injury present with periodic and explosive episodes of aggression and agitation.[59]

Other neurologic patients with bursts of aggressive behavior are those with mental retardation who present as management challenges for treating neurologists. Other neurologic disorders, such as Huntington disease, Wilson disease, Lafora disease, acute intermittent porphyria, Lesch-Nyhan syndrome, and neuroacanthocytosis may present with aggressive behavior as part of their clinical manifestations.

Assessment

Violent patients present a heterogeneous group of individual with various underlying pathologies and, in many cases, do not suffer from a mental or psychiatric disorder. Therefore, assessment of an aggressive patient requires a careful approach to identify any concurrent neuropsychiatric disorder, such as psychosis, depression, mania, or mood liability. In addition, patients should be evaluated for any intellectual impairment or learning disabilities because this may lead to discovery of a previously unrecognized disorder.

Treatment

Management of an aggressive patient in the emergency room poses a significant challenge to the on-call neurologist. Agitated and aggressive patient may attack the emergency department personnel and cause injuries to them. In patients with acute aggression, use of neuroleptics, benzodiazepines, and external restraints are among the first choices. Although neuroleptics and benzodiazepines rapidly calm the patient, they should not be used for the long-term management owing to their troublesome side effects, particularly when the underlying cause of acute aggression is unrecognized. Aggressive patients with psychotic behavior should be treated with neuroleptic agents, such as haloperidol, which can be administered orally, intramuscularly, or intravenously. Other treatment options for rapid reduction of aggression and assaultiveness include newer agents, such as risperidone, olanzapine, and ziprasidone.

Lorazepam, a rapidly absorbable benzodiazepine with rapid onset, is another treatment option that can be used in combination with antipsychotic medications for further efficacy. For less severe forms of acute aggression and agitation, lorazepam alone is an adequate treatment. Long-term treatment of aggressive patients requires identification of the underlying cause of aggression. Mood-stabilizing agents, such as lithium, carbamazepine, valproic acid, beta-blockers, and SSRIs, have been used for long-term treatment of violent patients.

AMNESTIC SYNDROMES

The cardinal feature of the amnestic syndromes is impairment of learning new information. As a group, amnestic disorders are characterized by profound impairment of forming new memories or recalling previously learned data while the patient is in a normal state of consciousness. Both short-term and long-term memory systems are affected. The amnestic syndromes significantly interfere with the patient's activities of daily living. Various disorders, such as head trauma, epilepsy, dementia, electroconvulsive therapy, use of benzodiazepines and alcohol, and Wernicke-Korsakoff syndrome, are associated with amnesia. These conditions are differentiated from each other based on the presence of other physical findings on the examination. The exact incidence and prevalence of amnestic disorders are not known because they are uncommon. Wernicke-Korsakoff syndrome due to thiamine (vitamin-B1) deficiency is an example of an amnestic syndrome in which patients demonstrate severely impaired anterograde amnesia during the episode. Other clinical features include ataxia, confusion, and ophthalmoplegia. Another amnestic syndrome is transient global amnesia (TGA), which begins suddenly and usually resolves in a day.[60] Patients with TGA demonstrate confusion and have both anterograde and retrograde amnesia, ask repetitive questions, and may be aware of their memory impairment. Several underlying causes, such as epilepsy, emotional stress, migrainous vasospasm, and occlusive cerebrovascular disease, have been implicated in the development of TGA. Existing evidence indicates that development of one episode of TGA does not increase the patient's chance of developing more prolonged memory impairment. Other causes of an amnestic syndrome include limbic encephalitis, head trauma, vascular diseases, cerebral anoxia, and neurodegenerative diseases.

Dissociative amnesia (also known as psychogenic amnesia) is one of a group of disorders called dissociative disorders. Patients with dissociative amnesia usually attempt to escape from certain information, usually associated with stressful, unpleasant, and traumatic events. A prominent loss of autobiographical memory and not remembering one's own name (in the absence of aphasic or any other cognitive disorders that affect other intellectual spheres) are observed in this type of amnesia. Patients who suffer from neurologically-based amnesia remember their name and identity.

Assessment

The diagnosis of amnestic syndrome cannot be made in the context of dementia or delirium. The diagnostic approach to a patient with amnestic syndrome includes two main objectives: to determine the extent of the memory impairment and to evaluate the nature of memory impairment and its roots in encoding, storage, and retrieval processes.

Treatment

Generally, treatment of amnestic syndrome rests on the identification and management of the underlying cause of the forgetfulness. Patients with Wernicke encephalopathy should be treated with thiamine and patients with Korsakoff amnesia should be placed on alcohol abstinence. There is no specific treatment of transient global amnesia and it usually resolves completely in a few hours. In patients with chronic progressive neurologic diseases, such as Alzheimer disease, cognitive and behavioral rehabilitation should be used. In cases of a psychiatric patient with amnestic syndrome who cannot be managed at home or who is at high risk for injury to self or others, admission to a psychiatric unit is necessary.

SOMATOFORM DISORDERS

Neurologists commonly evaluate patients with baffling and inexplicable complaints that are resistant to several therapeutic regimens, known as somatoform disorders.[61]

Somatoform disorders include somatization disorder, undifferentiated somatoform disorder, conversion disorder, pain disorder, hypochondriasis, body dysmorphic disorder, and somatoform disorder not otherwise specified. Of these, conversion disorder is the one most commonly seen by neurologists. Patients with factitious or malingering disorders intentionally complain of symptoms and do have primary and secondary gains, respectively. However, patients with somatoform disorders unintentionally complain of somatic complaints and do not possess secondary gains. In many instances, these patients pose a therapeutic challenge to the treating neurologist. Patients with somatization disorder are identified by the presence of pain in at least four different locations, two gastrointestinal, one sexual, and one pseudoneurological symptom. Diagnostic criteria for somatoform disorders are presented in **Box 3**. Patients with conversion disorder present with symptoms or deficits that involve motor or sensory systems and are not intentionally feigned. In many cases of conversion disorder, psychological factors or stressors are present. Clinically, patients with

Box 3
Diagnostic criteria for somatization disorder

A. A history of many physical complaints beginning before age 30 years that occur over a period of several years and result in treatment being sought or significant impairment in social, occupational, or other important areas of functioning.

B. Each of the following criteria must have been met, with individual symptoms occurring at any time during the course of the disturbance:

1. Four pain symptoms: a history of pain related to at least four different sites or functions (eg, head, abdomen, back, joints, extremities, chest, rectum, during menstruation, during sexual intercourse, or during urination)
2. Two gastrointestinal symptoms: a history of at least two gastrointestinal symptoms other than pain (eg, nausea, bloating, vomiting other than during pregnancy, diarrhea, or intolerance of several different foods)
3. One sexual symptom: a history of at least one sexual or reproductive symptom other than pain (eg, sexual indifference, erectile or ejaculatory dysfunction, irregular menses, excessive menstrual bleeding, vomiting throughout pregnancy)
4. One pseudoneurological symptom: a history of at least one symptom or deficit suggesting a neurologic condition not limited to pain (conversion symptoms such as impaired coordination or balance, paralysis or localized weakness, difficulty swallowing or lump in throat, aphonia, urinary retention, hallucinations, loss of touch or pain sensation, double vision, blindness, deafness, seizures; dissociative symptoms such as amnesia; or loss of consciousness other than fainting)

C. Either (1) or (2):

1. After appropriate investigation, each of the symptoms in Criterion B cannot be fully explained by a known general medical condition or the direct effects of a substance (eg, a drug of abuse, a medication)
2. When there is a related general medical condition, the physical complaints or resulting social or occupational impairment are in excess of what would be expected from the history, physical examination, or laboratory findings

D. The symptoms are not intentionally feigned or produced (as in Factitious Disorder or Malingering).

Reprinted from The diagnostic and statistical manual of mental disorders, 4th edition, Text Revision. American Psychiatric Association; 2000; with permission.

somatization and conversion disorders present with impaired coordination, paresis or paralysis, visual loss, hallucinations, deafness, and loss of pain sensation. The neurologic complaints presented by patients with somatoform disorders are resistant to treatment, which in turn leads to ordering several tests and using significant resources to exclude any possible underlying neurologic disorder.[62]

Assessment

Usually patients with somatoform disorders have a history of multiple visits to emergency departments; therefore, careful assessment of these patients, thorough neurologic examination, and mental status evaluation are required to make the correct diagnosis. Neurologists who assess these patients in the emergency room must initially exclude any underlying neurologic and medical disease. Then the evaluating neurologist should pay attention to certain coexisting comorbid psychiatric disorders, such as depression, dysthymia, use of illicit drugs, or personality disorders. In addition, malingering and factitious disorders must be excluded.

Treatment

The treating neurologist should avoid confronting these patients because this form of intervention is generally ineffective. Because the symptoms and complaints do not have a structural basis, the neurologist should avoid ordering several dangerous diagnostic interventions and polypharmacy. In addition, the number of treating physicians involved in the care of each patient should be limited. Building a trusting relationship with the patient leads to treatment that is more effective. Obtaining psychiatric consultation and using cognitive behavioral therapy are also useful in the management of somatoform disorders.[63]

ETHICAL AND LEGAL ISSUES: INVOLUNTARY CONFINEMENT (COMMITMENT)

The first issue confronting the neurologist who evaluates an individual with psychiatric issues is always the safety of the individual and others. Does the person pose a danger to himself or herself, or others? Can the patient adequately care for herself or himself on an outpatient basis? Careful assessment of suicide or violence risk is mandatory. If the evaluation reveals that the patient is suicidal or homicidal, or gravely disabled, the neurologist must take the necessary steps to provide for safe treatment. Depending on the evaluation, the treatment may involve inpatient or outpatient psychiatric care, or, at times, hospitalization on a medical ward with a sitter. The patient may decide to seek further treatment and hospitalization on a voluntary basis. If this is the case, the neurologist should facilitate admission to the most appropriate facility. Often, however, the patient lacks insight into his illness and may refuse to accept psychiatric treatment and/or hospitalization. In this case, the neurologist needs to be aware of state legal statutes that provide for involuntary treatment. States vary in these requirements. In most jurisdictions, a licensed physician may initiate initial involuntary treatment if the patient poses a danger to self, others, or is gravely disabled; longer stays usually require a judicial order.[64]

Involuntary commitment does pose an ethical dilemma to the physician. Involuntary confinement limits autonomy and the right of the individual to make his own decisions. The decision for involuntary commitment should not be taken lightly. Most physicians will choose to limit autonomy if the physician considers that it is necessary to save human life (ie, beneficence).[65] The physician must take care to provide carefully written documentation in the medical record of his or her decision and the rationale surrounding this choice.[66]

Informed Consent and Capacity

Informed consent and patient autonomy are essential elements of medical ethics in the twenty-first century. In order for an individual to give informed consent, several criteria must be met: adequate information, absence of coercion, and patient competence. Adequate information includes information about the procedure or medication, risks and benefits of the procedure or medication, any available alternatives, and consequences if the patient refuses the treatment or procedure.[67] Psychotropic medication package inserts list many untoward side effects, including suicide, blood dyscrasias, death, tardive dyskinesia, and fetal abnormalities if pregnant. Many medicines are commonly used for conditions yet lack US Food and Drug Administration (FDA) approval for that disease state. For instance, antipsychotics carry FDA approval for many illnesses but lack the indication of use as treatment of delirium. Written treatment plans should include a discussion of the elements of informed consent if at all possible. Many government agencies provide written information sheets to patients about medications and include the patient's signature to indicate that she or he received the information.[65]

Because informed consent includes the element of competence, all physicians make an informal decision about competence every time they present a patient with a new treatment or have the patient sign an informed consent form. Yet, misconceptions exist about the term.[68] First, physicians do not evaluate competence; competence is a legal determination that can be made only by a judge. Physicians assess capacity; that is, the ability to make a decision. The terms may be used interchangeably if the physician recognizes that there is a legal difference between the two. Second, competence is not an all-or-none decision. Forms of competence include the competence to drive, the competency to make legal or financial decisions, or the competence to make medical decisions. Physicians usually evaluate the capacity to make medical decisions. Another misconception is that the lack of capacity is permanent. Individuals frequently lack the capacity to make medical decisions if they are comatose or delirious. As the patient's condition improves, however, medical decision-making capacity should be reassessed. The patient should be allowed to make his or her own treatment decisions when the condition improves. In some cases, the patient may lose the capacity to make decisions regarding her or his medical care if the condition deteriorates. Once again, documentation in the medical record of the physician's assessment of capacity is essential.[68]

Ethical experts suggest that the physician should weigh the risks and benefits of a proposed treatment when evaluating capacity. A patient needs a greater degree of understanding to agree to a procedure that has a greater degree of risks relative to the proposed benefit. Alternatively, a patient needs a greater degree of understanding to refuse a treatment that has more benefits and fewer risks. For instance, an elderly patient with several medical illnesses who is unable to care for himself or herself at home and has no one to help provide care may lack the capacity to refuse nursing home placement because the perceived benefits far outweigh the risks. An individual with an unexplained fever and confusion may lack the capacity to refuse a lumbar puncture because the benefits outweigh the risks. A patient may lack the capacity to agree to certain cardiac or neurosurgical procedures, depending on the relative risks and benefits. A wise clinician will document the reasoning for her or his assessment of capacity in the medical record instead of a general statement of capacity.[69]

Another fallacy is using the Folstein Mini–Mental State Exam (MMSE) as a basis to assess capacity.[70] For instance, individuals without deficits on the MMSE may still lack the capacity to give consent if delusional. An individual may have deficits on the MMSE and still have the capacity to give consent based on the procedure or treatment risks and benefits.[70] Problems arise when the clinician only looks at the final decision and not the *process* that the patient uses to arrive at his or her conclusion.[68] Information from the family and ancillary services can provide advice. Physical therapists, occupational therapists, and neuropsychological testing reports can document additional information that is useful in assessing capacity.[71]

Problematic patients include those who are unwilling or unable to answer questions or speak with the physician. This may be due to catatonia, severe depression, psychosis, or personality disorder. The physician has a responsibility to attempt a discussion about the treatments involved. Family members, friends, or members of the treatment team trusted by the patient may help to open or improve communication. Though not all patients who refuse treatment and refuse to explain their rationale are incompetent, the physician is wise to again weigh the risks and benefits of the refusal to the patient. In potentially life-threatening situations in which the patient cannot or will not explain his or her reasoning, and attempts to find others to communicate with the patient are unsuccessful, the physician may choose to consider that the patient lacks the capacity and attempt to find surrogate decision makers.[72]

Against Medical Advice

What about the patient who threatens to leave the hospital against medical advice (AMA)? Some precipitants for requests to leave AMA include fear, anger, or psychosis.[73] The request to leave AMA should prompt careful discussion between the patient and her or his physician. The problem often lies in faulty communication. Additional time spent by the physician with the patient may reveal areas of misperception or miscommunication because many hospitalized patients are not aware of planned treatments and anticipated length of stay.[74] Improved communication may be sufficient to alleviate the request to leave AMA or pave the way for the patient to return for treatment later.[75]

The threat to leave AMA should also prompt a capacity evaluation. Does this person have the capacity to fully understand the risks associated with hospital departure? Competent patients may refuse treatment. Some patients who refuse treatment or request to leave AMA may actually exhibit maladaptive denial. Denial is a defense mechanism used by many healthy and unhealthy individuals. The courts recognize that individuals with maladaptive denial may lack the capacity to make medical decisions.[65]

Ethical Issues in Other Psychiatric Disorders

Numerous illnesses in the psychiatry or neurology interface raise ethical considerations. Although many practice guidelines exist about the disclosure of a diagnosis of dementia, studies show that physicians do not always follow the recommendations.[76] Voluntarily suggesting to a patient with psychogenic movements that "he (or she) will improve" may be unethical because it may be deleterious to the patient's health and the therapeutic relationship.[77] Because many patients react to a diagnosis of a conversion disorder with anger and mistrust, neurologists often vary their diagnostic discussion with patients and choose to not be completely frank.[78] Direct confrontation is often not advised for patients with malingering or factitious disorder (Munchausen syndrome) and legal consultation is prudent.[79]

SUMMARY: PROFESSIONALISM

Professionalism is "the obligation of the physician to uphold the primacy of patients' interests, to achieve and maintain medical competency, and to abide by high ethical standards."[80] Physicians should be aware of current ethical principles and controversies, continue to advance their scope of knowledge, educate others, and promote competent patient care. Competent patient care may mean referral to other specialists if the condition is beyond one's scope of expertise or if there are personality conflicts that undermine the therapeutic relationship. The American Academy of Neurology (AAN) policy promotes professionalism and ethical standards.[81]

REFERENCES

1. Katon W, Sullivan MD. Depression and chronic medical illness. J Clin Psychiatry 1990;51(Suppl):3–11.
2. Laurent SM, Simons AD. Sexual dysfunction in depression and anxiety: conceptualizing sexual dysfunction as part of an internalizing dimension. Clin Psychol Rev 2009;29(7):573–85.
3. Wuwongse S, Chang RC, Law AC. The putative neurodegenerative links between depression and Alzheimer's disease. Prog Neurobiol 2010;91(4):362–75.
4. DeMichele-Sweet MA, Sweet RA. Genetics of psychosis in Alzheimer's disease: a review. J Alzheimers Dis 2010;19(3):761–80.
5. Whang W, Shimbo D, Kronish IM, et al. Depressive symptoms and all-cause mortality in unstable angina pectoris (from the Coronary Psychosocial Evaluation Studies [COPES]). Am J Cardiol 2010;106(8):1104–7.
6. Zafar MU, Paz-Yepes M, Shimbo D, et al. Anxiety is a better predictor of platelet reactivity in coronary artery disease patients than depression. Eur Heart J 2010; 31(13):1573–82.
7. Habra ME, Baker B, Frasure-Smith N, et al. First episode of major depressive disorder and vascular factors in coronary artery disease patients: baseline characteristics and response to antidepressant treatment in the CREATE trial. J Psychosom Res 2010;69(2):133–41.
8. Pereira AM, Tiemensma J, Romijn JA. Neuropsychiatric disorders in Cushing's syndrome. Neuroendocrinology 2010;92(Suppl 1):65–70.
9. Tiemensma J, Kokshoorn NE, Biermasz NR, et al. Subtle cognitive impairments in patients with long-term cure of Cushing's disease. J Clin Endocrinol Metab 2010; 95(6):2699–714.
10. Finocchi C, Villani V, Casucci G. Therapeutic strategies in migraine patients with mood and anxiety disorders: clinical evidence. Neurol Sci 2010;31(Suppl 1): S95–8.
11. Paemeleire K. Brain lesions and cerebral functional impairment in migraine patients. J Neurol Sci 2009;283(1-2):134–6.
12. Farner L, Wagle J, Engedal K, et al. Depressive symptoms in stroke patients: a 13 month follow-up study of patients referred to a rehabilitation unit. J Affect Disord 2010;127(1–3):211–8.
13. Broomfield NM, Laidlaw K, Hickabottom E, et al. Post-stroke depression: the case for augmented, individually tailored cognitive behavioural therapy. Clin Psychol Psychother 2011;18(3):202–17.
14. Robinson RG, Spalletta G. Poststroke depression: a review. Can J Psychiatry 2010;55(6):341–9.
15. Jorge RE, Starkstein SE, Robinson RG. Apathy following stroke. Can J Psychiatry 2010;55(6):350–4.
16. House A, Knapp P, Bamford J, et al. Mortality at 12 and 24 months after stroke may be associated with depressive symptoms at 1 month. Stroke 2001;32(3): 696–701.

17. Pohjasvaara T, Vataja R, Leppävuori A, et al. Depression is an independent predictor of poor long-term functional outcome post-stroke. Eur J Neurol 2001; 8(4):315–9.
18. Olin JT, Schneider LS, Katz IR, et al. Provisional diagnostic criteria for depression of Alzheimer disease. Am J Geriatr Psychiatry 2002;10(2):125–8.
19. Zubenko GS, Zubenko WN, McPherson S, et al. A collaborative study of the emergence and clinical features of the major depressive syndrome of Alzheimer's disease. Am J Psychiatry 2003;160(5):857–66.
20. Pinkston JB, Kablinger A, Alekseeva N. Multiple sclerosis and behavior. Int Rev Neurobiol 2007;79:323–39.
21. Paparrigopoulos T, Ferentinos P, Kouzoupis A, et al. The neuropsychiatry of multiple sclerosis: focus on disorders of mood, affect and behaviour. Int Rev Psychiatry 2010;22(1):14–21.
22. McDonald WM, Richard IH, DeLong MR. Prevalence, etiology, and treatment of depression in Parkinson's disease. Biol Psychiatry 2003;54(3):363–75.
23. Paulsen JS, Nehl C, Hoth KF, et al. Depression and stages of Huntington's disease. J Neuropsychiatry Clin Neurosci 2005;17(4):496–502.
24. Bagary M. Epilepsy, antiepileptic drugs and suicidality. Curr Opin Neurol 2011; 24(2):177–82.
25. Litofsky NS, Farace E, Anderson F Jr, et al. Glioma outcomes project investigators. Depression in patients with high-grade glioma: results of the glioma outcomes project. Neurosurgery 2004;54(2):358–66 [discussion: 366–7].
26. Farrugia ME, Conway R, Simpson DJ, et al. Paraneoplastic limbic encephalitis. Clin Neurol Neurosurg 2005;107(2):128–31.
27. Shapshak P, Kangueane P, Fujimura RK, et al. Editorial neuroAIDS review. AIDS 2011;25(2):123–41.
28. Heath CA, Cooper SA, Murray K, et al. Validation of diagnostic criteria for variant Creutzfeldt-Jakob disease. Ann Neurol 2010;67(6):761–70.
29. Stoudemire A. New antidepressant drugs and the treatment of depression in the medically ill patient. Psychiatr Clin North Am 1996;19(3):495–514.
30. Blanchet P, Frommer GP. Mood change preceding epileptic seizures. J Nerv Ment Dis 1986;174(8):471–6.
31. Shulman LM, Taback RL, Rabinstein AA, et al. Non-recognition of depression and other non-motor symptoms in Parkinson's disease. Parkinsonism Relat Disord 2002;8(3):193–7.
32. Gonera EG, van't Hof M, Berger HJ, et al. Symptoms and duration of the prodromal phase in Parkinson's disease. Mov Disord 1997;12(6):871–6.
33. Siemers ER, Shekhar A, Quaid K, et al. Anxiety and motor performance in Parkinson's disease. Mov Disord 1993;8(4):501–6.
34. Frumin M, Chisholm T, Dickey CC, et al. Psychiatric and behavioral problems. Neurol Clin 1998;16(2):521–44.
35. Lim RF, Hilty DM, Jerant AF. An algorithm for treating psychotic disorders in primary care. Prim Psychiatry 2001;8:68–74.
36. Cummings JL. Organic delusions: phenomenology, anatomical correlations, and review. Br J Psychiatry 1985;146:184–97.
37. Almeida OP. Bipolar disorder with late onset: an organic variety mood disorder. Rev Bras Psiquiatr 2004;26:27–30 [in Portuguese].
38. Mendez MF. Mania in neurological disorders. Curr Psychiatry Rep 2000;2: 440–5.
39. Heinrich TW, Grahm G. Hypothyroidism presenting as psychosis: myxedema madness revisited. Prim Care Companion J Clin Psychiatry 2003;5:260–6.

40. Radhika SA, Sriram MS. Mania as a presentation of primary hypothyroidism. Singapore Med J 2009;50:65–7.
41. Oliveira JP, Araujo MD, Carlotti CG Jr, et al. Mood disorder due to a general medical condition with manic features. Case Report Med 2009;10:1–4.
42. Shulman KI. Disinhibition syndromes, secondary mania and bipolar disorder in old age. J Affect Disord 1997;46:175–82.
43. Arora M, Daughton J. Mania in the medically ill. Curr Psychiatry Rep 2007;9:232–5.
44. Botre F, Pavan A. Enhancement drugs and the athlete. Neurol Clin 2009;26: 149–67.
45. Schneck CD. Bipolar disorder in neurologic illness. Curr Treat Options Neurol 2002;4:477–86.
46. Mula M, Bell GS, Sander JW. Suicidality in epilepsy and possible effects of antiepileptic drugs. Curr Neurol Neurosci Rep 2010;10(4):327–32.
47. Wenzel A, Berchick ER, Tenhave T, et al. Predictors of suicide relative to other deaths in patients with suicide attempts and suicide ideation: a 30-year prospective study. J Affect Disord 2011;132(3):1–8, 375–82.
48. Mitchel AJ, Dennis M. Self harm and attempted suicide in adults. 10 practical questions and answers for emergency department staff. Emerg Med J 2006; 23:251–5.
49. Blasco-Fontecilla H, Alegria AA, Lopez-Castroman J, et al. Short self-reported sleep duration and suicidal behavior: a crosssectional study. J Affect Disord 2011;133(1-2):239–46.
50. Skegg K. Self harm. Lancet 2005;366:1471–83.
51. Rosenbush PT, Mazurek MF. Catatonia and its treatment. Schizophr Bull 2010;36: 239–42.
52. Margetić B, Aukst-Margetić B. Neuroleptic malignant syndrome and its controversies. Pharmacoepidemiol Drug Saf 2010;19(5):429–35.
53. Khaldi S, Kornreich C, Choubani Z, et al. Neuroleptic malignant syndrome and atypical antipsychotics: a brief review. Encephale 2008;34(6):618–24.
54. Dassa D, Drai-Moog D, Samuelian JC. Neuroleptic malignant syndrome with the addition of aripiprazole to clozapine. Prog Neuropsychopharmacol Biol Psychiatry 2010;34(2):427–8.
55. Ables AZ, Nagubilli R. Prevention, recognition, and management of serotonin syndrome. Am Fam Physician 2010;81(9):1139–42.
56. Caroff SN, Hurford I, Lybrand J, et al. Movement disorders induced by antipsychotic drugs: implications of the CATIE schizophrenia trial. Neurol Clin 2011; 29(1):127–48, viii.
57. Grover S, Aggarwal M. Long-term maintenance lorazepam for catatonia: a case report. Gen Hosp Psychiatry 2011;33(1):82.e1–3.
58. McShane RH. What are the syndromes of behavioral and psychological symptoms of dementia? Int Psychogeriatr 2000;12(Suppl 1):147–53.
59. Chew E, Zafonte RD. Pharmacological management of neurobehavioral disorders following traumatic brain injury–a state-of-the-art review. J Rehabil Res Dev 2009;46(6):851–79.
60. Kritchevsky M, Squire LR, Zouzounis JA. Transient global amnesia: characterization of anterograde and retrograde amnesia. Neurology 1988;38(2):213–9.
61. Fink P, Hansen MS, Sondergaard L, et al. Mental illness in new neurological patients. J Neurol Neurosurg Psychiatry 2003;74:817–9.
62. Smith GR Jr, Monson RA, Ray DC. Patients with multiple unexplained symptoms. Their characteristics, functional health, and health care utilization. Arch Intern Med 1986;146(1):69–72.

63. Kroenke K, Swindle R. Cognitive-behavioral therapy for somatization and symptom syndromes: a critical review of controlled clinical trials. Psychother Psychosom 2000;69(4):205–15.
64. Gutheil TG, Appelbaum PS. Legal issues in emergency psychiatry. In: Clinical handbook of psychiatry and the law. 3rd edition. Philadelphia: Lippincott Williams & Wilkins; 2000. p. 39–82.
65. Simon RI. Legal and ethical issues. In: Wise MG, Rundell JR, editors. Textbook of consultation-liaison psychiatry: psychiatry in the medically ill. 2nd edition. Washington, DC: American Psychiatric Publishing, Inc; 2002. p. 167–89.
66. Park JM, Donovan AL, Park L, et al. Emergency psychiatry. In: Stern TA, Fricchione GL, Cassem NH, et al, editors. Massachusetts general hospital handbook of general hospital psychiatry. 6th edition. Philadelphia: Saunders Elsevier; 2010. p. 529–40.
67. Committee on Medical Education. Summary and review of basic ethical concerns. In: Group for the Advancement of Psychiatry, Report No. 129. A Casebook in Psychiatric Ethics. New York: Brunner/Mazel; 1990. p. 79–94.
68. Ganzini L, Volicer L, Nelson W, et al. Pitfalls in assessment of decision-making capacity. Psychosomatics 2003;44(3):237–43.
69. Gutheil TG, Appelbaum PS. Competence and substitute decision making. In: Clinical handbook of Psychiatry and the law. 3rd edition. Philadelphia: Lippincott Williams & Wilkins; 2000. p. 215–60.
70. Etchells E, Shuchman M, Workman S, et al. Accuracy of clinical impressions and mini-mental state exam scores for assessing capacity to consent to major medical treatment: comparison with criterion-standard psychiatric assessments. Psychosomatics 1997;38(3):239–45.
71. Farnsworth MG. Competency evaluations in a general hospital. Psychosomatics 1990;31(1):60–6.
72. Hurst SA. When patients refuse assessment of decision-making capacity: how should clinicians respond? Arch Intern Med 2004;164:1757–60.
73. Albert HD, Kornfeld DS. The treat to sign out against medical advice. Ann Intern Med 1973;79:888–91.
74. O'Leary KJ, Kulkami N, Landler MP, et al. Hospitalized patients' understanding of their plan of care. Mayo Clin Proc 2010;85(1):47–52.
75. Schouten R, Brendel RW. Legal aspects of consultation. In: Stern TA, Fricchione GL, Cassem NH, et al, editors. Massachusetts General Hospital handbook of general hospital psychiatry. 6th edition. Philadelphia: Saunders Elsevier; 2010. p. 639–50.
76. Carpenter B, Dave J. Disclosing a dementia diagnosis: a review of opinion and practice, and a proposed research agenda. Gerontologist 2004;44(2):149–58.
77. Shamy MC. The treatment of psychogenic movement disorders with suggestion is ethically justified. Mov Disord 2010;25(3):260–4.
78. Kanaan R, Armstrong D, Wessely S. Limits to truth-telling: neurologists' communication in conversion disorder. Patient Educ Couns 2009;77(2):296–301.
79. Braun IM, Greenberg DB, Smith FA, et al. Functional somatic symptoms, deception syndromes, and somatoform disorders. In: Stern TA, Fricchione GL, Cassem NH, et al, editors. Massachusetts General Hospital handbook of general hospital psychiatry. 6th edition. Philadelphia: Saunders Elsevier; 2010. p. 173–87.
80. Larriviere D, Beresford HR. Invited article: professionalism in neurology, the role of law. Neurology 2008;71:1283–8.
81. American Academy of Neurology Code of Professional Conduct. Available at: http://www.aan.com/globals/axon/assets/3968.pdf. Accessed April 6, 2011.

Neurologic Emergencies: Case Studies

Alireza Minagar, MD[a,*], Alejandro A. Rabinstein, MD[b], Kourosh Rezania, MD[c], Marvin Sih, MD[c], Nadejda Alekseeva, MD[a,d], Rodica E. Petrea, MD[e], Abdulnasser Alhajeri, MD[f], Saeed Talebzadeh Nick, MD[a], Eduardo Gonzalez-Toledo, MD, PhD[a,g], Mohammad Ali Sahraian, MD[h], Roger E. Kelley, MD[i]

KEYWORDS

• Neurologic disease • Emergency • Visual • MRI • Stroke • Agitation • Shortness of breath • Coma

During the past 2 decades, the world has witnessed a significant improvement in the understanding of the pathogenesis and treatment of neurologic diseases, which present as emergencies. Every day neurologists are consulted for patients who present with neurologic emergencies to the emergency departments. In this article, we present a series of case reports about patients with acute neurologic problems and discuss their management briefly.

[a] Department of Neurology, Louisiana State University Health Sciences Center, 1501 Kings Highway, Shreveport, LA 71130, USA
[b] Department of Neurology, Mayo Clinic, 200 First Street SW - Mayo W8B, Rochester, MN 55905, USA
[c] Department of Neurology, The University of Chicago Medical Center, 5841 South Maryland Avenue, MC 2030, Chicago, IL 60637-1470, USA
[d] Department of Psychiatry, Overton Brooks VAMC, Shreveport, LA, USA
[e] Department of Neurology, University of Kentucky College of Medicine, 740 South Limestone, Suite L 445, Lexington, KY 40536-0284, USA
[f] Division of Neuroradiology, Department of Radiology and Neurosurgery, University of Kentucky, Lexington, KY, USA
[g] Departments of Radiology and Neurology, Louisiana State University Health Sciences Center, Shreveport, LA, USA
[h] Sina MS Research Center, Sina Hospital, Hassan Abad Square, Tehran, Iran
[i] Department of Neurology, Tulane University, New Orleans, LA, USA
* Corresponding author.
E-mail address: aminagar@gmail.com

Neurol Clin 30 (2012) 345–356
doi:10.1016/j.ncl.2011.10.002 **neurologic.theclinics.com**

CASE REPORTS

Case 1: Progressive Visual Loss

A 35-year-old healthy woman presents to the emergency room with decreased vision in her right eye. Two days before the development of right visual loss, she felt pain in her globe on eye movements. The patient has no significant past medical history and was not taking any medication. Neurologic examination revealed normal visual acuity of the left eye with visual acuity of 20/400 in the left eye with a central scotoma. Color perception of the right eye was impaired, and a relative afferent pupillary defect was present. Ocular movements were normal, whereas funduscopic examination showed left papillitis. Neurologic examination was unremarkable otherwise. Magnetic resonance imaging (MRI) of the brain and orbits revealed the presence of scattered hyperintense lesions on T2-weighted sequence with enhancement of the left optic sheath on postgadolinium T1-weighted images (**Fig. 1**). Analysis of the cerebrospinal fluid (CSF) demonstrated normal glucose levels with elevated protein levels and 18 lymphocytes per cubic millimeter. The CSF IgG index was elevated, and 4 oligoclonal bands were present only in the CSF and not in the concomitant serum. The visual evoked potential (VEP) was prolonged only in the right eye at 112 millisecond. The patient was treated with intravenous methylprednisolone, 1 g daily, for 3 days. Four weeks later, the vision of the right eye had improved much and the right visual field was within normal limits. The patient decided to start therapy with β-interferon to decrease the risk of developing clinically definite multiple sclerosis.

Comment

This patient represents a typical case of optic neuritis with other abnormal findings such as white matter lesions on brain MRI, the presence of oligoclonal bands only in the CSF, and prolonged VEP in the right eye. She did not have any other neurologic symptoms. However, because the patient was at higher risk for a second

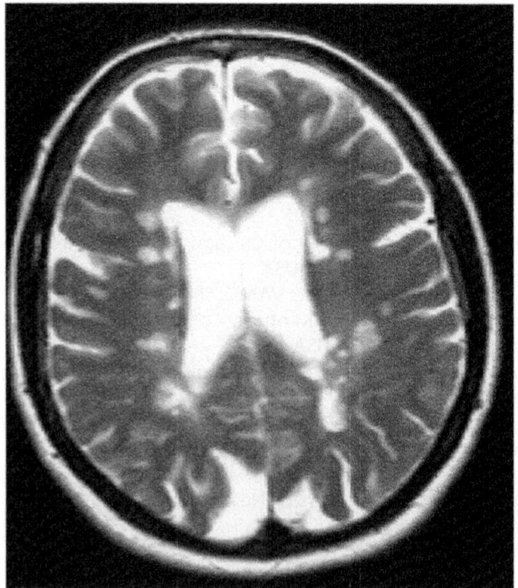

Fig. 1. MRI of the brain, axial view and T2-weighted sequence, demonstrating multiple white matter hyperintense signals consistent with a demyelinating disease.

demyelinating attack and development of multiple sclerosis, she opted to be treated with β-interferon to delay the onset of multiple sclerosis.[1,2]

Case 2: Eyes-Open Coma

A 29-year-old woman with congenital heart disease underwent a major cardiovascular surgery to correct her atrioventricular discordance from previously corrected vessel transposition. As a child, the patient had developed cerebral abscesses in the right frontal and temporal lobes as a complication of her cyanotic congenital heart disease, but she had recovered without sequelae after surgical resection and antibiotic therapy. Her neurologic condition was normal before the surgery. After the operation, the patient was kept sedated with propofol for 36 hours. On discontinuation of the infusion, the patient remained unresponsive. A neurology consultation was requested. The patient's examination showed that her eyes were open, but she was not fixating, tracking, or blinking to visual threat. Gaze was conjugate. No abnormal eye, facial, or limb movements were observed. The patient had no motor responses to pain. Computed tomographic (CT) scan of the brain only revealed areas of chronic encephalomalacia in the regions affected by the distant abscesses. Emergent electroencephalogram (EEG) demonstrated continuous seizure activity arising from the right temporal area. The patient was treated with lorazepam and fosphenytoin and the seizures resolved. The following day she was fully awake and lucid. The patient was discharged 7 days later on maintenance levetiracetam with no neurologic deficits.

Comment

Nonconvulsive status epilepticus must be considered in cases of unexplained coma, even in the absence of acute brain injury or history of epilepsy.[3] Subtle clinical manifestations may be present, such as nystagmus or low-amplitude rhythmic movements of fingers or toes, but electroencephalography is indispensable to make this diagnosis. As illustrated by this case, eyes open without any sign of reactivity to external stimulation should raise suspicion of this diagnosis. Although nonconvulsive seizures are probably more common in comatose patients with preexistent brain lesions (eg, strokes, tumors, neurosurgical scars), they are not rare in critically ill patients without previous brain disease, especially in cases of cardiac arrest, prolonged shock, and severe sepsis.[4]

Case 3: Extreme Agitation

A 66-year-old man with a history of several autoimmune diseases (diabetes mellitus, hypothyroidism, vitiligo, hypogonadism) began having sudden spells of right arm jerking. Concurrently, he developed progressive behavioral changes, with increasing irritability. Over the following 4 to 6 weeks, the spells became more frequent and were followed by periods of drowsiness. The patient underwent extensive evaluations at a local hospital without a definite diagnosis. He was started on antiepileptics after epileptiform abnormalities were identified on electroencephalography. The patient became completely disabled by his symptoms. Over the week before presentation to our hospital, the patient had begun to exhibit frank confusion and agitation. He was scheduled to be evaluated as outpatient in our center, but the night before the appointments he became so agitated that he had to be brought to the emergency department. On arrival, the patient's movements were extremely violent and his agitation proved refractory to regular sedatives (antidopaminergics and benzodiazepines). The situation demanded endotracheal intubation, mechanical ventilation, and initiation of a continuous infusion of midazolam.

Once in the intensive care unit (ICU), withdrawal of sedation was impossible because of the dangerous intensity of the abnormal movements, which had atypical choreiform features and at times seemed to be combined with myoclonus. Continuous electroencephalography showed no ongoing seizures. Brain imaging was unremarkable. The CSF was acellular but showed elevated protein content. The patient was treated empirically with high-dose methylprednisolone from first day, and plasma exchange was initiated on the second day for suspected autoimmune encephalitis. Four days later, the report of the autoimmune panel confirmed the presence of voltage-gated potassium channel (VGKC) antibodies in the serum and CSF. Workup results for malignancy were negative.

The patient required anesthetic doses of sedatives for control of severe agitation for more than 2 weeks. Only on the third week, he tolerated very gradual tapering of the sedation. The patient remained on methylprednisolone, 1 g daily, until his condition began to improve and underwent plasma exchange for a total of 7 sessions. On the third week, he was switched to prednisone, 100 mg daily; sedation was stopped; and he was liberated from mechanical ventilation. The patient left the ICU in a much improved condition after 21 days. He continued to improve in the general ward and was transferred to a rehabilitation facility to complete his recovery after 31 days in the hospital.

Comment

Extreme agitation can be the presenting manifestation of autoimmune encephalitis. We have seen these presentations associated with antibodies against VGKC and *N*-methyl-D-aspartate receptors.[5,6] Induction of anesthesia may be necessary to control the symptoms. Electroencephalography needs to be used to exclude seizures, because these disorders can cause epilepsy. Aggressive immune therapy with high-dose intravenous corticosteroids, often accompanied by plasma exchange or intravenous immunoglobulin (IVIG), is the mainstay of treatment, and it should not be tapered until the patient begins to show signs of improvement. Outcome can be favorable even in cases of prolonged, severe, and initially refractory symptoms.[5,6]

Case 4: Sudden Blindness and Confusion

A 41-year-old man was admitted for treatment of necrotizing pancreatitis and developed acute renal failure requiring dialysis. During one of his dialysis sessions, the patient became suddenly confused, nauseous, and tremulous. He complained he could not see. The physicians responding to the emergency call noted a blood pressure of 208/134 mm Hg. Neurologic examination revealed drowsiness, confusion, and cortical blindness. Shortly after, he had a generalized seizure that resolved spontaneously. The patient's CT scan of the brain showed areas of low attenuation consistent with edema in the posterior brain regions with small areas of hemorrhage in the occipital lobes. Brain MRI demonstrated typical findings of posterior reversible encephalopathy syndrome (PRES) (**Fig. 2**).

The patient was treated with gradual blood pressure reduction and levetiracetam for prevention of recurrent seizures. Within 5 days, his clinical condition was much improved. Three weeks later, the patient was neurologically intact except for a small right visual field deficit. Repeat brain MRI was normal, apart from the expected evolution of the previous areas of hemorrhage. The anticonvulsant was stopped after 4 weeks without recurrent seizures.

Comment

PRES is a clinical syndrome characterized by acute mental changes, often associated with visual disturbances, most typically cortical blindness (characterized by preserved

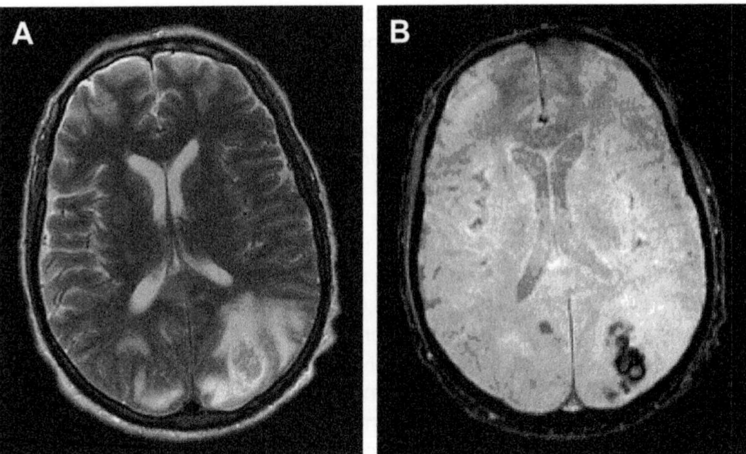

Fig. 2. MRI of the brain, T2-weighted sequence (*A*), showing areas of hyperintensity consistent with vasogenic edema in the posterior regions bilaterally with foci of occipital hemorrhage better visualized on the gradient recall echo T2* sequence (*B*).

vision but with inability to interpret the images acquired by the retina and transmitted by visual pathways), and seizures.[7]

(1) Radiologic findings of vasogenic edema predominantly affecting the posterior brain regions are confirmatory. However, atypical radiologic presentations are not rare and may include predominant anterior brain involvement, areas of cytotoxic edema (most often representative of infarction), and hemorrhage, as illustrated by this case.[8]
(2) The risk factors are acute hypertension, renal failure, cytotoxic drugs (especially calcineurin inhibitors), eclampsia, and probably autoimmune disorders.[9]
(3) Treatment consists of gradual blood pressure reduction and removal of any potential triggering factor, such as drugs. If seizures are present, antiepileptic therapy is indicated. In fact, PRES can present with status epilepticus.[10]
(4) Because these presentations may be clinically subtle, it is prudent to have a low threshold to obtain an EEG. The prognosis is generally, but not invariably, benign. The antiepileptic can be stopped within a month of the event. PRES may recur, especially among patients with poorly controlled hypertension undergoing hemodialysis and transplant recipients. Careful control of the blood pressure may decrease the risk of recurrences.

Case 5: Progressive Weakness and Gait Impairment

A 22-year-old man with no significant past medical history presented to the emergency department for progressive weakness and gait impairment. He started to have a tingling sensation and “tightness” in the toes and fingertips 1 week before the visit. Two days later, he noted difficulty with walking and inability to walk on the toes and heels, followed by impaired manual dexterity. The patient had an MRI study of the brain and cervical spine, which did not show any abnormalities. Examination showed that the mental status and cranial nerves were normal. Motor strength evaluation showed the following results: neck flexion and extension, 4+/5; hand interossei, 3/5; ankle dorsiflexion, 2/5 on the right and 4−/5 on the left side; and other muscles of the upper to lower limbs graded 4/5. Muscle bulk and tone were normal. The deep tendon reflexes were generally absent, and pathologic reflexes were not present. Sensory examination showed diminished pinprick and light touch sensation up to the ankles and fingertips and normal vibratory and position sense. The patient could not walk on the toes or heels and had difficulty with tandem walk.

Nerve conduction study and electromyography (EMG) were done immediately after the patient's clinic visit. It showed normal bilateral sural and absent right median and ulnar sensory responses. The right median and ulnar motor response had prolonged distal latencies and mildly low amplitudes. The conduction velocity of the right median motor response was markedly slow (37 m/s), and there was a partial conduction block with stimulation of the right ulnar nerve below the elbow. Right tibial motor response had a temporally dispersed compound motor action potential. F waves could not be elicited. Needle study showed early evidence for denervation in the right tibialis anterior and first dorsal interosseous. The patient was admitted, and a spinal tap was performed the same day. The CSF protein level was 105 mg/dL (normal<40 mg/dL), with normal glucose level and cell count and no oligoclonal bands. Complete blood cell count, chemistry panel, Lyme titer, serologic tests for collagen vascular diseases, and antibodies to gangliosides (including GM1) did not show any abnormality.

The patient was diagnosed with acute inflammatory demyelinating polyradiculopathy (AIDP) and was treated with IVIG, 2 g/kg, over a period of 3 days. He had partial improvement and was discharged for outpatient rehab. The patient reported increasing gait impairment and weakness of the hands 3 weeks after his discharge. Deterioration of leg and hand muscle strength compared with his discharge date was found on his follow-up examination. Another course of IVIG, 2 g/kg, was given (home infusion), with partial recovery of symptoms. The patient preferred not to be treated with IVIG when he had another mild relapse 1 month later. Six months after the initial admission, the gait had become normal and the patient was able to run, with mild weakness of the hand interosseous muscles.

Comments

AIDP is an acute immune-mediated polyradiculoneuropathy and is characterized by proximal and distal upper and lower limb weakness. Although sensory symptoms are common, the muscle weakness is the predominant aspect. Cranial nerves (especially facial nerve) and respiratory muscles are commonly involved. It can be fatal because of respiratory or bulbar dysfunction and dysautonomia. Immediate diagnosis and treatment of AIDP with IVIG or plasma exchange, as well as advances in the critical care management of these patients, has significantly decreased the fatal outcome. The course is often monophasic, but relapses are often encountered. In about 5% to 10% of patients with AIDP treated with IVIG, the condition relapses after initial improvement. A common practice is to treat the relapse with a subsequent course of IVIG. Some patients (like ours) have several relapses, raising the question of acute-onset chronic inflammatory demyelinating polyneuropathy (A-CIDP). A-CIDP should be specially suspected if patients with AIDP have 3 or more relapses or if there is evidence for deterioration after 9 weeks.[11,12] The diagnosis of AIDP should be suspected on the clinical grounds and supported by the CSF finding of albuminocytological dissociation. Nerve conduction study may also provide diagnostic evidence days after the onset of symptoms. Findings suggestive of AIDP include absent F waves and H reflexes, evidence for segmental demyelination (conduction block, temporal dispersion), and slowing of the conduction velocity (including distal and F wave latencies) in the demyelinating range. Sural responses are often spared, which is in contrast to most of the other neuropathies.[13]

Case 6: Increasing Shortness of Breath

An 81-year-old woman with a history of hypertension, congestive heart failure (CHF), and recently diagnosed diabetes was brought to the emergency room because of progressive shortness of breath (SOB). She developed mild right eyelid droopiness and blurring of vision 2 months before the admission, and progressive SOB and intermittent dysphagia started 1 month later. The patient had a brain MRI that showed T2-weighted image signal intensity abnormalities in the subcortical white matter and the brainstem. One day before the admission, she had increasing SOB and became lethargic. Medications included aspirin, metformin, atenolol, and ciprofloxacin that had been started one week before for a urinary tract infection. Physical examination revealed a lethargic elderly lady unable to support her head upright, with a slight right ptosis and full extraocular movements. There was 3/5 neck extension and 4/5 neck flexion weakness. No significant muscle weakness was noted in the upper and lower limbs. The reflexes were symmetrically present, and the sensory examination was normal. The patient's condition rapidly deteriorated over the next several hours, and she underwent tracheal intubation, and mechanical ventilation was started. An arterial blood gas analysis done immediately before intubation showed a pH of 7.31, partial pressure of carbon dioxide of 67 mm Hg, partial pressure of oxygen of 94 mm Hg, bicarbonate concentration of 33 mEq/L at a fraction of inspired oxygen of 30%. Creatinine kinase level was normal. Nerve conduction study and needle EMG were done at the bedside on the seventh day of the ICU stay. The motor and sensory nerve action potentials were normal. Low-frequency (3 Hz) repetitive stimulation of the ulnar nerve (recorded at adductor digiti minimi) did not show any decrement of the compound muscle action potential at the baseline. Postexercise repetitive stimulation could not be done because of sedation. Repetitive simulation of the facial nerve (recorded at nasalis) was suboptimal because of patient's movement. Needle EMG showed no spontaneous activity, and myopathic motor units were observed in the deltoid and iliopsoas. The EMG was interpreted to be suggestive for a myopathy. The serologic tests for myasthenia gravis (MG) came back with positive results when discontinuation of mechanical ventilation and comfort care was being considered by the family and the ICU team. The acetylcholine receptor binding antibody titer was 85 nmol/L (normal<0.02 nmol/L), and the titer of striational muscle antibody was 1/128,000. The patient then underwent treatment with IVIGs, 2 g/kg divided over 5 days, as well as prednisone and pyridostigmine. Other medical complications set in, and, after about 3 weeks, she was taken off mechanical ventilation and transferred to a rehabilitation facility with a tracheostomy. In a follow-up visit 3 months after discharge, the patient's tracheostomy had been discontinued, and she had normal strength and was ambulatory.

Comment

Generalized MG may present very late in life, and respiratory failure often occurs early in the course (MG crisis). Infections and some medications (ie, in our case, urinary tract infection and ciprofloxacin, respectively) are known to cause MG exacerbation and crisis. The diagnosis of MG may be delayed because of common comorbidities in the elderly individuals (ie, ptosis was attributed to brainstem small vessel disease and SOB to CHF in our case).[14,15] The presence of head drop may indicate concomitant respiratory muscle weakness and may herald a respiratory failure.

MG should be considered in patients with unexplained proximal and truncal muscle weakness, even in the case of a nondiagnostic repetitive nerve stimulation. That is specially the case when the test is done in the technically challenging ICU environment, where there is often lack of patient cooperation. Furthermore, repetitive nerve stimulation has a rather low sensitivity if the weakness predominantly affects the truncal and bulbar muscles.[16] Myopathic motor units may be present in the EMG of patients with MG or other diseases of neuromuscular junction transmission.

Case 7: New-Onset Gait Impairment

A 16-year-old previously healthy adolescent girl presented to the emergency department with 2 days' history of progressive gait ataxia, which began 12 days after a cold. The patient also complained of double vision and weakness of her left leg. Neurologic examination showed an ataxic girl with internuclear ophthalmoplegia and left hemiparesis, which was more severe in the left lower extremity. MRI of the brain revealed the presence of multiple T2-weigthted hyperintense periventricular lesions as well as an enhancing brainstem lesion affecting pontine tegmentum in the region of the medial longitudinal fasciculus (**Fig. 3**). Spinal cord MRI was unremarkable. Analysis of CSF demonstrated moderate elevation of protein level and lymphocytic pleocytosis (35 cells/mL) with an absence of oligoclonal bands. No evidence of viral or bacterial DNA in the CSF was found. Diagnostic workup excluded alternate causes of central nervous system demyelinating diseases such as sarcoidosis, vasculitis, and AIDS. Based on the history of recent common cold and neuroimaging findings, a diagnosis of acute disseminated encephalomyelitis (ADEM) was made, and the patient was treated with intravenous methylprednisolone, 1000 mg daily, for 5 days. The patient improved clinically and most of her symptoms resolved within 2 weeks. A second brain MRI 1 month after treatment revealed partial resolution of white matter lesions on T2-weighted images. The patient was followed up once every 6 months for 2 years and did not develop any new neurologic symptoms.

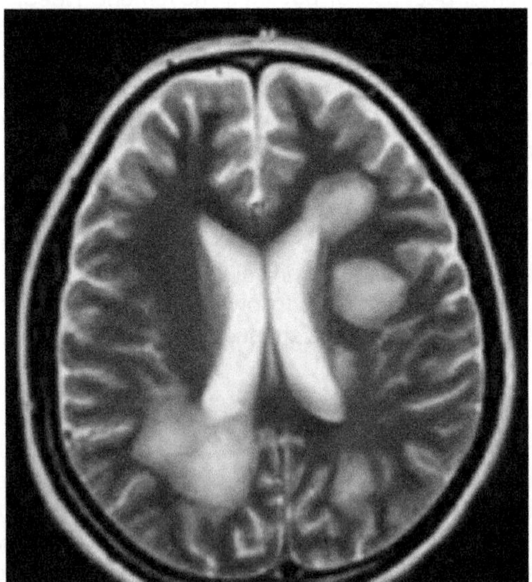

Fig. 3. MRI of brain, axial view and T2-weighted sequence, demonstrating multiple round and poorly defined hyperintense lesions of the white matter. Some of these lesions are at the gray-white matter, which are more suggestive of acute disseminated encephalomyelitis.

Comment

ADEM is usually a monophasic illness that affects children and young adults and occurs after a febrile illness or vaccination.[17,18] Patients with ADEM present with acute encephalopathy, headache, vomiting, seizures, altered level of consciousness, meningismus, as well as optic neuritis, which may be bilateral. Potential causes associated with ADEM include nonspecific upper respiratory tract infections as well as varicella. In addition, ADEM may occur following infection with mumps, rubella, adenovirus, human herpes virus 6, and influenza A and influenza B. ADEM must be differentiated from multiple sclerosis because their treatment and prognosis differ. In most cases, ADEM is monophasic and does not relapse.

Case 8: New-Onset Psychosis

A 32-year-old previously healthy man who works as an office manager presents to the emergency department disheveled, agitated, disoriented, and with headache. He also has paranoid delusions and visual hallucinations. He is reluctant to forward any information about himself and his relationship with others. After detailed interview, the patient mentions that for the past 3 days his coworkers have been manipulating his files and police cars were following him in the street. He is angry all the time, cannot sleep, and has lost 15 lb in the past 1 month. Psychiatric examination reveals a psychotic male with paranoia and visual hallucinations. The patient is delusional about his coworkers and thinks that they intend to hurt him. He is also afraid to open his mail because he is afraid they contain dangerous material. On further questioning, the patient mentions that he has been using crystal methamphetamine for the past 4 weeks.

Comment

This case presents an escalating social problem of use of methamphetamine in the society. Acute overdose with methamphetamine manifests with sympathetic overdrive, cardiovascular collapse, ventricular tachyarrhythmia, and death. Chronic use of methamphetamine is associated with hypertension, CHF, sepsis, periodontal disease, personality disorders, and cognitive decline. The patient may also develop new-onset seizures.[19] Psychiatric presentations of methamphetamine use include psychotic and anxiety disorder–like state, hyperactivity, inability to concentrate on mental tasks, and paranoid delusions. Treatment consists of cessation of use of methamphetamine, sedation, and supportive care.

Case 9: Sudden-Onset Hemiplegia Following Car Accident

A 20-year-old right-handed Caucasian man was brought from the scene of a motor vehicle accident to our hospital emergency department. He was found to have significant blunt trauma to the neck, chest, abdomen, and left femur. This included the presence of anterior mediastinal as well as abdominal hematomas. The patient also had a left femoral fracture. His neurologic condition deteriorated rapidly with acute left-sided weakness and hemisensory loss. Neurologic examination, at the time, was consistent with an NIH Stroke Scale (NIHSS) score of 16. However, the patient remained alert and fully oriented and followed commands. He had dysarthric speech and intact extraocular movements. However, there was decreased vision in the patient's left eye secondary to trauma. There was left-sided hemiplegia involving the face, arm, and leg along with left-sided hemisensory loss for all modalities. There was also visual and tactile inattention on the left as well as a positive left Babinski sign.

The head CT brain scan, without contrast, revealed a right middle cerebral artery (MCA) hyperdense sign (**Fig. 4**A) consistent with an intravascular luminal thrombus.

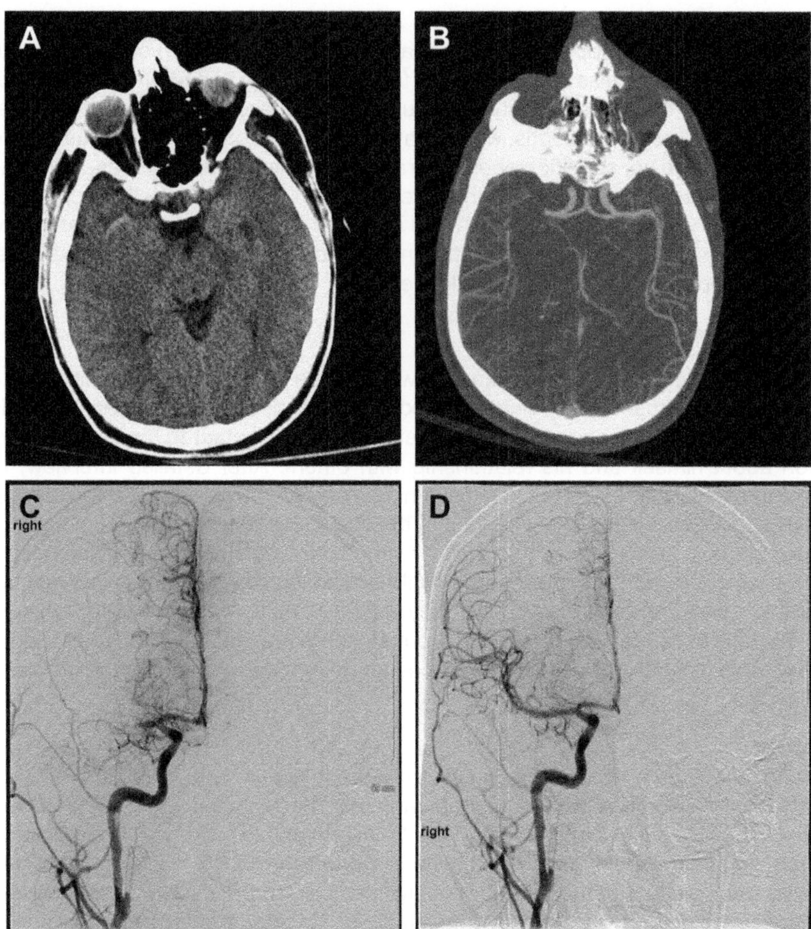

Fig. 4. (*A, B*). Right MCA sign with CT angiography correlate. (*C, D*) Cerebral angiography that demonstrated confirmed complete occlusion and thrombus of the right MCA (*A*) and recanalization and restoration of flow into the right MCA with the exception of a very distal M3 right MCA branch (*B*).

The CT angiogram of the head and neck (see **Fig. 4**B) showed the filling defect, which correlated the right MCA intravascular thrombus. This was seen in association with a right internal carotid artery (ICA) dissection with narrowing, but no occlusion, along with aneurysmal dilatation at the cervical level (see **Fig. 4**C). The patient was immediately taken for interventional angiography. The angiography confirmed complete occlusion and thrombus of the right MCA. One to 2 hours from the onset of neurologic symptoms, intra-arterial thrombolysis with tissue plasminogen activator (tPA) was administered. This was associated with recanalization and restoration of flow into the right MCA with the exception of a very distal M3 right MCA branch (see **Fig. 4**D). MRI of the brain without contrast, the following day, demonstrated a right basal ganglionic acute infarct with mild hemorrhagic transformation along with few foci of scattered right frontal and parietal signal changes reflective of ischemia. At 2- and 4-month follow-up, the patient was found with NIHSS scores of 6 and 2, respectively, and a Rankin score of 2. A follow-up CT angiography of his head and neck, at 3 months, showed persistence of normal intracranial vasculature as well as improvement in the luminal findings of the previously noted right ICA dissection. However, there was an increase in the pseudoaneurysm formation within the cervical right ICA.

Comment

This is an illustrative case of acute right MCA occlusion from a traumatic right ICA dissection. The patient was successfully treated with intra-arterial tPA, which was successful despite being in the setting of severe multiple trauma with carotid dissection as well as mediastinal and abdominal hematomas. The case demonstrates the potential of a beneficial effect of intra-arterial thrombolysis, for acute ischemic stroke, despite a significant contraindication to the use of intravenous thrombolysis with tPA.[20,21]

REFERENCES

1. Beck RW, Chandler DL, Cole SR, et al. Interferon beta-1a for early multiple sclerosis: CHAMPS trial subgroup analyses. Ann Neurol 2002;51:481–90.
2. CHAMPS Study Group. Interferon beta-1a for optic neuritis patients at high risk for multiple sclerosis. Am J Ophthalmol 2001;132:463–71.
3. Rabinstein AA. Management of status epilepticus in adults. Neurol Clin 2010;28: 853–62.
4. Oddo M, Carrera E, Claassen J, et al. Continuous electroencephalography in the medical intensive care unit. Crit Care Med 2009;37:2051–6.
5. Tan KM, Lennon VA, Klein CJ, et al. Clinical spectrum of voltage-gated potassium channel autoimmunity. Neurology 2008;70:1883–90.
6. Dalmau J, Gleichman AJ, Hughes EG, et al. Anti-NMDA-receptor encephalitis: case series and analysis of the effects of antibodies. Lancet Neurol 2008;7: 1091–8.
7. Hinchey J, Chaves C, Appignani B, et al. A reversible posterior leukoencephalopathy syndrome. N Engl J Med 1996;334:494–500.
8. Lee VH, Wijdicks EF, Manno EM, et al. Clinical spectrum of reversible posterior leukoencephalopathy syndrome. Arch Neurol 2008;65:205–10.
9. Fugate JE, Claassen DO, Cloft HJ, et al. Posterior reversible encephalopathy syndrome, 2010 posterior reversible encephalopathy syndrome: associated clinical and radiologic findings. Mayo Clin Proc 2010;85:427–32.
10. Kozak OS, Wijdicks EF, Manno EM, et al. Status epilepticus as initial manifestation of posterior reversible encephalopathy syndrome. Neurology 2007;69(9):894–7.
11. van Doorn PA, Ruts L, Jacobs BC. Clinical features, pathogenesis, and treatment of Guillain-Barre syndrome. Lancet Neurol 2008;7:939–50.
12. Ruts L, van Koningsveld R, van Doorn PA. Distinguishing acute-onset CIDP from Guillain-Barre syndrome with treatment related fluctuations. Neurology 2005;65: 138–40.
13. Vucic S, Cairns KD, Black KR, et al. Neurophysiologic findings in early acute inflammatory demyelinating polyradiculoneuropathy. Clin Neurophysiol 2004; 115:2329–35.
14. Vincent A, Clover L, Buckley C, et al. Evidence of underdiagnosis of myasthenia gravis in older people. J Neurol Neurosurg Psychiatry 2003;74:1105–8.
15. Alshekhlee A, Miles JD, Katirji B, et al. Incidence and mortality rates of myasthenia gravis and myasthenic crisis in US hospitals. Neurology 2009;72:1548–54.

16. Benatar M. A systematic review of diagnostic studies in myasthenia gravis. Neuromuscul Disord 2006;16:459–67.
17. Alper G, Heyman R, Wang L. Multiple sclerosis and acute disseminated encephalomyelitis diagnosed in children after long-term follow-up: comparison of presenting features. Dev Med Child Neurol 2009;51:480–6.
18. Lee YJ. Acute disseminated encephalomyelitis in children: differential diagnosis from multiple sclerosis on the basis of clinical course. Korean J Pediatr 2011;54: 234–40.
19. Sekine Y, Iyo M, Ouchi Y, et al. Methamphetamine-related psychiatric symptoms and reduced brain dopamine transporters studied with PET. Am J Psychiatry 2001;158:1206–14.
20. Choi JH, Bateman BT, Mangla S, et al. Endovascular recanalization therapy in acute ischemic stroke. Stroke 2006;37:419–24.
21. Kan PT, Orion D, Yashar P, et al. Intra -arterial thrombolysis and thrombectomy for acute ischemia stroke: technique and results. J Neurosurg Sci 2011;55(2): 151–60.

BONUS ARTICLE: Disorders of Consciousness Induced by Intoxication

Peter De Paepe, Sabine Lemoyne, Walter Buylaert

Edited by G. Bryan Young, MD, FRCP(C)

Disorders of Consciousness Induced by Intoxication

Peter De Paepe, MD, PhD[a,b,*], Sabine Lemoyne, MD[a], Walter Buylaert, MD, PhD[a]

KEYWORDS

• Coma • Delirium • Consciousness • Intoxication

Xenobiotics that induce alterations in mental status or consciousness can be divided into two groups.[1] The first group includes agents that produce neuroexcitation resulting in confusion, agitation, hallucinations, or seizures. The second group consists of agents producing neuroinhibition leading to decreased consciousness and coma. Intoxication is a frequent cause of coma accounting for approximately 30% of all patients presenting to an emergency department with coma of unknown origin.[2]

The prognosis of patients with altered consciousness is mainly determined by early diagnosis and appropriate therapeutic interventions and by the type of toxin. The potential causes of altered consciousness are many and may reflect systemic illness, isolated organ system dysfunction, drug intoxications or withdrawal, psychiatric illness, or neurologic disease. In this article, a comprehensive approach to patients with altered consciousness and suspected poisoning is discussed. This survey, however, does not intend to be a substitute for the need for consultation with a clinical toxicologist qualified in the diagnosis and treatment of poisoned patients.

PATHOPHYSIOLOGY

Neuroexcitatory agents enhance neurotransmission of excitatory amino acids or diminish inhibitory input from γ-aminobutyric acid (GABA) neurons.[2] A non limitative list of agents inducing agitation and/or delirium is shown in **Box 1**. Enhanced transmission can occur through inhibition of presynaptic metabolism (monoamine oxidase

No financial disclosures and/or conflicts of interest.

[a] Department of Emergency Medicine, Ghent University Hospital, De Pintelaan 185, B-9000 Ghent, Belgium

[b] Heymans Institute of Pharmacology, Ghent University, De Pintelaan 185, B-9000 Ghent, Belgium

* Corresponding author. De Pintelaan 185, B-9000 Ghent, Belgium.

E-mail address: peter.depaepe@ugent.be

Neurol Clin 30 (2012) 359–384
doi:10.1016/j.ncl.2011.10.003 **neurologic.theclinics.com**

Box 1
Nonlimitative list of agents that may induce agitation and/or delirium

Alcohols

Amantadine

Anticholinergics (eg, antihistamines, atropine, scopolamine, antiparkinson agents, antispasmodics, phenothiazines, and tricyclic antidepressants)

Carbon monoxide (CO)

Drug withdrawal states

Hallucinogens (eg, lysergic acid diethylamide [LSD], phencyclidine, mescaline, psilocybin, ketamine, and designer amphetamines)

Heavy metals

Hypoglycemic agents

Lithium

Local anesthetics

Salicylates

Sympathomimetics (eg, amphetamines, cocaine, caffeine, phenylpropanolamine, and theophylline)

inhibitors [MAOIs]), stimulation of neurotransmitter release (amphetamines), impairment of neurotransmitter reuptake (cocaine), or inhibition of synaptic degradation (acetylcholinesterase inhibitors). Central nervous system (CNS) excitation after anticholinergic poisoning is caused predominantly by blockade of central G protein–linked muscarinic receptors resulting in disinhibition. Methylxanthines, such as caffeine and theophylline, act in the CNS as adenosine antagonists as well as inhibitors of phosphodiesterase C, allowing an increased and prolonged response to other stimulatory hormones. Withdrawal states may also cause excitation. Chronic presence of ethanol causes increased numbers of *N*-methyl-d-aspartate (NMDA) receptors as well as increased sensitivity of NMDA receptors to glutamate, which explains the overexcitation of the CNS when alcohol is withdrawn. Withdrawal of ethanol is also associated with a decrease in GABAergic activity because persistent stimulation of the inhibitory GABA receptor-chloride channel complex by ethanol leads to down-regulation of the complex. Similar to frequent ethanol and benzodiazepine use, chronic γ-hydroxybutyric acid (GHB) use is believed to lead to tolerance associated with down-regulation of inhibitory GABA and GHB receptors. Subsequent decreased GHB consumption results in decreased GABA-mediated and GHB-mediated neuroinhibition, resulting in unopposed excitatory neurotransmission (glutamate, norepinephrine, and dopamine systems) and the onset of a withdrawal syndrome.[3] Neuroexcitation may also be caused by agents inducing metabolic derangements, such as hypoglycemia and hypoxia (discussed later).

Many substances are capable of producing coma and they can be classified into two groups: agents that produce coma through a direct effect on brain cells and agents for which coma is an indirect result of derangements involving other organ systems (**Table 1**).[4,5]

Examples of direct-acting neurotoxins include agents that increase GABA effects, such as benzodiazepines, alcohols, barbiturates, and GHB.[6] $GABA_A$ receptors are the primary mediators of inhibitory neurotransmission in the brain. The $GABA_A$ receptor is a pentameric structure composed of varying polypeptide subunits

Table 1
Non limitative list of substances that may be involved in coma due to poisoning classified according to their mechanism

Direct Effect on the Brain	Indirect Effect on the Brain
Anticholinergic agents	Antiarrhythmics
Barbiturates	Antihypertensives
Benzodiazepines	CO
Carbamazepine	Gases and fumes
CO	Insulin
Cyanide	Methemoglobin-forming agents
Ethanol	Oral hypoglycemic drugs
Ethylene glycol	
GHB	
Glutethimide	
H_1-antihistamines	
Hydrogen sulfide	
Lithium	
MAOIs	
Methanol	
Neuroleptics	
Opioids	
Organophosphates	
Phenytoin	
Presynaptic α2-receptor agonists	
Salicylates	
Selective serotonin reuptake inhibitors	
Trichloroethanol	
Tricyclic antidepressants	
Valproic acid	

associated with a chloride channel on the postsynaptic membrane. Sedative-hypnotics alter the function of the chloride channel by increasing either its frequency or duration of opening. Indirect-acting agonists, such as benzodiazepines, require the presence of GABA to affect the channel. Other agents, such as barbiturates, can directly open the channel at high doses without the presence of GABA. This may explain the high lethality seen with barbiturate overdoses as compared with benzodiazepine overdoses. Many sedative hypnotics, such as barbiturates, alcohols, and trichloroethanol, also decrease the effects of glutamate-mediated excitatory neurotransmission by interaction with the NMDA receptors.[7] GHB also has affinity for inhibitory presynaptic $GABA_B$ and opioid receptors. In addition, there is evidence to suggest that there are also specific GHB receptor sites.[8] Agents with anticholinergic properties like H1-antihistamines, tricyclic antidepressants and neuroleptics induce coma by antagonism at the central muscarinic acetylcholine receptors. H1-antihistamines and neuroleptics also produce central nervous system depression due to central histamine H1 receptor inhibition.[9–11]

Opioids produce sedation by their effect on μ receptors and κ receptors, which belong to the family of G protein–coupled receptors and inhibit adenylate cyclase, reducing the intracellular cyclic adenosine monophosphate content.[12] These receptors also exert effects on ion channels through a direct G protein coupling to the channel. By these means, opioids promote the opening of potassium channels and inhibit the opening of voltage-gated calcium channels. These membrane effects reduce both neuronal excitability and transmitter release, resulting in an overall inhibitory effect at the cellular level.

Cyanide causes direct neurotoxicity by binding to the ferric ions of cytochrome a_3, an integral component of the third and final cytochrome oxidase enzyme in the mitochondrial electron transport chain.[13] Once bound, the enzyme becomes inactivated and oxidative phosphorylation is blocked. Cells are thus deprived of their major energy source. The inhibition of oxidative phosphorylation results in widespread metabolic derangements. ATP is consumed by active cells, but little can be produced. Tissues quickly exhaust their supply of ATP. Furthermore, hydrogen ions that are generated by ATP hydrolysis begin to accumulate because they can no longer be recycled into the process of ATP formation resulting in metabolic acidosis. The result of these intracellular derangements is cellular dysfunction and ultimately cell death if cytochrome inhibition persists. Cyanide also induces cellular oxidative stress possibly through inhibition of antioxidant enzymes, such as catalase, glutathione dehydrogenase, glutathione reductase, or superoxide dismutase. Cyanide-induced lipid peroxidation occurs to the greatest extent in the brain, which explains the predominance of neurologic findings in patients with cyanide poisoning. There is also compelling evidence that cyanide neurotoxicity is mediated by glutamate release, leading to increased cytosolic calcium and cell death.

Hydrogen sulfide's toxicity results from its potent inhibition of cytochrome oxidase, thereby interrupting oxidative phosphorylation. Like cyanide, hydrogen sulfide binds to the ferric moiety of cytochrome a_3 oxidase complex. The resulting inhibition of oxidative phosphorylation produces cellular hypoxia.[14]

The second group of agents are those for which coma is an indirect result of derangements involving other organ systems. Examples of indirect agents include those causing hypoxia, such as methemoglobin-forming agents, or agents that decrease oxygen delivery to cells via hypoperfusion, such as antiarrhythmic and antihypertensive drugs.

CO is an example of a substance-producing coma via a combination of systemic effects and direct cellular toxicity.[15] CO's most obvious effect is binding to hemoglobin, rendering it incapable of delivering oxygen to the cells because the affinity for hemoglobin is 200 to 250 times greater than that of oxygen. Direct cellular toxicity is caused by cytochrome oxidase inactivation accompanied by ischemic-reperfusion injury. Animal studies suggest that CO poisoning may also cause glutamate increases in the brain, resulting in intracellular calcium release and neuronal cell death.

PRIMARY ASSESSMENTS

Safety

Before any rescue attempts are undertaken, the rescuer's safety should be guaranteed. This is especially important for gas intoxications (eg, CO and hydrogen sulfide) because there still may be gas present in the air. Some toxic agents, for instance, organophosphates, may be absorbed through the skin and mucosa and may intoxicate a health care provider when in contact with a patient without taking protective measures. In cases of an illegal drug overdose, the rescuer should always be alert for the presence of intravenous needles to avoid stick injuries. Managing patients with aggressive behavior due to altered consciousness may also pose a risk to the personal safety of health care professionals and may lead to mistakes in the assessment of a patient's presenting illness. Successful management of aggression requires an interdisciplinary management plan with an underlying philosophy that all health professionals accept responsibility for assessing, responding to, and managing aggression.

Primary Assessment and Resuscitation

Irrespective of the cause of altered consciousness, primary assessment requires identification and treatment of life-threatening conditions.[16–22] The primary assessment should be repeated after emergency treatment and with any further deterioration in the patient's condition. The importance of these measures cannot be overemphasized. In many cases, altered mental status induced by poisoning has a good prognosis provided secondary damage due to hypoxia, hypoperfusion, and sepsis is avoided.

In order not to overlook life-threatening conditions, a structured approach to patients with altered consciousness is provided. As discussed later, however, management is often also guided by the underlying cause. The aim of the primary assessment is to identify and treat all immediately life-threatening conditions.

Key components of the primary assessment (ABCDE) are

A—Airway and oxygen administration
B—Breathing
C—Circulation
D—Disability
E—Exposure

A—Airway and oxygen administration

All agents causing CNS depression may compromise airway patency. Improper or nonaggressive airway management may lead to anoxic brain injury and/or aspiration. Airway patency may be assessed by evaluating a patient's verbal response to questions. A patient answering appropriately indicates an open airway, the presence of breathing, and adequate cerebral perfusion. If a patient remains unresponsive, the airway should be opened with the head tilt–chin lift maneuver. If a neck injury cannot be excluded (discussed later), however, cervical immobilization should be maintained; the jaw thrust technique is then the safest approach to control the airway. The mouth should be inspected for foreign bodies. Removing liquid (blood, saliva, and gastric contents) from the upper airway using a suction device may be necessary to clear the airway. This should be done cautiously, however, if a patient has an intact gag reflex because the suction device can provoke vomiting. Oropharyngeal airway cannulas are curved plastic tubes that fit between the tongue and the hard palate and are often helpful to improve or maintain airway patency in an unconscious patient. These devices should not be used in patients with preserved glossopharyngeal and laryngeal reflexes because insertion may cause vomiting and laryngospasm.[20,21] The recovery position may be used in unresponsive and spontaneously breathing patients to avoid airway obstruction by the tongue or mucus and vomit. Indications for orotracheal intubation in comatose patients are the presence of apnea and bradypnea related to deep coma and/or vomiting.[21] Deep coma, often defined as the presence of a Glasgow Coma Scale (GCS) score lower than 8, is not an absolute criterion for intubation (see examples later) and the score intended for head trauma has never been validated in intoxications.[23] Clinical assessment by experienced medical staff rather than physiologic variables is the key to determining intubation requirements in poisoned patients with a reduced GCS score. GCS score alone is not a good predictor of intubation.[24] Once control of the airway has been achieved, supplemental oxygen should be delivered.

B—Breathing

To assess breathing, an open airway should be maintained and chest movements subsequently looked for, breathing sounds listened for, and expired air felt for.

If there are signs of inadequacy, ventilation through a mask and an orotracheal tube is needed.[16] Respiratory depression and bradypnea may occur in opiate and sedative-hypnotic overdose. Hyperventilation is observed in poisoning with salicylates and during the initial stage of any cause of hypoxia, such as CO and cyanide poisoning; if left untreated, these ultimately result in respiratory failure. Cheyne-Stokes respiration, defined as alternating hyperpnea and apnea, is rarely observed in poisoned patients; rather, it indicates the presence of a structural lesion at the level of the midbrain, infection, cardiopulmonary disease, or other metabolic disorders.

Hypoxemia can easily be detected with pulse oximetry. Pulse oxymeters, however, are unable to detect hypercarbia, which may result from hypoventilation. Pulse oxymeters are also totally unreliable in CO poisoning because the apparatus cannot distinguish between oxyhemoglobin and carboxyhemoglobin (COHb). Newer devices, called pulse CO-oximeters, allow immediate noninvasive COHb measurement.

C—Circulation

A patient's hemodynamic status should be assessed by checking for an arterial pulse, ideally the carotid, for rate, rhythm, and character. Blood pressure should be measured and peripheral perfusion should be assessed using capillary refill time. Patients should be connected to a cardiac monitor, and urinary catheterization is necessary for all unconscious patients to follow urine output.

In cases of cardiac arrest, resuscitation should be started at once. Cardiac arrest may be due to a direct toxic effect on the heart or a severe metabolic disturbance or may be secondary to a respiratory arrest. Examples of drugs that can cause a cardiac arrest through a direct effect on the heart include the tricyclic antidepressants, chloral hydrate, and the phenothiazines. Calcium antagonists, β-adrenergic antagonists, vasodilators and any negative inotropic drug in overdose may also cause cardiovascular collapse, leading to cardiac arrest. Resuscitation for a prolonged period should be considered because the poison may be metabolized or excreted during extended life-support measures.[21]

Hemodynamic shock can impair consciousness due to reduced cerebral perfusion. Malignant tachyarrhythmias resulting in hypotension may be observed in intoxications with tricyclic antidepressants or theophylline. Bradyarrhythmias and hypotension may result from an overdose of β-adrenoceptor antagonists, digoxin, and clonidine. Intravenous access has to be established and shock should be treated appropriately with, for instance, intravenous fluids and vasopressors to prevent secondary brain injury and other organ failures. Cardiovascular collapse after overdose with β-adrenergic or calcium antagonists requires specific antidote therapy (eg, glucagon and calcium).[25]

D—Disability

The initial neurologic assessment should be a rapid evaluation of the GCS score and the pupils (size, equality, and reaction to light). The alert/verbal/painful/unresponsive (AVPU) responsiveness scale provides a more rapid and simple alternative to the GCS score in assessing consciousness level in most poisoned patients.[26] Both scales are difficult to use in uncooperative patients (eg, ethanol-intoxicated patients).

During this phase, the crucial question should arise if the altered consciousness is really due to intoxication. Causes of altered consciousness may be of toxicologic, metabolic, infectious, neurologic with structural changes, or psychiatric nature. Life-threatening conditions should be looked for, such as hypoglycemia, meningitis, epilepsy, and opiate poisoning, and treated appropriately. Hypoglycemia may result not only from insulin and oral hypoglycemic poisoning but also from intoxication with ethanol (more common in young children), paracetamol (acetaminophen), and salicylates. Confirming hypoglycemia can easily be done and should be routine in every comatose patient. Rapid bedside tests are available but the apparatus may not always be accurate, with falsely elevated glucose levels. Furthermore, diabetic patients may experience glycopenic symptoms at lower but still normal glucose levels.[27] The treatment of hypoglycemia is discussed later.

Signs of recent head trauma (eg, abrasions, contusions, and hematoma) or the presence of lateralizing or asymmetric neurologic findings should prompt an immediate search for a structural lesion. Bilateral orbital hematoma (raccoon eyes) and ecchymosis behind the ear (Battle sign) may indicate a skull fracture. Focal findings on examination greatly reduce the likelihood of toxic etiology alone. Patients may have more than one cause of coma. For instance, poisoning with CNS depressants may result in a fall leading to a traumatic subdural hematoma.

The pupils may provide important information in establishing a diagnosis. Many medical textbooks state that in coma caused by a toxic-metabolic process, the integrity of the pupillary light reflex remains intact. Exceptions include anoxia, hypothermia, and intoxication with anticholinergics, barbiturates, cholinergics, glutethimide, or opioids.[5] In a prospective study, the loss of the light reflex and anisocoria were independent predictors for structural causes of coma, with sensitivity and specificity for loss of light reflex of 83% and 77%, respectively (likelihood ratio 3.56) and for anisocoria 39% and 96%, respectively (likelihood ratio 9); this means, however, that in 23% of patients with coma of metabolic-toxic origin light reflex was absent.[28] Pupils that are equal, pinpoint, and fixed may be observed in intoxications with opioids and organophosphates and should be differentiated from pontine lesions. Equal, dilated, and reactive pupils can be seen in methylenedioxymethamphetamine (MDMA) and amphetamine users but may also result from metabolic disturbances or midbrain lesions. Equal, dilated, and fixed pupils may occur in anticholinergic poisoning and also in hypoxemia, hypothermia, and in the peri-ictal phase. Meningeal irritation should be checked if there are no contraindications to mobilization of the spine.

E—Exposure

Patients must be fully exposed to allow complete assessment, and body temperature must be measured. Hypothermia is an important cause of coma. Factors predisposing to hypothermia are CNS depression and immobilization, which may be observed after an overdose with, for instance, sedatives. In an urban setting, alcohol intoxication is the most common predisposing factor to hypothermia. The mechanism by which ethanol predisposes to hypothermia is probably based on its depressive effects on the CNS, vasodilation, and blunting of behavioral responses to cold. Hyperthermia may indicate the presence of a serotonergic syndrome, a neuroleptic malignant syndrome, an anticholinergic syndrome, or intoxication with CNS stimulants (eg, cocaine and amphetamines). Important information can be obtained by contacting relatives and friends and by searching the patient's clothes for useful information, such as medical cards and drugs. Environmental manipulation (eg, quiet room and calm conversation) is important in patients with agitation.

At the end of the primary assessment, the potential lethality of the overdose should be assessed. This requires knowledge of the substance, the time of intake, and the dose. It often happens, however, that information about these 3 key elements is not available or not reliable; in these cases there should be a high suspicion of a potentially lethal intoxication.

Etiology-Oriented Approach

In comatose patients with respiratory depression, etiologic clues of a heroin overdose should immediately alert the rescuer to watch carefully for needles to avoid stick injuries. Initial airway management consists of oxygenation and bag mask ventilation followed by administration of the antidote naloxone rather than immediately performing an orotracheal intubation (discussed later).

A comatose, spontaneously breathing patient with a history of insulin-dependent diabetes mellitus should immediately prompt the rescuer to exclude hypoglycemia and, if needed, the intravenous administration of glucose (discussed later). Except for providing a patent airway, additional airway management maneuvers usually are not needed.

Respiratory insufficiency in patients with an organophosphate poisoning must be managed by immediate orotracheal intubation and appropriate antidotal treatment. Protective safety measures for the rescuer are important because organophosphates may be absorbed through the skin.

CO poisoning poses an important safety risk to the rescuers. Carrying CO detectors by rescuers is an important safety measure. The mainstay of treatment of comatose patients from CO poisoning is attention to the airway and oxygenation. As soon as possible, 100% oxygen should be provided by mask reservoir followed, if necessary, by endotracheal tube, and the patient should be transferred to a hospital with hyperbaric oxygen (HBO) therapy facilities (discussed later).

Most patients comatose from barbiturate poisoning require definite airway protection by orotracheal intubation and ventilatory support due to the expected prolonged, profound coma. Conversely, uncomplicated coma induced by benzodiazepines and/or alcohol can often be managed by providing oxygen, free airway, and positioning of patients in the recovery position under close monitoring. For benzodiazepines, the use of the antidote flumazenil can be considered under certain and rare conditions (discussed later).

SECONDARY ASSESSMENTS

The secondary assessment should only be done once the immediately life-threatening conditions have been treated. In most cases, a complete history taking and thorough clinical examination result in identification of the substance taken.[29] Important information can also be obtained by anamnesis of the patient's surroundings and by searching, for example, (empty) drug blisters. Identifying the toxic substance by clinical examination requires profound knowledge of the different toxidromes.

Neurologic Examination

Trying to determine the cause of altered consciousness should be part of the primary assessment, because a rapid diagnosis may be important for prognosis of a patient's neurologic outcome. Subsequently, during the secondary assessment, a careful neurologic assessment should be performed to further distinguish between a toxic-metabolic cause for altered consciousness and structural neurologic causes, for instance, a cerebrovascular accident or an epidural or subdural hematoma. At this stage, the role of a thorough neurologic clinical examination is of pivotal importance. Examination of pupillary reactivity, motor responses to noxious stimuli, and ocular movements is of paramount importance to differentiate between these two entities.[2,5,30]

As discussed previously, pupil size and reaction to light may provide valuable information. Dysconjugate gaze in the horizontal plane is normally observed in drowsiness and in various sedated states, including alcohol intoxication, with parallel ocular axes re-emerging when a patient awakens or slips deeper into coma. Dysconjugate gaze in the vertical plane, called skew deviation, generally results from pontine or cerebellar lesions. Sustained conjugate upward gaze is usually the result of hypoxic encephalopathy.

Focal or asymmetric findings in motor responses to a noxious stimulus should invoke a search for a structural lesion. There are, however, exceptions to this generalization. For instance, mass lesions of the brain may cause compression of the brainstem bilaterally resulting in bilateral and symmetric neurologic deficit. Some toxic-metabolic conditions, such as hyperosmolar nonketotic hyperglycemia or hypoglycemia, may produce focal deficits. Different metabolic demands in different brain regions and circulation defects have been suggested as the causes of hypoglycemia-related stroke-like episodes.[31] Focal neurologic signs observed in hyperosmolar nonketotic hyperglycemia have been hypothesized as secondary to effects of hyperosmolality on the brain, resulting in focal regions of brain edema and reactivation of previously resolved neurologic deficits.

The presence of oculocephalic and oculovestibular reflexes also helps in differentiating toxic from structural causes of coma. The oculocephalic reflex (doll's eye movements) implies conjugate eye movement away from the direction of rotation. This maneuver is strictly contraindicated when there is a possibility of cervical instability. The oculovestibular reflex, which involves cold-water irrigation of the tympanic membrane, produces transient conjugate slow deviation of gaze toward the side of the stimulus (brainstem mediated) followed by a quick saccadic correction back to midline (cortically mediated). Because the hallmark of a toxic-metabolic coma is a dissociation of findings, these reflexes should be paired with other findings, such as pupillary reactivity. For instance, with respect to pupillary reactivity, this means that pupillary reactivity is dissociated from other neuraxis dysfunction in a fashion that is not characteristic of structural brain disease. Thus, in addition to symmetric findings, patients whose coma originates from a toxicologic or metabolic cause typically have an intact and equal pupillary light reflex that may be paired with an absent oculovestibular response, an absent motor response to noxious stimuli, or hypoventilation requiring ventilatory support. This phenomenon of dissociation occurs with toxic-metabolic coma because other brainstem functions tend to be far more vulnerable to toxic and metabolic insult than are the pupillary light reflexes. In contrast with coma caused by structural disease, in coma caused by a toxic-metabolic process there is symmetry in either response or nonresponse to provocative maneuvers.

Seizures caused by drugs and toxins are mostly of the generalized tonic-clonic variety unless there is underlying focal neurologic disease or epilepsy. Seizures may result from a direct reduction of seizure threshold or from secondary events, such as hypoxia. Toxin-induced seizures are most commonly caused by tricyclic antidepressants or sympathomimetic or anticholinergic agents. Seizures as part of an alcohol or benzodiazepine withdrawal syndrome are also frequently observed.[32,33]

Clonus is caused by a variety of substances, most commonly sedative-hypnotics and anticonvulsants. Rigidity, clonus, hyperreflexia, and tremor are seen with lithium poisoning.

Serotonin syndrome and neuroleptic malignant syndrome typically have a motor component combined with altered mental status and hyperthermia. The key differences between the two syndromes are shown in **Table 2**. The serotonin syndrome is an adverse drug reaction resulting from excessive serotonergic neurotransmission after therapeutic drug use (rare when only one serotonergic drug is used), intentional self-poisoning, or inadvertent interactions between drugs, such as selective serotonin

Table 2
Key differences between serotonin and neuroleptic malignant syndrome

Feature	Serotonin Syndrome	Neuroleptic Malignant Syndrome
Neuroleptic drugs	0	+++
Serotonergic drugs	+++	0
Hyperactivity	+++	0
Clonus	+++	0
Tremor	+++	+
Shivering	+++	0
Hyperreflexia	+++	0
Rapid onset	+++	0
Leaden rigidity	0	+++
Bradykinesia	0	+++
Stupor/mutism	0	+++
Creatine kinase activity	++	+++
Hallucinations	+	++
Hyperthermia	++	++

Data from Richards D, Aronson J. Oxford handbook of practical drug therapy. Oxford: Oxford University Press; 2005.

reuptake inhibitors; serotonin precursors, such as tryptophan and serotonin agonists, such as the triptans; serotonin releasers, such as amphetamines; tricyclic antidepressants; and MAOIs.[34] Neuroleptic malignant syndrome (NMS) is an idiosyncratic reaction to antipsychotic agents. There are also case reports of other medications causing NMS, including venlafaxine, promethazine, metoclopramide, and prochlorperazine. NMS is believed to result from CNS dopamine receptor blockade or withdrawal of exogenous dopaminergic agonists. NMS can develop in patients with Parkinson disease after withdrawal of levodopa therapy. The probability of developing NMS is directly related to the antidopaminergic potency of the neuroleptic agent.

Toxidromes

The identification of specific toxidromes may be helpful in establishing a diagnosis when the exposure is not well defined.[18] These are grouped physiologically based on abnormalities of vital signs, general appearance, skin, eyes, mucous membranes, and pulmonary, cardiovascular, gastrointestinal, and neurologic systems, that are known to occur with specific classes of substances, such as anticholinergic, cholinergic, sympathomimetic, and opioid agents (**Table 3**). The list of representative agents in the table is not limitative. The actual clinical manifestations of an ingestion or exposure are far more variable than the syndromes described in the table.

Odors and Skin

Odors can provide useful hints. An odor of alcohol may indicate ethanol intoxication. An odor of acetone may accompany diabetic ketoacidosis, chloral hydrate, or isopropyl alcohol poisoning; the scent of bitter almonds with cyanide; and a garlic-like odor with organophosphates and arsenic.

Central cyanosis is a sign of hypoxia, but methemoglobinemia may also cause a similar color. The cherry pink skin color of COHb is not always obvious, and its absence does not exclude serious CO poisoning. Anticholinergics, alcohol, cocaine, cyanide, and borates may produce a flushed pink skin. The presence of track marks is often indicative of intravenous drug use and resultant opiate or sympathomimetic toxicity. Cutaneous bullae (coma blisters) may be found not only in barbiturate, glutethimide, and other sedative overdoses but also in tricyclic antidepressant and CO poisoning.

Bruises and hematoma indicate a traumatic injury, which may be due to violence. In this context, some drugs (eg, GHB, flunitrazepam, and ketamine) may be used to assist a sexual assault because of their sedative, muscle relaxant, and amnestic properties and are, therefore, called date rape drugs.

Patients who have been lying in coma for a long time on a hard surface may develop cutaneous bullae and rhabdomyolysis due to pressure necrosis of the skin and muscles. This particularly affects muscles in compartments leading to compartment syndrome and renal failure. The agents most often implicated are CO, alcohol, opioids, barbiturates, or other CNS depressants. Therefore, all extremities of coma patients should be inspected for edema, color change, or vascular deficit. Diagnosis of a compartment syndrome can be established by measuring compartment pressures. Some agents, such as cocaine and ethanol, may induce rhabdomyolysis by direct toxic effects on the sarcoplasmic reticulum.

DECONTAMINATION PROCEDURES

Decontamination procedures have to be considered in the treatment of poisoned patients. These procedures are discussed briefly based on the guidelines published by the American Academy of Clinical Toxicology and the European Association of Poison Centres and Clinical Toxicologists.

In cases of a potentially lethal overdose or if the exact nature of the overdose is not known, measures to prevent or reduce toxic drug levels should always be considered. This may be achieved by reducing drug absorption and/or by enhancing drug elimination. Methods used to decrease drug absorption in the gastrointestinal tract are activated charcoal, gastric lavage, whole-bowel irrigation, and therapeutic emesis. Procedures enhancing drug elimination include multiple doses of activated charcoal, therapeutic diuresis, urinary alkalinization, hemoperfusion, and hemodialysis.

Before initiating these procedures, consultation with a clinical toxicologist is advisable. In comatose patients, emesis is prohibited, and gastric lavage and the administration of activated charcoal are contraindicated unless a patient has a secured airway by means of an orotracheal tube with inflated cuff.

Reducing Absorption

Skin decontamination

Skin decontamination should always be considered on toxic exposure of the skin.[35] Removal of the clothes is an important measure to prevent direct effects and systemic absorption of certain toxins (eg, organophosphates). In general, a copious amount of water is the decontamination agent of choice for skin irrigation. Soap should be added when adherent materials are involved.

Gastrointestinal decontamination

Activated charcoal Charcoal works by adsorbing ingested drugs onto its large surface area and adsorbs 10% of its own weight. In most instances, 0.5 g/kg to 1 g/kg is an appropriate initial dose of activated charcoal; doses of 1.5 g/kg to 2 g/kg should be used after particularly massive or dangerous ingestions. In vitro studies show that ideal activated charcoal-to-drug ratios vary widely, but 10:1 is a representative value for many typical drugs and is, therefore, useful in theoretic consideration of optimal

Table 3
Toxidromes

Toxidrome	Mental Status	Pupils	Vital Signs	Other Symptoms	Representative Agents
Sympathomimetic	Hyperalertness Agitation Hallucinations Paranoia	Mydriasis	Hyperthermia Tachycardia Hypertension Tachypnea Hyperpnea	Diaphoresis Tremor Hyperreflexia Seizures	Cocaine Amphetamines Ephedrine Pseudoephedrine Phenylpropanolamine Theophylline Caffeine
Anticholinergic	Hyperalertness Agitation Hallucinations Delirium Mumbling speech Coma	Mydriasis	Hyperthermia Tachycardia Hypertension Tachypnea	Flushing Dry skin Dry mucosa Blurred vision Decreased bowel sounds Urinary retention Myoclonus Choreoathetosis Seizures	H_1-antihistamines Tricyclic antidepressants Antiparkinson drugs Antispasmodic drugs Phenothiazines Atropine Scopolamine Belladonna alkaloids
Hallucinogenic	Hallucinations Distortion of perception Depersonalization Agitation	Mydriasis (usually)	Hyperthermia Tachycardia Hypertension Tachypnea	Nystagmus	Phencyclidine LSD Mescaline Psilocybin Amphetamines (eg, 3, 4-Methylenedioxy-N-ethylamphetamine and *N*-methyldiethanolamine)
Opiates	CNS depression Coma	Miosis	Hypothermia Bradycardia Hypotension Hypopnea Bradypnea	Hyporeflexia Lung edema Decreased bowel sounds Needle track marks	Opiates (eg, heroin, morphine, methadone, oxycodone, and hydromorphone) Diphenoxylate

Hypnotic	Sedation Stupor Coma Slurred speech Ataxia	(usually)	Bradycardia Hypotension Hypopnea Bradypnea		Zolpidem Barbiturates Alcohol
	Combativeness interspersed with obtundation Sudden awakening	Variable			GHB
Cholinergic	Confusion Coma	Miosis	Bradycardia (initially tachycardia) Hypertension or hypotension Tachypnea or bradypnea	Salivation Urination Defecation (diarrhea) Diaphoresis Lacrimation Abdominal cramps Bronchoconstriction Bronchorrhea Muscle weakness and fasciculations Seizures	Organophosphates Nerve agents Nicotine Pilocarpine Physostigmine Edrophonium Bethanechol Urecholine
Serotonin syndrome	Confusion Agitation Coma	Mydriasis	Hyperthermia Tachycardia Hypertension Tachypnea	Tremor Myoclonus Hyperreflexia Clonus Diaphoresis Flushes Jaw stiffness Muscle stiffness Diarrhea	Selective serotonin reuptake inhibitors, serotonin precursors (tryptophan), serotonin agonists (eg, triptans), serotonin releasers (eg, MDMA), MAOIs, tricyclic antidepressants, others (eg, dextromethorphan and lithium)
Tricyclic antidepressants	Confusion Agitation Coma	Mydriasis	Hyperthermia Tachycardia Hypertension followed by hypotension Hypopnea	Seizures Myoclonus Choreoathetosis Arrhythmia Conduction disorders	Amitriptyline Nortriptyline Imipramine Clomipramine Desipramine Doxepin

Data from Burns MJ, Schwartzstein RM. General approach to drug poisoning in adults. UpToDate online 19.2; 2011.

activated charcoal dosing. Substances, such as toxic alcohols, lithium, and iron, are not effectively adsorbed by activated charcoal. Based on volunteer studies, the administration of activated charcoal should be considered if a patient has ingested a potentially toxic amount of a poison (which is known to be adsorbed to charcoal) up to 1 hour previously.[36,37] Although volunteer studies demonstrate that the reduction of drug absorption decreases to values of questionable clinical importance when charcoal is administered at times greater than 1 hour, the potential for benefit after 1 hour cannot be excluded, and it should therefore still be considered in intoxications where delayed gastrointestinal absorption is possible (eg, tricyclic antidepressants causing delayed gastric emptying due to anticholinergic effect or sustained-release preparations). In this respect, unless a patient has an intact or protected airway, the administration of charcoal is contraindicated because of the risk of lung aspiration. Activated charcoal is also contraindicated if its use increases the risk and severity of aspiration (eg, ingestion of a hydrocarbon with a high aspiration potential). Patients who are at risk of gastrointestinal hemorrhage or perforation due to medical conditions or recent surgery of the gastrointestinal tract could be further compromised by single-dose activated charcoal. Presence of activated charcoal in the gastrointestinal tract may obscure endoscopic visualization, but intoxication with a corrosive is not a contraindication for activated charcoal when it is administered for co-ingested agents that are systemic toxins.

Multiple-dose activated charcoal therapy involves the repeated administration (more than 2 doses) of oral activated charcoal to enhance the elimination of drugs already absorbed into the body. Multiple-dose activated charcoal is thought to produce its beneficial effect by interrupting the enteroenteric and, in some cases, the enterohepatic and the enterogastric circulation of drugs.[38] Based on experimental and clinical studies, multiple-dose activated charcoal should be considered only if a patient has ingested a life-threatening amount of carbamazepine, dapsone, phenobarbital, quinine, or theophylline. The use of multiple-dose charcoal in salicylate poisoning is controversial.

Finally when weighing the advantages of activated charcoal against its disadvantages, it should be stressed that there is no evidence from randomized controlled trials that the administration of activated charcoal improves clinical outcome.

Gastric lavage Gastric lavage should not be used routinely, if ever, in the management of poisoned patients.[39] The results of clinical outcome studies in overdose patients are weighted heavily on the side of showing a lack of beneficial effect. Serious risks of the procedure include hypoxia, arrhythmias, laryngospasm, perforation of the gastrointestinal tract or pharynx, fluid and electrolyte abnormalities, and aspiration pneumonitis. In comatose patients without a gag reflex, endotracheal or nasotracheal intubation should always precede gastric lavage. Contraindications for gastric lavage include ingestion of a strong acid or alkali, ingestion of a hydrocarbon with a high aspiration potential, or risk of gastrointestinal hemorrhage due to an underlying medical or surgical condition. In situations where the procedure may be a reasonable treatment option (eg, recent overdose with a life-threatening toxin, such as tricyclic antidepressants, lithium, and organophosphates), the clinician should carefully examine the risk-benefit ratio. Gastric lavage is usually followed by the administration of activated charcoal.

Whole-bowel irrigation Whole-bowel irrigation cleanses the bowel by the enteral administration of large amounts of an osmotically balanced polyethylene glycol electrolyte solution, which induces a liquid stool. It reduces drug absorption by decontaminating the entire gastrointestinal tract by physically expelling intraluminal contents. Whole-bowel irrigation should be considered for potentially toxic ingestions of sustained-release or enteric-coated drugs, particularly for those patients presenting more than 2 hours after drug ingestion.[40] It should also be considered for the removal of ingested packets of illicit drugs in body packers. In cases of a ruptured cocaine packet, however, emergency surgery is required whereas in cases of a ruptured heroin packet, patients may be treated by a continuous naloxone infusion awaiting spontaneous elimination. Whole-bowel irrigation is contraindicated in patients with bowel obstruction, perforation, or ileus and in patients with hemodynamic instability or compromised unprotected airways. The concurrent administration of activated charcoal and whole-bowel irrigation may decrease the effectiveness of the charcoal.

Emesis Apomorphine and saltwater are outdated and dangerous emetics and should no longer be used.

Syrup of ipecac has been used to promote active vomiting.[41] There is, however, no evidence from clinical studies that ipecac improves the outcome of poisoned patients and its routine administration in the emergency department should be abandoned. Ipecac may delay the administration or reduce the effectiveness of activated charcoal, oral antidotes, and whole-bowel irrigation. Ipecac should not be administered to patients who have a decreased level or impending loss of consciousness or who have ingested a corrosive substance or hydrocarbon with high aspiration potential.

Increasing Elimination

Measures to increase elimination include therapeutic diuresis, urinary alkalinization, hemoperfusion, and hemodialysis.

Forced diuresis by administration of large volumes of isotonic fluids and diuretics to increase renal excretion of a drug or metabolite is of limited clinical value. It is not recommended because of potential volume overload and electrolyte abnormalities.

Urinary alkalinization to enhance excretion of weak acids is achieved by the administration of intravenous sodium bicarbonate to produce urine with a pH greater than or equal to 7.5 and may be beneficial for compounds, such as salicylates and phenobarbital/primidone.[42] Side effects of urinary alkalinization are alkalemia and electrolyte disturbances, such as hypokalemia and hypocalcemia.

Invasive techniques, such as hemodialysis and hemoperfusion, are reserved for elimination of specific life-threatening toxins.[43] Hemodialysis is particularly suited for drugs or metabolites that are water soluble, have a low volume of distribution, have a molecular weight less than 500 Da, and have low plasma protein binding (eg, methanol, ethylene glycol, lithium, and salicylates). Hemoperfusion involves the passage of blood through an adsorptive-containing cartridge (usually resin or charcoal). This technique removes substances that have a high degree of plasma protein binding. Charcoal hemoperfusion may be indicated for intoxications with carbamazepine, phenobarbital, phenytoin, and theophylline. There are limited data available on drug removal by continuous arteriovenous or continuous venovenous hemofiltration. Hemofiltration has been used to enhance elimination of aminoglycosides, vancomycin, and metal chelate complexes, but the technique does not remove highly protein-bound drugs effectively. It may also be of benefit for intoxications with drugs that have a large volume of distribution, tight tissue binding, or slow intercompartmental transfer.

FURTHER DIAGNOSTIC APPROACH

ECG

A 12-lead ECG should be recorded in all patients with a potential risk of cardiac effects from their overdose or if rhythm disturbances are observed on cardiac monitoring. The ECG should be examined for rate and rhythm disturbance, ST changes indicative of ischemia, atrioventricular(AV) block, QRS and QT interval prolongation, and right axis deviation. For instance, prolongation of the QRS duration greater than100 milliseconds and/or right axis deviation of the terminal 40 milliseconds of the QRS complex (terminal S wave in lead I and elevated R wave in lead aVR) after tricyclic antidepressant intoxication is a sign of potential cardiac toxicity.[44] Poisoning with cardiac glycosides can present with almost any type of rhythm disturbance but frequently express a bradycardic rhythm with AV block similar to intoxication with calcium channel or β-blocking agents. Cocaine use may be associated with myocardial ischemia and dysrhythmias. Unfortunately, in the setting of cocaine-associated chest pain, the ECG has neither the sensitivity nor the specificity necessary to permit exclusion or confirmation of cardiac injury.

Blood and Urine Analysis

A glucose level should be obtained during the primary assessment to rule out hypoglycemia. Blood should be taken for complete blood count, renal and liver function, electrolyte tests, clotting studies, and osmolality. Cardiac markers are always required when considering myocardial ischemia after cocaine use. A creatine kinase level should be obtained when rhabdomyolysis is suspected. The possibility of pregnancy should be ruled out in every woman presenting with coma. Hypokalemia may indicate salbutamol, theophylline, or salicylate poisoning. Raised osmolality suggests ethanol, methanol, ethylene glycol, or isopropanol poisoning. Arterial blood gases help with quantifying any respiratory compromise and also indicate an acid-base disturbance. If an acidosis is present, a serum lactate level and calculation of the serum anion gap (anion gap = sodium – [chloride + bicarbonate], normal value 13 ± 4 meq/L) help assess the type of acid-base disorder. Metabolic acidosis may result from poisoning with, for example, salicylates, paracetamol (acetaminophen), ethanol, methanol, and ethylene glycol or also from circulatory shock. Any poison causing seizure, hypoxemia, shock (hypotension), cellular anoxia, or rhabdomyolysis results in a high anion gap metabolic acidosis from increased lactic acid concentrations. Poisoning with CO or the presence of methemoglobin can be ruled out by measuring COHb and methemoglobin levels, respectively. As discussed previously, pulse oximetry is unable to distinguish between oxyhemoglobin and COHb because of their spectrophotometric similarities. Urinalysis can assist in the evaluation of ketosis, hemolysis, and renal injury. Microscopy of urine may reveal calcium oxalate crystals, suggesting ethylene glycol poisoning.

Toxicologic Testing

Toxicology screening on blood and/or urine may be ordered depending on the clinical picture.[45,46] It is obvious that when clinically indicated, therapy for patients with suspected poisoning should never be postponed until the toxicologic results are known. In practice, however, many clinicians, emergency physicians, and neurologists believe that toxicologic testing is useful. When, for instance, in patients with altered consciousness, doubt remains about the cause, toxicologic data are of great help even when they are negative. This aspect is rarely studied. Furthermore, identifying the toxic substance influences therapy and prevents morbidity and mortality in a few percentages of patients. For instance, knowing that a coma is due to lithium poisoning may point to the necessity of hemodialysis. Finally for documentation and liability concerns, confirmation of a suspected poisoning with a toxicologic analysis is preferred by most clinicians. A more important issue than whether or not to order tests is how to order the tests. Clinicians treating patients with altered consciousness and suspected poisoning should know the limitation of a "comprehensive tox-screen." The number of drugs detected in a screen varies from laboratory to laboratory and can be falsely negative or reassuring. Moreover a comprehensive screen demands a lot of work in a laboratory and may not be cost effective. To increase efficiency and reduce the cost of toxicologic analysis, it is important that clinicians provide information on the suspected drugs and consult with a clinical toxicologist.

The possibility of (co-)intoxication with paracetamol (acetaminophen) and salicylate poisoning should always be considered in patients presenting with an overdose because these drugs are widely available, potentially lethal, and treatable in the early phase of intoxication.[47] Salicylates by themselves can cause coma through cerebral edema, and paracetamol (acetaminophen) and combination preparations, for instance, paracetamol (acetaminophen) and codeine, in massive overdose have been associated with coma.[48,49]

For some drugs and poisons, quantitative concentration measurements may be useful because they may guide treatment (**Box 2**). For some coma-inducing substances, such as anticonvulsants, lithium, and methemoglobin, there is a good correlation between the concentration and the clinical symptoms. Levels of alcohol and benzodiazepines usually do not correlate well with depth of coma due to the large interindividual variability; chronic users, for instance, exhibit CNS depression at significantly higher blood concentrations than nontolerant individuals. The problem with using COHb levels is that there is wide variation in clinical manifestations with identical COHb levels and that particular COHb levels are not predictive of symptoms or final outcome.[50] Also for salicylates, the severity of toxicity poorly correlates with serum levels. Quantitative levels of tricyclic antidepressants also have little correlation with clinical symptoms and fail to predict the risk of seizures or ventricular dysrhythmias

Box 2
Some examples of compounds for which quantitative analysis may be useful in guiding treatment

Antiepileptics: carbamazepine, phenytoin, and valproic acid

COHb

Digoxin

Ethylene glycol

Heavy metals: iron, lead, and mercury

Lithium

Methanol

Methemoglobin

Paracetamol

Paraquat

Salicylates

Theophylline

and are therefore rarely indicated. Timing of measuring blood concentrations may be important; for example, concentrations measured during the absorption phase may lead to underestimation of the risk and to potentially fatal errors. Sometimes repeated drug concentrations should be determined to look for trends, because drug absorption in overdose may be delayed or erratic.

Radiography

A chest radiograph is indicated in patients presenting with coma to evaluate for an infectious source of coma or aspiration pneumonia. All suspected body packers should undergo radiographic evaluation of the abdomen; packets can be visualized as multiple radiodense foreign bodies.

Cranial CT should be performed if a concern for an intracranial lesion exists or if cerebral edema is suspected (eg, in acetaminophen-induced liver failure). If indicated, a lumbar puncture should be considered to rule out subarachnoid bleed, meningitis, or encephalitis.

URGENT SPECIFIC ANTIDOTES

Some of the most frequently used antidotes that may be considered during initial management of patients with altered consciousness are reviewed. Antidotes for cyanides, organophosphates, tricyclic antidepressants, and methemoglobin-forming agents are not discussed and readers are referred to specialized textbooks in toxicology.[51] Normobaric oxygen (NBO) should be delivered to all comatose patients and in cases of CO poisoning the administration of HBO may be considered. The value of the antidotes dextrose and thiamine and the opiate antagonist naloxone used as a "coma cocktail" is discussed later.[52] More recently, the benzodiazepine receptor antagonist flumazenil has also been considered an urgent antidote. Benzodiazepines have an important role in the treatment of substance-induced agitation.

Hyperbaric Oxygen

HBO involves exposing patients to 100% oxygen under supra-atmospheric conditions. This results in a decrease in the half-life of carboxyhemoglobin (COHb), from 40 to 80 minutes on 100% NBO to 15 to 30 minutes during HBO. HBO may be beneficial in preventing the late neurocognitive deficits associated with severe CO poisoning; however, the quality and results of clinical trials have varied widely.[53–55]

A well-designed double-blind controlled trial randomly assigned 152 patients with symptomatic CO intoxication within 24 hours of presentation to HBO or NBO.[56] Treatment was administered during 3 sessions in a hyperbaric chamber. Six weeks after presentation, cognitive sequelae were more common in the group treated with NBO (46 vs 25%). This advantage of HBO was maintained at 1 year after initial presentation. In 31% of the patients in the study by Weaver and colleagues,[56] CO intoxication was related to a suicide attempt.

Another study randomly assigned 343 patients without initial impairment of consciousness in a nonblinded way to either 6 hours of NBO or 2 hours of HBO at 2 atm plus 4 hours of NBO.[57] No difference in mortality or in the incidence of delayed neurologic sequelae was observed. Critics of the study noted, however, that many patients in the HBO group did not receive treatment until more than 6 hours from the time of poisoning and that patients were treated with only one HBO session.

Similar findings were noted in a double-blind randomized trial of 191 patients with CO poisoning referred to a tertiary center, which failed to document benefit for patients who received HBO.[58] On the contrary, delayed neurologic sequelae and poor performance on neuropsychiatric tests after 1 month were significantly more common among HBO-treated patients. In this study, although people with all levels of CO were included, a high proportion (73%) of patients with severe CO poisoning was presented. Moreover, cluster randomization was used for patients presenting simultaneously, which may have engendered the risk of bias. Also, mean time interval to treatment was high (>6 hours), and it is therefore possible that a significant proportion of the patients were treated at a time after CO exposure when HBO is unlikely to be effective. Annane and colleagues[59] randomized patients with transient loss of consciousness due to CO poisoning to HBO (2 ATA for 2 hours followed by 100% oxygen at atmospheric pressure for 4 hours) versus NBO; no benefit from HBO over NBO was found. The investigators, however, only permitted less severely poisoned patients to be randomized to HBO or NBO. Because interventions are, in general, most likely to show benefit in patients with more severe disease, the possibility of type II error in these trials is high. Consequently, this trial does not disprove a benefit of HBO, particularly in more severely poisoned patients.

Despite the uncertainty in identifying patients who will benefit from HBO therapy, most authorities favor HBO in the presence of COHb greater than 25%, metabolic acidosis, a history of loss of consciousness, or neurologic or cardiovascular dysfunction or in pregnant women with COHb greater than 15% or evidence of fetal distress. All patients selected to receive HBO should have at least 1 treatment at 2.5 atm to 3.0 atm as soon as possible to reverse the acute effects of CO intoxication, possibly with additional hyperbaric sessions directed toward limitation or prevention of delayed neurologic sequelae.

Glucose and Glucagon

Any patients with an altered mental status should be suspected of hypoglycemia. Clinical diagnosis of hypoglycemia is not easy. Symptoms may range from agitation to deep coma with diaphoresis and tachycardia. Other neurologic symptoms, however, such as decerebrate and decorticate posturing may occur and even focal signs with, for instance, hemiplegia. In most cases a glucose dose of 10 g to 15 g in adults (as hypertonic glucose 50%) is sufficient to reverse hypoglycemic coma; however, in some cases doses as high as 0.5 g/kg to 1 g/kg are needed (for instance in deliberate insulin overdose). Glucagon (adult dose 1–2 mg) may be used as a temporizing measure in patients who have no intravenous access because it can be administered intramuscularly.

Thiamine

Although Wernicke encephalopathy is rare, thiamine (100 mg intravenously or intramuscularly) should be given in any patient with an altered mental state.[60] Adverse effects seldom occur after administration of thiamine, but hypersensitivity reactions have occurred, mainly after parenteral administration ranging in severity from very mild to, rarely, fatal anaphylactic shock. It only rarely immediately improves the mental state but its routine use reminds us of potential nutritional deficiencies in many patients, especially chronic alcoholics who are at risk of Wernicke encephalopathy. Administration of intravenous glucose to severely malnourished patients can exhaust their supply of thiamine and precipitate Wernicke-Korsakoff syndrome. Therefore, glucose and thiamine should be given as a cocktail for comatose patients.

Naloxone

Naloxone is an antagonist with a high affinity for μ, κ, and σ opioid receptors.[61] It antagonizes, therefore, the opiate effects, such as sedation and the life-threatening respiratory depression, which makes it of great value in cases of intoxication. It is less effective in poisoning with d-propoxyphene, pentazocine, and buprenorphine. It is a pure antagonist, which means that it does not produce opiate effects by itself and is specific for opiate poisoning.

Naloxone is a competitive antagonist, which implies that the dose needed to reverse the opiate effects depends on the amount of the opiate present in a poisoned patient, which is of course rarely known in acute poisoning.

Initially, and especially in the United States, naloxone was propagated in the coma cocktail for diagnostic and therapeutic use in any patient with decreased consciousness. This indiscriminate use is questioned now, however, because of the poor yield of beneficial effects (only in approximately 3% of comatose patients) and because studies indicate that clinical diagnosis of opiate poisoning based on respiratory rate and pupil size is reliable.[62] Therefore, naloxone is only indicated now in coma and/or respiratory depression (rate <12/min) in patients showing signs of opiate poisoning. The side effects, such as pulmonary edema, are rare.

Potentially severe withdrawal problems may occur in opiate addicts. Therefore, when naloxone is used in potentially dependent patients, the use of incremental doses intravenously is recommended based on the clinical response, such as reversal of respiratory depression and decreased consciousness. A practical starting dose in most adult patients is 0.05 mg, increasing to 0.4 mg, then to 2 mg, and finally to 10 mg.[61] If there is no response to 10 mg, then an opioid is unlikely responsible for the coma and/or respiratory depression.

Recurrent toxicity is common after an initial good response because the half-life of naloxone is short (20–30 minutes), which obviates a continuous infusion or a repeat bolus administration (eg, after 15 minutes). Naloxone can also be administered by the intramuscular, subcutaneous, intralingual, and intratracheal route.

Flumazenil

Flumazenil is a competitive antagonist of the benzodiazepine receptor in the CNS, which facilitates gabaminergic transmission, giving rise to the classical effects of benzodiazepines, such as sedation, anxiolytic, anticonvulsive, and hypnotic properties.[63] Flumazenil reverses the effects, such as sedation, and also the anticonvulsant properties of the benzodiazepines. Although the use of flumazenil is well established to counteract the effects of benzodiazepines used in diagnostic procedures, such as endoscopy, where benzodiazepines are used for sedation, its use in patients with acute poisoning is still the subject of debate.

Opponents of the use of flumazenil in patients with benzodiazepine poisoning stress that benzodiazepines rarely cause morbidity and mortality. The latter is often not due to respiratory depression (which is not always reversed by flumazenil) but to aspiration pneumonia, which already occurred before admission to the hospital. They emphasize the importance of the risk of inducing seizures, which can be due to co-ingested drugs (eg, tricyclic antidepressants) or to the acute withdrawal provoked in patients chronically taking benzodiazepines.

Proponents of the use of flumazenil stress the benefit of avoiding procedures carrying their own risks in the diagnostic work-up of a coma patient. Furthermore, they mention the benefits of avoiding the risks of endotracheal intubation and ventilation.[64]

Flumazenil is better avoided, or even contraindicated, in patients with a history of seizures or current treatment for seizures. History of intake or ingestion of substances capable of provoking seizures or provoking cardiac arrhythmias (eg, tricyclic antidepressants, theophylline, carbamazepine, chloroquine, and chlorinated hydrocarbons) is also a contraindication. Long-term use of benzodiazepines is also a contraindication. Finally flumazenil should never be used in patients with abnormal vital signs.

If needed, flumazenil should be given slowly and by titration (0.1 mg/min in adults) without exceeding a total dose of 1 mg. Relapse of the sedation may occur after 20 or more minutes due to the short half-life of flumazenil.

In summary, many investigators agree that the indications for flumazenil in the overdose setting are pure benzodiazepine poisoning in individuals who are not tolerant to benzodiazepines, who have CNS depression, normal vital signs, normal ECG, otherwise normal neurologic examination, and no history of epilepsy.[65] Such cases are rare in adults with benzodiazepine poisoning.

Benzodiazepines

Benzodiazepines are used as first-line anticonvulsants for virtually all xenobiotic-induced seizures; as the sedatives of choice for most forms of xenobiotic-induced agitation and for withdrawal from ethanol, GHB, and a variety of sedatives; and as muscle relaxant for disorders, such as serotonin syndrome and NMS.[66] Cocaine-associated myocardial ischemia and infarction are also indications for benzodiazepines. For the treatment of agitation induced by xenobiotics, it is important to titrate the benzodiazepines until the patient is calm. Cumulative benzodiazepine dosages required in the initial 30 minutes to achieve adequate sedation frequently exceed 100 mg of diazepam or its equivalent. Antipsychotics are not recommended for the treatment of xenobiotic-induced agitation because they may lower the seizure threshold, alter temperature regulation, and cause acute dystonia and cardiac dysrhythmias.

DISPOSITION

All patients with altered consciousness should be closely observed with frequent controls of blood pressure, heart rate, respiratory rate, body temperature, GCS score, and pupils. ECG monitoring is required in all patients intoxicated with potential cardiotoxic agents. Continuous pulse oximetry is recommended in comatose patients because all agents causing CNS depression may compromise airway patency. Depending on end-organ toxicity, toxin characteristics, requirements for physiologic monitoring and specialized treatment, and patient factors, admission to an intensive care unit is indicated.

In a retrospective study, a set of criteria was established to identify those poisoned patients needing intensive care unit admission without taking into account the specific toxin ingested.[67] Criteria defining high-risk patients were need for intubation, unresponsiveness to verbal stimuli, seizures, P_{CO_2} greater than 45 mm Hg, systolic blood pressure less than 80 mm Hg, QRS duration greater than 0.12 seconds, or any cardiac rhythm except normal sinus rhythm, sinus tachycardia, or sinus bradycardia.

Intensive care unit admission is always warranted for patients with expected serious toxic effects from an ingested poison. This is especially true for those toxins known to be deadly, such as calcium channel blockers, cocaine, cyanide, cyclic antidepressants, and salicylates. Indicators of toxicity should be identified for individual toxins so that high-risk patients may be closely monitored and aggressively treated.

The intensive care unit setting provides a nurse-to-patient ratio that allows for frequent or continuous monitoring of basic physiologic parameters. The intensive care units are also most equipped to provide supportive care measures to treat respiratory failure and hemodynamic shock. Extracorporeal methods for eliminating toxins and most antidotal therapy are also best performed in the intensive care unit.

Pre-existing medical conditions increase a patient's risk for developing toxicity and may, therefore, require intensive care unit admission. For instance, patients with underlying cardiac disease are more susceptible to myocardial ischemia from CO poisoning. Renal and hepatic disease may alter drug metabolism and elimination resulting in prolonged toxicity.

PSYCHOSOCIAL APPROACH

Most intoxications presenting to the emergency department result from autointoxication. Therefore, psychosocial factors are significant in the evaluation and treatment of patients with toxicologic emergencies.[68] The acute event of an intoxication offers opportunity to initiate well-coordinated care management with particular attention to continuity and follow-up. Integrated health care systems include formal and informal linkages to community-based health, mental health, substance abuse treatment, and social service agencies, all of which interact with interdisciplinary teams in their management of toxicologic emergencies. Even with the highest levels of clinical and technologic expertise applied in the diagnosis and treatment of poisoned or overdosed patients, successful outcomes may be compromised by inadequacies in aftercare and follow-up. Therefore, it is important to identify and cultivate appropriate referral resources for a wide range of continuing-care services.

Self-poisoning prompts immediate referral for further psychosocial, social, and psychiatric assessment and poses unique problems for clinicians who must make appropriate assessment and management decisions.[68–70] The assessor should at least have received specific training and have access to support from a psychiatrist.[71] Identifying risk factors for suicide can aid clinicians in using preventive or early intervention strategies. Important risk factors for suicidal behavior include past history of suicide attempts, comorbid mental illness, substance intoxication, young age groups, and absence of a social/family support network. Mental status examination for suicidal risk should focus on extrinsic factors, such as current ideation, intent, lethality of the plan, and current life stressors as well as intrinsic vulnerability factors, such as comorbid mental illness, feelings of hopelessness, and impulsivity. Early detection and rapid intervention for patients at risk for suicide are the best means for preventing injury or death.[72]

Appropriate interventions should also be offered to patients with hazardous or harmful alcohol drinking.[73] In general, health care providers tend to have an overly pessimistic view of the benefits of treating alcoholism. This view is not in line with psychosocial interventional strategies, however, which have proved effective.

Optimal psychosocial care of patients with substance abuse is also challenging. A compassionate and nonjudgmental approach is important to gain their confidence and enhance the care rendered. Providing access to programs that support detoxification is essential.

SUMMARY

Patients with altered consciousness and suspected poisoning are a challenge to the clinicians involved in the management of these patients. The approach of these patients should start with stabilization of vital parameters and the judicious use of antidotes. Clinicians should be alert not only for specific clinical signs of acute poisoning but also for other causes of decreased consciousness. They should always be suspicious for associated traumatic injuries in poisoned patients. Thorough knowledge of toxidromes, clinical neurologic examination, decontamination procedures, and toxicologic testing are of major importance in the management of these patients.

Therefore, early consultation between the neurologist and the clinical toxicologist is of utmost importance as is communication with the toxicology laboratory. Attention should be paid to optimal psychosocial support of poisoned patients, especially in autointoxications.

REFERENCES

1. Meehan TJ, Bryant SM, Aks SE. Drugs of abuse: the highs and lows of altered mental states in the emergency department. Emerg Med Clin North Am 2010; 28:663–82.
2. Rao RB. Neurologic principles. In: Nelson LS, Lewin NA, Howland MA, et al, editors. Goldfrank's toxicologic emergencies. 9th edition. New York: McGraw-Hill; 2011. p. 275–84.
3. Dyer JE, Roth B, Hyma BA. Gamma-hydroxybutyrate withdrawal syndrome. Ann Emerg Med 2001;37:147–53.
4. De Paepe P, Calle PA, Buylaert WA. Coma induced by intoxication. Handb Clin Neurol 2008;90:175–91.
5. Kostic MA, Dart RC. Coma of unclear etiology. In: Dart RC, editor. Medical toxicology. Philadelphia: Lippincott Williams & Wilkins; 2004. p. 66–8.
6. Chebib M, Johnston GA. The 'ABC' of GABA receptors. A brief review. Clin Exp Pharmacol Physiol 1999;26:937–40.
7. Zhu H, Cottrell JE, Kass IS. The effect of thiopental and propofol on NMDA- and AMPA-mediated glutamate excitotoxicity. Anesthesiology 1997;87:944–51.
8. Wong CG, Chan KF, Gibson KM, et al. Gamma-hydroxybutyric acid: neurobiology and toxicology of a recreational drug. Toxicol Rev 2004;23:3–20.
9. Simons FE, Simons KJ. The pharmacology and use of H1-receptor-antagonist drugs. N Engl J Med 1994;330:1663–70.
10. Parsons M, Buckley NA. Antipsychotic drugs in overdose: practical management guidelines. CNS Drugs 1997;6:427–41.
11. Bateman DN. Tricyclic antidepressant poisoning: central nervous system effects and management. Toxicol Rev 2005;24:181–6.
12. Dhawan BN, Cesselin F, Raghubir R, et al. Classification of opioid receptors. Pharmacol Rev 1996;48:567–92.
13. Gracia R, Shepherd G. Cyanide poisoning and its treatment. Pharmacotherapy 2004;24:1358–65.
14. Smith RP, Gosselin RE. Hydrogen sulfide poisoning. J Occup Med 1979;21:93–7.
15. Jaffe FA. Pathogenicity of carbon monoxide. Am J Forensic Med Pathol 1997;18: 406–10.
16. Advanced Life Support Group. Acute medical emergencies. London: BMJ Books; 2010.
17. Greene SL, Dargan PI, Jones AL. Acute poisoning: understanding 90% of cases in a nutshell. Postgrad Med J 2005;81:204–16.
18. Hack JB, Hoffman RS. General management of poisoned patients. In: Tintinalli JE, Kelen GD, Stapczynski JS, editors. Emergency medicine. A comprehensive study guide. New York: McGraw-Hill; 2004. p. 1015–22.
19. Huff JS. Altered mental status and coma. In: Tintinalli JE, Kelen GD, Stapczynski JS, editors. Emergency medicine. A comprehensive study guide. New York: McGraw-Hill; 2004. p. 1390–7.
20. Koster RW, Baubin MA, Bossaert LL, et al. European Resuscitation Council Guidelines for Resuscitation 2010. Section 2. Adult basic life support and use of automated external defibrillators. Resuscitation 2010;81:1277–92.

21. Deakin CD, Nolan JP, Soar J, et al. European Resuscitation Council Guidelines for Resuscitation 2010. Section 4. Adult advanced life support. Resuscitation 2010;81:1305–52.
22. Mokhlesi B, Leiken JB, Murray P, et al. Adult toxicology in critical care. Part I: general approach to the intoxicated patient. Chest 2003;123:577–92.
23. Chan B, Gaudry P, Grattan-Smith TM, et al. The use of Glasgow Coma Scale in poisoning. J Emerg Med 1993;11:579–82.
24. Donald C, Duncan R, Thakore S. Predictors of the need for rapid sequence intubation in the poisoned patient with reduced Glasgow coma score. Emerg Med J 2009;26:510–2.
25. Dewitt CR, Waksman JC. Pharmacology, pathophysiology and management of calcium channel blocker and beta-blocker toxicity. Toxicol Rev 2004;23:223–38.
26. Kelly CA, Upex A. Comparison of consciousness level assessment in the poisoned patient using the alert/verbal/painful/unresponsive scale and the Glasgow Coma Scale. Ann Emerg Med 2004;44:108–13.
27. Boyle PJ, Schwartz NS, Shah SD, et al. Plasma glucose concentrations at the onset of hypoglycemic symptoms in patients with poorly controlled diabetes and in nondiabetics. N Engl J Med 1988;318:1487–92.
28. Tokuda Y, Nakazato N, Stein GH. Pupillary evaluation for differential diagnosis of coma. Postgrad Med J 2003;79:49–51.
29. Olson KR, Pentel PR, Kelley MT. Physical assessment and differential diagnosis of the poisoned patient. Med Toxicol 1987;2:52–81.
30. Cooke JL. Depressed consciousness and coma. In: Marx JA, Hockberger RS, Walls RM, et al, editors. Rosen's emergency medicine. Concepts and clinical practice. St Louis (MO): Mosby; 2010. p. 106–12.
31. Gold AE, Marshall SM. Cortical blindness and cerebral infarction associated with severe hypoglycemia. Diabetes Care 1996;19:1001–3.
32. Pétursson H. The benzodiazepine withdrawal syndrome. Addiction 1994;89: 1455–9.
33. Schuckit MA, Tipp JE, Reich T, et al. The histories of withdrawal convulsions and delirium tremens in 1648 alcohol dependent subjects. Addiction 1995;90:1335–47.
34. Boyer EW, Shannon M. The serotonin syndrome. N Engl J Med 2005;352: 1112–20.
35. Lewin NA, Nelson LS. Dermatologic principles. In: Nelson LS, Lewin NA, Howland MA, et al, editors. Goldfrank's toxicologic emergencies. 9th edition. New York: McGraw-Hill; 2011. p. 410–22.
36. American Academy of Clinical Toxicology, European Association of Poison Centres, Clinical Toxicologists. Position paper: single-dose activated charcoal. Clin Toxicol 2005;43:61–87.
37. Isbister GK, Kumar VV. Indications for single-dose activated charcoal administration. Curr Opin Crit Care 2011;17:351–7.
38. American Academy of Clinical Toxicology, European Association of Poison Centres, Clinical Toxicologists. Position statement and practice guidelines on the use of multi-dose activated charcoal in the treatment of acute poisoning. Clin Toxicol 1999;37:731–51.
39. American Academy of Clinical Toxicology, European Association of Poison Centres, Clinical Toxicologists. Position paper: gastric lavage. Clin Toxicol 2004;42:933–43.
40. American Academy of Clinical Toxicology, European Association of Poison Centres, Clinical Toxicologists. Position paper: whole bowel irrigation. Clin Toxicol 2004;42:843–54.

41. American Academy of Clinical Toxicology, European Association of Poison Centres, Clinical Toxicologists. Position paper: ipecac syrup. Clin Toxicol 2004; 42:133–43.
42. Proudfoot AT, Krenzelok EP, Vale JA. Position paper on urine alkalinization. Clin Toxicol 2004;42:1–26.
43. Cutler RD, Forland SC, Hammond PG. Extracorporeal removal of drugs and poisons by hemodialysis and hemoperfusion. Annu Rev Pharmacol Toxicol 1987;27:169–91.
44. Liebelt EL. Cyclic antidepressants. In: Nelson LS, Lewin NA, Howland MA, et al, editors. Goldfrank's toxicologic emergencies. 9th edition. New York: McGraw-Hill; 2011. p. 1049–59.
45. Rainey PM. Laboratory principles and techniques for evaluation of the poisoned or overdosed patient. In: Nelson LS, Lewin NA, Howland MA, et al, editors. Goldfrank's toxicologic emergencies. 9th edition. New York: McGraw-Hill; 2011. p. 70–89.
46. Wu AH, McKay C, Broussard LA, et al. National academy of clinical biochemistry laboratory medicine practice guidelines: recommendations for the use of laboratory tests to support poisoned patients who present to the emergency department. Clin Chem 2003;49:357–79.
47. Hartington K, Hartley J, Clancy M. Measuring plasma paracetamol concentrations in all patients with drug overdoses; development of a clinical decision rule and clinicians willingness to use it. Emerg Med J 2002;19:408–11.
48. Schiodt FV, Rochling FA, Casey DL, et al. Acetaminophen toxicity in an urban county hospital. N Engl J Med 1997;337:1112–7.
49. Yip L, Dart RC, Gabow PA. Concepts and controversies in salicylate toxicity. Emerg Med Clin North Am 1994;12:351–64.
50. Myers RA. Carbon monoxide poisoning. J Emerg Med 1984;1:245–8.
51. Nelson LS, Lewin NA, Howland MA, et al, editors. Goldfrank's toxicologic emergencies. 9th edition. New York: McGraw-Hill; 2011.
52. Hoffman RS, Goldfrank LR. The poisoned patient with altered consciousness. Controversies in the use of a 'coma cocktail'. JAMA 1995;274:562–9.
53. Clardy P, Manaker S, Perry H. Carbon monoxide poisoning. UpToDate online 19.2; 2011.
54. Phin N. Carbon monoxide poisoning (acute). Clin Evid 2010;10:2103.
55. Buckley NA, Juurlink DN, Isbister G, et al. Hyperbaric oxygen for carbon monoxide poisoning. Cochrane Database Syst Rev 2011;4:CD002041.
56. Weaver LK, Hopkins RO, Chan KJ, et al. Hyperbaric oxygen for acute carbon monoxide poisoning. N Engl J Med 2002;347:1057–67.
57. Raphael JC, Elkharrat D, Jars-Guincestre MC, et al. Trial of normobaric and hyperbaric oxygen for acute carbon monoxide intoxication. Lancet 1989;19: 414–9.
58. Scheinkestel CD, Bailey M, Myles PS, et al. Hyperbaric or normobaric oxygen for acute carbon monoxide poisoning: a randomised controlled clinical trial. Med J Aust 1999;170:203–10.
59. Annane D, Chadda K, Gajdos P, et al. Hyperbaric oxygen therapy for acute domestic carbon monoxide poisoning: two randomized controlled trials. Intensive Care Med 2011;37:486–92.
60. Zubaran C, Fernandes JG, Rodnight R. Wernicke-Korsakoff syndrome. Postgrad Med J 1997;73:27–31.
61. Howland MA, Nelson LS. Antidotes in depth—opioid antagonists. In: Nelson LS, Lewin NA, Howland MA, et al, editors. Goldfrank's toxicologic emergencies. 9th edition. New York: McGraw-Hill; 2011. p. 579–85.

62. Hoffman JR, Schriger DL, Luo JS. The empiric use of naloxone in patients with altered mental status: a reappraisal. Ann Emerg Med 1991;20:246–52.
63. Howland MA. Antidotes in depth—flumazenil. In: Nelson LS, Lewin NA, Howland MA, et al, editors. Goldfrank's toxicologic emergencies. 9th edition. New York: McGraw-Hill; 2011. p. 1072–7.
64. Höjer J, Baehrendtz S, Matell G, et al. Diagnostic utility of flumazenil in coma with suspected poisoning: a double blind, randomised controlled study. BMJ 1990; 301:1308–11.
65. Gueye PN, Hoffman JR, Taboulet P, et al. Empiric use of flumazenil in comatose patients: limited applicability of criteria to define low risk. Ann Emerg Med 1996; 27:730–5.
66. Hoffman RS, Nelson LS, Howland MA. Antidotes in depth. Benzodiazepines. In: Nelson LS, Lewin NA, Howland MA, et al, editors. Goldfrank's toxicologic emergencies. 9th edition. New York: McGraw-Hill; 2011. p. 1109–14.
67. Brett A, Rothchild N, Gray R, et al. Predicting the clinical course in intentional drug overdose: implications for use of the intensive care unit. Arch Intern Med 1987;147:133–7.
68. National Institute for Health, Clinical Excellence. Self-harm. The short-term physical and psychological management and secondary prevention of self-harm in primary and secondary care. London: NICE; 2004.
69. Hawton K, Arensman E, Townsend E, et al. Deliberate self harm: systematic review of efficacy of psychosocial and pharmacological treatments in preventing repetition. BMJ 1998;317:441–7.
70. Sinclair J, Green J. Understanding resolution of deliberate self harm: qualitative interview study of patients' experiences. BMJ 2005;330:1112–5.
71. Skegg K. Self-harm. Lancet 2005;366:1471–83.
72. Gunnell D, Ho D, Murray V. Medical management of deliberate drug overdose: a neglected area for suicide prevention? Emerg Med J 2004;21:35–8.
73. Ritson B. Treatment for alcohol related problems. BMJ 2005;330:139–41.

Index

Note: Page numbers of article titles are in **boldface** type.

Neurol Clin 30 (2012) 385–404
doi:10.1016/S0733-8619(11)00120-4
neurologic.theclinics.com
0733-8619/12/$ – see front matter

B

F

G

H

Printed and bound by CPI Group (UK) Ltd, Croydon, CR0 4YY
03/10/2024
01040449-0011

R

S

U

V

W

X